Dentofacial and Occlusal Asymmetries

Dentofacial and Occlusal Asymmetries

Edited by

Birte Melsen, D.D.S., Dr. Odont., Dr. h.c.
Visiting Professor of Orthodontics, College of Dentistry, New York University, New York, NY, USA
Former Professor and Head of Orthodontics, Department of Dentistry and Oral Health,
Aarhus University, Aarhus, Denmark

Athanasios E. Athanasiou, D.D.S., M.S.D., Dr. Dent.
Dean and Professor of Orthodontics, School of Dentistry, European University Cyprus, Nicosia, Cyprus
Honorary Professor of Orthodontics, Mohammed Bin Rashid University of Medicine and Health Sciences
Dubai, UAE
Former Dean, Professor and Head of Orthodontics, School of Dentistry, Aristotle University of Thessaloniki
Thessaloniki, Greece

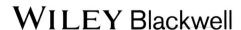

This edition first published 2025

© 2025 John Wiley & Sons Ltd

Registered Offices

John Wiley & Sons, Inc., 111 River Street, Hoboken, NJ 07030, USA

John Wiley & Sons Ltd, The Atrium, Southern Gate, Chichester, West Sussex, PO19 8SQ, UK

For details of our global editorial offices, customer services, and more information about Wiley products visit us at www.wiley.com.

Wiley also publishes its books in a variety of electronic formats and by print-on-demand. Some content that appears in standard print versions of this book may not be available in other formats.

Library of Congress Cataloging-in-Publication Data applied for:

ISBN 9781119794813 (hardback)

Cover Design: Wiley

Cover Images: Courtesy of George Anka, Ioannis Latrou, Ute Schneider-Moser

Set in 9.5/12.5pt STIXTwoText by Straive, Pondicherry, India

Printed in Singapore

M115814_190824

Contents

List of Contributors

Aron Aliaga-Del Castillo, D.D.S., M.Sc., Ph.D.
Clinical Assistant Professor, Department of Orthodontics
and Pediatric Dentistry School of Dentistry
University of Michigan
Ann Arbor, MI
USA

George Anka, D.D.S., M.S.
Private Practice of Orthodontics
Tokyo
Japan

Athanasios E. Athanasiou, D.D.S., M.S.D., Dr. Dent.
Dean and Professor of Orthodontics, School of Dentistry
European University Cyprus
Nicosia
Cyprus

Honorary Professor of Orthodontics
Mohammed Bin Rashid University of Medicine and
Health Sciences
Dubai
UAE

Former Dean, Professor and Head of Orthodontics
School of Dentistry
Aristotle University of Thessaloniki
Thessaloniki
Greece

Zakaria Bentahar, D.M.D., M.D.Sc., M.Sc., Ph.D.
Professor of Orthodontics
Hassan II University
Casablanca
Morocco

Joseph Bouserhal, D.D.S., M.D.S., Ph.D.
Professor and Acting Chair, Department of Orthodontics
Faculty of Dental Medicine
Saint Joseph University of Beirut
Beirut
Lebanon

Director, Craniofacial Research Laboratory
Faculty of Dental Medicine
Saint Joseph University of Beirut
Beirut
Lebanon

Adjunct Clinical Professor, Department of Orthodontics and
Dentofacial Orthopedics, Henry Goldman School of Dentistry
Boston University
Boston
USA

Lea J. Bouserhal, DDS, M.S.
Private Practice of Orthodontics
Beirut
Lebanon

Philippe J. Bouserhal, D.D.S., M.D.S.
Private Practice of Orthodontics
Beirut, Lebanon and Leuven
Belgium

*Eugene Chan, B.D.S., M.D.Sc., M.Orth.R.C.S.Ed.,
M.R.A.C.D.S.(Ortho), Ph.D.*
Clinical Professor, Discipline of Orthodontics
School of Dentistry Faculty of Medicine and Health
University of Sydney
Sydney
Australia

Kwangchul Choy, D.D.S., M.S., Ph.D.
Clinical Professor, Department of Orthodontics
School of Dentistry
Yonsei University
Seoul
South Korea

Lucia H. Soares Cevidanes, D.D.S., M.S., Ph.D.
Thomas and Doris Graber Endowed Professor of Dentistry
and Associate Professor, Department of Orthodontics
School of Dentistry
University of Michigan
Ann Arbor, MI
USA

M. Ali Darendeliler, B.D.S., Ph.D., Dip. Orth., Certif. Orth.,
Priv. Doc, F.I.C.D., M.R.A.C.D.S. (Orth.)
Professor and Chair, Discipline of Orthodontics
School of Dentistry
Faculty of Medicine and Health
University of Sydney
Sydney
Australia

Head, Department of Orthodontics
Sydney Dental Hospital
Sydney
Australia

Karine Evangelista, D.D.S., M.S., Ph.D.
Assistant Professor, Division of Orthodontics
School of Dentistry
Federal University of Goiás
Goiás
Brazil

Giampietro Farronato, M.D., D.D.S.
Professor Emeritus of Orthodontics, School of Dentistry
University of Milan
Milan
Italy

Padhraig S. Fleming, B.Dent.Sc.(Hons.), M.Sc., Ph.D.,
F.D.S.(Orth.), F.F.D.(Orth.), F.H.E.A.
Chair and Professor of Orthodontics and Programme
Lead, Doctorate in Orthodontics, Division of Public and
Child Dental Health
Dublin Dental University Hospital, The University of
Dublin, Trinity College Dublin
Ireland

Honorary Professor of Orthodontics
Queen Mary University of London
London
UK

Joseph G. Ghafari, D.M.D.
Professor and Chair, Department of Dentofacial Medicine
American University of Beirut Medical Center
Beirut
Lebanon

Hans Gjørup, DDS, PhD
Specialist in Orthodontics
Ikast
Denmark

Ismaeel Hansa, B.D.S., M.D.S.
Private practice of Orthodontics
Durban
South Africa

David C. Hatcher, D.D.S., M.Sc., M.R.C.D. (C)
Specialist in Oral and Maxillofacial Radiology
University of California Los Angeles, University of
California San Francisco, University of California Davis
and University of Pacific
California
USA

Dorte Haubek, D.D.S., Ph.D., Dr. Odont.
Professor, Department of Dentistry and Oral Health
Aarhus University
Aarhus
Denmark

Ioannis Iatrou, D.D.S., M.D., Ph.D.
Professor Emeritus of Oral and Maxillofacial Surgery
School of Dentistry
National and Kapodistrian University of Athens
Athens
Greece

Guilherme Janson, D.D.S., M.Sc., Ph.D. (deceased)
Professor and Head, Department of Orthodontics
Bauru Dental School
University of São Paolo
Bauru, São Paolo
Brazil

Eleftherios G. Kaklamanos, D.D.S., Cert., Cert., M.Sc.,
M.A., Ph.D.
Associate Professor, School of Dentistry
Aristotle University of Thessaloniki
Thessaloniki
Greece

Adjunct Associate Professor of Orthodontics, Hamdan Bin
Mohammed College of Dental Medicine
Mohammed Bin Rashid University of Medicine and
Health Sciences
Dubai
UAE

Associate Professor, School of Dentistry
European University Cyprus
Nicosia
Cyprus

Stavros Kiliaridis, D.D.S., Odont. Dr. / Ph.D.
Professor Emeritus of Orthodontics, School of Dental
Medicine, Faculty of Medicine
University of Geneva
Geneva
Switzerland

Adjunct Professor, Department of Orthodontics and
Dentofacial Orthopedics, School of Dental Medicine
Faculty of Medicine
University of Bern
Bern
Switzerland

Steven J. Lindauer, D.M.D., M.Dent.Sc.
Paul Tucker Goad Professor and Chair, Department of
Orthodontics, School of Dentistry
Virginia Commonwealth University
Richmond, VA
USA

Cesare Luzi, D.D.S., M.Sc.
Visiting Professor, Department of Orthodontics
University of Ferrara, Ferrara and University Cattolica
Rome
Italy

Camila Massaro, D.D.S., M.S.D., Ph.D.
Bauru Dental School
University of São Paulo
Bauru
Brazil

School of Dentistry
University of Michigan
Ann Arbor, MI
USA

Maria Costanza Meazzini di Seyssel, D.M.D., M.Med.Sci.
Scientific Director, Cleft Lip and Palate Regional Center
Operation Smile S. Paolo Hospital
Milan
Italy

Consultant for Craniofacial Anomalies, Department of
Maxillo-Facial Surgery
S. Gerardo Hospital
Monza
Italy

Adjunct Professor in Craniofacial Anomalies
University of Milan
Milan
Italy

Birte Melsen, D.D.S., Dr. Odont., Dr. h.c.
Visiting Professor of Orthodontics, College of Dentistry
New York University
New York, NY
USA

Former Professor and Head of Orthodontics
Department of Dentistry and Oral Health
Aarhus University
Aarhus
Denmark

Lorenz Moser, M.D., D.D.S.
Visiting Professor, Department of Orthodontics
University of Ferrara
Ferrara
Italy

Thomas Klit Pedersen, D.D.S., Ph.D.
Clinical Professor, Consultant Orthodontist
Department of Oral and Maxillofacial Surgery
Aarhus University Hospital and Section of Orthodontics
Department of Dentistry and Oral Health
Aarhus University
Aarhus
Denmark

Pertti Pirttiniemi, D.D.S., Ph.D., Dr. Orthod.
Professor Emeritus of Oral Development and
Orthodontics, Faculty of Odontology
University of Oulu
Oulu
Finland

Antonio Carlos de Oliveira Ruellas, Ph.D.
Universidade Federal do Rio de Janeiro
Rio de Janeiro
Brazil

Ute E.M. Schneider-Moser, D.D.S., M.S.
Visiting Professor, Department of Orthodontics
University of Ferrara
Ferrara
Italy

Department of Orthodontics
University of Pennsylvania
Philadelphia, PA
USA

Bhavna Shroff, D.D.S., M.Dent.Sc., M.P.A.
Norborne Muir Professor and Graduate Program Director
Department of Orthodontics, School of Dentistry
Virginia Commonwealth University
Richmond, VI
USA

Steven M. Siegel, D.M.D.
Private Practice of Orthodontics
Glen Burnie, MD
USA

Peter B. Stoustrup, D.D.S., Ph.D.
Associate Professor and Head, Section of Orthodontics
Director of Postgraduate Orthodontic Program
Department of Dentistry and Oral Health
Aarhus University
Aarhus
Denmark

Emese Szabò, D.D.S.
Private Practice of Orthodontics
Rome
Italy

**Nadia Theologie-Lygidakis, D.D.S., M.Sc.(Med),
M.Sc.(Dent), Ph.D.**
Associate Professor, Department of Oral and Maxillofacial
Surgery School of Dentistry
National and Kapodistrian University of Athens
Athens
Greece

**Nikhillesh Vaiid, B.D.S., M.D.S., Ph.D., F.D.T.F.(Ed.),
M.F.D.S. R.C.S.(Glasgow)**
Adjunct Professor, Department of Orthodontics
Saveetha Dental College
Saveetha Institute of Medical and Technical Sciences
Saveetha University
Chennai
India

Vidhya Venkateswaran, B.D.S., M.P.H., Ph.D.
DATA Scholar, National Institute of Dental and
Craniofacial Research
Bethesda, MD
USA

Larry M. Wolford, D.M.D.
Clinical Professor, Departments of Oral and Maxillofacial
Surgery and Orthodontics
Texas A&M University College of Dentistry
Baylor University Medical Center
Dallas, TX
USA

1

Introduction

Birte Melsen and Athanasios E. Athanasiou

CHAPTER MENU

References, 3

Although each person shares with the rest of the population many characteristics, there are enough differences to make each human being a unique individual. Such limitless variation in the size, shape, and relationship of the dental, skeletal, and soft tissue facial structures are important in providing each individual with their identity (Bishara et al. 2001).

Dorland's Medical Dictionary defines symmetry as "the similar arrangement in form and relationships of parts around a common axis or on each side of a plane of the body" (*Dorland's Illustrated Medical Dictionary* 2000).

The absence of symmetry is asymmetry and is frequently experienced by man in their facial features, both structurally and functionally.

The term symmetry is generally used in two different contexts:

The first meaning is a precise and well-defined concept of balance or "patterned self-similarity" that can be demonstrated or proved according to the rules of a formal system, namely geometry, physics, or otherwise.

The second meaning is an imprecise sense of harmonious or esthetically pleasing proportionality and balance reflecting beauty or perfection. As such, symmetry was demonstrated within art by Leonardo Da Vinci in his Vitruvian Man in 1492 (Figure 1.1) (Baudouin and Tiberghien 2004).

Asymmetry has, on the other hand, been part of the features characterizing the unpleasant and the unharmonious (Edler 2001; Rhodes et al. 2001).

Whereas symmetry in art is used to express harmony, beauty, and peace, asymmetrical layouts are generally more dynamic, and by intentionally ignoring balance, the designer can generate tension, express movement, or convey a mood such as anger, excitement, joy, or casual amusement (Komoro et al. 2009).

Facial asymmetry, being a common phenomenon, was probably first observed by the artists of early Greek statuary who recorded what they had found in nature – normal facial asymmetry (Lundstrom 1961).

A perfect facial symmetry is extremely rare and practically all normal faces exhibit a degree of asymmetry (Figure 1.2). As in art, where the side has an importance in the interpretation of a movement displayed on a painting, the two sides of the face may express feelings (Schirillo 2000).

The left side of the face is considered more emotionally expressive and more often connotes more negative emotions than the right side. Also interestingly, artists tend to expose more of their models left cheek than their right. This is significant, in that artists also portray more females than males with their left cheek exposed. These psychological findings lead to explanations for the esthetic leftward bias in portraiture (Schirillo 2000; Powell and Schirillo 2009).

The studies of asymmetry of the craniofacial region can be divided into two categories. One is focusing on facial asymmetry in various populations and its impact on perception of the individual's attractiveness and health. The second category is dealing with the influence of asymmetry on treatment of patients receiving orthodontic treatment or craniofacial surgery.

Studies of various populations belong to the first category, and facial symmetry has been associated with health, physical attractiveness, and beauty of a person. It is also hypothesized as a factor in interpersonal attraction, and relevant research indicates that bilateral symmetry is an important indicator of freedom from disease and worthiness for mating (Edler 2001).

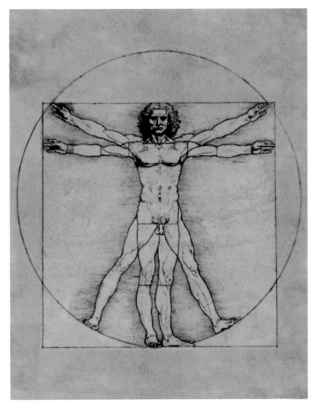

Figure 1.1 Vitruvian Man drawn by Leonardo Da Vinci in 1492 demonstrating the symmetry of the ideal body.

Most facial asymmetries among nonpatients are, however, fluctuating meaning that they have no significant influence on the attractiveness of the face. The perception of a face as attractive is more influenced by averageness meaning: what do the persons I like in "my tribe" look like. The beauty ideal is clearly changing with time and between various populations (Rhodes et al. 2001). The impact of averageness was studied by Komoro et al. (2009) who let laypeople evaluate the effect of symmetry and averageness on photographs and found that symmetry had a limited if any influence on attractiveness, thus confirming earlier findings by Baudouin and Tiberghien (2004). In a more recent study, it was found that symmetry on one hand reduced attractiveness by decreasing perceived normality, but on the other hand could also increase attractiveness by promoting the perceived symmetry (Zheng et al. 2021). Furthermore, it has been suggested that completely symmetrical faces might appear unemotional and thus less attractive (Swaddle and Cuthill 1995).

The second category of studies deal with asymmetry in relation to treatment. In reference to the need for treatment, it should be noted that the point at which normal asymmetry becomes abnormal cannot be easily defined and is often determined by the clinician's sense of balance and the patient's perception of the imbalance (Bishara et al. 2001). Minor asymmetry of the craniofacial skeleton and in the dentoalveolar region is often not easily detected. This can be the reason for which the optimal result of an orthodontic treatment cannot be reached since the asymmetry will often interfere with a satisfactory finishing.

The true prevalence of asymmetries in a population has never been described. Methodological limitations related to etiological factors, timing of appearance, degree of severity, progressing characteristics, and individuals' age, have enabled relevant studies only in subgroups of patients with facial asymmetry (i.e. hemofacial

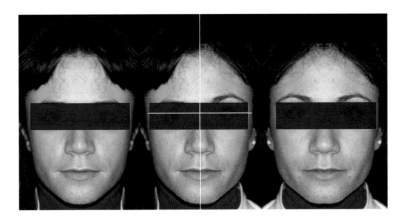

Figure 1.2 Three images where the right face is composed of two right sides, the middle one is the real face, and the left one is composed of two left sides.

microsomia) or dentofacial deformities in university orthodontic clinics.

When studying dentofacial deformity patients at the University of North Carolina, it was found that 34% demonstrated an apparent facial asymmetries. When present, asymmetry affected the upper face in only 5%, the midface (primarily the nose) in 36%, and the chin in 74% (Severt and Proffit 1997).

Recently, Evangelista et al. (2022) performed a review of the prevalence of mandibular asymmetry in different skeletal sagittal patterns and found that there was a significant difference between findings reported from different studies varying from 17.43 to 72.95%, and indicated that the more severe malocclusions exhibited more severe chin deviations than the nonorthodontic population.

Whereas most of the relevant studies have been focusing on facial asymmetry, Sheats et al. (1998) looked into the occlusal status of patients being treated in a graduate clinic and found that in 62% of the patients, the mandibular midline deviated from the facial midline.

An important part of this book will focus on the treatment of patients with various types of facial and dentoalveolar asymmetry focusing on interception, correction, or camouflage. The interception can only be performed for asymmetries related to functional deviations or/and eruption of teeth. Corrections and camouflage in some patients with skeletal asymmetries start at an early age and often continue for the remaining growth period. In adult patients, treatment comprises displacement of teeth and dentoalveolar modeling with goal-oriented biomechanics and orthognathic surgery when needed. For asymmetries with different localization, their etiology and the possible treatment modalities from a biological, biomechanical, and surgical viewpoints will be discussed. In relation to management, generating symmetry is among the goals of most treatment plans. However, when the outcome of orthodontics is assessed, even minor asymmetries are frequently impossible to generate a result that is compatible with ideal morphology and function.

The challenges in dealing with problems related to facial asymmetry are numerous and, to the knowledge of the editors, many of them have not been dealt with systematically. The purpose of this book is to satisfy the need for a comprehensive text on etiology, localization, and treatment of asymmetries within the craniofacial region. It is our hope that this books will cover all aspects of asymmetry starting with localization followed by etiology, congenital, or acquired through disease or trauma. In addition, it is crucial to verify if what is detected is reflecting a static or a developing deviation. Not only the localization and the morphological characteristics are important when categorizing the different types of asymmetries, but also the etiology should be established before a treatment plan can be worked out.

All contributing authors of this publication are prominent colleagues recognized as experts each within their specialization and the assigned subject within face asymmetries. It is our hope that this book will serve as inspiration for the colleague to approach a goal-oriented therapy based on all-inclusive diagnoses, localization of the asymmetry, and the definition of a comprehensive treatment goal.

References

Baudouin J, Tiberghien G. Symmetry, averageness, and feature size in the facial attractiveness of women. Acta Psychol. 2004;117:313–332.

Bishara SE, Burkey PS, Kharouf JG, Athanasiou AE. Dental and facial asymmetries. In: Bishara SE, ed. Textbook of Orthodontics. Philadelphia: WB Saunders Company, 2001:532–544.

Dorland's Illustrated Medical Dictionary. Philadelphia: WB Saunders, 2000.

Edler RJ. Background considerations to facial aesthetics. J Orthod. 2001;28:159–168.

Evangelista K, Teodoro AB, Bianchi J, Cevidanes LHS, de Oliveira Ruellas AC, Silva MAG, Valladares-Neto J. Prevalence of mandibular asymmetry in different skeletal sagittal patterns. Angle Orthod. 2022;92:118–126.

Komoro M, Kawamura S, Ishihara S. Averageness or symmetry: which is more important for facial attractiveness? Acta Psychol. 2009;131:136–142.

Lundstrom A. Some asymmetries of the dental arches, jaws, and skull, and their etiological significance. Am J Orthod. 1961;47:81–106.

Powell WR, Schirillo JA. Asymmetrical facial expressions in portraits and hemispheric laterality: a literature review. Laterality. 2009;14:545–572.

Rhodes G, Zebrowitz LA, Clark A, Hightower A, McKay R. Do facial averageness and symmetry signal health? Evol Hum Behav. 2001;22:31–46.

Schirillo JA. Hemispheric asymmetries and gender influence Rembrandt's portrait orientations. Neuropsycologia. 2000;38:1593–1606.

Severt TR, Proffit WR. The prevalence of facial asymmetry in the dentofacial deformities population at the University of North Carolina. Int J Adult Orthodon Orthognath Surg. 1997;12:171–176.

Sheats RD, McGorray SP, Musmar Q, Wheeler TT, King GJ. Prevalence of orthodontic asymmetries. Semin Orthod. 1998;3:138–145.

Swaddle JP, Cuthill IC. Asymmetry and human facial attractiveness: symmetry may not always be beautiful. Proc Biol Sci. 1995;261:111–116.

Zheng R, Ren D, Xie C, Pan J, Zhou G. Normality mediates the effect of symmetry on facial attractiveness. Acta Psychol. 2021;217:103311.

Part I

Etiology

2

The Etiology of Dentofacial and Occlusal Asymmetries – An Overview

Birte Melsen

Introduction

Before generating a treatment plan, the etiology of the asymmetry should be determined.

Asymmetries can be congenital or acquired. The congenital asymmetries will be either deformation or malformation occurring prenatally, some of which may be part of various syndromes. Some of the etiologies related to congenital asymmetries have been reviewed in the past (Bishara et al. 1994; Cohen 1995a, 1995b, 1995c), but almost 30 years later a lot of their aspects remain unclear (Medina-Rivera 2016).

Congenital

The deformation generated prenatally will be dependent on the space available and, therefore, more frequent in the case of twins or triplets or after a hard delivery. Mild plagiocephaly is routinely diagnosed at birth as it may be the result of a restrictive environment (Flannery et al. 2012; Looman and Flannery 2012).

The congenital deformation will have strong tendency to self-correct postnatal and this is underlined when advising the importance of the sleeping posture. Among the congenital deformations that led to an asymmetry of the craniofacial skeleton, in the side of the skull, the sleeping posture is considered important. A mild and widespread form is characterized by a flat spot on the back or on one side of the head caused by remaining in a supine position for prolonged periods (Laughlin et al. 2011). Plagiocephaly is a diagonal asymmetry across the head shape. Often it is a flattening of one side at the back of the head that will lead to some facial asymmetry. Depending on whether a synostosis is involved, plagiocephaly can be divided into two groups: If there is premature union of skull bones, this is more properly called craniosynostosis (malformation) or nonsynostotic (deformational) (Kadom and Sze 2010). Surgical treatment of these groups includes the deference method; however, the treatment of deformational plagiocephaly is controversial.

The incidence of deformational plagiocephaly has increased dramatically since the advent of recommendations for parents to keep their babies sleeping on their backs. Data also suggest that the rates of plagiocephaly are higher for twins and multiple births, premature babies, babies who were positioned in the breech position or back-to-back, as well as for babies born after a prolonged labor (Ditthakasem and Kolar 2017).

The most frequently seen asymmetry visible at birth is cleft palate followed by some kind of plagiocephaly or hemifacial microsomia. Hemifacial microsomia is the asymmetry the cause of which is mostly unknown. Chen et al. (2018) suggested different etiologies for a disruption which occur during the first weeks of gestation. One would be external factors as various types of medication, or maternal intrinsic factors as maternal diabetes or genetic factors. In addition, three other causes have been proposed for hemifacial microsomia including a physical damage to the Meckel's cartilage, an abnormal development of the cranial neural crest cells, and a vascular abnormality and hemorrhage model. However, none of these proposed etiological factors can account for the asymmetry and the related deformation. The impact of the vascularization is, however, stressed also when analyzing the effect of maternal factors either genetic or related to disease as diabetes or medication. Contributing to some of the congenital asymmetries may be expression of genetically determined malformations that attack only tissues on one side. This abnormality may be of all tissues, cleft palate and hemifacial microsomia being the most prevalent. The abnormal growth may be of all parts of the craniofacial skeleton. It may be the size of all the tissues or only the skin. However, according to Tingaud-Sequeira et al. (2022) none of these etiologies account for the abnormal development of the first and second branchial arches described by Kjær (2017).

Postnatally

Thumb Sucking

The etiology of asymmetry developed postnatally will, if not related to a congenital disease, be the result of lifestyle or trauma to hard or soft tissues. The most frequent lifestyle cause of asymmetries is the nonnutritional sucking either by pacifier or thumb sucking. During the nonnutritional sucking, the mandible is kept back and the baby does not have to move the mandible forward, a movement as is normally done when sucking and swallowing take place simultaneously. The nonnutritional sucking has been found to be related to open bite and lateral crossbite. The latter may lead to asymmetry and crowding (Dimberg et al. 2010). Apart from the narrow upper arch, an asymmetrical arch form can also be the result of a prolonged thumb sucking (Figure 2.1).

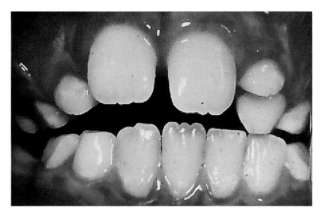

Figure 2.1 Asymmetric anterior open bite generated by prolonged thumb sucking.

Mandibular Fractures

A frequent etiology postnatally can be that trauma both in relation to birth or during early childhood will influence the growth. The most prevalent fractures resulting in asymmetry are the unilateral condylar fractures (Figure 2.2). According to the literature between 25% and 40% of all mandibular fractures are condylar fractures (Enghoff and Siemssen 1956; Müller 1963; Rowe and Milley 1968; Zachariades et al. 2006). In addition, epidemiological studies indicate that the majority of the fractures occur in growing individuals (Lautenbach 1967). The literature comprised description of patients with unilateral fractures where the fractures led to reduced growth on the fracture side whereas others demonstrated the opposite effect, an overgrowth of the fracture side. On this background, Lund (1974) decided to perform a cephalometric radiographic registration on both sagittal and frontal images taken with small intervals in order to be able to describe the changes occurring shortly after the trauma. The age of the 38 patients ranged from 4 to 17 years. He performed an examination of individuals who had been seen in the emergency hospital clinic following severe accidents. He realized that in a major part of the patients, the fractured condyle demonstrated not only healing, but also regeneration toward a normal morphology. He developed a classification of the condylar fractures based on their localization. They were categorized as high when they involved the condylar head or the condylar neck or as low if located in the condylar process. He also classified the fractures according to the position of the head in type 1 where the condylar head was situated in contact with the articular fossa and type 2 where the condylar head was displaced outside the articular fossa. It was demonstrated that type 2 was dominant in relation to high fractures whereas type 1 was seen more frequently in relation to low fractures. Type 2 fracture was also the only one seen in the

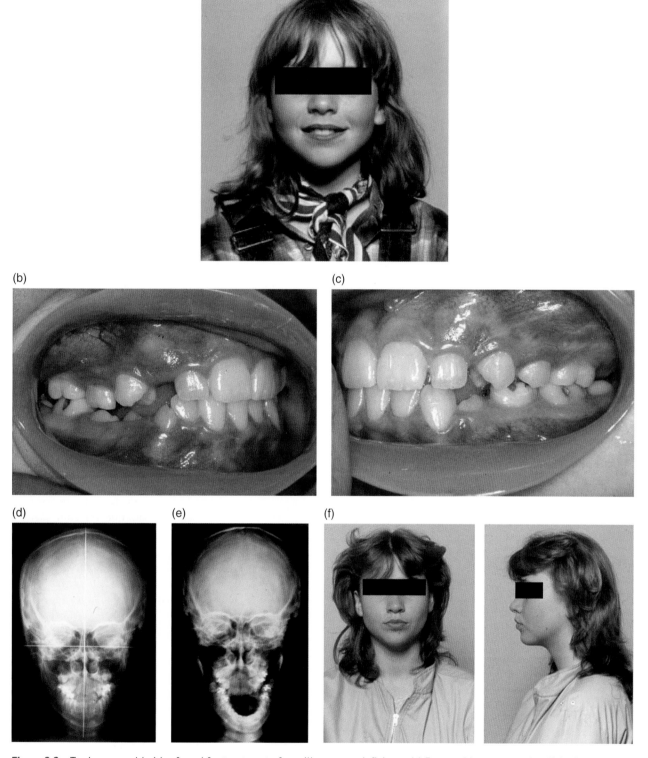

Figure 2.2 Twelve-year-old girl referred for treatment of maxillary space deficiency. (a) Extraoral images reveal a slight face asymmetry; (b and c) intraoral images exhibiting neutral molar occlusion bilaterally, normal overjet, and overbite. There was a midline discrepancy of the lower midline almost one tooth width to the left and space deficiency especially in relation to the upper left canine. The lower arch was characterized by moderate crowding; (d) frontal cephalometric radiograph disclosing an asymmetry, the lower midline displaced to the left; (e) frontal radiograph of the patient with an open mouth. There is an obvious deviation of the mandible to the left; (f) extraoral images of the patient after two years of treatment. The asymmetry is less visible.

older age group. The conclusion drawn from this thorough report was that the changes, namely compensation, occurring following the fracture led to growth that in many cases was larger than that of the healthy side so that an asymmetry characterized by midline displacement to the healthy side was observed. Unfortunately, the classification of the fractures and the systematic way of analyzing the changes occurring after the fracture were not followed up in the multitude of reports on condylar fractures published later. When Strobl et al. (1999) followed 55 patients aged between 2.6 and 9.9 years with the same combination of cephalogram and orthopantomogram as Lund (1974) they found that within the first year there was a very varying reaction to a treatment with a myofunctional appliance, but generally the younger patients (4–7 years old) had no or only minor condylar deformity at the end of the observation period whereas the 7–10 years old children exhibited everything from moderate deformity with reduced height to increase growth and hypertrophy. Unfortunately, this publication did not focus on the influence on the facial asymmetry and midline discrepancy.

Later epidemiological studies collecting data from patients with condylar fractures only assembled information obtained at one point of time. Based on a review of 466 cases seen in an emergency hospital clinic Zachariades et al. (2006) concluded that most fractures occurred between 21 and 30 years of age and, thus did not interfere with growth. Most fractures were exhibiting a displacement of the condylar head but had still contact between the mandible and the fractured condyle. In these cases, it seemed as if the best treatment was done with a functional treatment or intermaxillary fixation. The authors formulated a conclusion regarding type of fracture and need for surgical treatment, but none of their observations or their references who also described fractures in children focused on the midlines or the asymmetries nor at the fracture moment or at the end of growth.

When adult individuals present at a hospital after an accident which may involve several organs the focus is rarely at the occlusion, but later the patient may complain over changes in the way he/she bites, e.g. a gradual opening of the bite and an asymmetry. The panoramic radiograph does not render very much information while cone-beam computed tomography (CBCT) images providing sagittal and frontal images make it obvious that a condylar fracture has taken place (Figure 2.3). An interference with normal development that may lead to asymmetry can be a fracture that actually does not get detected until the consequences,

(a)

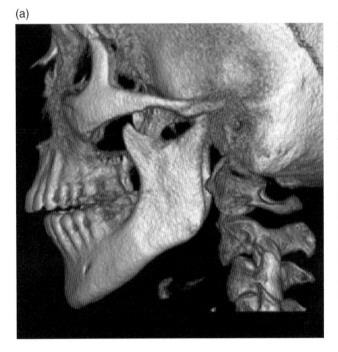

(b)

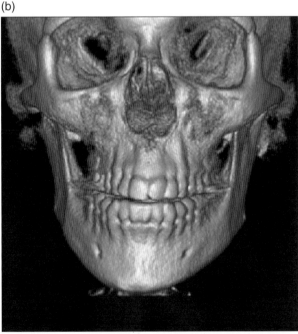

Figure 2.3 (a–c) Radiographs of a patient who days after a trauma detected an opening of the bite and an asymmetry, the reason being a condyle fracture on the right side. (a and b) CBCT images of the patient. A midline discrepancy toward the right side can be observed; (c) the panoramic radiograph does not clearly illustrate what happened to the condyle, but sift of the mandibular midline toward the trauma side can be observed; (d and e) lateral image observed from the traumatized side. It can be observed that the posterior border of the traumatized condyle is pulled back; (f and g) focus on the traumatize condyle on the CBCT image does however illustrate an abnormal morphology; (h) the result of the tomogram clearly illustrate the displacements of the fractured condyle. These images explain why the fracture cannot always be verified on the panoramic radiograph.

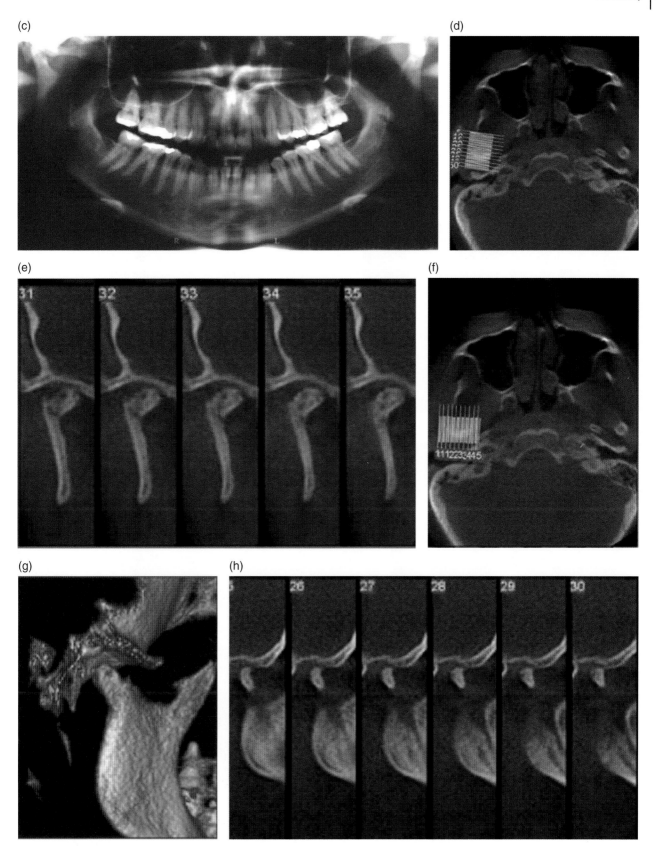

Figure 2.3 (Continued)

in terms of asymmetry in the occlusion and an open bite become obvious.

Soft Tissue Burning

Soft tissue trauma can result in asymmetry. The patient in Figure 2.4 was referred to the orthodontist for crowding in the canine region and minor midline discrepancy. The etiology was a soft tissue burning when the child was playing with an electric cord and contacted the facial soft tissues. This resulted in a scar that influenced the development of the alveolar process of the mandible and a midline discrepancy occurred. Since the result of this kind of trauma, the electric cords have been changed in Denmark so that this kind of damage cannot occur.

(a)

(b)

(c)

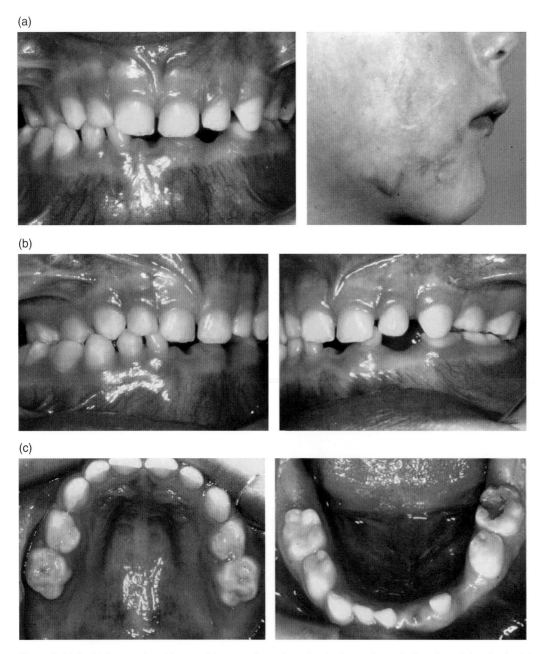

Figure 2.4 (a–b) Extraoral and intraoral images of a patient that had experienced a burning of the check with an electric cord. On the right cheek, a scar can be observed; Intraoral image of the "scar side" demonstrating a cross bite and a severe mandibular midline displacement towards the scar side; (c) Occlusal views demonstrating dentoalveolar asymmetry.

Iatrogenic Trauma

The orthodontist has to be aware of the fact that asymmetries may be generated by orthodontic treatments. Both intra- and inter-arch appliances can generate asymmetries (Grippaudo et al. 2020). If a leveling with super elastic wires is performed in an arch with crowding, the occlusal plane can be influenced (Figure 2.5). Such a standard appliance can easily be part of the etiology of an asymmetry when used for leveling without taking into consideration the effect of the applied force system on the dentoalveolar region (Figures 2.6 and 2.7).

Late Maxillary Expansion

An expansion of the upper dental arch when the midpalatal suture has become interdigitated, as described by Melsen (1975), will lead to a fracture the healing of which prevents further widening of the airways and the patients become mouth breathers. When correction of this situation is attempted, a dentoalveolar asymmetry with periodontal problems may develop.

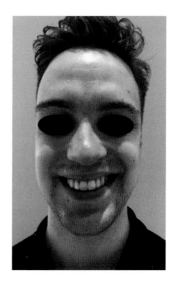

Figure 2.5 Result of a straight-wire treatment with unilateral Class II elastics.

(a)

(b)

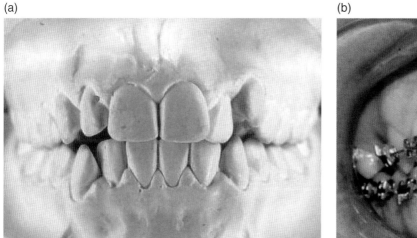
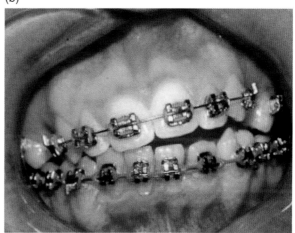

Figure 2.6 (a) Plaster model of a patient with a canine with high labial position; (b) patient where an indiscriminant leveling with Ni–Ti wires had taken place.

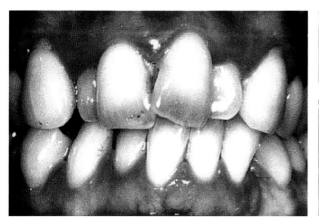
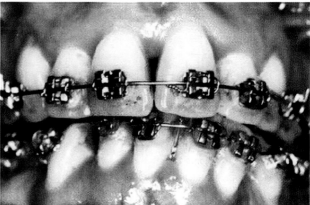

Figure 2.7 A patient who has been treated with a straight-wire appliance.

References

Bishara SE, Burkey PS, Kharouf GF. Dental and facial asymmetries: a review. Angle Orthod. 1994;64:89–98.

Chen Q, Zhao Y, Shen G, Dai J. Etiology and pathogenesis of hemifacial microsomia. J Dent Res. 2018;97:1297–1305.

Cohen MM Jr. Perspectives on craniofacial asymmetry. I. The biology of asymmetry. Int J Oral Maxillofac Surg. 1995a;24:2–7.

Cohen MM Jr. Perspectives on craniofacial asymmetry. II. Asymmetric embryopathies. Int J Oral Maxillofac Surg. 1995b;24:8–12.

Cohen MM Jr. Perspectives on craniofacial asymmetry. III. Common and /or well-known causes of asymmetry. Int J Oral Maxillofac Surg. 1995c;24:127–133.

Dimberg L, Bondemark L, Söderfeldt B, Lennartsson B. Prevalence of malocclusion traits and sucking habits among 3-year-old children. Swed Dent J. 2010;34:35–42.

Ditthakasem K, Kolar JC. Deformational plagiocephaly: a review. Pediatr Nurs. 2017;43:59–64.

Enghoff A, Siemssen SO. Kæbefracturer gennem 10 år. Tandlaegebladet. 1956;11:851–854.

Flannery AB, Looman WS, Kemper KJ. Evidence-based care of the child with deformational plagiocephaly, part II: management. J Pediatr Health Care. 2012;26:320–331.

Grippaudo MM, Quinzi V, Manai A, Paolantonio EG, Valente F, La Torre G, Marzo G. Orthodontic treatment need and timing: assessment of evolutive malocclusion conditions and associated risk factors. Eur J Paediatr Dent. 2020;21:203–208.

Kadom N, Sze RW. Radiological reasoning: a child with posterior plagiocephaly. AJR Am J Roentgenol. 2010;194(3 Suppl): WS5–WS9.

Kjær I. Etiology-based Dental and Craniofacial Diagnostics. Oxford: Wiley-Blackwell, 2017.

Laughlin J, Luerssen TG, Dias MS, Committee on Practice Ambulatory Medicine, Section on Neurological Surgery. Prevention and management of positional skull deformities in infants. Pediatrics. 2011;128:1236–1241.

Lautenbach E. Effects of temporomandibular joint fractures in children and adolescents. Fortschr Kiefer Gesichtschir. 1967;12:78–85.

Looman WS, Flannery AB. Evidence-based care of the child with deformational plagiocephaly. Part I: assessment and diagnosis. J Pediatr Health Care. 2012;26:242–250.

Lund K. Mandibular growth and remodelling processes after condylar fracture. A longitudinal roentgencephalometric study. Acta Odontol Scand Suppl. 1974;32:3–117.

Medina-Rivera JM. Craniofacial asymmetry: a literature review. Int J Orthod Milwaukee. 2016;27:63–65.

Melsen B. Palatal growth studied on human autopsy material. A histologic microradiographic study. Am J Orthod. 1975;68:42–54.

Müller W. Die Frakturen des Gesichtschädels. Dtsch Zahn-Mund- u Kieferheilk. 1963;39:115–128.

Rowe NL, Milley HC. Fractures of the Facial Skeleton. Edinburgh: Livingstone, 1968.

Strobl H, Emshoff R, Röthler G. Conservative treatment of unilateral condylar fractures in children: a long-term clinical and radiologic follow-up of 55 patients. Int J Oral Maxillofac Surg. 1999;28:95–98.

Tingaud-Sequeira A, Trimouille A, Sagardoy T, Lacombe D, Rooryck C. Oculo-auriculo-vertebral spectrum: new genes and literature review on a complex disease. J Med Genet. 2022;59:417–427.

Zachariades N, Mezitis M, Mourouzis C, Papadakis D, Spanou A. Fractures of the mandibular condyle: a review of 466 cases. Literature review, reflections on treatment and proposals. J Craniomaxillofacial Surg. 2006;34:421–432.

3

Congenital

3.1

Distortion/Malformation

Pertti Pirttiniemi

Etiology – Definition

A malformation is a condition where some body part is not properly formed and usually has existed so from the birth, at least so to some degree. A synonym to malformation can be distortion or deformity. These descriptions do not include the etiology of the condition. Therefore, the etiology can be genetic, multifactorial, or due to external conditions for example during the intrauterine period.

When it comes to asymmetric growth of the face, or possible effects on occlusion, various malformations can cause disturbances in normal growth. Therefore, the proper diagnosis and the etiology of the condition are very important, also from the clinical point of view.

The following division does not include cleft lip or palate, or specific syndromes.

Craniosynostosis

Craniosynostosis is a congenital condition where one or several sutures between cranial bones have been prematurely closed. Craniosynostoses are the second most common craniofacial anomaly after the clefts.

Craniosynostosis can be linked to a specific syndrome or it can be separate, with different and often unknown origin. The condition causes abnormal cranial growth and facial dysmorphism. In some cases, the dental occlusion is affected, depending on the location of the premature fusion of the suture (Kreiborg and Björk 1981; Arvystas et al. 1985).

At the moment, about 85% of the craniosynostoses are not linked to any known syndrome. However, this number is continuously decreasing due to advances in genetics (McKusick 2017).

The fusion of craniofacial sutures or the existence of a functional suture is dependent on a group of cytokines, growth factor receptors, and transcription factors. Especially in syndromic craniosynostoses specific mutations in gene coding have been revealed. There are, however, some findings of nonsyndromic craniosynostoses with genetic background, usually with incomplete penetrance (Heuzé et al. 2014).

Single suture craniosynostosis is the most common involvement, being found in 85–90% in all craniosynostoses. Of the single suture craniosynostoses, the most common involvement is the sagittal suture. The next in prevalence are metopic and coronal sutures (Kolar 2011). Premature fusion of cranial suture, as a single suture fusion

Dentofacial and Occlusal Asymmetries, First Edition. Edited by Birte Melsen and Athanasios E. Athanasiou.
© 2025 John Wiley & Sons Ltd. Published 2025 by John Wiley & Sons Ltd.

comprises about half of all single fusions. No asymmetric occlusal involvement has been reported with this type of craniosynostosis. Typically, asymmetric dentofacial growth when linked to nonsyndromic craniosynostosis, has been reported in association with unilateral fusion of coronal suture. In unilateral craniosynostosis of the coronal suture the midface often shifts to the affected side and the mandible does not shift to the same degree, the condition causing a midline shift in the occlusion. However, the dental midlines may be coinciding, due to compensatory mechanisms in the orofacial region, especially in the mandible. The functional occlusion is important in maintaining the symmetry, especially in the oral region (Kreiborg and Björk 1981; Arvystas et al. 1985; Pelo et al. 2011).

Plagiocephaly

The term plagiocephaly is used when there is flattening or bossing of the skull anteriorly or posteriorly. This can be either unilateral or bilateral. Plagiocephaly can be associated with craniosynostosis, or it can be caused by outer forces (Valkama et al. 2019), when it is called positional plagiocephaly. Anterior or frontal plagiocephaly, when linked to craniosynostosis, is usually linked to fusion of the coronal suture and posterior plagiocephaly linked to premature fusion of the lambdoid suture.

Pelo et al. (2011) examined the occlusion and craniofacial structures of 21 patients with unilateral coronal craniosynostosis. They found many craniofacial and dental alterations. The overbite and the overjet were increased in the craniosynostosis group and the lower midline deviation, when compared to the upper midline, was significant. However, as the authors state, the real asymmetry was difficult to measure, as nearly all the structures in the patient group were to some degree asymmetric and a clear reference line in cephalometry is difficult to find. Their conclusion was that the found mandibular asymmetry in the craniosynostosis group with the unilateral coronal synostosis would primarily be dependent on the altered position of the glenoid fossa on the affected side. Thus, the mandibular asymmetry is the consequence of the skull base asymmetry in these cases. Lebuis et al. (2015) did a study on a group of patients with scaphocephaly, where the premature fusion of the sagittal suture causes craniofacial alterations. They found an increase in the prevalence of Class II malocclusion. There was not any increase in asymmetry of the face or lateral malocclusions in these patients and the lateral cephalometric values were mostly within the limits of normal range, which finding could be related to the fact that the primary premature fusion of the suture in these cases was symmetric in the midsagittal plane and not affecting the symmetry of the developing skull or occlusion.

Deformation Plagiocephaly

Deformation plagiocephaly can frequently occur in healthy infants, the highest frequency being found at about three months of age. Deformation plagiocephaly can arise from unevenly distributed external forces on the head of the child which causes the growth direction asymmetrically. Deformation plagiocephaly can be expressed as occipital flattening or unilateral frontal baossing and anterior shifting of the ear. One possible etiological factor has been suggested to be congenital muscular torticollis. However, a high risk for the development of the condition has been shown to be the one-sided positioning and the infant positional preference of the child during the first months of life (Aarnivala et al. 2016). In this respect, it is interesting that it has been shown that by giving parental guidance on the infant sleeping positions, a significant resolution of the condition has been shown to occur (Aarnivala et al. 2015).

Muscular Torticollis

Congenital muscular torticollis is relatively common congenital condition causing asymmetry of the growth, the incidence being reported from 0.3 to 1.3% in newborn population. In muscular torticollis, abnormal cervical muscle function causes abnormality in head posture but also affects orofacial structures which in turn are related to the development of occlusal asymmetry. The etiology of muscular torticollis is multifactorial, but often thought to be a trauma or developmental disorder during the intrauterine period that causes tightness or dysfunction in the sternocleidomastoid muscle. In most cases, head is tilted and the mandible is shifted to the opposite side. When it comes to the increased risk of malocclusions, a high prevalence of lateral crossbites has been reported in the cases of congenital muscular torticollis (Pirttiniemi et al. 1989; Kawamoto et al. 2009). Typically, if the condition is left without treatment in the early childhood, the asymmetric development in the orofacial area is advancing with more severe asymmetry, with many structures distorted. Then the occlusal plane in the frontal view becomes tilted and the mandible becomes asymmetric, which condition is difficult to correct without surgery. In early childhood, the treatment may include operative actions on the affected muscle or physiotherapy only, but most essential is to facilitate the normal balanced muscular function in the neck region.

Developmental Dysplasia of the Hip

Developmental dysplasia (DDH) of the hip is a common musculoskeletal disorder with a hip subluxation and dislocation in newborns with an incidence of 0.1–1%. The etiology of DDH is multifactorial, and like in the cases of muscular torticollis, often thought to be associated with difficulties in intrauterine position, like breech presentation and development of facial asymmetry. One possible risk factor for cranial molding is suggested to be the common treatment method of hip dislocation, where the children are held on their back for a long time to fix the hip to immobilize the hip when using a splint therapy of the joint. In addition, female sex and genetic factors are listed as risk factors (Hanis et al. 2010; de Hundt et al. 2012; Launonen et al. 2018).

By using a stereophotogrammetric method, it has been shown that there is distinct facial asymmetry linked to congenital hip dislocation, which is advancing in nature during growth (Hanis et al. 2010; Tolleson et al. 2010; Launonen et al. 2018). The found asymmetry in the cases of hip dislocation is associated with occlusal asymmetry. There were three times more lateral crossbites in the hip dislocation cases than in the controls and there were significantly more crossbites on the right side and a significant preference for girls (Harila et al. 2012).

Scoliosis

Idiopathic scoliosis is a rather common condition affecting about 3% of adolescent youth. The exact etiology is multifactorial and according to a recent systematic review, there is moderate evidence that there is no known distinct genetic cause of idiopathic scoliosis (Maqsood et al. 2020; Sarwark et al. 2021). However, there is some evidence that in some cases scoliosis may be genetically determined, as a recent GWAS study demonstrated various unknown genetic loci that could explain over 4% of the phenotypic variance of idiopathic scoliosis (Kou et al. 2019).

An increase in facial asymmetry associated with idiopathic scoliosis has been shown in many studies. Because there is a close anatomical relationship between the cervical column and the mandible, it can easily be suspected functional consequences in the orofacial region, if the symmetric development in the spine or trunk is affected.

Most typical findings, associated with scoliosis, concerning asymmetry are midline deviation in the upper and lower dental arch, mandibular deviation, as well as differences in bilateral molar occlusion (Huggare et al. 1991; Ben-Bassat et al. 2006; Saccucci et al. 2011; Nakashima et al. 2017). The found mandibular deviation has been shown to correlate with the degree and direction of the scoliosis curve. Most often reported finding associated with scoliosis, in addition to the occlusal midline shift or differences in molar occlusion, is lateral crossbite (Saccucci et al. 2011). There is also evidence that when the degree of scoliosis becomes more severe, the frequency of lateral crossbite becomes more frequent, while the side of the crossbite being opposite to the deviation in the curve of spine (Sambataro et al. 2019). In many studies, a spine curvature of 10° or over has been considered to be significant in respect to the development of dentofacial asymmetry. Korbmacher et al. (2007) studied a group of children with orthopedic diagnoses. They selected a group with lateral malocclusions and a group with normal lateral occlusion. They found that in the lateral malocclusion group, there were significantly more pathological orthopedic findings, like scoliosis, in the children with crossbite. Based on the occlusal findings with frequent crossbite and unilateral Class II malocclusion, the review of Saccucci et al. (2011) suggests regular orthodontic screening for this patient group, to avoid further development of asymmetry in the dentofacial area.

Hemifacial Hyperplasia

Hemifacial hyperplasia is a condition, which can be diagnosed at birth and thus is a congenial malformation with manifest overgrowth of the half of the soft and bony facial tissues, the other half remaining normally developing. It is interesting that also teeth on the affected side can be enlarged, which fact could point to a genetic origin in these cases. The affected side grows with higher rate than the nonaffected side worsening the asymmetry during growth. Hemifacial hyperplasia must be distinguished from hemimandibular elongation and unilateral condylar hyperplasia, which conditions develop much later and therefore cannot be considered in most cases congenital (Pirttiniemi et al. 2009; Dattani and Heggie 2021).

The etiology of hemifacial hypertrophy has mostly remained unresolved. Recently, Nolte et al. (2020) in a case study revealed mosaicism mutation in condylar tissue of a patient with hemifacial hyperplasia. There are many other attempts to explain the etiology of hemifacial hypertrophy. Most of these studies have a low level of evidence and most of them are based on case presentations (Dattani and Heggie 2021). One explanation for the etiology has been presented by Pollock et al. (1985) where they suggest that there is an increased number of neural crest cells on the affected side in the neural tube area during embryonic development.

The clinical severity of the hemifacial hypertrophy depends on the extent of the growth rate of the involved tissues, as well as the region of the affected tissues. The overgrowth in affected tissues, however, ceases when somatic growth is over (Dattani and Heggie 2021).

References

Aarnivala H, Vuollo V, Harila V, Heikkinen T, Pirttiniemi P, Valkama AM. Preventing deformational plagiocephaly through parent guidance: a randomized, controlled trial. Eur J Pediatr. 2015;174:1197–1208.

Aarnivala H, Vuollo V, Harila V, Heikkinen T, Pirttiniemi P, Holmström L, Valkama AM. The course of positional cranial deformation from 3 to 12 months of age and associated risk factors: a follow-up with 3D imaging. Eur J Pediatr. 2016;175:1893–1903.

Arvystas MG, Antonellis P, Justin AF. Progressive facial asymmetry as a result of early closure of the left coronal suture. Am J Orthod. 1985;87:240–246.

Ben-Bassat Y, Yitschaky M, Kaplan L, Brin I. Occlusal patterns in patients with idiopathic scoliosis. Am J Orthod Dentofac Orthop. 2006;130:629–633.

Dattani A, Heggie A. Hemifacial hyperplasia: a case series and review of the literature. Int J Oral Maxillofac Surg. 2021;50:341–348.

Hanis SB, Kau CH, Souccar NM, English JD, Pirttiniemi P, Valkama M, Harila V. Facial morphology of Finnish children with and without developmental hip dysplasia using 3D facial templates. Orthod Craniofacial Res. 2010;13:229–237.

Harila V, Valkama M, Sato K, Tolleson S, Hanis S, Kau CH, Pirttiniemi P. Occlusal asymmetries in children with congenital hip dislocation. Eur J Orthod. 2012;34:307–311.

Heuzé Y, Holmes G, Peter I, Richtsmeier JT, Jabs EW. Closing the gap: Genetic and genomic continuum from syndromic to nonsyndromic craniosynostoses. Curr Genet Med Rep. 2014;2:135–145.

Huggare J, Pirttiniemi P, Serlo W. Head posture and dentofacial morphology in subjects treated for scoliosis. Proc Finn Dent Soc. 1991;87:151–158.

de Hundt M, Vlemmix F, Bais JM, Hutton EK, de Groot CJ, Mol BW, Kok M. Risk factors for developmental dysplasia of the hip: a meta-analysis. Eur J Obstet Gynecol Reprod Biol. 2012;165:8–17.

Kawamoto HK, Kim SS, Jarrahy R, Bradley JP. Differential diagnosis of the idiopathic laterally deviated mandible. Plast Reconstr Surg. 2009;12:1599–1609.

Kolar JC. An epidemiological study of nonsyndromal craniosynostoses. J Craniofac Surg. 2011;22:47–49.

Kou I, Otomo N, Takeda K, Momozawa Y, Lu HF, Kubo M, Kamatani Y, Ogura Y, Takahashi Y, Nakajima M, Minami S, Uno K, Kawakami N, Ito M, Yonezawa I, Watanabe K,

Kaito T, Yanagida H, Taneichi H, Harimaya K, Taniguchi Y, Shigematsu H, Iida T, Demura S, Sugawara R, Fujita N, Yagi M, Okada E, Hosogane N, Kono K, Nakamura M, Chiba K, Kotani T, Sakuma T, Akazawa T, Suzuki T, Nishida K, Kakutani K, Tsuji T, Sudo H, Iwata A, Sato T, Inami S, Matsumoto M, Terao C, Watanabe K, Ikegawa S. Genome-wide association study identifies 14 previously unreported susceptibility loci for adolescent idiopathic scoliosis in Japanese. Nat Commun. 2019;10:3685.

Korbmacher H, Koch L, Eggers-Stroeder G, Kahl-Nieke B. Associations between orthopaedic disturbances and unilateral crossbite in children with asymmetry of the upper cervical spine. Eur J Orthod. 2007;29:100–104.

Kreiborg S, Björk A. Craniofacial asymmetry of a dry skull with plagiocephaly. Eur J Orthod. 1981;3:195–203.

Launonen A, Maikku M, Vuollo V, Pirttiniemi P, Valkama AM, Heikkinen T, Kau CH, Harila V. 3D follow-up study of facial asymmetry after developmental dysplasia of the hip. Orthod Craniofacial Res. 2018;21:146–152.

Lebuis A, Bortoluzzi P, Huynh N, Bach N. Occlusal relations in patients with scaphocephaly. J Craniofac Surg. 2015;26:1893–1899.

Maqsood A, Frome DK, Gibly RF, Larson JE, Patel NM, Sarwark JF. IS (idiopathic Scoliosis) etiology: Multifactorial genetic research continues. A systematic review 1950 to 2017. J Orthop. 2020;21:421–426.

McKusick V. Online medelian inheritance in man (OMIM). Retrieved from www.omim.org, 2017.

Nakashima A, Nakano H, Yamada T, Inoue K, Sugiyama G, Kumamaru W, Nakajima Y, Sumida T, Yokoyama T, Mishiama K, Mori Y. The relationship between lateral displacement of the mandible and scoliosis. Oral Maxillofac Surg. 2017;21:59–63.

Nolte JW, Alders M, Karssemakers LHE, Becking AG, Hennekam RCM. Molecular basis of unilateral condylar hyperplasia? Int J Oral Maxillofac Surg. 2020;49:1397–1401.

Pelo S, Marianetti TM, Cacucci L, Di Nardo F, Borrelli A, Di Rocco C, Tamburrini G, Moro A, Gasparini G, Deli R. Occlusal alterations in unilateral coronal craniosynostosis. Int J Oral Maxillofac Surg. 2011;40:805–809.

Pirttiniemi P, Lahtela P, Huggare J, Serlo W. Head posture and dentofacial asymmetries in surgically treated muscular torticollis patients. Acta Odontol Scand. 1989;47:193–197.

Pirttiniemi P, Peltomäki T, Müller L, Luder HU. Abnormal mandibular growth and the condylar cartilage. Eur J Orthod. 2009;31:1–11.

Pollock RA, Newman MH, Burdi AR, Condit DP. Congenital hemifacial hyperplasia: an embryologic hypothesis and case report. Cleft Palate J. 1985;22:173–184.

Saccucci M, Tettamanti L, Mummolo S, Polimeni A, Festa F, Tecco S. Scoliosis and dental occlusion: a review of the literature. Scoliosis. 2011;6:15.

Sambataro S, Bocchieri S, Cervino G, La Bruna R, Cicciù A, Innorta M, Benedetto Torrisi B, Cicciù M. Correlations between malocclusion and postural anomalies in children with mixed dentition. J Funct Morphol Kinesiol. 2019;4:45.

Sarwark JF, Castelein RM, Lam TP, Aubin CE, Maqsood A, Moldovan F, Cheng J. Elucidating the inherent features of IS to better understand idiopathic scoliosis etiology and progression. J Orthop. 2021;26:126–129.

Tolleson SR, Kau CH, Lee RP, English JD, Harila V, Pirttiniemi P, Valkama M. 3-D analysis of facial asymmetry in children with hip dysplasia. Angle Orthod. 2010;80:519–524.

Valkama AM, Aarnivala HI, Sato K, Harila V, Heikkinen T, Pirttiniemi P. Plagiocephaly after neonatal developmental dysplasia of the hip at school age. J Clin Med. 2019;9:21.

3.2

Syndromes and Rare Diseases with Asymmetry in the Craniofacial and Dental Regions

Hans Gjørup and Dorte Haubek

Syndromes and Rare Diseases

Syndromes and rare diseases might be associated with facial asymmetry and/or asymmetry of the oral cavity, the dental arches, or the dentition. The present chapter demonstrates examples of syndromes and rare diseases, which in different ways may cause asymmetry. The presentation is mainly restricted to inherited conditions, and it is not the intention to cover all syndromes with asymmetry.

In the medical world, a syndrome is defined as a recognizable complex of symptoms and physical findings, which indicate a specific condition deviating from normal, and for which a direct cause is not necessarily understood (Spranger et al. 1982). However, nowadays the genetic background for many syndromes has been discovered,

e.g. Apert syndrome, which is associated with a pathologic variant of a specific gene, *FGFR2* (Hamm and Robins 2014). Other syndromes are characterized by a diversity of genetic associations, e.g. Cornelia de Lange syndrome, which is associated with pathologic variants of one out of six different genes (Goldenberg and Vera 2021).

The definition of a rare disease varies according to national or regional criteria. According to EU regulations, a disease is rare, if the prevalence is equal to or less than 5 in 10,000 inhabitants (European Commission 1999). In the present context, we use the Danish/Scandinavian definition (Danish Health Authority 2014). According to this, a rare disease is defined as a congenital, complex, and serious disease or condition, which requires access to professionals with special knowledge and expertise. In addition, the rare disease needs well-coordinated and highly

Table 3.2.1 Overview of conditions included in the chapter.

Unilateral overgrowth of craniofacial and/or oro-dental structures		Unilateral underdevelopment of craniofacial and/or oro-dental structures				
Overgrowth syndromes	*Hamartoneoplastic syndromes*	*Branchial arch and oral-acral disorders*	*Syndromic cranio-dysostosis*	*Syndromes affecting skin and mucosa*	*Syndromes with unusual facies*	*Rare dental anomalies*
Primary condylar hyperplasia	Klippel–Trenauneau syndrome (KTS)	Oculo-auriculo-vertebral spectrum	Saethre–Chotzen syndrome (SCS)	Focal dermal hypoplasia (Goltz syndrome)	Progressive hemifacial atrophy	Regional odontodys-plasia
Congenital infiltrating lipomatosis of the face (CIL-F)	Proteus syndrome	Hypoglossia-hypodactyly syndrome		Incontinentia pigmenti		Oligodontia
Segmental odonto-maxillary dysplasia (SOD)				Hypohidrotic ectodermal dysplasia		

specialized diagnostic setting, where relevant procedures, treatments, follow-ups, and controls are carried out. Furthermore, the prevalence of a rare disease has to be equal to or less than 1–2/10,000 inhabitants.

Basically, the craniofacial and dental asymmetries, which may develop in syndromes and rare diseases, are associated with either unilateral overgrowth or unilateral underdevelopment of the structures (Table 3.2.1). Thus, the following description of syndromes is divided into these two main categories, and each of them is subdivided according to a modification of Gorlin's classification of syndromes with impact on head and neck (Gorlin et al. 2001). The diseases and syndromes are defined according to definitions by Orphanet® ("Orphanet: an online database of rare diseases and orphan drugs" 1997).

Unilateral Overgrowth of Craniofacial or Dental Structures

Syndromes with unilateral overgrowth can be divided into overgrowth and hamartoneoplastic syndromes. Selected conditions within these two main groups will be addressed in the following text and illustrations (Table 3.2.1).

Primary Condylar Hyperplasia

Primary condylar hyperplasia is a rare temporomandibular joint anomaly characterized by progressive, nonneoplastic overgrowth of a mandibular condyle. Normally, it is unilateral and leads to progressive facial asymmetry with the chin of the mandible deviating to the nonaffected side. It is hard to delineate bilateral condylar overgrowth from the development of mandibular prognathism, and bilateral cases are seldom reported (Obwegeser 2001). In the present context, only unilateral occurrence is of relevance. Previously, the condition was suggested to be divided into two types: hemimandibular hyperplasia affecting the whole ramal and corporal part of the mandible in the affected side and hemimandibular elongation with an extended vertical dimension of the condyle only (Obwegeser and Makek 1986). The etiology of the condition remains unclear, but it has been associated with excessive formation of articular cartilage or an extended zone of the proliferation zone of the condyle (de Bont et al. 1985; Pirttiniemi et al. 2009).

Craniofacial and Dental Characteristics

The maxilla adapts to the asymmetric development of the mandible and becomes asymmetric as well. A severe canting of the occlusal plane evolves in addition to malocclusion with midline-shift to the unaffected side and a tendency for lateral open bite in the affected side (Arora et al. 2019). In addition to facial disfigurement, the patients may experience severe attrition of the teeth in the nonaffected side because of the unbalanced occlusion. The recommended treatment in the active phase of the condition is high condylectomy, articular repositioning, and orthognathic surgery as alternatives to orthognathic surgery alone (Wolford et al. 2002, 2009). Recontouring of the mandibular inferior border by osteotomy is a treatment option in cases with moderate facial asymmetry and minor or no malocclusion.

Congenital Infiltrating Lipomatosis of the Face (CIL-F)

Congenital infiltrating lipomatosis of the face (CIL-F) is a very rare disorder in which mature unencapsulated lipocytes invade muscle and soft tissues of the facial region (Slavin et al. 1983). It is a unilateral facial condition, characterized by hypertrophy of both soft and hard structures on the affected side and the absence of malignancy. The hypertrophy of the affected side evolves gradually, and the resulting facial asymmetry becomes clearly visible during childhood (Frimpong et al. 2018; Li et al. 2018). The etiology of CIL-F is unknown. However, it has been suggested that the condition might share its pathogenesis with other overgrowth syndromes, i.e. pathologic variants of gene *PIK3CA* (Couto et al. 2017; Maclellan et al. 2014; Sun et al. 2019).

Craniofacial and Dental Characteristics

In addition to the marked facial asymmetry, macrodontism, early eruption of teeth, maxillary and mandibular hypertrophy, macroglossia, and the proliferation of parotid gland on the affected side have been described. Furthermore, some case reports mention agenesis of permanent teeth (MacMillan et al. 1990; Padwa and Mulliken 2001; Sun et al. 2013). The unilateral overgrowth may be extreme and the dental midline of affected jaws can move dramatically to the contralateral side in addition to an obvious vertical effect with canting of the occlusal plane and rima oris (Figure 3.2.1).

Surgical treatment of the soft tissue is controversial because of the infiltrating nature of the condition, and recurrence of facial hypertrophy is common. Surgical treatment might include excision and liposuction (Kamal et al. 2010; Padwa and Mulliken 2001). Extraction of macrodontic teeth, orthodontic treatment, and orthognathic surgery might be indicated to solve the dental problems. Reports on outcome of dental treatment are, however, absent in the scientific literature.

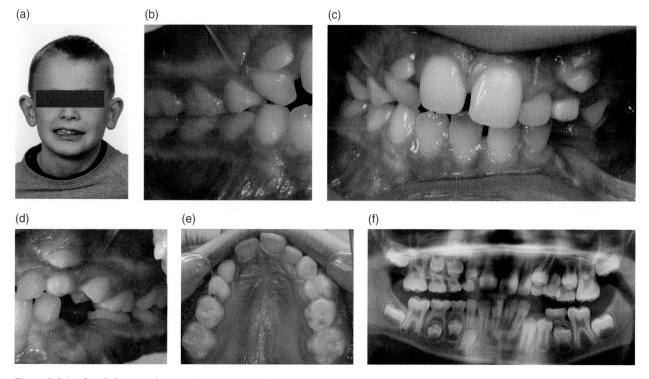

Figure 3.2.1 Boy 9, 3 years of age with congenital infiltrating lipomatosis of the face (CIL-F). (a) Facial asymmetry because of infiltration of lipocytes into soft tissues of the face in left side; (b–d) occlusion with canting of occlusal plane; (e) upper dental arch demonstrating hypertrophic left side processus alveolaris; (f) panoramic radiograph showing asymmetric in dental maturation and eruption, the left side being advanced compared to right side.

Segmental Odontomaxillary Dysplasia

Segmental odontomaxillary dysplasia (SOD) is a rare disorder characterized by unilateral enlargement of the right or left maxillary alveolar bone and gingiva in the region from the back of the canines to the maxillary tuberosity, including dental abnormalities (Danforth et al. 1990). The term SOD was introduced in 1990 as a specification of the term "hemi-maxillofacial dysplasia" (HMFD), which previously was the denomination (Miles et al. 1987).

Craniofacial and Dental Characteristics

In the enlarged region, dental abnormalities, such as missing premolars, abnormal spacing, and delayed dental eruption, occur. Deciduous as well as the permanent molars of the affected region have an abnormal morphology: An enlarged crown, enamel hypoplasia, and widely spread roots of the deciduous molars, which typically present with primary or secondary retention; irregular outer contours and enamel hypoplasia of the permanent molars, which also may be retained or erupted very late.

The bone of the affected area appears dense and sclerotic on radiographs. Histologically, the bone is irregular and immature. SOD has been reported in a limited number of case reports, some of them with reviews of cases (Alakeel 2020; Becktor et al. 2002b; González-Arriagada et al. 2012; Prusack et al. 2000; Whitt et al. 2011) (Figure 3.2.2).

In addition to the symptoms in bone, teeth, and mucosa, facial asymmetry and symptoms of the skin may also be present. Often, the facial asymmetry is moderate, and the facial appearance cannot be characterized as syndromic. The skin symptoms have been reported as unilateral erythema, hypertrichosis, hairy nevus, or Becker nevus. Thus, the condition has by some authors been denominated HATS (*H*emifacial enlargement, *A*symmetry of the face, *T*ooth abnormalities) (Alakeel 2020; Welsch and Stein 2004).

The etiology of SOD is unknown. A vascular theory has been suggested. Recently, a genetic background to SOD has been suggested: Mosaicism with a pathologic variant of *PIK3CA* gene expressed in the affected region (Gibson et al. 2021).

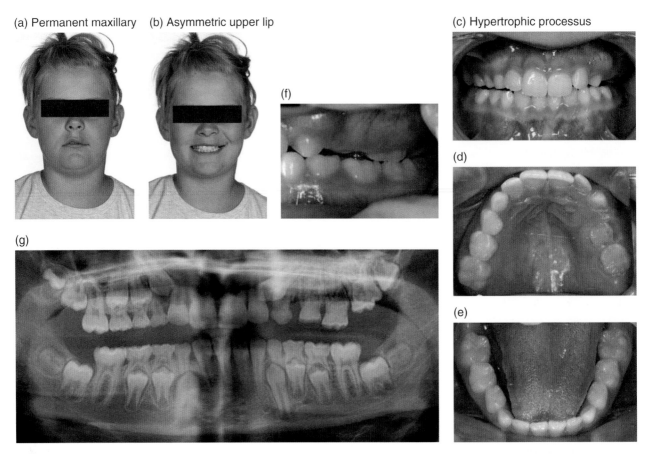

(a) Permanent maxillary (b) Asymmetric upper lip (c) Hypertrophic processus (f) (d) (e) (g)

Figure 3.2.2 A boy, 10.5 years of age with segmental odontodysplasia (SOD). (a and b) Two en face pictures; (c) frontal view of dentition in occlusion; (d) dentition in upper jaw; (e) dentition in lower jaw; (f) occlusion left side; (g) panoramic radiograph showing enlarged left deciduous maxillary molars, aplasia of 34,35, dysplastic permanent molars 26,27, and impacted permanent maxillary canines. Note asymmetric upper lip and hypertrophic processus alveolaris in left side of the maxilla.

The prognosis of the malformed teeth in the affected side is less favorable and implant-supported prosthesis to replace missing teeth is a prevalent need in young adults with SOD. However, the number of reports on the outcome of implant treatment is very limited (Whitt et al. 2011). With lack of eruption and/or early loss of teeth in the affected side, there is a risk of over-eruption of mandibular teeth and a succeeding canting of the mandibular occlusal plan. Reports on the outcome of orthodontic interventions are nonexistent.

Proteus Syndrome and Klippel–Trenauneau Syndrome

Proteus syndrome (PS) is a rare and complex hamartomatous overgrowth disorder, characterized by progressive overgrowth of the skeleton, skin, adipose, and central nervous systems. Normally, the onset of PS occurs from 6 to 18 months of age, and the disease is characterized by asymmetric overgrowth mainly of the hands or feet, but may in addition include unilateral overgrowth of other structures, e.g. facial structures. The skeletal overgrowth occurs rapidly and progressively resulting in the development of distorting and irregular calcified overgrowth in the tubular bones of the limbs, the skull, and vertebral bodies. PS has been reported to be associated with pathologic mutations in one of two components of the phosphatidylinositol 3-kinase (PI3K)-AKT signaling pathway: *PTEN* and *AKT1*. The gene deviations may occur as either a *de novo* mutation or a somatic mosaic mutation (Keppler-Noreuil et al. 2016).

Klippel–Trenaueau syndrome (KTS) (Synonyms: Klippel–Trenaunay–Weber syndrome or Angio-osteohypertrophic syndrome) is a congenital vascular bone syndrome (CVBS) characterized by the presence of an arteriovenous malformation in a limb, which results in overgrowth of the affected limb (You et al. 1983). The disease is associated with deviation in *PIK3CA* (John 2019). Craniofacial and oro-dental involvement in terms of overgrowth and venous varicosities and skeletal and dental hypertrophy may occur (Auluck et al. 2005; Fakir et al. 2009).

Craniofacial and Dental Characteristics
PS, and in some cases also KTS, may be associated with a severely asymmetric development of both craniofacial and oro-dental structures. The result is an obvious disfigurement of the face due to a unilateral overgrowth of skeletal structures and soft tissue. In addition, the maturation of the dentition in the affected side is accelerated, and the physical dimensions of the teeth increase in comparison to teeth of the unaffected side. Furthermore, the patients develop dental crowding and malocclusion with obvious midline-shift toward unaffected side and a canting of the

occlusal plane (Munhoz et al. 2021). Idiopathic root resorptions and dysfunction of the temporomandibular joint have also been described in cases with PS (Becktor et al. 2002a) (Figure 3.2.3).

Unilateral Underdevelopment of Craniofacial or Dental Structures

The second overall topic, being unilateral underdevelopment of craniofacial and/or dental structures, can be divided into many subgroups as illustrated in Table 3.2.1, where an overview of the conditions addressed in the present chapter is given.

Oculo-Auriculo-Vertebral Spectrum

Branchial arch disorders include oculo-auriculo-vertebral spectrum (OAV), previously denoted "hemifacial microsomia" (HFM) or Goldenhar syndrome. The phenotypic spectrum of OAV ranges from isolated mild facial asymmetry to severe bilateral craniofacial microsomia and additional multiple extracranial abnormalities. The craniofacial involvement is in most cases unilateral and includes auricular abnormalities, preauricular appendages and/or fistulas, hypoplasia of the mandible, the maxilla, the malar bone, and/or the zygomatic arch, and epibulbar dermoids. The extent of involvement varies from mild and hardly recognizable to severe with socially handicapping dysmorphic appearance (Rath 2017). Next to cleft lip and palate, OAV is the most common facial anomaly affecting one in 5000 births. Unilateral occurrence in terms of HFM is much more prevalent than bilateral occurrence, and it is a well-known background for facial asymmetry. The etiology of OAV/HFM is debatable, but it is suggested to be associated with incidents occurring during the development and migration of neural crest cells, responsible for the mandibular arch formation (the first branchial arch). In the more severe cases, the second branchial arch is also affected (Gorlin et al. 2001). Embryonic vascular abnormality or hemorrhage might be another explanation to HFM (Hartsfield 2007).

Craniofacial and Dental Characteristics
The variation in severity is the background for a classification according to the degree of mandibular hypoplasia. In mildly affected cases, the contour of the mandibular ramus and condyle is fairly normal, but reduced in size, and the facial asymmetry is moderate. In the most severely affected cases, the condyle and most of the ramus are absent, and the facial asymmetry is severe (Kaban et al. 1988).

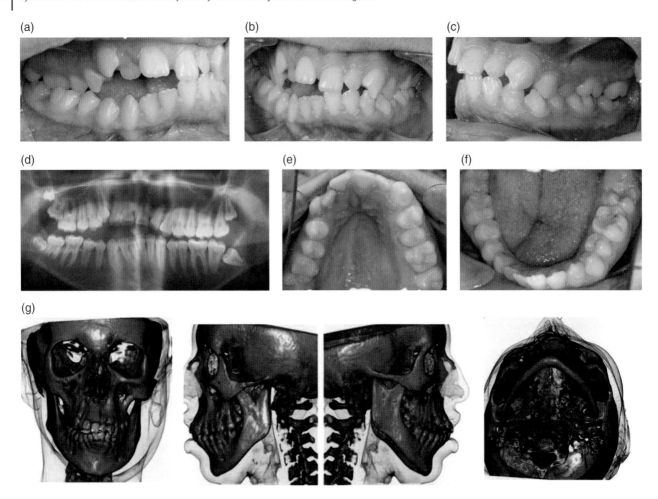

Figure 3.2.3 Clinical photos of a 16-year-old girl with Klippel–Weber–Trenaunay syndrome, including orthopantomography and CBCT of the cranium. (a) Right side of dentition; (b) frontal view of upper and lower jaws with teeth in occlusion; (c) left side of dentition; (d) panoramic radiograph; (e) dentition in upper jaw; (f) dentition in lower jaw; (g) CBCT of cranium. Pictures (a–g) show left-side over-growth of jaws and tongue, increased dimension and advanced maturation of teeth in left side compared to right side. Malocclusion develops in right side, contralateral to the over-growth side.

Agenesis of mandibular teeth is prevalent in individuals with HFM compared to unaffected individuals, and the occurrence of dental anomaly in the affected side seems to be associated with the severity of HFM (Maruko et al. 2001; Silvestri et al. 1996). Further, dental eruption and maturation might be delayed (Farias and Vargervik 1988).

The deviation in mandibular growth induces malocclusion in terms of distal molar relationship and unilateral crossbite in the affected side, and furthermore, a canting of the occlusal plane develops. The vertical development of both the mandibular ramus and the maxilla of the affected side is diminished. Thus, the occlusal plane cants cranially in the affected side.

The majority of children with HFM undergo craniofacial surgery. The mandible becomes reconstructed by distractions-osteogenesis, costochondral rib craft or other bone-graft, or by conventional mandibular sagittal split osteotomy. Additional correction of the maxilla is often requested, and it is performed as a Le Fort I osteotomy or surgically assisted rapid maxillary expansion. In the severe cases with absence of outer ear, a multistage reconstruction with the usage of costo-chondral graft is an option nowadays (Pluijmers et al. 2019).

Saethre–Chotzen Syndrome (SCS)

The most common type of syndromic cranio-synostosis, Crouzon syndrome is normally not associated with asymmetries in the oral and craniofacial structures. In contrast, Saethre–Chotzen syndrome (SCS) presents with unilateral or bilateral synostosis of coronal, eventually in conjunction with sagittal, metopic, or lambdoid, sutures resulting in abnormal skull shape and facial asymmetry, ptosis, and small ears, especially in unilateral cases. Digital abnormalities are also often present. Intelligence is normal in most cases. Some may experience conductive and/or sensorineural hearing loss. Less common manifestations include short stature, hypertelorism, cleft palate, bifid uvula, maxillary hypoplasia, lacrimal duct stenosis, parietal foramina, vertebral anomalies, radio-ulnar synostosis, obstructive sleep apnea, and congenital heart malformations (Gallagher et al. 1993). SCS is due to point mutations or deletions involving the *TWIST1* gene (7p21), which encodes a basic helix-loop-helix (bHLH) transcription factor responsible for cell lineage determination and differentiation (Howard et al. 1997).

Craniofacial and Dental Characteristics

In unilateral cases, asymmetries of the neurocranium may be reflected in the craniofacial region and predispose for dental malocclusion in terms of mandibular overjet and lateral crossbite. The relevant treatments during the period of growth may be different types of neurocranial procedures (fronto-orbital advancement, monobloc biparticipation, forehead cranioplasty) followed by orthognathic procedures (e.g. Le Fort I maxillary expansion and advancement) (Abulezz et al. 2020).

Focal Dermal Hypoplasia (Goltz Syndrome)

Focal dermal hypoplasia (FDH), also called Goltz syndrome, is a rare dysmorphic syndrome characterized by abnormalities in ectodermal- and mesodermal-derived tissues. The classical symptoms are skin abnormalities, limb defects, ocular malformations, and facial dysmorphism (Lombardi 2019). The skin abnormalities include patchy skin hypoplasia, subcutaneous fat herniation, hypoplastic nails, sparse hair and peri-orificial skin, and mucous membranes papilloma. Typical ocular abnormalities include congenital microphthalmia (occasionally anophthalmia), cataracts and iris, and chorioretinal colobomas. Finally, FDH may include craniofacial deviations and dental anomalies (Bostwick et al. 1993).

FDH is caused by mutations in *PORCN,* located at the X-chromosome (Xp11.23), which encodes the porcupine *O*-acyltransferase, involved in the secretion and signaling of WNT proteins. A number of different mutations and deletions have been described (Wang et al. 2014). The inheritance is X-linked dominant, which normally is associated with lethality in boys. However, due to the presence of post-zygotic mosaicism in *PORCN,* FDH has also been reported in boys (Happle 2016).

Craniofacial and Dental Characteristics

Craniofacial dysmorphism includes facial asymmetry, notched nasal alae, small, underfolded pinnae, low-set and protruding ears, mid-facial hypoplasia, and a pointed chin. Dental anomalies in terms of enamel hypoplasia with longitudinal grooving and irregularity of enamel surface are common. Microdontia, peg-shaped teeth, and other irregularities in dental morphology may occur. The irregularities include talon cusps or marked incisal notching of incisors and canines, and molars may have anomalous forms with supernumerary cusps. Hypodontia with dental agenesis is common, and some of the teeth may be delayed in eruption (Murakami et al. 2011). In general, the clinical signs on FDH are more severe on one side than on the other. Interestingly, the asymmetric pattern of symptoms is reflected in the dentition, being most severely affected in one side (Murakami et al. 2011) (Figure 3.2.4).

Incontinentia Pigmenti

Incontinentia pigmenti (IP) is an X-linked syndromic multi-systemic ectodermal disease, which neonatally in females present with a bullous rash along Blaschko's lines (BL), followed by verrucous plaques and hyperpigmented swirling patterns. Furthermore, IP is characterized by abnormalities in other ectodermal tissues, which may include alopecia, nail dystrophy, and tooth anomalies. Ophthalmologic anomalies in terms of microphtalmia or retinal detachment may also be present in addition to central nervous system (CNS) abnormalities (Scheuerle 2019). The neonatally bullous rash evolves from stage I to a verrucous stage II and further to stage III with hyperpigmentation along BL. In adulthood, the skin symptoms remain as hypo-pigmented, hairless regions following BL. IP is caused by mutations of the NF-kappaB essential modulator gene *IKBKG* (formerly *NEMO*), and the inheritance is X-linked dominant (Smahi et al. 2000). Primarily females are affected because of the dominant X-linked inheritance. However, due to the presence of post-zygotic mosaicism, males with IP have also been reported (Gregersen et al. 2013).

Craniofacial and Dental Characteristics

Dental anomalies are described as major diagnostic criteria in line with the dermatologic characteristics and pathologic variant of *IKBKG* (Bodemer et al. 2020). The main dental anomalies are agenesis of multiple teeth in both dentitions (90% of cases have absence of multiple permanent teeth), deviations in crown morphology (in approximately 70% of cases), delayed dentition, and various types of dental malocclusion, arched palate, and eventually an orofacial cleft. In the permanent dentition, the pattern of agenesis follows the pattern in other patients with hypodontia, i.e. absence of the lateral incisors, second maxillary premolars, and mandibular premolars being the dominant

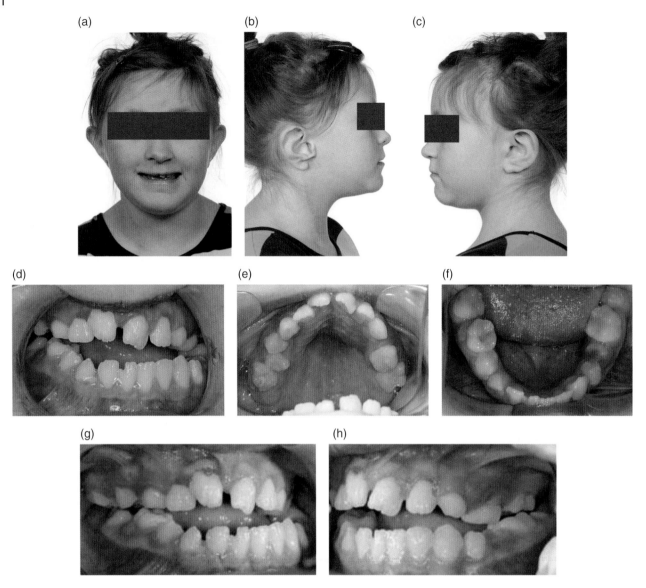

Figure 3.2.4 14-year-old female with focal dermal hypoplasia (FDH). (a) En face picture; (b) right side of face; (c) left side of face; (d) frontal view of upper and lower jaw with teeth in occlusion; (e) dentition in upper jaw; (f) dentition in lower jaw; (g) dental occlusion from right perspective; (h) dental occlusion from left perspective. Notice asymmetry of external facial structures (nose and outer ears) and oro-dental structures. The morphology of teeth is most irregular in right side.

trait (Santa-Maria et al. 2017). The clinical crown of the incisors is frequently peg-shaped or with other morphological abnormalities. Molars may appear with fewer cusps than normal. Clinical variability is marked in IP, and especially in IP-males, asymmetry in the dental arches may occur, as consequence of the mosaic nature of the condition in boys. An example of a boy with IP demonstrates the absence of four permanent maxillary teeth (22,25,26,27) in the left side and only two absent teeth in the right side (12,17) (Figure 3.2.5). In relation to the retained mandibular deciduous canines, the permanent successors erupt distally to the deciduous canine in the right side and mesially

in the left side. In left side only, the deciduous molars (65,75) are retained both in the upper and the lower jaw. It is noteworthy that the right-left asymmetry in the dental symptoms, being most severe in left side, mirrors the asymmetry of the ophthalmologic symptoms, the boy being blind at the left eye and having normal vision in right eye.

Hypohidrotic Ectodermal Dysplasia

Hypohidrotic ectodermal dysplasia (HED) is a genetic disorder of ectoderm development, characterized by hypotrichosis (underdevelopment of scalp and body hair),

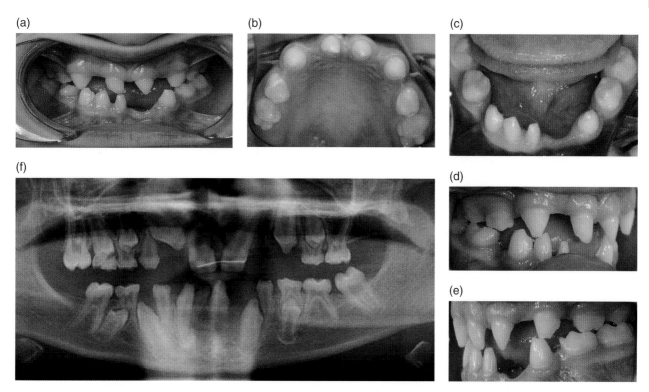

Figure 3.2.5 Boy (5 years of age) with incontinentia pigmentia (IP) and with agenesia of 12 permanent teeth. (a) Frontal view of upper and lower jaw with teeth in occlusion; (b) dentition in upper dental arch; (c) dentition in lower dental arch; (d) dental occlusion (right side); (e) dental occlusion (left side); (f) panoramic radiographs at the age of 11 years of age showing agenesis of multiple (5) permanent maxillary teeth in left side and of few missing teeth in right side (2), ectopic position of canine in left side of upper jaw and fully preserved roots of primary molars in left side of jaws. Notice abnormal shape of incisors.

hypohidrosis (underdevelopment of sweat glands), and hypodontia (underdevelopment of teeth). It comprises three clinically subtypes with impaired sweating as the key symptom: X-linked HED (synonym: Christ-Siemens-Touraine syndrome), autosomal recessive (AR), and autosomal dominant (AD) HED. Furthermore, a fourth subtype of HED with immunodeficiency as an additional symptom exists (HED with immunodeficiency). X-linked HED is the classical and most prevalent type of HED. The prevalence of HED has been estimated to be 1/15,000 (Schneider 2012). In a Danish register study, the prevalence of molecular confirmed X-linked HED was 1.6:100,000 (Nguyen-Nielsen et al. 2013). Children with HED have a decreased or absent ability to sweat (hypohidrosis), which leads to heat intolerance, which may cause recurrent, potentially life-threatening hyper-thermic episodes. Dry eyes, nasopharyngeal furness, and hyposalivation are common characteristics. In X-linked HED, males are more severely affected than females, in whom the symptoms may be mild and in some females even remain unrecognized. HED is caused by mutations in genes of the ectodysplasin/NF-kappaB pathway, which is necessary for the development of ectodermal structures. Mutations in *EDA*, which is

located at the X-chromosome (Xq12-q13.1), explain X-linked HED. Mutations in *EDAR* (2q13), encoding the EDA-receptor, or *EDAR-ADD* (1q42.3), encoding the EDAR-associated death domain (EDAR-ADD) protein, cause AR as well as AD HED. Mutations in *IKBKG* (Xq28) mutations cause HED with immunodeficiency. Some few HED cases are associated with mutations in other genes (Wright et al. 2017).

Craniofacial and Dental Characteristics

Agenesis of teeth and deviations in tooth morphology are cardinal symptoms of HED. Congenital absence of nearly all deciduous and permanent teeth or even absence of all teeth (anodontia) is a dominant symptom in males with X-linked HED. Typically, the crown of the present anterior teeth is conical and widely spaced (Bergendal 2014). The few deciduous molars, if present, may be retained for many years and support the prosthodontic replacement of missing teeth. In general, females with X-linked HED have a much higher number of natural teeth in both dentitions, eventually nearly all teeth are present, and they are described as carriers of the disease. However, some females may have severe dental symptoms equivalent to symptoms

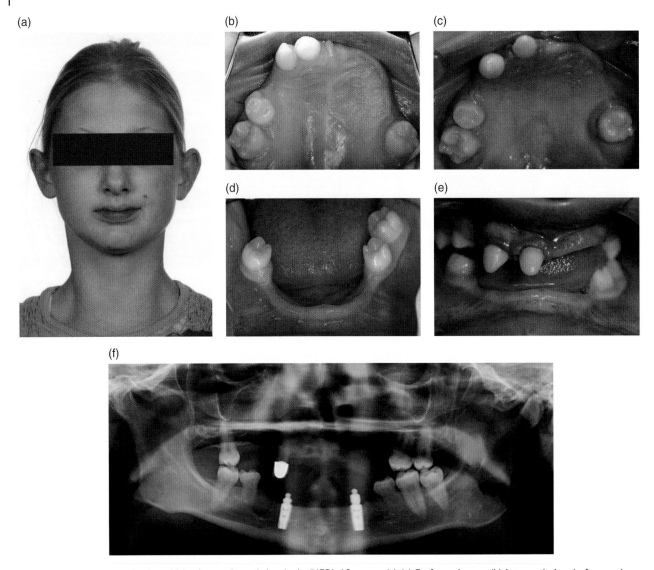

Figure 3.2.6 Female with hypohidrotic ectodermal dysplasia (HED), 10 years old. (a) En face picture; (b) intraoral view before and (c) after orthodontic separation of two pegshaped maxillary incisors (11,51); (d) lower dental arch; (e) anterior occlusal view; and (f) panoramic X-rays after implant insertion at 13 years of age. The deciduous incisor (51) is exfoliated and the 55 has been extracted because of infraposition.

of males, presumably because of a high degree of inactivation of the normal allele (Lexner et al. 2008). Figure HED shows a girl with X-linked HED and demonstrates how the dental arches in addition to absence of teeth is affected by asymmetry. In the upper dental arch, one permanent and one deciduous peg-shaped incisor was developed in the right side and none in the left side. Posteriorly, the right side contained one permanent and one deciduous molar, and the left side contained two permanent molars. In the lower arch, the asymmetry was minor: The right side contained one permanent and one deciduous molar in contrast to two permanent and one deciduous molar in left side.

The treatment of the children with HED exhibiting severe phenotypes of oligodontia or anodontia may call for implant-supported prosthesis at a very early stage, long before growth has ceased. However, not younger than seven years of age and primarily in the anterior mandibular region (Wright et al. 2017) (Figure 3.2.6).

Progressive Hemifacial Atrophy

Parry in 1825 and Romberg in 1845 first described progressive hemifacial atrophy (PHA), synonymously Parry–Romberg syndrome. It is a rare acquired disorder, characterized by unilateral progressive atrophy of the skin and soft tissues of half of the face (Tolkachjov et al. 2015). Muscles, cartilage, and the underlying bony structures may also be involved in addition to neurological symptoms, like seizures (Chen et al. 2020). The unilateral atrophy includes the territory of one or more branches of the fifth cranial nerve and develops slowly during the first two decades of life. The condition is self-limiting. In many ways, PHA and "morphea en coup de sabre" are alike, and PHA may be considered as a facial subtype of localized scleroderma (Paprocka et al. 2006). The etiology of PHA is unknown, but autoimmunity has been suggested, and treatment with methotrexate and other immune-suppressing drugs is common. Other potential etiologies to PHA are localized vascular dysfunction, trauma, or infection (Tolkachjov et al. 2015).

Craniofacial and Dental Characteristics

It is of relevance for the dental function to be aware of the common presence of unilateral tongue atrophy and hypoplastic masticatory muscles of the affected side. In addition, the salivary glands may be absent or hypoplastic, which is a caries risk factor. To a varying degree, both the maxilla and the mandible are underdeveloped in the HPA affected side, e.g. with a reduced ramal height of the mandible. Depending on the degree of underdevelopment, the face becomes more or less asymmetric. In the affected side, short roots, missing teeth, and crowding of teeth may be present. In addition, deviations in dental occlusion (crossbite) may occur (Al-Aizari et al. 2015; O'Flynn and Kinirons 2006).

Conjunctional to the pharmacological treatment of PHA, surgical treatment has to be considered.

Regional Odontodysplasia (ROD)

Regional odontodysplasia (ROD) is a localized developmental anomaly of the dental tissues. In the affected region of the jaw, the teeth are usually hypoplastic, small, and atypically shaped with irregular and discolored surfaces. ROD is more common in the maxilla than in the mandible, and the condition is generally unilateral. Other common features include eruption failure or delay, and abscesses or fistulae in the absence of caries. Radiographically, ROD is characterized by ghost-like teeth with large irregular pulp chambers and absence of the normal contrast between the irregular layers of dentin and enamel. Histologically, the affected teeth are characterized by mixed areas of cellular, amorphous, and interglobular dentin in addition to a hypoplastic and hypocalcified enamel. The surrounding bone is unaffected. The etiology of the condition is unknown, but circulatory disorders, viral infections, and local trauma have been suggested as causative (Cahuana and Gonzalez 2007).

Craniofacial and Dental Characteristics

In general, the overall bony craniofacial structures are unaffected or only mildly affected by ROD. In contrast, the abnormal and missing teeth may influence both the psychosocial and the masticatory function of the dentition. Due to the unilateral nature of ROD, varying degrees of dental arch asymmetry and malocclusion may also evolve: Examples given are tipping of teeth adjacent to the affected region, midline shift towards the affected side, and overeruption of antagonists (Nijakowski et al. 2022) (Figure 3.2.7). Furthermore, the patient with ROD needs prosthodontic treatment starting with provisional solutions during childhood. When the patient has grown up, the treatment continues with fixed partial dentures, which nowadays typically are implant supported (Abdel-Kader et al. 2019; Hess et al. 2020).

Oligodontia

Clinical features of nonsyndromic oligodontia include six or more missing teeth, lack of development of maxillary and mandibular alveolar bone height, and reduced lower facial height. Deviation in tooth morphology is also observed along with problems in tooth development, eruption, and exfoliation (Bloch-Zupan and Clauss 2013). Oligodontia may be associated with pathogenic variants in one of the genes *PAX9, MSX, WNT10A, EDA, LTBP3,* or others ["Online Mendelian Inheritance in Man (OMIM)" 2022]. The prevalence of oligodontia in Denmark has been estimated to be 0.16% (Rølling and Poulsen 2001), which is in accordance with the reporting (prevalence = 0.14%) in the meta-analysis by Polder et al. (2004).

In cases with oligodontia, the pattern of dental agenesis seems to be associated with the genetic background (Arzoo et al. 2014; Bergendal et al. 2011). According to meta-analysis on hypodontia, unilateral agenesis of the respective tooth types occurs nearly as often as bilateral agenesis (Polder et al. 2004). Unilateral agenesis introduces asymmetry in the dental arch in relation to the dental midline. In rare oligodontia cases, the asymmetry can take extreme forms, e.g. by the congenital absence of all teeth in the left side of the mandible in addition to both mandibular central incisors (Figure 3.2.8). A similar case, including their management of the patient, has been reported by others (Ephraim et al. 2015).

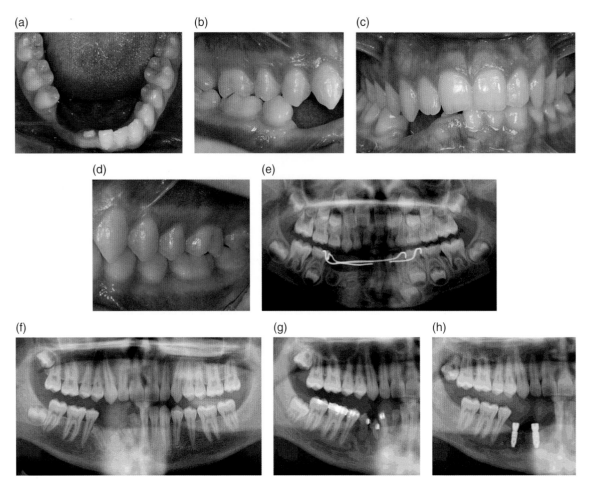

Figure 3.2.7 Male 18 years old with regional odontodysplasia. (a–d) Clinical view demonstrating three absent mandibular teeth (44,43,42) in right side and one dysplastic incisor (41); (e–g) panoramic radiographs showing the unilateral presence of dysplastic, ghost-like mandibular teeth at age seven years (e), at 18 years before initiation of multidiciplinary treatment (f), at age 21 years after orthodontic treatment (g), and after insertion of implants (h).

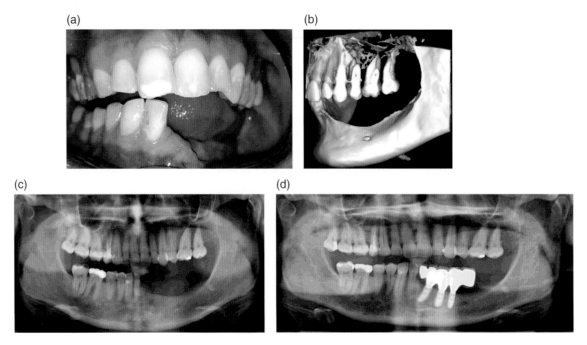

Figure 3.2.8 Male with agenesis of all mandibular teeth in left side. (a) Intraoral photo showing edentulous left side of mandible and absent 41; (b) CBCT-scanning left side of jaws; (c and d) panoramic radiographs before and after treatment with implant-supported fixed partial denture in lower left side.

References

Abdel-Kader MA, Abdelazeem AF, Ahmed NEB, Khalil YM, Mostafa MI. Oral rehabilitation of a case with regional odontodysplasia using a regenerative approach - A case report and a review of literature. Spec Care Dentist. 2019;39:330–339.

Abulezz TA, Allam KA, Wan DC, Lee JC, Kawamoto HK. Saethre–Chotzen syndrome: a report of 7 patients and review of the literature. Ann Plast Surg. 2020;85:251–255.

Al-Aizari NA, Azzeghaiby SN, Al-Shamiri HM, Darwish S, Tarakji B. Oral manifestations of Parry–Romberg syndrome: a review of literature. Avicenna J Med. 2015;5:25–28.

Alakeel A. Hemimaxillary enlargement, asymmetry of the face, tooth abnormalities, and skin findings (HATS) syndrome: a case report and review of the literature. Cureus. 2020;12:e8159.

Arora KS, Bansal R, Mohapatra S, Pareek S. Review and classification update: unilateral condylar hyperplasia. BMJ Case Rep. 2019;12:e227569.

Arzoo PS, Klar J, Bergendal B, Norderyd J, Dahl N. WNT10A mutations account for (1/4) of population-based isolated oligodontia and show phenotypic correlations. Am J Med Genet A. 2014;164A: 353–359.

Auluck A, Suhas S, Pai KM. Klippel–Trenaunay syndrome. Oral Dis. 2005;11:255–258.

Becktor KB, Becktor JP, Karnes PS, Keller EE. Craniofacial and dental manifestations of Proteus syndrome: a case report. Cleft Palate Craniofac J. 2002a;39:233–245.

Becktor KB, Reibel J, Vedel B, Kjaer I. Segmental odontomaxillary dysplasia: clinical, radiological and histological aspects of four cases. Oral Dis. 2002b;8:106–110.

Bergendal B. Orodental manifestations in ectodermal dysplasia – a review. Am J Med Genet A. 2014;164A: 2465–2471.

Bergendal B, Klar J, Stecksen-Blicks C, Norderyd J, Dahl N. Isolated oligodontia associated with mutations in EDARADD, AXIN2, MSX1, and PAX9 genes. Am J Med Genet A. 2011;155A:1616–1622.

Bloch-Zupan A, Clauss F. Oligodontia. Orphanet encyclopedia. Retrieved from https://www.orpha.net/consor/cgi-bin/Disease_Search.php?lng=EN&data_id=14371&Disease_Disease_Search_diseaseGroup=Oligodontia&Disease_Disease_Search_diseaseType=Pat&Disease(s)/group%20of%20diseases=Oligodontia&title=Oligodontia&search=Disease_Search_Simple, 2013.

Bodemer C, Diociaiuti A, Hadj-Rabia S, Robert MP, Desguerre I, Manière MC, Steffann J. Multidisciplinary consensus recommendations from a European network for the diagnosis and practical management of patients with incontinentia pigmenti. J Eur Acad Dermatol Venereol. 2020;34:1415–1424.

de Bont LG, Blankestijn J, Panders AK, Vermey A. Unilateral condylar hyperplasia combined with synovial chondromatosis of the temporomandibular joint. Report of a case. J Maxillofac Surg. 1985;13:32–36.

Bostwick B, Van den Veyver IB, Sutton VR. Focal dermal hypoplasia. In: Adam MP, Ardinger HH, Pagon RA, Wallace SE, Bean LJH, Mirzaa G, Amemiya A, eds. GeneReviews(®). Seattle: University of Washington, 1993.

Cahuana A, Gonzalez Y. Regional odontodysplasia. Orphanet Encyclopedia. Retrieved from https://www.orpha.net/consor/cgi-bin/Disease_Search.php?lng=EN&data_id=11569&Disease_Disease_Search_diseaseGroup=odontodysplasia&Disease_Disease_Search_diseaseType=Pat&Disease(s)/group%20of%20diseases=Regional-odontodysplasia&title=Regional%20odontodysplasia&search=Disease_Search_Simple, 2007.

Chen GC, Chen MJ, Wei WB, Hao YB. Parry–Romberg syndrome with hemimasticatory spasm: a rare combination. J Craniofac Surg. 2020;31:e205–e208.

Couto JA, Konczyk DJ, Vivero MP, Kozakewich HPW, Upton J, Fu X, Greene AK. Somatic PIK3CA mutations are present in multiple tissues of facial infiltrating lipomatosis. Pediatr Res. 2017;82:850–854.

Danforth RA, Melrose RJ, Abrams AM, Handlers JP. Segmental odontomaxillary dysplasia. Report of eight cases and comparison with hemimaxillofacial dysplasia. Oral Surg Oral Med Oral Pathol. 1990;70:81–85.

Danish Health Authority. National Strategy on Rare Diseases. Retrieved from Copenhagen, Denmark, 2014.

Ephraim R, Rajamani T, Feroz TM, Abraham S. Agenesis of multiple primary and permanent teeth unilaterally and its possible management. J Int Oral Health. 2015;7:68–70.

European Commission. Regulation (EC) No 141/2000 of the European Parliament and of the Council of 16 December 1999 on orphan medicinal products. Retrieved from https://www.gmp-compliance.org/guidelines/gmp-guideline/ec-141-2000-regulation-ec-no-141-2000-of-the-european-parliament-and-of-the-council-of-16-december-1999-on-orphan-medicinal-prod. 1999, 2000.

Fakir E, Roberts T, Stephen L, Beighton P. Klippel–Trenaunay-Weber syndrome: orodental manifestations and management considerations. Oral Surg Oral Med Oral Pathol Oral Radiol Endod. 2009;107:754–758.

Farias M, Vargervik K. Dental development in hemifacial microsomia. I. Eruption and agenesis. Pediatr Dent. 1988;10:140–143.

Frimpong GAA, Aboagye E, Amamoo M, Obiri-Yeboah S, Olesu JT. Congenital infiltrating lipomatosis of the face with hyperplastic mandibular, maxillary and pterygoid bones: case report and a review of literature. Int Med Case Rep J. 2018;11:233–238.

Gallagher ER, Ratisoontorn C, Cunningham ML. Saethre–Chotzen syndrome. In: Adam MP, Ardinger HH, Pagon RA, Wallace SE, Bean LJH, Mirzaa G, Amemiya A, eds. GeneReviews(®). Seattle: University of Washington, 1993.

Gibson TM, Rafferty K, Ryan E, Ganguly A, Koutlas IG. Segmental ipsilateral odontognathic dysplasia (mandibular involvement in segmental odontomaxillary dysplasia?) and identification of PIK3CA somatic variant in lesional mandibular gingival tissue. Head Neck Pathol. 2021;15:368–373.

Goldenberg A, Vera G. Cornelia de Lange syndrome. Orphanet Encyclopedia. Retrieved from https://www.orpha.net/consor/cgi-bin/Disease_Search.php?lng=EN&data_id=299&Disease_Disease_Search_diseaseGroup=Cornelia-de-Lange&Disease_Disease_Search_diseaseType=Pat&Disease(s)/group%20of%20diseases=Cornelia-de-Lange-syndrome&title=Cornelia%20de%20Lange%20syndrome&search=Disease_Search_Simple, 2021.

González-Arriagada WA, Vargas PA, Fuentes-Cortés R, Nasi-Toso MA, Lopes MA. Segmental odontomaxillary dysplasia: report of 3 cases and literature review. Head Neck Pathol. 2012;6:171–177.

Gorlin RJ, Cohen MM, Hennekam RC. Syndromes of the Head and Neck. New York: Oxford University Press, 2001.

Gregersen PA, Sommerlund M, Ramsing M, Gjørup H, Rasmussen AA, Aggerholm A. Diagnostic and molecular genetic challenges in male incontinentia pigmenti: a case report. Acta Derm Venereol. 2013;93:741–742.

Hamm A., Robins N. Apert syndrome. Orphanet encyclopedia. Retrieved from https://www.orpha.net/consor/cgi-bin/Disease_Search.php?lng=EN&data_id=261&Disease_Disease_Search_diseaseGroup=Apert-syndrome&Disease_Disease_Search_diseaseType=Pat&Disease(s)/group%20of%20diseases=Apert-syndrome&title=Apert%20syndrome&search=Disease_Search_Simple, 2014.

Happle R. Goltz syndrome and PORCN: a view from Europe. Am J Med Genet C: Semin Med Genet. 2016;172C:21–23.

Hartsfield JK. Review of the etiologic heterogeneity of the oculo-auriculo-vertebral spectrum (hemifacial microsomia). Orthod Craniofacial Res. 2007;10:121–128.

Hess P, Lauridsen EF, Daugaard-Jensen J, Worsaae N, Kofod T, Hermann NV. Treatment strategies for patients with regional odontodysplasia: a presentation of seven new cases and a review of the literature. Oral Health Prev Dent. 2020;18:669–681.

Howard TD, Paznekas WA, Green ED, Chiang LC, Ma N, Ortiz de Luna RI, Jabs EW. Mutations in TWIST, a basic helix-loop-helix transcription factor, in Saethre–Chotzen syndrome. Nat Genet. 1997;15:36–41.

John PR. Klippel–Trenaunay syndrome. Tech Vasc Interv Radiol. 2019;22:100634.

Kaban LB, Moses MH, Mulliken JB. Surgical correction of hemifacial microsomia in the growing child. Plast Reconstr Surg. 1988;82:9–19.

Kamal D, Breton P, Bouletreau P. Congenital infiltrating lipomatosis of the face: report of three cases and review of the literature. J Craniomaxillofac Surg. 2010;38:610–614.

Keppler-Noreuil KM, Parker VE, Darling TN, Martinez-Agosto JA. Somatic overgrowth disorders of the PI3K/AKT/mTOR pathway and therapeutic strategies. Am J Med Genet C: Semin Med Genet. 2016;172:402–421.

Lexner MO, Bardow A, Juncker I, Jensen LG, Almer L, Kreiborg S, Hertz JM. X-linked hypohidrotic ectodermal dysplasia. Genetic and dental findings in 67 Danish patients from 19 families. Clin Genet. 2008;74:252–259.

Li Y, Chang G, Si L, Zhang H, Chang X, Chen Z, Wang X. Congenital Infiltrating lipomatosis of the face: case report and literature review. Ann Plast Surg. 2018;80:83–89.

Lombardi MP. Focal dermal hypoplasia. Orphanet encyclopedia. Retrieved from https://www.orpha.net/consor/cgi-bin/Disease_Search.php?lng=EN&data_id=2004&Disease_Disease_Search_diseaseGroup=Focal-dermal-hypoplasia&Disease_Disease_Search_diseaseType=Pat&Disease(s)/group%20of%20diseases=Focal-dermal-hypoplasia&title=Focal%20dermal%20hypoplasia&search=Disease_Search_Simple, 2019.

Maclellan RA, Luks VL, Vivero MP, Mulliken JB, Zurakowski D, Padwa BL, Kurek KC. PIK3CA activating mutations in facial infiltrating lipomatosis. Plast Reconstr Surg. 2014;133:12e–19e.

MacMillan AR, Oliver AJ, Reade PC, Marshall DR. Regional macrodontia and regional bony enlargement associated with congenital infiltrating lipomatosis of the face presenting as unilateral facial hyperplasia. Brief review and case report. Int J Oral Maxillofac Surg. 1990;19:283–286.

Maruko E, Hayes C, Evans CA, Padwa B, Mulliken JB. Hypodontia in hemifacial microsomia. Cleft Palate Craniofac J. 2001;38:15–19.

Miles DA, Lovas JL, Cohen MM Jr. Hemimaxillofacial dysplasia: a newly recognized disorder of facial asymmetry, hypertrichosis of the facial skin, unilateral enlargement of the maxilla, and hypoplastic teeth in two patients. Oral Surg Oral Med Oral Pathol. 1987;64:445–448.

Munhoz L, Arita ES, Nishimura DA, Watanabe PCA. Maxillofacial manifestations of Proteus syndrome: a systematic review with a case report. Oral Radiol. 2021;37:2–12.

Murakami C, de Oliveira Lira Ortega A, Guimarães AS, Gonçalves-Bittar D, Bönecker M, Ciamponi AL. Focal dermal hypoplasia: a case report and literature review. Oral Surg Oral Med Oral Pathol Oral Radiol Endod. 2011;112:e11–e18.

Nguyen-Nielsen M, Skovbo S, Svaneby D, Pedersen L, Fryzek J. The prevalence of X-linked hypohidrotic ectodermal dysplasia (XLHED) in Denmark, 1995–2010. Eur J Med Genet. 2013;56:236–242.

Nijakowski K, Woś P, Surdacka A. Regional odontodysplasia: a systematic review of case reports. Int J Environ Res Public Health. 2022;19:1683.

Obwegeser HL. Mandibular Growth Anomalies: Terminology, Aetiology, Diagnosis, Treatment. Berlin: Springer-Verlag, 2001:2001.

Obwegeser HL, Makek MS. Hemimandibular hyperplasia - hemimandibular elongation. J Maxillofac Surg. 1986;14:183–208.

O'Flynn S, Kinirons M. Parry–Romberg syndrome: a report of the dental findings in a child followed up for 9 years. Int J Paediatr Dent. 2006;16:297–301.

Online Mendelian Inheritance in Man (OMIM). Tooth agenesis, selective. Retrieved from https://www.omim.org/phenotypicSeries/PS106600, 2022.

Orphanet: an online database of rare diseases and orphan drugs. Retrieved 15.07.2021, from http://www.orpha.net, 1997.

Padwa BL, Mulliken JB. Facial infiltrating lipomatosis. Plast Reconstr Surg. 2001;108:1544–1554.

Paprocka J, Jamroz E, Adamek D, Marszal E, Mandera M. Difficulties in differentiation of Parry–Romberg syndrome, unilateral facial sclerodermia, and Rasmussen syndrome. Childs Nerv Syst. 2006;22:409–415.

Pirttiniemi P, Peltomäki T, Müller L, Luder HU. Abnormal mandibular growth and the condylar cartilage. Eur J Orthod. 2009;31:1–11.

Pluijmers BI, Caron C, van de Lande LS, Schaal S, Mathijssen IM, Wolvius EB, Dunaway DJ. Surgical correction of craniofacial microsomia: evaluation of interventions in 565 patients at three major craniofacial units. Plast Reconstr Surg. 2019;143:1467–1476.

Polder BJ, Van't Hof MA, Van der Linden FP, Kuijpers-Jagtman AM. A meta-analysis of the prevalence of dental agenesis of permanent teeth. Community Dent Oral Epidemiol. 2004;32:217–226.

Prusack N, Pringle G, Scotti V, Chen SY. Segmental odontomaxillary dysplasia: a case report and review of the literature. Oral Surg Oral Med Oral Pathol Oral Radiol Endod. 2000;90:483–488.

Rath A. The portal for rare diseases and orphan drugs. Retrieved from http://www.orphanet.fr/, 2017.

Rølling S, Poulsen S. Oligodontia in Danish schoolchildren. Acta Odontol Scand. 2001;59:111–112.

Santa-Maria FD, Mariath LM, Poziomczyk CS, Maahs MAP, Rosa RFM, Zen PRG, Kiszewski AE. Dental anomalies in 14 patients with IP: clinical and radiological analysis and review. Clin Oral Investig. 2017;21:1845–1852.

Scheuerle A. Incontinentia pigmenti. Orphanet encyclopedia. Retrieved from https://www.orpha.net/consor/cgi-bin/Disease_Search.php?lng=EN&data_id=360&Disease_Disease_Search_diseaseGroup=Incontinentia-pigmenti&Disease_Disease_Search_diseaseType=Pat&Disease(s)/group%20of%20diseases=Incontinentia-pigmenti&title=Incontinentia%20pigmenti&search=Disease_Search_Simple, 2019.

Schneider H. Hypohidrotic ectodermal dysplasia. Orphanet encyclopedia. Retrieved from https://www.orpha.net/consor/cgi-bin/Disease_Search.php?lng=EN&data_id=19266&Disease_Disease_Search_diseaseGroup=Hypohidrotic-ectodermal-dysplasia&Disease_Disease_Search_diseaseType=Pat&Disease(s)/group%20of%20diseases=Hypohidrotic-ectodermal-dysplasia&title=Hypohidrotic%20ectodermal%20dysplasia&search=Disease_Search_Simple, 2012.

Silvestri A, Natali G, Fadda MT. Dental agenesis in hemifacial microsomia. Pediatr Dent. 1996;18:48–51.

Slavin SA, Baker DC, McCarthy JG, Mufarrij A. Congenital infiltrating lipomatosis of the face: clinicopathologic evaluation and treatment. Plast Reconstr Surg. 1983;72:158–164.

Smahi A, Courtois G, Vabres P, Yamaoka S, Heuertz S, Munnich A, Nelson DL. Genomic rearrangement in NEMO impairs NF-kappaB activation and is a cause of incontinentia pigmenti. The International Incontinentia Pigmenti (IP) Consortium. Nature. 2000;405:466–472.

Spranger J, Benirschke K, Hall JG, Lenz W, Lowry RB, Opitz JM, Smith DW. Errors of morphogenesis: concepts and terms. Recommendations of an international working group. J Pediatr. 1982;100:160–165.

Sun L, Sun Z, Zhu J, Ma X. Tooth abnormalities in congenital infiltrating lipomatosis of the face. Oral Surg Oral Med Oral Pathol Oral Radiol. 2013;115:e52–e62.

Sun R, Sun L, Li G, Sun Z, Zhao Y, Ma X, Sun C. Congenital infiltrating lipomatosis of the face: a subtype of hemifacial hyperplasia. Int J Pediatr Otorhinolaryngol. 2019;125:107–112.

Tolkachjov SN, Patel NG, Tollefson MM. Progressive hemifacial atrophy: a review. Orphanet J Rare Dis. 2015;10:39.

Wang L, Jin X, Zhao X, Liu D, Hu T, Li W, Chen Q. Focal dermal hypoplasia: updates. Oral Dis. 2014;20:17–24.

Welsch MJ, Stein SL. A syndrome of hemimaxillary enlargement, asymmetry of the face, tooth abnormalities, and skin findings (HATS). Pediatr Dermatol. 2004;21:448–451.

Whitt JC, Rokos JW, Dunlap CL, Barker BF. Segmental odontomaxillary dysplasia: report of a series of 5 cases with long-term follow-up. Oral Surg Oral Med Oral Pathol Oral Radiol Endod. 2011;112:e29–e47.

Wolford LM, Mehra P, Franco P. Use of conservative condylectomy for treatment of osteochondroma of the mandibular condyle. J Oral Maxillofac Surg. 2002;60:262–268.

Wolford LM, Morales-Ryan CA, García-Morales P, Perez D. Surgical management of mandibular condylar hyperplasia type 1. Proc Baylor Univ Med Cent. 2009;22:321–329.

Wright JT, Grange DK, Fete M. Hypohidrotic ectodermal dysplasia. GeneReviews® [Internet]. Retrieved from https://www.ncbi.nlm.nih.gov/books/NBK1112/, 2017.

You CK, Rees J, Gillis DA, Steeves J. Klippel–Trenaunay syndrome: a review. Can J Surg. 1983;26:399–403.

4

Acquired

4.1

Acquired Dentofacial Deformity and Asymmetry

Peter B. Stoustrup and Thomas Klit Pedersen

Introduction

The growth of the mandible and maxilla hinge on sound development of the soft tissue function and the jaw function. Any condition interfering with the development of the functional matrices or directly affecting bone formation may cause changes in the growth (size) and development (morphology) of the mandible and maxilla, termed dentofacial deformity. By definition, acquired dentofacial deformities occur after birth. Dentofacial deformities may vary in expression and severity and often involve an element of skeletal and dental asymmetry.

Diseases causing disturbances in dentofacial growth and development may originate from local or systemic conditions and often involve soft tissue and/or the temporomandibular joint (TMJ). Various underlying pathologies may lead to a similar morphological expression of dentofacial deformity. In order to understand the underlying etiologies of acquired dentofacial and dental asymmetries, it is important to first understand the unique properties of TMJ development to appreciate how different conditions may impact dentofacial growth. This chapter, therefore, begins with a description of TMJ growth and development and its association with asymmetric dentofacial development.

The Temporomandibular Joint (TMJ) and Its Association with Asymmetric Dentofacial Development

The TMJ is a synovial joint with unique properties related to histology, anatomy, biology, and function (Owtad et al. 2013). These unique properties are important for normal TMJ growth and function but are also critical in situations in which acquired conditions interfere with normal dentofacial development.

TMJ Prenatal Development

The mandible is developed from intramembranous ossification, but the condyle is formed independently. Until approximately the 15th week of gestation, the condylar ossification is intramembranous; hereafter, endochondral ossification appears (Mérida Velasco et al. 2009). The fusion of what later becomes the mandibular bone and the condyle occurs in this period. In contrast to other synovial joints, the TMJ condyle is covered with secondary cartilage, fibrocartilage, which appears later in embryonic life than hyaline cartilage does in the synovial joints of the appendicular skeleton. The fibrocartilage

is characterized by a high content of type I collagen normally characteristic of cutis, tendons and vessels.

Temporomandibular Joint (TMJ) and Mandibular Postnatal Growth and Development

In the long bones of the appendicular skeleton, the bone forms in the epiphysis situated near both ends of the bone, whereas the cartilage in the developing joint derives from the original hyaline cartilage model of the developing bone. Hyaline is a primary cartilage and consists mainly of type II collagen. During compression and inactivity, hyaline cartilage will remain largely intact and unaffected because of its high type II collagen content, whereas fibrocartilage will potentially degenerate because of its high type I collagen content. Furthermore, the fibrocartilage on the TMJ condyle serves as a basis for generating bone by appositional proliferation. Hence, the fibrocartilage is an important mandibular growth site. The TMJ condyle develops by remodeling, apposition, and resorption, based on cartilage proliferation, whereas the ramus and mandibular body grow and develop by periosteal appositional and resorptive activity. The bone-forming activity related to the mandibular condyle is characterized as endochondral ossification. Endochondral ossification also occurs in the epiphyseal plates of the long bones. However, the complex process of the endochondral ossification is somewhat different between condylar growth and growth of the long bones because of the anatomical position of the calcifying zones (Enlow and Hans 1996).

Environmental and genetic factors impact the epigenetic expression of hormones, growth factors, and cytokines within the growth cartilage that orchestrates the condylar and ramus ossification. This intra-articular position makes the condylar growth cartilage vulnerable to environmental changes such as compression (e.g. after orthognathic surgery or trauma) or pathological conditions (e.g. inflammation, infections, and disc displacements). Such environmental changes will affect the epigenetic expression within the condylar cartilage which may, in turn, impact mandibular morphology by interfering with "normal" dentofacial growth and development (Figure 4.1.1). When such a condition occurs in one side only or the timing of the condition is different for the right and left side, the result is a mandibular dentofacial asymmetry, which often has a secondary impact on maxillary growth and development.

Dentofacial asymmetry may also occur in skeletally mature patients if they experience local conditions leading to unilateral TMJ degeneration (e.g. arthritis or

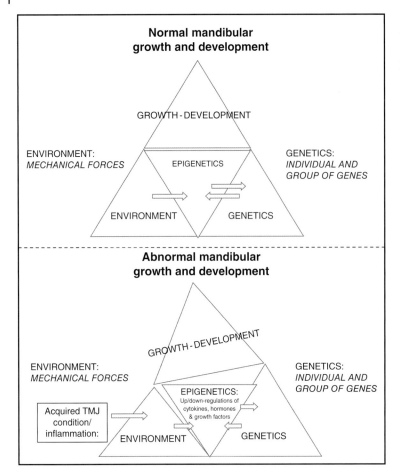

Figure 4.1.1 Normal and abnormal mandibular growth and development. Interplay between environmental and genetic factors in normal and abnormal mandibular growth and development following acquired temporomandibular condition.

osteoarthritis). TMJ degeneration may change the mandibular position and cause dentofacial deformity and asymmetry (Tanaka et al. 2008).

Dental Occlusion and Acquired Skeletal and Dental Asymmetries

Dental occlusion is formed by a complex interplay of various morphological, physiological, genetic, and functional components. The contributing factors influencing occlusal development are listed in Table 4.1.1. Acquired conditions interfering with any of these factors may foster the development of malocclusion. Dental asymmetries are often caused by an underlying skeletal mandibular asymmetry. These asymmetries are often more pronounced in the lower third of the face involving primarily the mandible and, to some extent, the maxilla. Maxillary asymmetries are often secondary to mandibular asymmetries. Dentofacial deformity and skeletal asymmetries may lead to soft-tissue asymmetries. A close relation and similarity exists between facial hard-tissue and soft-tissue asymmetries (Economou et al. 2018).

Table 4.1.1 Contributing factors with an impact on the development of dental occlusion.

- Dentoalveolar growth and development
- Facial growth
- Soft-tissue matrix
- Masticatory function
- Oral habits
- Tongue posture/habits
- Mode of respiration
- Genetics
- Epigenetics

Acquired Dentofacial and Dental Asymmetries

The etiological conditions that can lead to acquired dentofacial deformity and asymmetry are listed in Table 4.1.2. These conditions may occur in both growing patients and in skeletally mature patients. Acquired asymmetries typically originate from dentofacial undergrowth/degeneration of one side

Table 4.1.2 Etiological conditions that may cause dentofacial deformity and asymmetry.

Etiological conditions	Skeletally immature subjects	Skeletally mature subjects
Autoimmune diseases and conditions	***Undergrowth/degeneration*** – Juvenile idiopathic arthritis (JIA) – Idiopathic condylar resorption (ICR) – Systemic lupus erythematosus (SLE) – Mixed connective tissue disease (MCTD)[a] – Scleroderma[a] – Chronic recurrent multifocal osteomyelitis (CRMO)	***Degeneration*** – Rheumatoid arthritis (RA) – Osteoarthritis (OA) – Idiopathic condylar resorption (ICR)
Skeletal growth diseases	***Undergrowth/degeneration*** – Hemimandibular hypoplasia – Hemifacial microsomia[a] – Fibrous dysplasia – Radiotherapy ***Overgrowth*** – Hemimandibular hyperplasia – Tumours	***Degeneration*** — ***Overgrowth*** – Acromegaly
Soft-tissue conditions	***Undergrowth/degeneration*** – Parry–Romberg Syndrome – Tumours – Myopathies	***Undergrowth/degeneration*** — ***Overgrowth*** —
Temporomandibular joint (TMJ) conditions	***Undergrowth/degeneration*** – TMJ ankyloses – Disc displacement – Trauma to the condyle – Idiopathic condylar resorption (ICR) – Septic infection	***Degeneration*** – Disc displacement – Idiopathic condylar resorption (ICR) – Septic infection

[a] May also be grouped in the "soft-tissue condition" category.

compared with the contralateral side. However, in specific conditions, overgrowth may act as an underlying factor causing asymmetric development. Four general categories exist of acquired conditions leading to dentofacial deformity and asymmetry: (i) Autoimmune diseases and conditions, (ii) skeletal growth diseases, (iii) soft-tissue conditions, and (iv) TMJ conditions (Pirttiniemi et al. 2009). The four general categories and their subcategories are listed in Table 4.1.2 and will be elucidated below. The table should be seen as an attempt to summarise acquired conditions leading to dentofacial asymmetry. It should be noted, however, that the division into subcategories is not mutually exclusive, as some of the subtypes are represented in more than one of the general categories.

Autoimmune Conditions

Autoimmune diseases may cause dentofacial deformity and asymmetry in growing individuals and skeletally mature patients alike. In growing patients, autoimmune diseases may impact dentofacial development through condylar growth reduction and deformity. Through involvement of the TMJs, conditions like juvenile idiopathic arthritis (JIA) and systemic lupus erythematosus (SLE) can impact dentofacial growth and development. Scleroderma and, to some degree, mixed connective tissue disease (MCTD) may cause the development of underlying skeletal asymmetry due to abnormal hardening and inflexible cutis in growing individuals. The common features of these conditions in growing patients are that an autoimmune reaction interferes with normal dentofacial growth and development through (i) inflammation of the synovial lining of the TMJ in close contact with the condylar growth cartilage, leading to growth reduction and degeneration; (ii) affection of the soft-tissue matrices and normal joint function; (iii) a direct impact on the remodeling of the mandibular and maxillary bodies; and (iv) an indirect impact on maxillary development secondary to impaired mandibular growth (Tanaka et al. 2008; Arnett et al. 1996a, 1996b; Stoustrup et al. 2020).

Rheumatoid arthritis (RA), idiopathic condylar resorption (ICR), and osteoarthritis (OA) involving the TMJ are conditions that may lead to dentofacial deformity and asymmetry in skeletally mature subjects (Table 4.1.2). Idiopathic condylar resorption and OA have traditionally both been considered "low-inflammatory" TMJ conditions with condylar degeneration related to micro trauma. The autoimmune category of acquired conditions in skeletally immature subjects also involves ICR. In fact, controversy reigns over the ICR condition which is, by some, perceived as a local form of OA with a juvenile or adolescent onset. Others consider ICR to be an isolated form of TMJ arthritis that is different from JIA. Finally, others consider that this isolated TMJ condition belongs to the TMJ conditions category as it is thought to occur due to mechanical functional overloading in predisposed individuals. The ICR condition is therefore listed in both the autoimmune category and the TMJ condition category of acquired conditions in Table 4.1.2.

Juvenile Idiopathic Arthritis (JIA)

JIA is the most common autoimmune disease in childhood affecting 12.8–15/100,000 children annually in the Nordic European countries (Berntson et al. 2003). A high risk exists of TMJ involvement where inflammation causes condylar deformity and impaired condylar and mandibular development. JIA most often presents with several joints involved. However, in rare cases, JIA may occur in a form involving only the TMJ(s). The inflammatory cytokine-driven process influences normal endochondral ossification, changing the morphology of the condyle and affecting the normal development of the mandible and, secondarily, the development of the maxilla. JIA-related dentofacial deformity should be seen as the outcome of a complex process involving decreased bone formation, TMJ dysfunction, and degeneration of TMJ components (Stoustrup et al. 2020) (Figure 4.1.2).

Unilateral TMJ involvement will often cause development of dentofacial asymmetry with a typical morphology consisting of a short condyle and ramus on the affected side and thereby mandibular rotation according to the *z*-axis (Figure 4.1.3). The chin deviates toward the affected side, but the incisal dental midline will often deviate to the contralateral side since the point of rotation according to the *z*-axis will be located between the pogonion and the incisal midpoint. Furthermore, the occlusal plane is canted upward to the affected side. Although asymmetry is more pronounced in cases with unilateral TMJ involvement, asymmetry may also be seen in bilateral cases because of a timely difference in involvement. Deformation of the joint

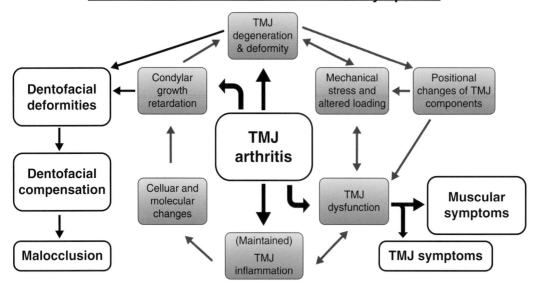

Figure 4.1.2 From temporomandibular joint (TMJ) arthritis to malocclusion in individuals with juvenile idiopathic arthritis. Explanatory model for the arthritis-initiated processes causing malocclusion and orofacial symptoms in skeletally immature subjects. TMJ arthritis may directly impact condylar cartilage homeostasis causing mandibular growth retardation/TMJ degeneration and TMJ dysfunction (black arrows). In turn, this may alter TMJ function (mechanical stress and loading), initiating a progressive inflammatory cycle and promoting further mandibular growth retardation and degeneration (blue boxes). The net result is dentofacial deformity followed by dentofacial compensation and malocclusion (black arrows). TMJ dysfunction may also initiate TMJ and orofacial muscular symptoms. *Suboptimal joint function may induce continuous progression of dentofacial deformity through the low-grade inflammatory cycle (blue boxes) despite successful anti-inflammatory treatment. *Source:* Stoustrup et al. (2020)/with permission of Elsevier.

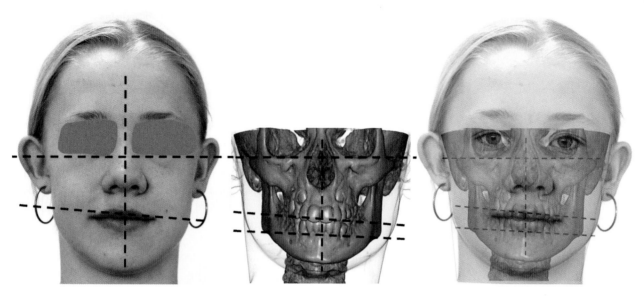

Figure 4.1.3 Autoimmune condition. A 10-year-old girl with juvenile idiopathic arthritis in the right temporomandibular joint causing reduced vertical mandibular development of the right side with dentofacial deformity and asymmetry. The occlusal plane canting towards the right side.

components may cause suboptimal joint function giving rise to pain, decreased jaw mobility, and TMJ dysfunction in the form of a reduced mouth-opening capability (Glerup et al. 2020; Stoustrup et al. 2018).

Idiopathic Condylar Resorptions

A considerable overlap exists between clinical and radiological findings in patients with ICR and patients with JIA (Alimanovic et al. 2021). The two conditions may cause similar manifestations of dentofacial deformity and asymmetry. Whether ICR should be seen as an isolated form of TMJ arthritis or if it may be classified as a unique disease is a subject of discussion, and a certain overlap of the two conditions must be accepted. ICR has previously been named "cheerleader syndrome" because of its characteristics: predilection in teenage females with a history of TMJ internal derangements (Wolford 2001). In addition, the influence of estrogen and general joint hypermobility are considered factors predisposing for ICR (Ji et al. 2020). According to the Diagnostic Criteria for Temporomandibular Disorders (TMD), ICR is a separate diagnosis in the group of TMJ disorders and a subgroup of joint diseases (Schiffman et al. 2014). Even so, it may be speculated that ICR is a juvenile form of OA (degenerative joint disease) occurring due to micro-trauma caused by internal derangements in exposed individuals predisposed by an enhanced hormonal imbalance (Ji et al. 2020). It has been debated if ICR is necessarily a bilateral incident or if it may present unilaterally (Pedersen and Stoustrup 2021); although asymmetric development is

seen in bilateral cases because of a timely difference in onset of the condition, unilateral cases may present with pronounced dentofacial asymmetries. In growing individuals, ICR is believed to impact dentofacial development through growth reduction and degeneration of TMJ components. In patients whose disease onset occurs after they have reached skeletal maturity, progressive dentofacial deformity and asymmetry are caused by TMJ degeneration and subsequent positional changes of the TMJ components.

Systemic Lupus Erythematosus (SLE), Mixed Connective Tissue Disease (MCTD), and Scleroderma

SLE is an autoimmune disease that can affect almost every organ in the body. It is characterized by an autoimmune reaction with widespread inflammation and tissue damage in the affected organs (Kaul et al. 2016). Scleroderma and MCTD are two other autoimmune conditions characterized as a connective tissue disorder where MCTD includes features from SLE, scleroderma, and polymyositis. Common to the three conditions is that they may all lead to TMJ inflammation and affect the surrounding soft tissue which, in turn, may lead to progressive development of TMJ condylar deformity and dentofacial deformity and asymmetry. Morphea en coup de sabre ("sword wound") is a local form of scleroderma that typically manifests in the frontoparietal area of the head. The condition may cause atrophy of the underlying soft tissue and bony structures leading to progressive facial hemiatrophy (Ullman et al. 2021) (Figure 4.1.4).

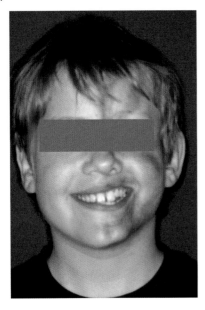

Figure 4.1.4 Scleroderma. Patient with facially localized scleroderma and left-sided coup de sabre.

Chronic Recurrent Multifocal Osteomyelitis (CRMO)

Chronic recurrent multifocal osteomyelitis (CRMO) is a rare autoimmune disease causing nonbacterial inflammation (osteomyelitis) in the bone. The condition is characterized by intermittent periods of pain and swelling of the affected bone followed by periods with symptom remission. The condition mostly involves the long bones. However, involvement of facial bones such as the mandible may occur, leading to mandibular signs and symptoms such as pain, trismus, and related dentofacial asymmetry caused by expansion of the cortical bone (Timme et al. 2020).

Rheumatoid Arthritis (RA)

RA is the most common form of arthritis worldwide. It is an adult autoimmune condition with a typical onset at 30–50 years of age. RA is a chronic inflammatory condition causing pain, stiffness, swelling, and a reduced range of motion of the affected joint (Campos et al. 2021). RA may involve the TMJ and promote degeneration and TMJ deformity, leading to subsequent loss of condylar height and positional changes of the condyle-fossa relationship and unstable occlusion (Campos et al. 2021). Undergoing these changes, the mandible rotates in a posterior direction indicated by a progressive anterior opening of the bite. In patients with unilateral TMJ involvement of RA, asymmetric dentofacial development may occur due to progressive unilateral degeneration and loss of condylar height in the affected side.

Osteoarthritis (OA)

OA of the TMJ is a progressive degenerative synovial joint disease caused by imbalance between anabolic and catabolic intraarticular processes due to mechanical loading. OA may occur due to a decrease in the adaptive capacity of the condylar articular surfaces and/or due to an excessive overloading and stress of joint components exceeding the adaptive capacity of the articular surfaces. Age, systemic conditions, and hormonal factors are believed to play a role in OA. Also, mechanical factors such as trauma, parafunction, unstable occlusion, increased overloading, and joint friction are aetiological factors believed to contribute to the development of the condition (Martel-Pelletier et al. 2016).

TMJ osteoarthritis is characterized by a loss of cartilage and inflammatory response in periarticular bone. The result is a collapse of the joint where the bone surfaces are directly articulating followed by pain and joint sounds (Valesan et al. 2021). Radiologically, a loss of bone substance will be evident. TMJ OA is seen mainly in women, and cases with juvenile or adolescent-onset OA might manifest similar to ICR. When TMJ OA occurs before dentofacial growth has ceased, the condition may result in asymmetric mandibular development.

Skeletal Growth Diseases

Skeletal growth diseases are a group of conditions characterized by abnormal dentofacial growth and development related to bone formation processes. The conditions may cause undergrowth/degeneration or overgrowth (Table 4.1.2). Most of the conditions are diagnosed in childhood and adolescence.

Conditions with Skeletal Undergrowth

Hemimandibular Hypoplasia

Hemimandibular hypoplasia is characterized by unilateral mandibular undergrowth with underdeveloped condylar and coronoid processes. The conditions are of unknown etiology and share great similarities with the congenital condition coined hemifacial/craniofacial microsomia, and distinguishing between the two diseases may be challenging. In contrast to patients with hemifacial/craniofacial microsomia, patients with hemimandibular hypoplasia have no soft-tissue, ear or nerve defects and soft-tissue matrix and masticatory muscles are rather well-developed (Meazzini et al. 2011). Usually, patients with hemimandibular hypoplasia have no history of trauma to the jaws. Differentiation between hemimandibular hypoplasia and hemifacial/craniofacial microsomia seems important for therapeutic reasons. Of the two conditions, hemimandibular hypoplasia has been found to have a better therapeutic prognosis during growth-stimulating treatment with an orthopedic functional appliance.

Fibrous Dysplasia

This is a rare condition causing benign fibro-osseous lesions characterized by replacement of normal bone with abnormal fibro-osseous tissue. Facial bones are common sites affected in patients with this condition. Fibrous dysplasia usually leads to pain, dentofacial deformity, and pathologic fractures. The etiology of the condition is related to genetic mutations. The diagnosis of fibrous dysplasia is based on clinical, radiological, and histopathological examinations. Other fibrous lesions that may involve the dentofacial area are ossifying fibromas and benign cemento-osseous dysplasias (MacDonald-Jankowski 2009; Toyosawa et al. 2007).

Conditions with Skeletal Overgrowth

Hemimandibular Hyperplasia (HMH)

Hemimandibular hyperplasia (HMH) is a developmental condition of the mandible of unknown etiology. The condition causes excessive enlargement of one side of the face. Affected structures may involve the condyle, i.e. the condylar neck. Furthermore, the ramus and also the total unilateral part of the mandibular may be enlarged by overgrowth.

Prenatal and acquired etiological factors have been proposed along with genetic mutation (Nolte et al. 2020). Clinically, the condition is characterized by high metabolic activity and dysplastic condylar formation (Figure 4.1.5). After general skeletal maturity is reached, continuous growth in the condylar area may continue to hamper decisions on the timing of treatment of the asymmetry issue.

Mandibular growth may continue long into adulthood (Obwegeser and Makek 1986; Vernucci et al. 2018). Continuous mandibular growth has been reported in patients up to 45 years of age (Jensen et al. 2017). The condition also presents in a less severe form where overgrowth affects only the condyle, coined condylar hyperplasia (CH). The etiology might be different between the two conditions; HMH presents with diffuse orientation of the subchondral trabeculae, and cartilage may be present in the bony structures. In contrast, CH presents with a more normal bone–cartilage structure (Pirttiniemi et al. 2009).

HMH is a relevant differential diagnosis in continuous late-growing patients presenting with progressive mandibular excess and a prognathic mandibular appearance. From a therapeutic point of view, it is important to distinguish between genuine HMH and asymmetric development in patients with a Class III molar relationship. Approximately 70% of Class III patients are found to have mandibular asymmetry, and it is important to bear in mind the possibility of HMH when planning orthognathic surgery (Haraguchi et al. 2002). To reach skeletal stability, it is critical to ensure long-term success after surgical correction of HMH has been initiated.

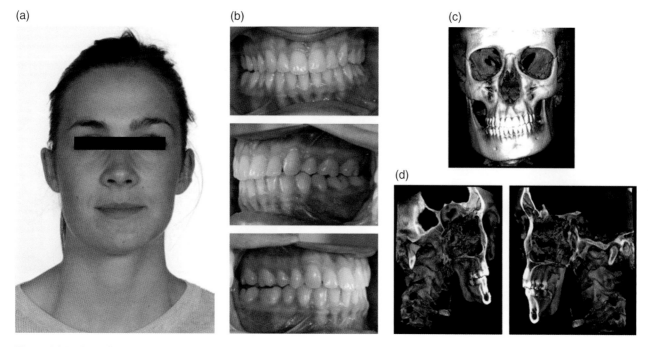

Figure 4.1.5 Hemifacial hyperplasia, (a) asymmetric mandible, longer ramus and higher corpus right side, (b) occlusal plane inclined up towards left side due to partly compensation with eruption of maxillary teeth in the right side, note tendency for open bite on the right side, (c) CBCT 3D reconstruction depicting a larger scale of all bony structures of the right mandible, (d) right sided condylar deformity, the condyle is large with anterior apposition of bone, on the left side the condyle is normal.

Acromegaly

Acromegaly is a differential diagnosis to HMH in which progressive asymmetric development may be seen after normal growth has ceased. Acromegaly is a rare condition caused by hypersecretion of growth hormone by the anterior lobe of the pituitary gland, i.e. pituitary gland tumor. If left untreated, growth of the mandible, the tongue, hands, and feet will continue and the mandibular development may cause dentofacial asymmetry (Meng et al. 2020; Mizuno and Motegi 1988).

Soft-tissue Conditions

The conditions listed in this category are characterised by a developmental disturbance in the surrounding soft-tissue matrix leading to abnormal dentofacial growth and development. Most of the conditions are rare and they may cause both dentofacial undergrowth and overgrowth.

Parry–Romberg Syndrome

Parry–Romberg syndrome is a rare, acquired condition with unknown etiology presenting in early childhood in subjects born with normal facial proportions. The condition is characterized by a unilaterally progressive atrophy (shrinkage) of the subcutaneous tissue, muscles, osseous, and cartilaginous structures of the face, gradually leading to facial asymmetry and malocclusion. The clinical manifestation of this condition may vary from mild to severe, and it has certain similarities with localized scleroderma/morphea. Occasionally, the condition may lead to developmental disturbances of the teeth and the tongue.

Tumors

Tumors and tumor-like lesions may affect the orofacial area. They can be of odontogenic and fibro-osseous origin and may cause swelling and facial asymmetry. Soft-tissue tumors may also directly impact dentofacial growth and development (Figure 4.1.6). The manifestations depend on location and tumor type. It is beyond the scope of this chapter to provide a detailed description of the various types of tumors (Iatrou et al. 2013).

Temporomandibular Joint (TMJ) Conditions

TMJ conditions are characterized by acquired and local TMJ conditions leading to dentofacial deformity and asymmetry. In skeletally immature subjects, these conditions may cause undergrowth/degeneration. The impact on dentofacial growth and development of these conditions vary with the severity and the timing of onset in relation to the growth trajectory.

Temporomandibular Joint (TMJ) Ankyloses

TMJ ankylosis is a condition characterized by a pathological fusion of TMJ components leading to a reduced TMJ range of motion and immobility. The condition

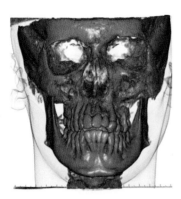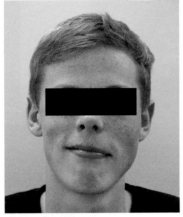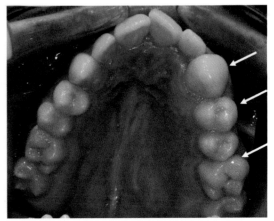

Figure 4.1.6 Soft-tissue condition (Tumor). A 17-year-old boy diagnosed with a benign tumor (infiltrating lipomatosis) of the left side of the face in early childhood. Congenital infiltrating lipomatosis of the face is a rare condition characterized by benign diffuse overgrowth of the adipose tissue into the adjacent tissues with subsequent impact on dental and skeletal development. The patient presents with facial asymmetry due to diffuse, painless enlargement of the left cheek. Only minor mandibular asymmetry is present. Intraorally, the patient displays bony hypertrophy and notable regional macrodontia of the maxillary left canine, premolars, and molars. On exam, his tongue and lower jaw presented with normal morphology.

may impact dentofacial growth and development and cause associated malocclusion if it occurs before skeletal maturity is reached. Trauma and infections (local or systemic) are the most frequent causes of TMJ ankyloses. However, autoimmune conditions, neoplasms, radiation exposure, and previous TMJ surgery may also cause TMJ ankyloses. Ankyloses are grouped based on the location of the condition (true/false condition), the type of tissue involved, and the extent of fusion. "True" ankyloses originate from fusion of intra-articular components. "False" ankyloses are caused by extra-articular pathological conditions not directly related to the TMJ structures (e.g. fusion of coronoid process with zygomatic bone). Furthermore, ankyloses may be complete or partial and occur as a bony form, a fibrous form, or as a combined fibrous-bony form. Fibrous ankylosis may eventually progress into bony ankylosis. The exact pathological pathways leading to ankyloses have yet to be fully elucidated. Intra-articular hematoma caused by previous trauma, fracture healing, and dislocated condylar fracture and also damage to the articular disc may all be contributing factors. It seems relevant to assume that several different pathological pathways may lead to the same clinical manifestation of TMJ ankyloses (Upadya et al. 2021).

Temporomandibular (TMJ) Disc Displacement (Internal Derangement)

Disc displacement may lead to intra-articular functional mechanical overload and inflammation which may, in turn, cause degeneration of TMJ components and reduced mandibular vertical dimension in the affected side. Suggested pathological factors leading to TMJ degeneration include conditions causing TMJ functional overloading and increased joint friction exceeding the host's adaptive capacity (e.g. trauma and disc displacement) (Tanaka et al. 2008).

Studies using magnetic resonance imaging (MRI) techniques have documented that TMJ disc displacement without reduction may cause TMJ inflammation comparable to the inflammation seen in subjects with TMJ JIA (Kellenberger et al. 2019). Disc displacement occurring in growing subjects may become more pronounced because it involves aspects of degeneration and growth reduction comparable to what is seen in JIA. Longitudinal studies have shown that teenage subjects with unilateral TMJ disc displacement have a significantly higher prevalence of dentofacial asymmetry than pediatric subjects without unilateral TMJ disc displacement (Xie et al. 2015, 2016).

Trauma

Facial trauma may lead to dentofacial deformity and asymmetry by impacting the growth potential within the condylar cartilage and by condylar fracture. One-sided trauma to the mandible may lead to asymmetric dentofacial mandibular development in growing subjects. The relationship between facial trauma and dentofacial asymmetry is elucidated elsewhere in this book.

Management of Acquired Dentofacial Deformity and Asymmetry

The objectives of optimal management are to provide a timely diagnosis of the condition, normalize local TMJ conditions (e.g. by reducing TMJ inflammation and internal derangement), alleviate orofacial symptoms and dysfunction if present, and address dentofacial deformity and asymmetry. Optimal treatment planning depends on careful diagnostics and hinges on an understanding of the pathological mechanisms of the underlying condition causing the dentofacial deformity and asymmetry. Common to all of the conditions described in this chapter, there is limited evidence to guide the treatment of dentofacial deformity and asymmetry. Management strategies remain based primarily on conviction and tradition rather than on high-level evidence. The diverse etiological mechanisms and manifestations of conditions leading to dentofacial deformity and asymmetry highlight the importance of an interdisciplinary management approach.

From Diagnosis to Management

Understanding the pathophysiology of the underlying acquired condition is important to build an understanding of the etiology, diagnosis, and treatment. The logical management sequence involves: (i) clinical, radiological, and imaging examination, (ii) diagnostic workup of the pathological mechanism leading to dentofacial deformity and asymmetry, (iii) treatment planning, (iv) treatment and, finally, (v) post-treatment follow-ups. The specific individual components that should be included in this sequence are dictated by the manifestation of the underlying disease. Moreover, the treatment approach to dentofacial deformity varies with the patient's age (growing/nongrowing individual), the type of underlying condition, and the severity of the dentofacial deformity and asymmetry. It is therefore difficult to issue recommendations that are valid and applicable for all conditions causing dentofacial deformity and asymmetry. Most literature has focused on management of conditions that lead to reduced dentofacial growth and development.

Imaging

Imaging of the TMJ and other related structures is an important element in the total diagnostic workup of dentofacial deformity. Traditionally, orthopantomograms (OPG) have been used to diagnose TMJ deformity and other dentoalveolar and dental aspects of importance for treatment planning. Cone-beam computerized tomography (CBCT) is the choice for hard-tissue imaging of dentofacial deformity/asymmetry. CBCTs with a large field of view provide radiological information of TMJ status and facilitate assessment of dentofacial deformity and asymmetry. MRI may be used to assess soft tissue, bone, and functional issues related to facial and TMJ components. When used in combination with intravenous administration of a gadolinium-based contrast medium, MRI may display an increase in T1-weighted signaling in inflamed tissue, which is of great importance for detection of TMJ inflammation (synovial enhancement) (Moe et al. 2016). However, caution is warranted as contrast medium enhancement may be seen both in normal TMJ tissue and in patients with TMD. A minor degree of enhancement may also be present in the normal pediatric TMJ.

Treatment of Dentofacial Deformity in Growing Individuals

In skeletally immature patients, orthopedic and functional treatment is a suggested modality aiming to normalize dentofacial growth and development. This approach has mostly been studied in patients with dentofacial deformities related to JIA and hemifacial/unilateral crania microsomia (Silvestri et al. 1996; Stoustrup et al. 2013). However, we have no reason to believe that the approach may not also be suitable for growing patients with mild to moderate deformities and asymmetry due to conditions such as ICR and internal derangements. Different types of orthopedic functional appliances have been suggested in the form of activators and occlusal splint types. It is important to recognize that mandibular growth and development will continue despite the onset of an acquired TMJ conditions such as JIA and ICR. It is precisely this growth potential that treatment with orthopedic appliances intends to exploit (González et al. 2016). The efficacy of the orthopedic treatment depends on early diagnosis of the dentofacial deformity, timely initiation of treatment, the presence of dentofacial growth potential and good patient cooperation. Treatment modalities are often long of duration and complex.

One way to normalize dentofacial growth and reduce dentofacial asymmetric development is by using a distraction splint (Stoustrup et al. 2013; Pedersen et al. 1995). The distraction splint is an orthopedic, removable appliance constructed to control the occlusal plane development and prevent z-axis asymmetry (Figure 4.1.7). Management is less effective when distraction splint treatment is initiated after mandibular asymmetry has been established. Early diagnosis of dentofacial deformity/asymmetry and timely initiation of treatment with a distraction splint are, therefore, of crucial importance for a successful outcome. The distraction splint is constructed from a flat acrylic splint covering the posterior teeth. The splint has balanced occlusion and after some weeks of use, small impressions are made in the splint corresponding to the habitual muscular occlusion. Hereafter, an acrylic layer is added to the affected side (Figure 4.1.7). Hence, the procedure is repeated, increasing the height of the splint on the affected side with time (Pedersen and Norholt 2011). Use of a distraction splint will create an open bite on the affected side,

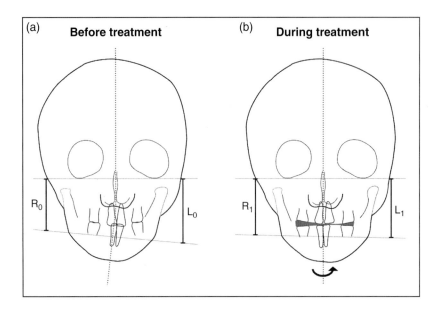

Figure 4.1.7 Distraction splint treatment of unilateral TMJ involvement in skeletally immature subjects. (a) Before distraction splint treatment. Unilateral TMJ involvement (right side) has led to reduced vertical right-sided mandibular development, dentofacial asymmetry, and a canted occlusal plan. Dentofacial asymmetry is illustrated by the reference lines R_0 and L_0; (b) during distraction splint treatment, the height of the splint is gradually increased in the right side. This distraction normalizes mandibular skeletal and dentofacial development in the right side and repositions the mandible in a more symmetric position. Long-term treatment will reduce dentofacial asymmetry as illustrated by the reference lines R_1 and L_1. *Source:* Stoustrup et al. (2020)/with permission of Elsevier.

(a) **Before treatment**   (b) **During treatment**

R_0 L_0 R_1 L_1

and the use of the splint should be changed to an activator once the premolars are erupting. The activator should be designed to mainly allow eruption from the upper jaw on the affected side. In adolescence, fixed orthodontic appliances may be necessary to establish occlusion.

In growing subjects, orthognathic surgery may also be considered if treatment with orthopedic appliances fails to normalize dentofacial development to an acceptable level. Distraction osteogenesis may be considered in growing patients with moderate to severe dentofacial deformity/ asymmetry (Figure 4.1.8). This modality may be used in both growing and nongrowing individuals. When used in growing subjects, residual post-surgical growth and development are controlled by means of individually planned orthopedic and orthodontic treatment. To finalize treatment, maxillary surgery may be required after skeletal maturity has been reached.

Orthodontic treatment alone (e.g. a fixed appliance) has limited effect on an underlying skeletal asymmetry. This modality may be used to correct minor dental discrepancies or to settle the occlusal asymmetry after orthopedic/ surgical-orthodontic correction.

Treatment of Nongrowing Individuals

Surgical modalities should be considered in skeletally mature patients with moderate to severe dentofacial deformity and asymmetry. Surgical options include: (i) distraction osteogenesis, (ii) surgical-orthodontic procedures, and (iii) total alloplastic joint replacement with or without costochondral grafting.

Distraction osteogenesis and orthognathic surgery require TMJ stability before treatment can be initiated (e.g. in patients with JIA, ICR, or internal derangement). No evident guidelines exist for this assessment. However, it is recommended to monitor the stability of the condylar morphology, symptoms, and clinical findings before initiating surgical management. The use of a flat splint with minor impressions from the occluding teeth is one manner in which the mandibular position may be monitored over time. In combination with subsequent CBCT assessments of TMJ components, this approach seems to be valid for assessment of TMJ stability before initiating surgery. In patients with autoimmune conditions, quiescence of the underlying disease should be obtained for a period of 2 years with or without medication before orthognathic

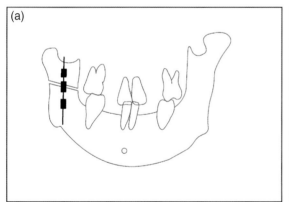
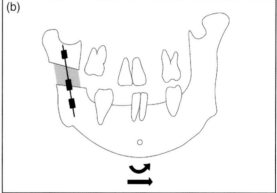
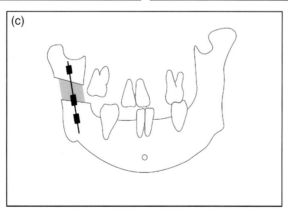

Figure 4.1.8 Surgical distraction osteogenesis. (a) Correction of dentofacial deformity and mandibular asymmetry by distraction osteogenesis (DO) vertically elongating the ramus on the right side; (b) the major mandibular segment rotates according to the *z*-axis and *y*-axis, correcting the occlusal plane cant and shifting the midline, skeletally and dentally, toward the left side; (c) the open bite caused by the vertical component of the DO allows for autorotation of the mandible to first contact on the left side. The maxillary occlusal plane now needs to be corrected by extrusion from the maxilla on the right side either by orthodontics or by orthognathic surgery.

surgery is considered. Insecurity regarding TMJ stability is an argument for dividing the surgical treatment into more than one procedure. Distraction osteogenesis may be used to address skeletal asymmetries at an early age (12–15 years) by ramus elongation on the short ramus side using a surgically inserted intraoral appliance (Pedersen and Norholt 2011). It is important to consider residual mandibular vertical growth individually to overcorrect the asymmetry, thereby achieving a symmetric result after growth has ceased. Once growth has ceased and stability of the TMJ has been obtained, residual skeletal and occlusal discrepancies may be treated orthodontically or through surgical-orthodontic treatment of the maxilla alone, addressing any residual deformity. The potential TMJ instability and condylar alterations throughout the remaining period of growth will be limited and can be addressed in a final surgical-orthodontic treatment at a later stage.

Treatment of Individuals with Continuous Mandibular Overgrowth

In conditions characterized by continuous mandibular or condylar hyperplasia (e.g. hemimandibular hyperplasia and acromegaly), a technetium-enhanced scan (bone scintigraphy) may be used to assess condylar metabolic activity although the result is not specific to growth but may also indicate functional TMJ overloading. In patients with mandibular excess and continued condylar growth, a partial condylectomy may be considered.

Conclusion

The TMJ is a unique joint and acquired TMJ conditions may have a negative impact on dentofacial development, causing deformities and asymmetry. Multiple acquired conditions exist that may lead to dentofacial deformities and asymmetry. They may be divided into four general groups: (i) autoimmune diseases and conditions, (ii) skeletal growth diseases, (iii) soft-tissue conditions, and (iv) TMJ conditions. Acquired conditions are often seen in growing subjects where dentofacial deformity occurs due to a mandibular growth reduction in combination with condylar degeneration (e.g. JIA, ICR, or internal derangement). Acquired diseases that lead to dentofacial deformity and asymmetry with adulthood onset are often caused by conditions leading to condylar degeneration (e.g. RA, OA, or ICR). In rare cases, acquired diseases may also lead to mandibular overgrowth (e.g. hemimandibular hyperplasia).

Treatment of dentofacial deformity varies with the patient's age (growing/nongrowing individual), the type of acquired condition, and the severity of dentofacial deformity and asymmetry. Optimal treatment depends on a careful diagnostic setup with elucidation of the pathological mechanisms causing skeletal asymmetry. In growing subjects, nonsurgical treatment modalities with orthopedic appliances may be considered in subjects with minor to moderate dentofacial deformity/asymmetry. Distraction osteogenesis and orthognathic surgical treatment modalities may be considered in patients with moderate to severe dentofacial deformity and asymmetry. However, both surgical modalities require stable TMJ conditions before treatment can be initiated. Distraction osteogenesis may be applied before skeletal maturity is reached as an early step in the total treatment sequence.

Acknowledgment

The authors want to acknowledge Sven Erik Nørholt, professor, and consultant maxillofacial surgeon, Aarhus University Hospital, Denmark for the management of the DO case presented in Figure 4.1.9.

(a) (b) (c)

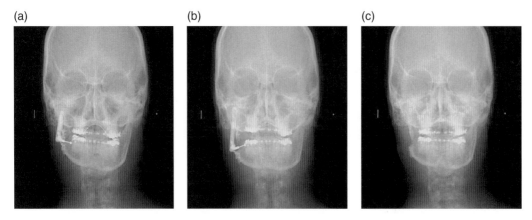

Figure 4.1.9 Unilateral surgical distraction osteogenesis (DO). DO: A 17-year-old girl with JIA and a history of arthritis of the right TMJ was treated with intraoral vertical DO of the ramus. (a) Frontal cephalogram of the device inserted; (b) after 18 mm of distraction; (c) at the time of removal of the device (3 months after insertion), a Le Fort I osteotomy was performed to level the maxilla. TMJ, temporomandibular joint. *Source:* Stoustrup et al. (2020)/Reproduced with permission from Elsevier.

References

Alimanovic D, Pedersen TK, Matzen LH, Stoustrup P. Comparing clinical and radiological manifestations of adolescent idiopathic condylar resorption and juvenile idiopathic arthritis in the temporomandibular joint. J Oral Maxillofac Surg. 2021;79:774–785.

Arnett GW, Milam SB, Gottesman L. Progressive mandibular retrusion—idiopathic condylar resorption. Part I. Am J Orthod Dentofac Orthop. 1996a;110:8–15.

Arnett GW, Milam SB, Gottesman L. Progressive mandibular retrusion-idiopathic condylar resorption. Part II. Am J Orthod Dentofac Orthop. 1996b;110:117–127.

Berntson L, Andersson GB, Fasth A, Herlin T, Kristinsson J, Lahdenne P, Marhaue G, Nielsen S, Pelkonen P, Rygg M, Nordic Study Group. Incidence of juvenile idiopathic arthritis in the Nordic countries. A population based study with special reference to the validity of the ILAR and EULAR criteria. J Rheumatol. 2003;30:2275–2282.

Campos DES, de Araújo Ferreira Muniz I, de Souza Villarim NL, Ribeiro ILA, Batista AUD, Bonan PRF, Oliveira MA. Is there an association between rheumatoid arthritis and bone changes in the temporomandibular joint diagnosed by cone-beam computed tomography? A systematic review and meta-analysis. Clin Oral Investig. 2021;25:2449–2459.

Economou S, Stoustrup P, Kristensen KD, Dalstra M, Kuseler A, Herlin T, Pedersen TK. Evaluation of facial asymmetry in patients with juvenile idiopathic arthritis: correlation between hard tissue and soft tissue landmarks. Am J Orthod Dentofac Orthop. 2018;153:662–672.e1.

Enlow DH, Hans MG, eds. Growth of the mandible. In: Essential of Facial Growth. Philadelphia: Saunders, 1996:57–78.

Glerup M, Stoustrup P, Matzen LH, Rypdal V, Nordal E, Frid P, Arnstad ED, Rygg M, Thorarensen O, Ekelund M, Berntson L, Fasth A, Nilsson H, Peltoniemi S, Aalto K, Arte S, Toftedal P, Nielsen S, Kreiborg S, Herlin T, Pedersen TK. Long-term outcomes of temporomandibular joints in juvenile idiopathic arthritis: 17 years of followup of a Nordic Juvenile Idiopathic Arthritis Cohort. J Rheumatol. 2020;47:730–738.

González MF, Pedersen TK, Dalstra M, Herlin T, Verna C. 3D evaluation of mandibular skeletal changes in juvenile arthritis patients treated with a distraction splint: a retrospective follow-up. Angle Orthod. 2016;86:846–853.

Haraguchi S, Takada K, Yasuda Y. Facial asymmetry in subjects with skeletal Class III deformity. Angle Orthod. 2002;72:28–35.

Iatrou I, Theologie-Lygidakis N, Tzerbos F, Schoinohoriti OK. Oro-facial tumours and tumour-like lesions in Greek children and adolescents: an 11-year retrospective study. J Craniomaxillofac Surg. 2013;41:437–443.

Jensen SØ, Eskildsen AF, Nørholt SE, Pedersen TK. Hemimandibular hyperplasi Danish. Dent J. 2017;7:602–607.

Ji YD, Resnick CM, Peacock ZS. Idiopathic condylar resorption: a systematic review of etiology and management. Oral Surg Oral Med Oral Pathol Oral Radiol. 2020;130:632–639.

Kaul A, Gordon C, Crow MK, Touma Z, Urowitz MB, van Vollenhoven R, Ruiz-Irastorza G, Hughes G. Systemic lupus erythematosus. Nat Rev Dis Primers. 2016;2:16039.

Kellenberger CJ, Bucheli J, Schroeder-Kohler S, Saurenmann RK, Colombo V, Ettlin DA. Temporomandibular joint magnetic resonance imaging findings in adolescents with anterior disk displacement compared to those with juvenile idiopathic arthritis. J Oral Rehabil. 2019;46:14–22.

MacDonald-Jankowski D. Fibrous dysplasia: a systematic review. Dentomaxillofac Radiol. 2009;38:196–215.

Martel-Pelletier J, Barr AJ, Cicuttini FM, Conaghan PG, Cooper C, Goldring MB, Goldring SR, Jones G, Teichtakl AJ, Pelletier J-P. Osteoarthritis. Nat Rev Dis Primers. 2016;2:16072.

Meazzini MC, Brusati R, Caprioglio A, Diner P, Garattini G, Giannì E, Lalatta F, Poggio C, Sesenna E, Silvestri A, Tomat C. True hemifacial microsomia and hemimandibular hypoplasia with condylar-coronoid collapse: diagnostic and prognostic differences. Am J Orthod Dentofac Orthop. 2011;139:e435–e447.

Meng T, Guo X, Lian W, Deng K, Gao L, Wang Z, Huang J, Wang X, Long X, Xing B. Identifying facial features and predicting patients of acromegaly using three-dimensional imaging techniques and machine learning. Front Endocrinol (Lausanne). 2020;11:492.

Mérida Velasco JR, Rodríguez Vázquez JF, De la Cuadra Blanco C, Campos López R, Sánchez M, Mérida Velasco JA. Development of the mandibular condylar cartilage in human specimens of 10–15 weeks' gestation. J Anat. 2009;214:56–64.

Mizuno A, Motegi K. Treatment of an asymmetric mandibular prognathism in an acromegalic patient. J Oral Maxillofac Surg. 1988;46:314–320.

Moe JS, Desai NK, Aiken AH, Soares BP, Kang J, Abramowicz S. Magnetic resonance imaging of temporomandibular joints of children. J Oral Maxillofac Surg. 2016;74:1723–1727.

Nolte JW, Alders M, Karssemakers LHE, Becking AG, Hennekam RCM. Unilateral condylar hyperplasia in hemifacial hyperplasia, is there genetic proof of overgrowth? Int J Oral Maxillofac Surg. 2020;49:1464–1469.

Obwegeser HL, Makek MS. Hemimandibular hyperplasia—hemimandibular elongation. J Maxillofac Surg. 1986;14:183–208.

Owtad P, Park JH, Shen G, Potres Z, Darendeliler MA. The biology of TMJ growth modification: a review. J Dent Res. 2013;92:315–321.

Pedersen TK, Norholt SE. Early orthopedic treatment and mandibular growth of children with temporomandibular joint abnormalities. Semin Orthod. 2011;17:235–245.

Pedersen TK, Stoustrup P. How to diagnose idiopathic condylar resorptions in the absence of consensus-based criteria? J Oral Maxillofac Surg. 2021;79:1810–1811.

Pedersen TK, Grønhøj J, Melsen B, Herlin T. Condylar condition and mandibular growth during early functional treatment of children with juvenile chronic arthritis. Eur J Orthod. 1995;17:385–394.

Pirttiniemi P, Peltomäki T, Müller L, Luder HU. Abnormal mandibular growth and the condylar cartilage. Eur J Orthod. 2009;31:1–11.

Schiffman E, Ohrbach R, Truelove E, Look J, Anderson G, Goulet JP, List T, Svensson P, Gonzalez Y, Lobbezoo F, Michelotti A, Brooks SL, Ceusters W, Drangsholt M, Ettlin D, Gaul C, Goldberg LJ, Haythornthwaite JA, Hollender L, Jensen R, John MT, De Laat A, de Leeuw R, Maixner W, van der Meulen M, Murray GM, Nixdorf DR, Palla S, Petersson A, Pionchon P, Smith B, Visscher CM, Zakrzewska J, Dworkin SF; International RDC/TMD Consortium Network, International Association for Dental Research; Orofacial Pain Special Interest Group, International Association for the Study of Pain. Diagnostic criteria for temporomandibular disorders (DC/TMD) for clinical and research applications: recommendations of the International RDC/TMD Consortium Network and Orofacial Pain Special Interest Group. J Oral Facial Pain Headache 2014;28:6-27.

Silvestri A, Natali G, Iannetti G. Functional therapy in hemifacial microsomia: therapeutic protocol for growing children. J Oral Maxillofac Surg. 1996;54:271–278. discussion 8–80.

Stoustrup P, Kuseler A, Kristensen KD, Herlin T, Pedersen TK. Orthopaedic splint treatment can reduce mandibular asymmetry caused by unilateral temporomandibular involvement in juvenile idiopathic arthritis. Eur J Orthod. 2013;35:191–198.

Stoustrup P, Iversen CK, Kristensen KD, Resnick CM, Verna C, Norholt SE, Abramowicz S, Kõseler A, Cattaneo PM, Herlin T, Pedersen TK. Assessment of dentofacial growth deviation in juvenile idiopathic arthritis: reliability and validity of three-dimensional morphometric measures. PLoS One. 2018;13:e0194177.

Stoustrup P, Pedersen TK, Norholt SE, Resnick CM, Abramowicz S. Interdisciplinary management of dentofacial deformity in juvenile idiopathic arthritis. Oral Maxillofac Surg Clin North Am. 2020;32:117–134.

Tanaka E, Detamore MS, Mercuri LG. Degenerative disorders of the temporomandibular joint: etiology, diagnosis, and treatment. J Dent Res. 2008;87:296–307.

Timme M, Bohner L, Huss S, Kleinheinz J, Hanisch M. Response of different treatment protocols to treat chronic non-bacterial osteomyelitis (CNO) of the mandible in adult patients: a systematic review. Int J Environ Res Public Health. 2020;17:1737.

Toyosawa S, Yuki M, Kishino M, Ogawa Y, Ueda T, Murakami S, Konishi E, Iida S, Kogo M, Komori T, Tomita Y. Ossifying fibroma vs fibrous dysplasia of the jaw: molecular and immunological characterization. Mod Pathol. 2007;20:389–396.

Ullman S, Danielsen PL, Fledelius HC, Daugaard-Jensen J, Serup J. Scleroderma en Coup de Sabre, Parry–Romberg hemifacial atrophy and associated manifestations of the eye, the oral cavity and the teeth: a Danish follow-up study of 35 patients diagnosed between 1975 and 2015. Dermatology (Basel). 2021;237:204–212.

Upadya VH, Bhat HK, Rao BHS, Reddy SG. Classification and surgical management of temporomandibular joint ankylosis: a review. J Korean Assoc Oral Maxillofac Surg. 2021;47:239–248.

Valesan LF, Da-Cas CD, Réus JC, Denardin ACS, Garanhani RR, Bonotto D, Januzzi E, Mendes de Souza BD. Prevalence of temporomandibular joint disorders: a systematic review and meta-analysis. Clin Oral Investig. 2021;25:441–453.

Vernucci RA, Mazzoli V, Galluccio G, Silvestri A, Barbato E. Unilateral hemimandibular hyperactivity: clinical features of a population of 128 patients. J Craniomaxillofac Surg. 2018;46:1105–1110.

Wolford LM. Idiopathic condylar resorption of the temporomandibular joint in teenage girls (cheerleaders syndrome). Proc (Baylor Univ Med Cent). 2001;14:246–252.

Xie Q, Yang C, He D, Cai X, Ma Z. Is mandibular asymmetry more frequent and severe with unilateral disc displacement? J Craniomaxillofac Surg. 2015;43:81–86.

Xie Q, Yang C, He D, Cai X, Ma Z, Shen Y, Abdelrehem A. Will unilateral temporomandibular joint anterior disc displacement in teenagers lead to asymmetry of condyle and mandible? A longitudinal study. J Craniomaxillofac Surg. 2016;44:590–596.

Part II

Localization and Problem List

5

Examination of Special Features in Patients with Dentofacial and Occlusal Asymmetries

Athanasios E. Athanasiou and Birte Melsen

CHAPTER MENU

Introduction

Minor asymmetry is a desirable variation of the craniofacial structures because these little inconsistencies are perceived as esthetically pleasing (Peck et al. 1991). Laterality in the normal asymmetry of the face is consistently found in humans and it is likely to be a hereditary rather than an acquired trait (Haraguchi et al. 2008).

A considerable number of patients suffer from noticeable asymmetry expressed in the face, jaws, and occlusion. However, there is no consensus concerning its degree, side prevalence, or localization. In a survey at a university dentofacial clinic, 34% of the patients were found to have clinically apparent facial asymmetry. When present, asymmetry affected the upper face in only 5%, the midface (primarily the nose) in 36%, the chin in 74%, and with the occlusal plane tilted in 41% (Severt and Proffit 1997).

Dentofacial and occlusal asymmetries can be found in children, adolescents, and adults and their categorization is limitless.

Classification based on etiology and time of appearance includes (a) congenital malformations with associated growth disorders, (b) primary growth disorders, and (c) acquired diseases or trauma with associated growth disorders (Pirttiniemi et al. 2009).

If syndromes and rare diseases with asymmetry in the craniofacial and dental regions are excluded, there is still a plethora of groups of patients characterized by mild, moderate, and severe manifestations of asymmetries affecting hard and soft tissues of the face and the dentoalveolar regions. They include cases with hemifacial microsomia (craniofacial microsomia), hemimandibular elongation, hemimandibular hyperplasia, condylar fractures, ankylosis of the temporomandibular joint, functional mandibular displacement, rheumatoid arthritis, muscle pathology, benign tumors, cleft lip and/or palate, craniosynostosis, temporomandibular disorders, etc. (Figure 5.1).

In an attempt for a systematic classification of facial asymmetry the skeletal structures of this kind of patients were analyzed and classified according to their structural characteristics using three-dimensional computed tomography (Baek et al. 2012). The two main groups consisted of patients with asymmetry caused by a shift or lateralization of the mandibular body (44%) or significant difference between the left and right ramus height with menton deviation to the short side (39%).

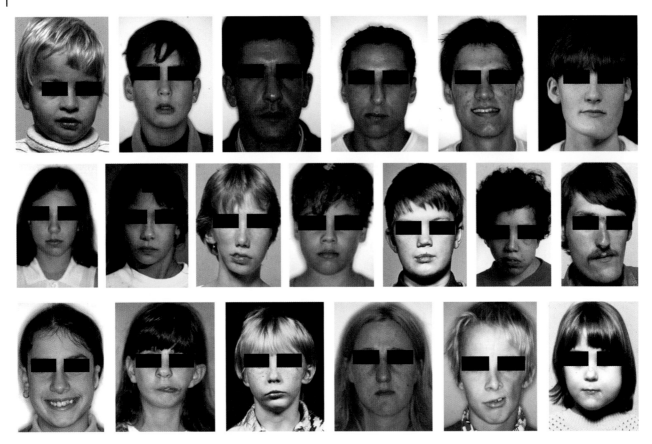

Figure 5.1 Collection of children, adolescent, and adult patients with face asymmetry of different categorization and severity.

When an investigation was undertaken for evaluating how severity of asymmetries affecting the mandible and chin point influence perceived attractiveness, asymmetry of 10 mm is perceived as being significant, but at 5 mm and below, it is largely unnoticed. The greater than 10 mm the degree of asymmetry, the more noticeable and the greater the desire was for correction. Clinician and patient ratings were similar and more critical than ratings of laypeople (Naini et al. 2012).

In general, the approach to diagnosis and treatment planning is the same for patients with asymmetries as for those with other malocclusions or dentofacial deformities (Proffit and Turvey 1990). However, it is important to realize that the word "asymmetry" comprises innumerable morphological variations as teeth, dental arches, skeletal components, and soft tissues may in theory be displaced and rotated in three planes of space leaving six degrees of freedom to every component. In the Chapter "Rotational diagnosis and treatment of dental asymmetries" of this book, a comprehensive presentation of the three-dimensional assessment is described. In this section, the examination of special features in patients with dentofacial and occlusal asymmetries will be addressed and only in relation to head posture, stomatognathic function, face evaluation, and malocclusion.

Head Posture

Before getting into the facial, oral, and occlusal clinical examination, it is important to verify whether the head posture is influenced by factors outside the stomatognathic region that either can be taken care of before focusing on the dentoalveolar asymmetry or have to be accepted and compensated for.

An example of a deviation that should be taken care of as early as possible is *torticollis* that is shortening of the sternocleidomastoids muscle leading to a torsion of the neck and affecting physiologic head posture. This is a dystonic condition defined by an abnormal asymmetrical head or neck position, which may be due to a variety of causes. The head becomes persistently turned to one side, often associated with painful muscle spasms. Being untreated this pathological condition will lead to marked craniofacial and dental asymmetries (especially in Class III malocclusions) (Pirttiniemi et al. 1989; Kawamoto et al. 2009; Yuan et al. 2012).

The younger the patients are when the affected sternocleidomastoid is cut the easier it is to correct the asymmetry, but even in older patients dentoalveolar corrections can be obtained without the need of

(a)

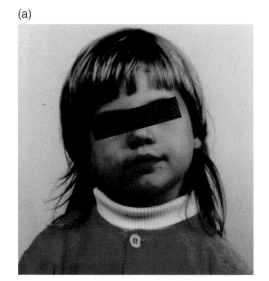

(b)

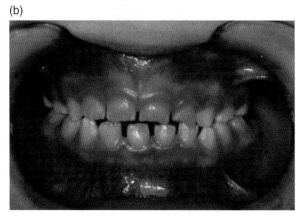

Figure 5.2 (a) Patient with a torticollis where the cervical muscle is contracted and forcing a rotation of the head and; (b) consequently a modeling of the dentoalveolar tissues.

orthognathic surgery (Do 2006; Sargent et al. 2019) (Figure 5.2). On the other hand, there are cases of torticollis in which the effect on facial appearance and occlusion are very moderate (Figure 5.3).

A more severe condition that influences the head posture is the *Sprengel's deformity* (also known as high scapula or congenital high scapula). It is a rare congenital skeletal abnormality where a person has one shoulder blade that sits higher on the back than the other. The deformity is due to a failure in early fetal development where the shoulder fails to descend properly from the neck to its final position. This deviation is characterized by a small and undescended scapula often associated with scapular winging and scapular hypoplasia. The diagnosis is made clinically with a high-riding, medially rotated, triangular-shaped scapula, with associated limitations in shoulder abduction and flexion leading to an asymmetric position of the head and the dentition (Harvey et al. 2012) (Figure 5.4).

Another example of a condition outside the stomatognathic region that may influence the head posture and cause asymmetrical dentoalveolar development is *scoliosis*. This is a sideways curvature of the spine that most often is diagnosed in adolescents. While scoliosis can occur in people with conditions such as cerebral palsy and muscular dystrophy, the etiology of most cases of scoliosis in children remains unknown. In this pathological condition, a lateral curvature of the spinal column can influence the position of the shoulders and the head posture (Zhou et al. 2013; Furlanetto et al. 2016) (Figure 5.5).

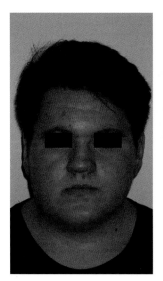
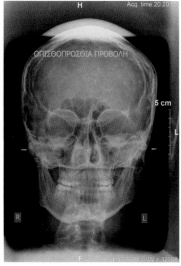
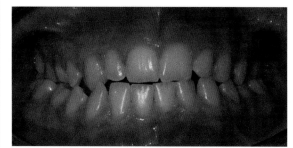

Figure 5.3 Patient with a torticollis with mild face asymmetry as appears in the extraoral photograph of the face, the posteroanterior cephalometric radiograph, and the intraoral photograph of occlusion.

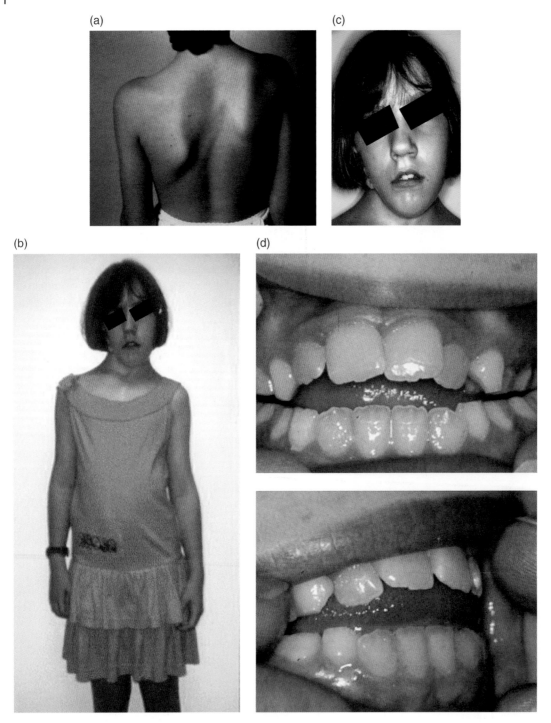

Figure 5.4 (a) Patient with Sprengel's deformity which influences the inclination of the shoulders and; (b) consequently the posture of the body; (c) the head posture in the frontal plane of space, and; (d) is associated with occlusal disharmonies.

Functional Assessment

Once the factors having an influence of the head posture are taken into consideration the clinical examination can be performed and the asymmetry should be classified as functional or morphological.

The first step when identifying an asymmetry is to verify whether an abnormal function, namely a forced bite, is contributing to the asymmetry (Figure 5.6). This can be verified by letting the patient open widely keeping the tongue in the palate. If the symmetry observed in relation to occlusion is less pronounced when opening it is a sign

Figure 5.5 (a) Radiograph of the column of a young boy; (b) the scoliosis influences the position of the shoulders leading to a tilting of the head and the shoulders as well as to an asymmetric position of the hip.

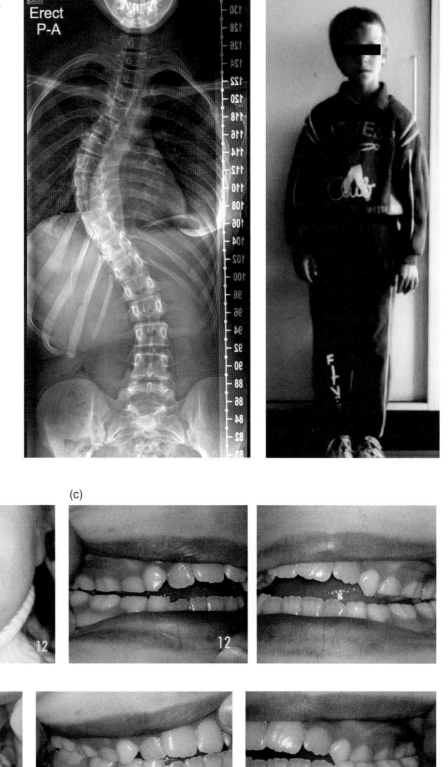

Figure 5.6 (a) An 8-year-old girl with a functional displacement of the mandible to the left resulting to; (b) a left deviation of the lower midline, to a crossbite on the left side, and to distal occlusion on the left side; (c) when asking the patient to open wide and close slowly in the midline to the first posterior contact there is no deviation to the left.

that a functional guidance of the mandible is contributing to the discrepancy.

The asymmetry caused by displacement, where the mandible will be rotating around the condyle on the crossbite side will result in an asymmetric displacement of the mandible in all three planes of space. It often develops during the deciduous or mixed dentition as a consequence of a narrow maxilla and a low posture of the tongue often seen as a result of a nonnutritive sucking habit e.g. pacifier or thumb sucking (Figure 5.7). When the deciduous canines are erupting the mandible will deviate to one side leading to an asymmetric occlusion. When opening wide the midlines will coincide and an open bite will be the result. Characteristic for the forced bite is that when closing the mandible rotates around the condyle on the crossbite side and the occlusion will be distal on the crossbite side and mesial on the contralateral side. A jaw tracking will indicate whether the primary contact is met close to the occlusion, meaning that it will be easy to correct with a minor expansion or occlusal adjustment if the teeth are deciduous. The jaw tracking may on the other hand also indicate that the closure is asymmetric from the start and a guidance may be necessary (Ackerman et al. 2007) (Figure 5.8).

In mixed dentition or in early permanent dentition cases, the longer an asymmetric function is maintained, due to a forced bite, the more morphological deviations of the dentoalveolar region will develop. The purpose of the functional clinical examination should be to define the intermaxillary position where the condyles are centered and which presents the malocclusion that has to be corrected with orthopedic or orthodontic means.

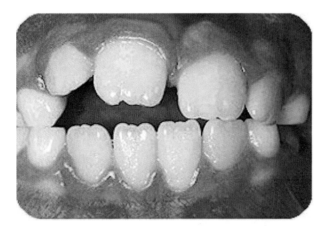

Figure 5.7 Right canine crossbite developed during the mixed dentition as a consequence of a narrow maxilla and a low posture of the tongue often seen as a result of a nonnutritive sucking habit.

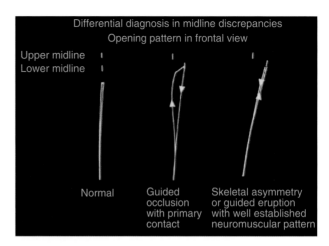

Figure 5.8 Differential diagnosis in midline discrepancies. Opening and closing patterns in the frontal view (Ackerman et al. 2007).

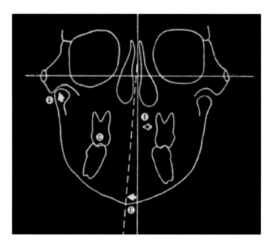

Figure 5.9 Asymmetry in bicondylar position is correlated with the occlusal asymmetry. Subjects with lateral malocclusions showed a more asymmetric position of the condyles with respect to their position within the glenoid fossa.

Crossbite that causes lateral mandibular shift must be immediately corrected in order to avoid detrimental dentoalveolar and basal mandibular asymmetry. It has been shown that the asymmetry in bicondylar position is correlated with the occlusal asymmetry. Subjects with lateral malocclusions showed a more asymmetric position of the condyles with respect to the posterior wall of the glenoid fossa (Figure 5.9). This may be of clinical importance and stresses the necessity for early correction of such malocclusions, as complete adaptation does not seem to occur in these cases (Pirttiniemi et al. 1991; Hesse et al. 1997). In addition, modifications of mandibular posture, activity of the muscles of mastication, lips, cheeks, supra- and infra-hyoid, and occlusal plane are also associated with functional crossbites.

In adult patients, the physiologic mandibular position can be found by using in the beginning a flat totally balanced hard acrylic splint with the condyles in a symmetrical posterior superior position. After a while, the occlusal contacts are no longer balanced and the splint has to be rebased. This process is repeated until the mandibular position no longer changes, the precise occlusal relationships can be observed and the necessary orthodontic tooth movements can be defined, planned, and performed (Figure 5.10).

If on the other hand, the asymmetry is more pronounced in relation to maximal opening it indicates that the occlusal asymmetry is reflecting a skeletal asymmetry that is combined with difference in the mobility of the condyles of the two sides (Figure 5.11).

The influence of function is elucidated by observing the skull in Figure 5.12a. When looking at the frontal view of the skull, it is obvious that there is no major asymmetry, no crossbite, and no midline discrepancy. When removing the mandible and looking at the skull it is obvious that the positions of the fossae articularis are in very asymmetrical position and that the width of the maxilla is different on the two sides (Figure 5.12b). By observing the mandible and the skull separated it is obvious that there is a major asymmetry which has been compensated for by asymmetrical growth of the condyles. This skull thereby demonstrates that even major differences in condylar growth will take place over time when the function is normal. The compensation illustrated by the observation of the skull has taken place during the major part of the postnatal growth period as the asymmetry probably was there at birth or generated artificially right after birth as part of a ritual (Figure 5.12c)

Photographic Assessment

When the clinical examination is performed, it is important to describe the face and the occlusion in all three planes of space. This can be done by taking extra-oral and intra-oral photographs in three planes of space (Figures 5.13–5.16). In addition to the sagittal, vertical, and transversal assessment of the face in identifying the topographic manifestations of the asymmetry, photographs should be also used in documenting soft tissue defects. They may include skin tags, facial clefts, cranial nerve

function, soft palate function, ear abnormalities, bulk of subcutaneous soft tissue, muscles of mastication and facial expression, macrostomia, and skin tags (Tuin et al. 2015) (Figures 5.13, 5.15, and 5.16).

Following clinical examination and photographic extra-oral assessment, the latter images can be used in deciding whether a cone beam computed tomography (CBCT) would be indicated (Figure 5.17). The chapters of this book "Imaging: Craniofacial asymmetries", "Cephalometric radiographic assessment of facial asymmetries" and "Localization and problem list - 3-D face reconstruction" present in detail all relevant information regarding radiographs and imaging.

Conclusion

To facilitate communication, all asymmetries should be expressed in a 3-dimensional coordinate system. When agreeing on a common language, the various professions involved in the detailed description of the problems then the treatment approaches can be more efficiently communicated. This is however has not been always the case as the coordinate system defined by Burstone (1998) varied from the one proposed by Kim et al. (2014). Different reference systems make communication difficult.

Adding asymmetry to the problem list is very important. Perfect facial symmetry is extremely rare, and in reality, all normal faces have a varying degree of asymmetry. The degree of asymmetry that is perceived as acceptable varies considerably between patients (Sargent et al. 2019) and most facial asymmetries cannot be completely corrected. Nevertheless, even minor occlusal asymmetries should be part of a problem list as they may be the reason why the optimal treatment result cannot be obtained. With the clinical examination, all aspects of asymmetry should be covered starting with those related to an abnormal function followed by the ones related to mandibular displacement or of congenital nature and focusing on their quantification and localization in the three planes of space. An important part will focus on treatment approaches of interception, correction, or camouflage. Within each heading, large variety will be presented elucidating the biological, the biomechanical, and the surgical possibilities. Of course, the limitations will be also dealt with and finally, the medical, social, and psychological aspects will determine how the major problems can be handled within the families.

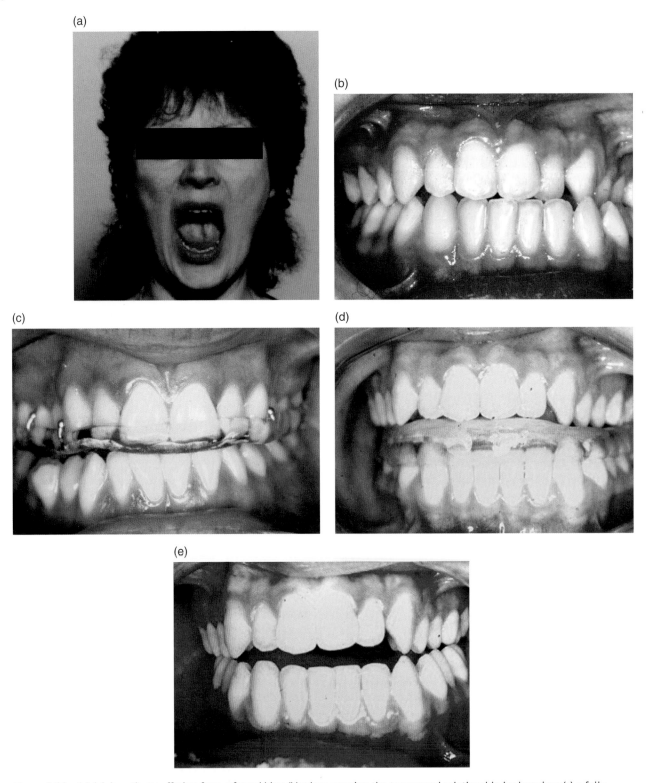

Figure 5.10 (a) Adult patient suffering from a forced bite; (b) when opening the transversal relationship is changing; (c) a fully balanced splint is inserted and continuously adapted when the contact points are changing; (d) a second occlusal coverage rendering a balanced contact may be necessary; (e) at the end, the occlusal relationship that needs to be corrected is different from the initial. In the new one, the mandibular position is reflecting a symmetrical position of the condyles.

Figure 5.11 Pronounced deviation of the mandible to the left during maximal opening due to condylar fracture of the left condyle.

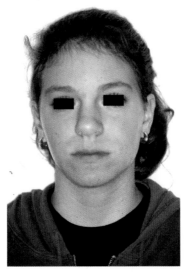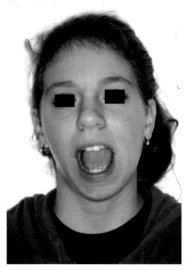

Figure 5.12 (a) Frontal image of a skull from the 15th century. It can be seen that there is no major asymmetry in the dentoalveolar region; (b) when removing the mandible and looking at the base of the skull it is obvious that the positions of the fossae articularis are in very asymmetrical position and that the width of the maxilla is different on the two sides; (c) the horizontal view clearly demonstrates how much asymmetrical growth can compensate in the case of normal function.

(a)

(b)

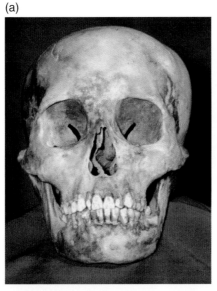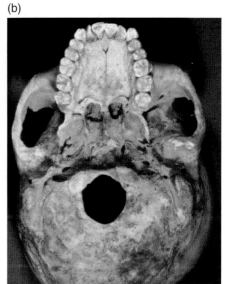

(c)

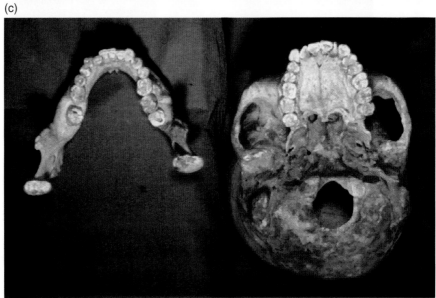

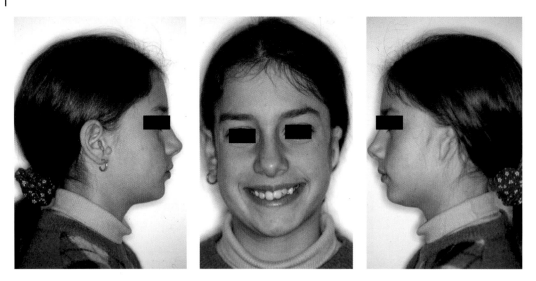

Figure 5.13   A 9-year-old girl with hemifacial microsomia and with ear and soft tissue defects.

(a)

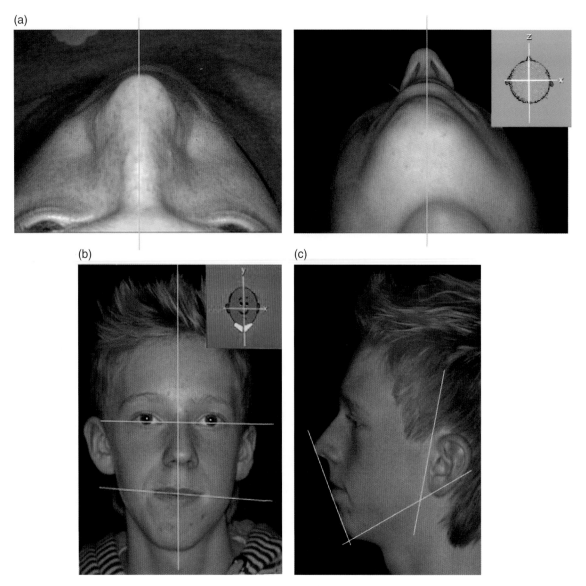

Figure 5.14   Photos taken at the three planes of space indicated in the corners of the image. (a) superoinferior view (left) and inferosuperior view (right); (b) frontal view; and (c) lateral view. The deviations can be expressed by the coordinates.

(a)

(b)

(c)

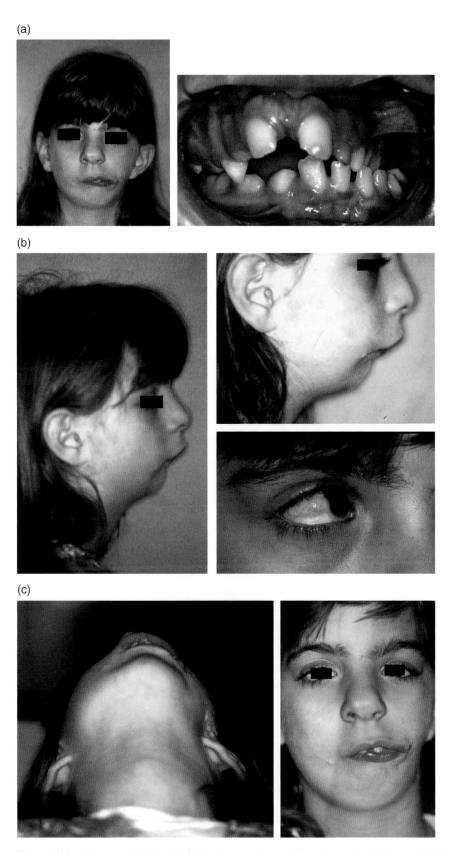

Figure 5.15 A 8-year-old girl with Goldenhar syndrome with extra-oral and intra-oral photographs in three planes of space showing. (a) Severe asymmetry expressed in the face, occlusion, and soft tissues; (b) significantly convex profile due to severe mandibular retrognathism, and with soft tissues and eye abnormalities, and; (c) asymmetrical base of the mandible, asymmetrical position of the ears, and dysfunction of the lips; (d) patient is characterized by missing the left condyle, coronoid process, and significant portion of the ramus thus resulting not only to the asymmetry but also to the severe mandibular retrognathism.

(d)

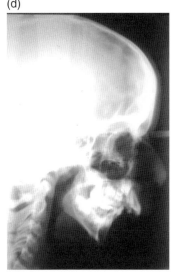
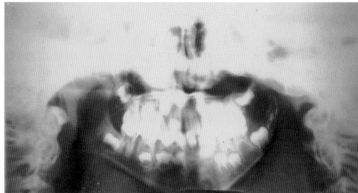

Figure 5.15 (Continued)

(a)

(b)

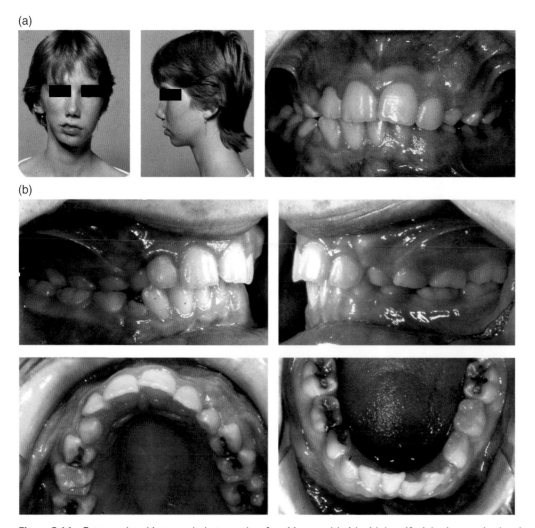

Figure 5.16 Extra-oral and intra-oral photographs of an 11-year-old girl with hemifacial microsomia showing. (a) Face asymmetry with chin deviation to the left, convex profile, retrognathic mandible, lower midline deviation to the left, left posterior crossbite, and tilting of the occlusal plane; (b) intraoral photographs present the dysplastic development of the occlusal and dentoalveolar structures due to the mandibular asymmetry.

Figure 5.17 A CBCT image of a 17-year-old female with face asymmetry due to hemimandibular elongation of the left side.

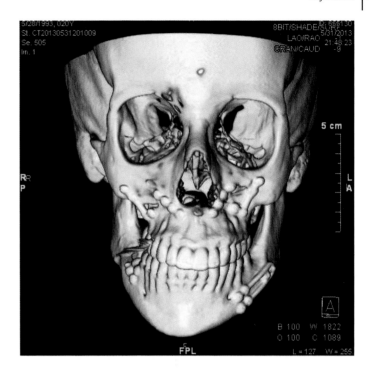

References

Ackerman JL, Proffit WR, Sarver DM, Ackerman MB, Kean MR. Pitch, roll, and yaw: describing the spatial orientation of dentofacial traits. Am J Orthod Dentofac Orthop. 2007;131:305–310.

Baek C, Paeng J-Y, Lee JS, Hong J. Morphologic evaluation and classification of facial asymmetry using 3-dimensional computed tomography. J Oral Maxillofac Surg. 2012;70:1161–1169.

Burstone CJ. Diagnosis and treatment planning of patients with asymmetries. Semin Orthod. 1998;4:153–164.

Do TT. Congenital muscular torticollis: current concepts and review of treatment. Curr Opin Pediatr. 2006;18:26–29.

Furlanetto TS, Sedrez JA, Candotti CT, Loss JF. Photogrammetry as a tool for the postural evaluation of the spine: a systematic review. World J Orthop. 2016;18(7):136–148.

Haraguchi S, Iguchi Y, Takada K. Asymmetry of the face in orthodontic patients. Angle Orthod. 2008;78:421–426.

Harvey JE, Bernstein M, Desy NM, Saran N, Ouellet JA. Sprengel's deformity: pathogenenis and management. J Am Acad Orthop Surg. 2012;20:177–186.

Hesse KL, Artun J, Joondeph DR, Kennedy DB. Changes in condylar position and occlusion associated with maxillary expansion for correction of functional unilateral posterior crossbite. Am J Ortohod Dentofacial Orthop. 1997;111:410–418.

Kawamoto HK, Kim SS, Jarrahy R, Bradley JP. Differential diagnosis of the idiopathic laterally deviated mandible. Plast Reconstr Surg. 2009;124:1599–1609.

Kim JY, Jung HD, Jung YS, Hwang CJ, Park HS. A simple classification of facial asymmetry by TML system. J Craniomaxillofac Surg. 2014;42:313–320.

Naini FB, Donaldson ANA, McDonald F, Cobourn MT. Assessing the influence of asymmetry affecting the mandible and chin point on perceived attractiveness in the orthognathic patient, clinician, and layperson. J Oral Maxillofac Surg. 2012;70:192–206.

Peck S, Peck L, Kataja M. Skeletal asymmetry in esthetically pleasing faces. Angle Orthod. 1991;61:43–48.

Pirttiniemi P, Lahtela P, Huggare J, Serio W. Head posture and dentofacial asymmetries in surgically treated muscular torticollis patients. Acta Odontol Scand. 1989;47:193–197.

Pirttiniemi P, Peltomäki T, Müller L, Luder HU. Abnormal mandibular growth and the condylar cartilage. Eur J Orthod. 2009;31:1–11.

Pirttiniemi P, Raustia A, Kantomaa T, Pyhtinen J. Relationships of bicondylar position to occlusal asymmetry. Eur J Orthod. 1991;13:441–445.

Proffit WR, Turvey TA. Dentofacial asymmetry. In: Proffit WR, White RP Jr, eds. Surgical – Orthodontic Treatment. St. Louis: Mosby Year Book, 1990:483–549.

Sargent B, Kaplan SL, Coulter C, Baker C. Congenital muscular torticollis: bridging the gap between research and clinical practice. Pediatrics. 2019;144:e20190582.

Severt TR, Proffit WR. The prevalence of facial asymmetry in the dentofacial deformities population at the University of North Carolina. Int J Adult Orthodon Orthognath Surg. 1997;12:171–176.

Tuin J, Tahiri Y, Paliga JT, Taylor JA, Bartlett SP. Distinguishing Goldenhar syndrome from craniofacial microsomia. J Craniofac Surg. 2015;26:1887–1892.

Yuan JT, Teng E, Heller JB, Kawamoto HK, Bradley JP. Asymmetric Class III malocclusion: association with cranial base deformation and occult torticollis. J Craniofac Surg. 2012;23:1421–1424.

Zhou S, Yan J, Hu D, Yang Y, Wang DY, Sun S. A correlational study of scoliosis and trunk balance in adult patients with mandibular deviation. PLoS One. 2013;8:e59929.

6

Imaging: Craniofacial Asymmetries

David C. Hatcher and Vidhya Venkateswaran

Introduction

A facial or craniofacial asymmetry is a significant sign or phenotype of deviant facial growth that has the potential to negatively impact facial appearance, occlusion, airway dimensions, and jaw function (Dadgar-Yeganeh et al. 2021; Phi et al. 2022; Trypkova et al. 2000). The emphasis of this chapter is to provide methods and strategies to identify the underlying cause and quantify a craniofacial asymmetry thus leading to a precise diagnosis. A precise diagnosis can be folded into the clinical decision process addressing the therapy options and prognosis.

There is a wide range of congenital, developmental, and acquired conditions that can evolve into a craniofacial asymmetry. A precise diagnosis of an asymmetry can aid in predicting the clinical course of the condition. It is anticipated that therapy outcomes will be improved when tailored to the unique behavior and expression of underlying conditions over time.

The craniofacial structures are composed of a series of interconnected anatomic elements, including jaws, teeth, temporomandibular joints (TMJs), and muscles. Numerical modeling has shown that the functional interaction of the anatomic elements generates and propagates stresses and strains throughout craniofacial structures (Faulkner et al. 1987; Hatcher et al. 1986; Korioth and Hannam 1990). These stresses and resulting strains provide functional signals that can modulate tissue differentiation, growth, development, modeling, remodeling, and failure. Variability of neuromuscular interactions combined with the

Dentofacial and Occlusal Asymmetries, First Edition. Edited by Birte Melsen and Athanasios E. Athanasiou.
© 2025 John Wiley & Sons Ltd. Published 2025 by John Wiley & Sons Ltd.

individual genetic and epigenetic influences on facial growth may contribute to a range of morphologic outcomes generated by apparently similar force stimuli.

The craniofacial structures contributing to asymmetry can be divided into two components – local and regional. Hard and soft tissues will be considered as local environments when they are related to the source of the asymmetry and as regional environments when they are adjacent to and biomechanically influenced by the local environment.

Asymmetry

Stress is an engineering term that expresses the force per unit area (Stress = Force/Area) while strain is the deformation of the structure during the application of force (Strain = change in size/original size). The functional interactions between components of anatomic environments lead to tissue stress and strain, subsequently inducing adaptive responses in the involved tissues. The adaptive tissue responses include changes in size and shape, structure, and 3D spatial position. The adaptive responses progress until an equilibrium is achieved between the functional demands and the capacity of the involved tissues (Carter and Beaupré 2007a, 2007b; Sommerfeldt and Rubin 2001).

Craniofacial asymmetry is a presenting sign for a wide variety of underlying biological causes. A selected group of diagnostic categories that are most relevant to the orthodontic community, primarily influencing the mandible

and occlusion will be featured in this chapter. The local environment for most of these mandibular-based asymmetries originate in the TMJ(s) and the regional environments extend to the remainder of the mandible, maxilla, skull base, occlusion, and airway.

Differential Diagnosis and Decision Tree for a Craniofacial Asymmetry

Differential diagnosis is a list of diagnostic possibilities for a given sign or symptom. In the case of a craniofacial asymmetry or phenotype (anatomic sign), it is diagnostically practical and efficient to organize the differential diagnosis into a decision tree. A decision tree presents decision points in a specific sequence that can be answered with discriminatory observations or applied tests and lead to a working radiographic diagnosis (Figure 6.1).

Imaging for Asymmetry

Choosing the Right Imaging Modality

Designing the optimal imaging study is a thoughtful process that begins with the decision to image and creating imaging objectives before selecting the imaging modality and imaging parameters. For example, in the case scenario of a clinically apparent facial asymmetry along with associated history, the clinician needs to decide if imaging will lead to clinically relevant findings. The best imaging studies are

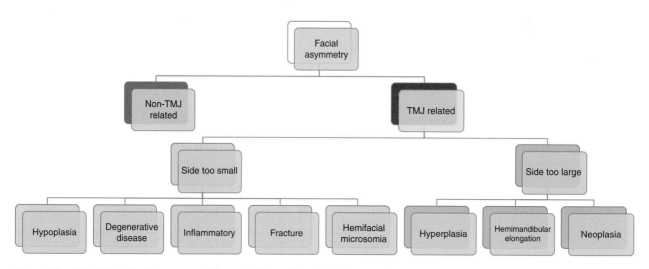

Figure 6.1 *DDx.* This table illustrates a differential diagnosis and decision tree for common and selected disorders primarily of TMJ origin are responsible for the development of mandibular asymmetries. There are many other disorders leading to a mandibular asymmetry that are not portrayed on this table.

achieved when the clinician decides precisely what they desire the imaging study to reveal about the patient's anatomy. Once imaging goals are known then the preferred imaging modality can be selected to achieve the desired diagnostic information while maintaining an acceptable cost and risk to the patient. Imaging methods have expanded and evolved to static and dynamic 2D and 3D methods. These methods include photo documentation, magnetic resonance imaging (MRI), and computed tomography (CT). In the case of craniofacial asymmetries, the field of view needs to encompass the involved local and regional environments. This field of view generally includes all of the maxilla, mandible, midface, TMJs, and temporal bone. The ideal imaging of skeletal asymmetry will allow for a metric quantification of the asymmetry. This can best be achieved with a three-dimensional imaging method, such as conebeam CT (CBCT) and multidetector CT (MDCT). The resolution needs to be sufficient to assess the anatomic detail of the temporal bone, dentition, and TMJs.

A CBCT is often preferred over MDCT because a CBCT has the most favorable value proposition including, cost, risk, spatial resolution, and acceptable tissue contrast. The usefulness of the imaging study is proportional to the appropriateness of the selected imaging modality, imaging quality, and the quality of the interpretation.

Volume Preparation for Analysis

Orientation: Image orientation is recommended prior to the imaging evaluation. When CBCT and MDCT scans are acquired, the scanner transfers its cartesian coordinate orientation to the produced image or voxel volume and this orientation is influenced by patient positioning. Post-acquisition viewing software, such as Anatomage InVivo 6.0, is available to optimize the volume orientation, i.e. perform a Cartesian coordinate transformation to align it with specific anatomic structures. This orientation process allows for optimized visualization of the right and left sides of the skeleton to assess and compare the size, shape, and positional differences. The reorientation is performed with six degrees of freedom (*X*, *Y*, *Z*, Yaw, Pitch, and Roll) (Figure 6.2). Yaw is adjusted by viewing the skull base using an inferior view and aligning the coronal plane to two points on the skull base such as foramen spinosum. Pitch can be adjusted in the lateral view aligning the sagittal plane to porion and orbitale landmarks (Frankfurt plane). Roll is adjusted in the frontal view by aligning the axial plane it to the right and left orbital rims.

Similarly, evaluation of specific anatomy, such as the TMJs, requires optimization of the plane of section in order to accurately determine the size, shape, quality, and spatial relationships. The optimized TMJ views create oblique sagittal and

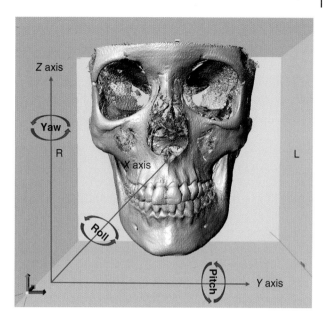

Figure 6.2 *Cartesian co-ordinates (6 DOF)*: The orientation process allows for optimized visualization of the right and left sides of the skeleton to assess and compare the size, shape, and positional differences. The re-orientation is performed with 6 DOF (*X*, *Y*, *Z*, Yaw, Pitch, and Roll). Yaw is adjusted viewing the skull base using an inferior view and aligning the coronal plane to 2 points on the skull base such as foramen spinosum. Pitch can be adjusted in the lateral view aligning the sagittal plane to porion and orbitale landmarks (Frankfurt plane). Roll is adjusted in the frontal view by aligning the axial plane it to the right and left orbital rims.

oblique coronal views that are aligned perpendicular or parallel to the mediolateral long axis of the condyle.

Analysis

CBCT volumes offer unique visualization and analysis opportunities when applied to the diagnosis and quantification of craniofacial skeletal asymmetries. Most of the encountered asymmetries display dimensional differences in size, shape, and spatial orientation when the right and left halves of the face are mirrored about the mid-sagittal plane. The local and regional expression of a disorder are important to identify, visualize, and quantify in order to establish a baseline anatomy for future comparison and to arrive at a final radiographic diagnosis.

The initial step in craniofacial analysis is three-dimensional landmarking of key anatomic features resulting in 3D coordinates for each landmark. The landmarking coordinates can be applied to various analysis strategies including generalized procrustes analysis (GPA), euclidean distance matrix analysis (EDMA), and principal component analysis (PCA).

Generalized Procrustes Analysis

GPA uses a 3D matrix of coordinate values for all of the local and regional anatomical landmarks of various individuals under study. As a first step, the shape of the structure under study can be mapped after removing confounding attributes of size, location, and rotation. This coordinate matrix of multiple individuals can then be compared to determine shape differences independent of size, location, and spatial orientation. For each patient under study, a landmark centroid is calculated using the coordinates values from the landmark matrix. Shape comparisons can be achieved by aligning all data sets onto the same coordinate system. This is achieved by superimposing the centroids, translating, rotating, and scaling the data matrices to minimize the distance between the corresponding landmarks. The aggregated cloud of data points for each landmark can be averaged to determine the mean location for each landmark. Subsequent Procrustes analysis can be performed to compare the average landmark locations with any given subject to help identify deviant anatomy.

Euclidian Distance Matrix Analysis (EDMA)

Euclidean distance involves calculating the distance between any two landmarks in 2D or 3D coordinate space using the Pythagorean theorem. The EDM for relevant anatomic elements associated with an asymmetry can be created for all components, for example, the length of the condylar process.

Principal Component Analysis

This is a method to reduce the dimensionality of data while retaining its primary characteristics. PCA isolates the landmarks that have the most significant influence of the data variance. PCA analysis includes computing the covariance matrix and eigenvectors and eigenvalues. Covariance measures how much two variables change together. Eigenvectors show the direction of the spread of data. Eigenvalues show the magnitude of the spread. Once the principal components are formed, PC1 will represent the variable with the greatest variance while PC2 will represent the variable with second most variance and so on. The greater the variance of a landmark location, the heavier its influence it has on the PCA analysis. Thus, the principal components with the greatest effect can be retained in the analysis, eliminating the others. Other variables with less influence can be eliminated in the subsequent analysis.

Examples of Asymmetrical Individuals

There are many conditions responsible for craniofacial asymmetry (Rathi and Hatcher 2019; Tamimi et al. 2017). This chapter will address selected disorders that initiate in the TMJ during the period of growth and development and lead to an asymmetry. In an orthodontic practice, the disorders of TMJ-associated facial asymmetry are the most frequently encountered asymmetries. The local environmental changes are characteristic of an initiating TMJ disorder and aid in a radiographic diagnosis. The regional adaptive changes are common among most of the various initiating disorders and are considered to be adaptations to the functional demands. The radiographic features of selected commonly encountered TMJ disorders will be discussed in this chapter. Since the regional changes are common among several disorders they will be discussed and illustrated separately as a group.

Overall Regional Changes Associated with the Developmental Onset of TMJ Disorders

In general, the severity of the asymmetry is indirectly proportional to the age of onset of the *underlying* TMJ disorder and directly proportional to the severity of the *underlying TMJ* disorder (Bryndahl et al. 2006; Legrell and Isberg 1998, 1999; Legrell et al. 1999; Kurita et al. 2002). The initiation of an asymmetrical mandible can begin with TMJ anomalies responsible for enlargement or reduction in size of the osseous TMJ components. The regional expression of an asymmetry of an underdeveloped side can be described as a comparison to the contralateral side as follows (Figure 6.3). Small condylar process (condyle and neck), shorter ascending ramus, vertical shortening of the body of the mandible, diminished lateral development of the mandible, change in mandibular posture, elevation of the occlusal plane on the ipsilateral side, steepening of the mandibular plane and shift the osseous midline of the mandible to the short side. Conversely, there is enlargement of the ipsilateral half of the mandible in individuals with conditions that enlarge the condyle, particularly condylar hyperplasia (Figure 6.6). There is a continuum of shape changes associated with mandibular size. In general, the convexity of the lower and posterior borders of the mandible are directly proportional to the size of the mandible. At the size extremes, the antegonial notch will be exceptionally concave in individuals with a small mandible and convex in individuals with very large mandibles. Similarly, in small mandibles, there is a tendency toward steep mandibular plane angles and obtuse gonial angles. The vertical dimensions of anterior region of the mandible in individuals with a steep mandibular plane are large while the labiolingual dimensions of the alveolar bone are small. The osseous midline of asymmetrical mandible is shifted to the short side.

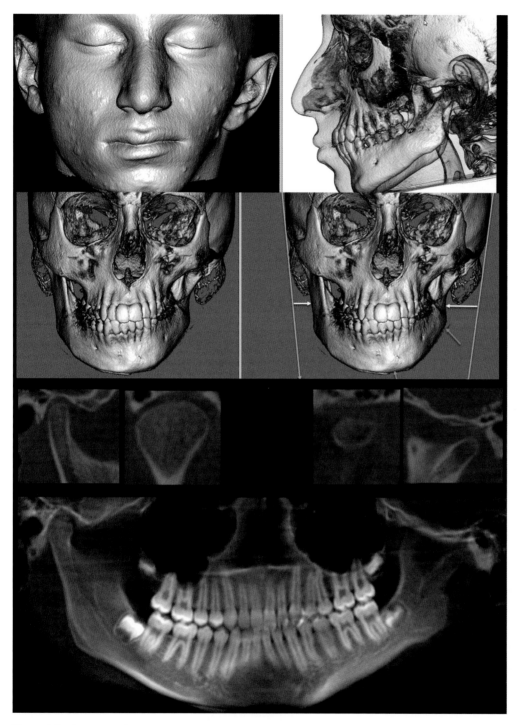

Figure 6.3 *Asymmetry features*: oriented and rendered CBCT volume of a 14 year old male with a neonatal subcondylar fracture (Hatcher and Petrikowski 2016a). The differential diagnosis for a neonatal subcondylar fracture includes hemifacial microsomia (HFM) (Hatcher 2016b). HFM is a congenital anomaly of unknown origin involving structures derived from the first and second branchial arches. HFM, unlike neonatal fractures, can be expressed in the underdevelopment of the ipsilateral mastoid process, internal and external ear, malar bone, zygomatic arch and orbit. *Local changes*: The left condylar process is anteroinferiorly displaced and has attached to the surface of the ramus. The repositioning of the proximal segment changes the size and shape of the sigmoid notch creating the impression of "crossing scissor blades." The articular portion of the left condyle has not formed a contact with the opposing temporal bone and therefore not stimulated growth of the fossa/eminence complex. *Regional features*: The left ascending ramus and body of the mandible are less than the right side. The left TMJ and cranial base are inferiorly positioned when compared to the right. The yellow arrows form a tangent to the squamous portion of the temporal bone. The lateral development of the left half of the mandible is less than the right (white arrows). The osseous midline of the mandible is shifted to the short side (green arrow). The left angle of the mandible is elevated (blue arrow). The occlusal plane is elevated on the left side.

Common Disorders and Associated Local and Regional Changes

Progressive Condylar Resorption (PCR)

PCR synonyms include idiopathic condylar resorption (ICR) and juvenile form of degenerative joint disease (DJD). PCR is a localized noninflammatory degenerative disorder localized to the TMJs and characterized by lysis and repair of the articular fibrocartilage and underlying subchondral bone (Alsabban et al. 2018; Dahl Kristensen et al. 2017; Hatcher 2013; Mizoguchi et al. 2013; Pirttiniemi et al. 2009). PCR occurs around the time of puberty and primarily affects females.

Natural History

Soft tissue changes, such as a disc displacement, often precede the osseous changes. PCR can be unilateral or bilateral. Unilateral and bilateral expression of PCR can create a facial asymmetry if either the PCR onset timing or severity is not symmetrical. PCR goes through an active or destructive stages that is followed by repair and disease stability stages. Since PCR occurs during the active facial growth there is the potential to influence limited growth of the ipsilateral condylar process, ascending ramus, and body of the mandible. Compensations may occur in the occlusion, maxilla, cranial base, and airway. The associated occlusal changes can include elevation of the posterior occlusal plane on the ipsilateral side, posterior open bite on the contralateral side, and anterior open bite (Figure 6.4).

Differential Diagnosis

The differential diagnosis includes condylar hypoplasia and juvenile idiopathic arthritis (JIA) (Shah and

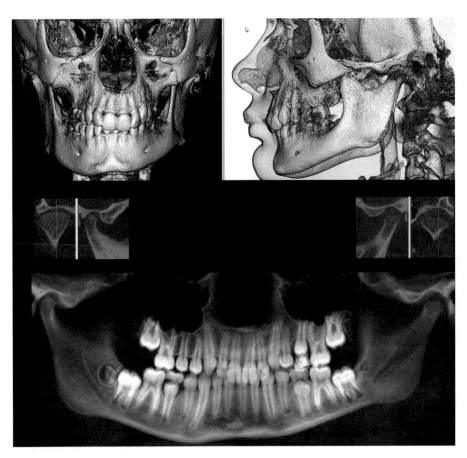

Figure 6.4 *Progressive condylar resorption* (Alsabban et al. 2018; Dahl Kristensen et al. 2017; Hatcher 2013): Oriented and rendered CBCT volume of an 11-year-old female with left TMJ PCR in the repair stage. *Local changes*: There is a size reduction and associated shape changes occurring from the superior surface of the left condyle. The osseous components of the right TMJ have a normal size, shape, and quality. The superior joint space in the left TMJ is relatively large. *Regional changes*: The vertical dimensions of the left condylar process, ascending ramus and body of the mandible are less than the contralateral side. The lateral development of the left half of the mandible is less than the right side. The posterior occlusal plane is elevated on the left side. The osseous midline of the mandible is shifted to the left. In contrast, condylar hypoplasia will have a normal shape and no evidence of a destructive process (Shah and Hatcher 2016).

Hatcher 2016). The onset of JIA occurs at an age earlier than PCR is bilaterally symmetrical and has a different pattern of destruction. PCR can heal without significant evidence of a destructive process that can make it difficult to differentiate from condylar hypoplasia. The confirmation goal for PCR is to identify prior evidence of a destructive process.

Condylar Hypoplasia

A hypoplastic condyle is a developmental disorder characterized by a small condyle that has normal anatomic architecture and shape (Figure 6.5). The regional changes include all of those associated with an underdeveloped condyle (Hatcher et al. 2016). Condylar hypoplasia is thought to be secondary to a joint insult, such as a trauma or displaced disc that occurs during the period of growth and development.

Natural History: The differential growth between the normal and hypoplastic sides only occurs during the period of somatic growth.

Differential Diagnosis: The differential diagnosis includes a normal variation, progressive condylar resorption, neonatal subcondylar fracture (Hatcher and Petrikowski 2016a), and juvenile idiopathic arthritis (Shah and Hatcher 2016). Condylar hypoplasia and PCR at a young age can trigger similar overall shape and size changes in the mandible. However, the history of disease progression, evidence of prior destruction, age of onset, and certain local and regional changes can help contrast the two.

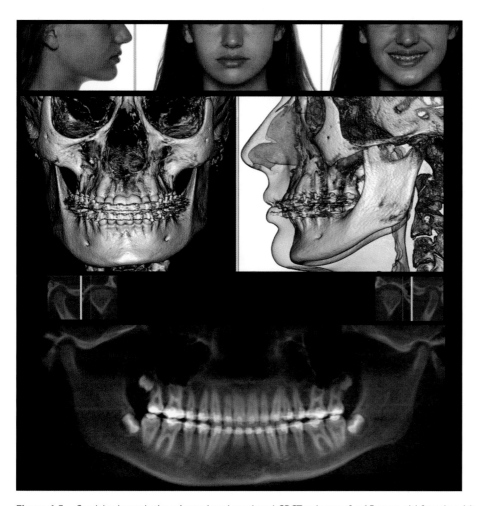

Figure 6.5 *Condylar hypoplasia*: oriented and rendered CBCT volume of a 15-year-old female with a left-side condylar hypoplasia (Shah and Hatcher 2016). *Local changes*: The osseous components of the right TMJ have a normal size, shape, quality, and spatial relationships. The left condyle has a normal shape and quality but is relatively small when compared to the contralateral side. *Regional changes*: The vertical dimensions of the left condylar process, ascending ramus, and body of the mandible are less than the right side. The lateral development of the left half of the mandible is slightly less than the right side. The left TMJ is inferiorly located on the cranial base when compared to the right. The posterior occlusal plane is elevated on the left side. The osseous midline of the mandible is shifted to the left.

Hemifacial Microsomia (HFM)

Synonyms include oculoauriculoverbral dysplasia, Goldenhar syndrome, first and second arch syndrome, lateral facial dysplasia, and craniofacial syndrome. HFM is a congenital anomaly of unknown origin unilaterally affecting first and second branchial arch derivatives including face, ear, mandible, teeth, zygoma, zygomatic arch, masticatory muscles, orbit, and facial nerve (Figure 6.6) (Hatcher 2016b). The osseous midline of the mandible is shifted to the ipsilateral side. Small or absent condyle, small ramus, elevated occlusal plane, reduced lateral development of the mandible. The ear findings may include microtia, preauricular ear tags or pits, and aural atresia.

Natural History: Failure or reduced growth of ipsilateral side.

Differential Diagnosis: The differential diagnosis includes a neonatal fracture and condylar hypoplasia. HFM can be differentiated from other conditions by identifying involvement orbit, ear, zygomatic bone, and muscles of mastication.

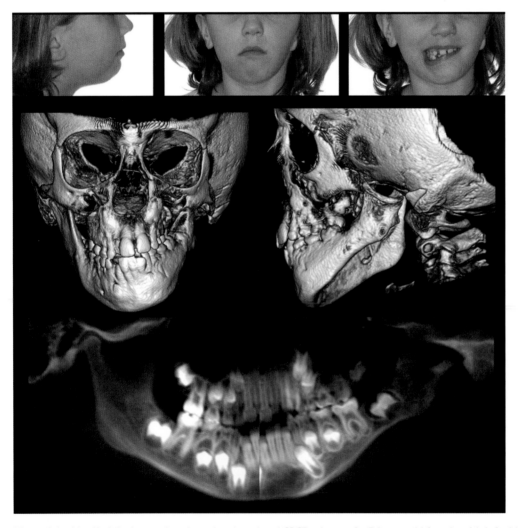

Figure 6.6 *Hemifacial microsomia*: oriented and rendered CBCT volume of a 7.6-year-old female with left side hemifacial microsomia. The left condylar process is very small and does not articulate with the temporal bone. The left side articular eminence has not formed. The vertical dimensions of the left ramus and body of the mandible are short. The left side mandibular plane angle is steep and the left gonial angle is obtuse. The left side occlusal plane is elevated. The osseous midline of the mandible is shifted to the left. The lateral development of the mandible is less than the right. The skull base is depressed on the left side. The left mastoid process is hypoplastic and there is photographic evidence of VII palsy. There is a dehiscence in the left zymotic arch. The left side ossicles and ear canal are not present.

Condylar Hyperplasia

Synonyms include hemimandibular hyperplasia and hemifacial hypertrophy. Condylar hyperplasia is characterized by a large condyle when compared to the dimensions of the ipsilateral fossa and contralateral condyle (Hatcher and Koening 2016). The size changes primarily occur in a vector associated with vertical dimension. The condylar process, ascending ramus, and body of the mandible are greater than the contralateral side (Figure 6.7). The osseous midline is shifted to the contralateral side but the maxillary and mandibular dental midline remain coincident. The vertical growth of the ipsilateral half of the mandible inferiorly displaces the lower border of the mandible. The posterior teeth on the involved side may passively erupt and result in posterior occlusal contact or remain as an open bite. The mandibular canal on the involved side will maintain the same spatial relationships to the lower border of the mandible as observed on the contralateral side. The ipsilateral half of the mandible will demonstrate shape changes including: lateral bowing the ramus, convex

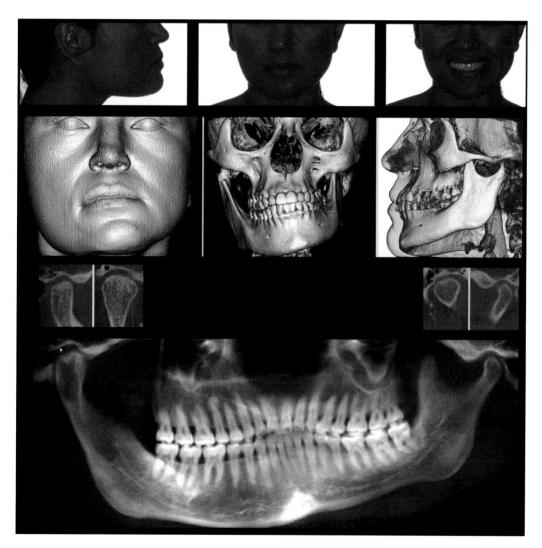

Figure 6.7 *Condylar hyperplasia*: oriented and rendered CBCT volume of an adult female with a right-side condylar hyperplasia (Hatcher and Koening 2016). *Local changes:* The right condyle is relatively large when compared to the dimensions of the left condylar and the ipsilateral fossa. The right condyle demonstrates superior surface flattening but is otherwise normal. *Regional changes:* The vertical dimensions of the right condylar process, ascending ramus and body of the mandible are greater than the left side. There is lateral bowing of the right side of the mandible. The posterior surface of the right ascending ramus and antegonial notch are less concave than the contralateral side. The right TMJ is superiorly positioned on the cranial base when compared to the left side. The posterior occlusal plane is depressed on right side. The osseous midline of the mandible is shifted to the left and the dental midlines are coincident.

shape of the posterior and inferior borders of the mandible and the vertical long axis of mandibular body will have a vertical orientation on the involved side. The temporal component of the TMJ may be elevated when compared to the uninvolved side.

Natural History: The onset of condylar hyperplasia is rare before the age of 9 and the period of active growth may extend beyond the period of somatic growth and in rare cases up to the age of 30. Since the eminence development is progressive from birth and is influenced by the functional interactions between the condyle and eminence, the relative size and shape of the involved fossa/eminence will start to deviate from the contralateral TMJ at time the onset of the condylar hyperplasia.

Differential Diagnosis: The differential diagnosis includes hemimandibular elongation (HME) (Hatcher 2016a), osteochondroma (Hatcher and Petrikowski 2016b), and hypoplasia (Hatcher and Petrikowski 2016a) of the contralateral condyle. Condylar hyperplasia can be differentiated from HME by the occlusal findings and distribution of the mandibular size changes. An osteochondroma is an add-on mass and not a global enlargement of the condyle, and it is localized to the cartilage portion of the condyle (Figure 6.9). An osteochondroma will not change dimensions of the neck, body, or ramus of the mandible. A minor expression of condylar hyperplasia is difficult to differentiate from a condylar hypoplasia of the contralateral side.

Hemimandibular Elongation (HME)

HME is characterized by vertical elongation of the condylar process (condyle and neck) without significant elongation of the ipsilateral ramus and body of the mandible (Hatcher 2016a). The anteroposterior distance from the condylion to the menton is largest on the involved side (Figure 6.8). The gonial angle may be more obtuse on the involved side. The osseous midline of the mandible is shifted to the contralateral side. The vector of mandibular growth is often associated with several of the following occlusal changes: Subdivision super class III on the involved side, posterior crossbite on the contralateral side, reduced or negative anterior overjet, and reduced overbite, shift of the mandibular dental midline to the contralateral side.

Natural History: The differential growth between the normal and involved sides may initiate in late mixed dentition, peaks prior to the pubertal growth spurt and continues up until the completion of somatic growth. It is prudent to confirm completion of mandibular growth prior to initiation of therapeutic remedies. It is not uncommon for the contralateral condyle to lose volume secondary to a degenerative disorder presumable secondary to altered mechanics during function.

Differential Diagnosis: The differential diagnosis includes condylar hyperplasia (Hatcher and Koening 2016) and an osteochondroma (Hatcher and Petrikowski 2016b). A condylar hyperplasia typically does not have a shift of the dental midline and crossbite of the contralateral posterior teeth. Condylar hyperplasia unlike HME is associated with vertical elongation of the ipsilateral ramus and body of the mandible. In contrast, HME demonstrates an AP elongation not seen in condylar hyperplasia. An osteochondroma exhibits the same occlusal changes as observed in HME but enlargement an "add on like enlargement, of the condyle is localized to the articular cartilage region (Figure 6.9).

Conclusions

Craniofacial asymmetries can pose a diagnostic challenge to the treating practitioner. Treatment considerations such as the timing and type of therapy depend upon a precise clinical diagnosis. An understanding of the underlying causes of asymmetry, coupled with advanced imaging, and careful quantification will aid in arriving at the right diagnosis.

True asymmetries can arise from various causes, ranging from syndromes affecting the entire body to local neoplasms. This chapter, however, limits the discussion to asymmetries arising from the TMJ which affect the shape and size of the craniofacial skeleton. Advanced imaging such as a CBCT can capture nuances in local and regional changes that can be missed in a clinical setting. In addition to visualizing the asymmetry, imaging can help in quantifying the variations in individual components.

Some asymmetries described in this chapter can have overlapping features and similar overall presentation. However, careful consideration of local and regional changes such as changes to the occlusion, skeletal midline, dental midline, and axis of mandibular growth can help in arriving at the correct diagnosis.

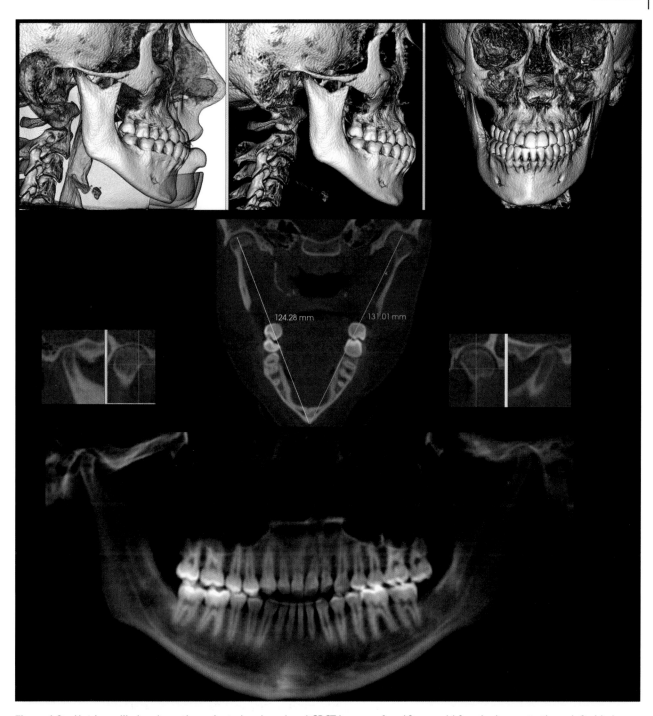

Figure 6.8 *Hemimandibular elongation*: oriented and rendered CBCT images of an 18-year-old female demonstrating a left sided hemimandibular elongation (Hatcher 2016a). *Local changes*: The left condylar process demonstrates a greater vertical dimension than the right side. The anteroposterior dimensions of the left half of the mandible are greater than the right as shown on the oblique axial view. *Regional changes*: The dental and osseous midlines of the mandible are shifted to the right. There is a left side subdivision super class III occlusion, right posterior cross bite and anterior end-to-end occlusion. The vertical dimensions of the right and left ascending rami and body of the mandible are nearly equal.

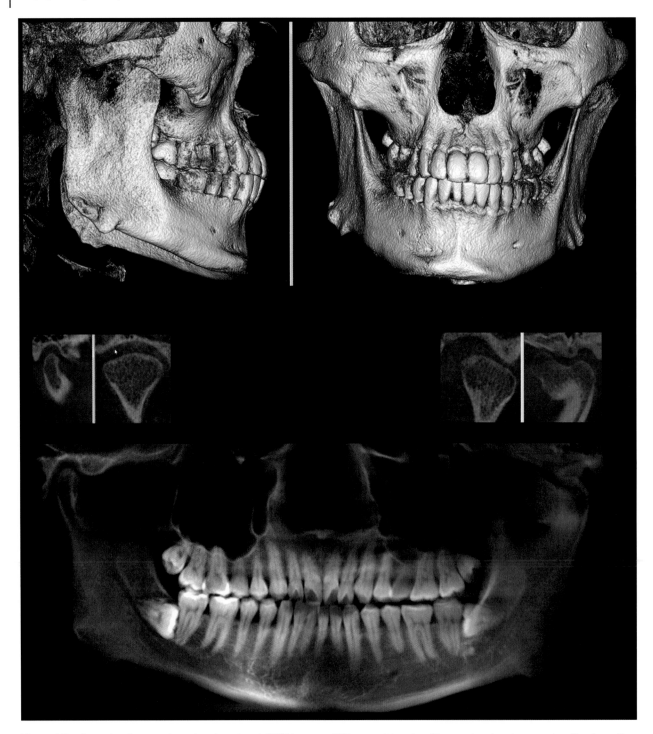

Figure 6.9 *Osteochondroma*: oriented and rendered CBCT images of 31-year-old male with an osteochondroma extending from the anterior surface of the left condyle (Hatcher and Petrikowski 2016b). *Local changes*: an osseous mass is extending anteriorly from fovea area of the left condyle. The outer margin of the osseous mass is well defined and corticated. The osteochondroma mass has formed a pseudo-articulation with the eminence crest. The mass has displaced the left condyle anteriorly and inferiorly within the fossa. The articular surface of the native portion of the left condyle has normal, size, shape and quality. *Regional changes*: The osseous and dental midlines of the mandible are shifted to the right. The left posterior occlusal plane is slightly depressed and the left side opposing teeth do not fully interdigitate. There is a right sided posterior crossbite. The vertical dimensions of the ascending rami and body of the mandible are the same.

References

Alsabban L, Amarista FJ, Mercuri LG, Perez D. Idiopathic condylar resorption: a survey and review of the literature. J Oral Maxillofac Surg. 2018;76:2316.e1–2316.e13.

Bryndahl F, Eriksson L, Legrell PE, Isberg A. Bilateral TMJ disk displacement induces mandibular retrognathia. J Dent Res. 2006;85:1118–1123.

Carter DR, Beaupré GS. Skeletal Function and Form: Mechanobiology of Skeletal Development, Aging, and Regeneration. Cambridge: Cambridge University Press, 2007a:1–31.

Carter DR, Beaupré GS. Skeletal Function and Form: Mechanobiology of Skeletal Development, Aging, and Regeneration. Cambridge: Cambridge University Press, 2007b:31–52.

Dadgar-Yeganeh A, Hatcher DC, Oberoi S. Association between degenerative temporomandibular joint disorders, vertical facial growth, and airway dimensions. J World Fed Orthod. 2021;10:20–28.

Dahl Kristensen K, Schmidt B, Stoustrup P, Pedersen TK. Idiopathic condylar resorptions: 3-dimensional condylar bony deformation, signs and symptoms. Am J Orthod Dentofac Orthop. 2017;152:214–223.

Faulkner MG, Hatcher DC, Hay A. A three-dimensional investigation of temporomandibular joint loading. J Biomech. 1987;20:997–1002.

Hatcher DC. Progressive condylar resorption: pathologic processes and imaging considerations. Semin Orthod. 2013;19:97–105.

Hatcher DC. Hemimandibular elongation. In: Tamimi D, Hatcher DC, eds. Specialty Imaging: Temporomandibular Joint. Philadelphia: Amirsys – Elsevier, 2016a:428–431.

Hatcher DC. Hemifacial macrosomia. In: Tamimi D, Hatcher DC, eds. Specialty Imaging: Temporomandibular Joint. Philadelphia: Amirsys – Elsevier, 2016b:404–407.

Hatcher DC, Faulkner MG, Hay A. Development of mechanical and mathematic models to study temporomandibular joint loading. J Prosthet Dent. 1986;55:377–384.

Hatcher DC, Koening LJ. Condylar hyperplasia. In: Tamimi D, Hatcher DC, eds. Specialty Imaging: Temporomandibular Joint. Philadelphia: Amirsys – Elsevier, 2016:418–423.

Hatcher DC, Koening LJ, Petrikowski CG. Condylar hypoplasia. In: Tamimi D, Hatcher DC, eds. Specialty Imaging: Temporomandibular Joint. Philadelphia: Amirsys – Elsevier, 2016:414–417.

Hatcher DC, Petrikowski CG. TMJ fracture, adult and neonatal. In: Tamimi D, Hatcher DC, eds. Specialty Imaging: Temporomandibular Joint. Philadelphia: Amirsys – Elsevier, 2016a:438–443.

Hatcher DC, Petrikowski CG. Osteochondroma. In: Tamimi D, Hatcher DC, eds. Specialty Imaging: Temporomandibular Joint. Philadelphia: Amirsys – Elsevier, 2016b:540–545.

Korioth TW, Hannam AG. Effect of bilateral asymmetric tooth clenching on load distribution at the mandibular condyles. J Pros Dent. 1990;64:62–73.

Kurita H, Ohtsuka A, Kobayashi H, Kurashina K. Alteration of the horizontal mandibular condylar size associated with temporomandibular joint internal derangement in adult females. Dentomaxillofac Radiol. 2002;31:373–378.

Legrell PE, Isberg A. Mandibular height asymmetry following experimentally induced temporomandibular joint disk displacement in rabbits. Oral Surg Oral Med Oral Pathol Oral Radiol Endod. 1998;86:280–285.

Legrell PE, Isberg A. Mandibular length and midline asymmetry after experimentally induced temporomandibular joint disk displacement in rabbits. Am J Orthod Dentofac Orthop. 1999;115:247–253.

Legrell PE, Reibel J, Nylander K, Hörstedt P, Isberg A. Temporomandibular joint condyle changes after surgically induced non-reducing disk displacement in rabbits: a macroscopic and microscopic study. Acta Odontol Scand. 1999;57:290–300.

Mizoguchi I, Toriya N, Nakao Y. Growth of the mandible and biological characteristics of the mandibular condylar cartilage. Japan Dent Scie Rev. 2013;49:139–150.

Phi L, Albertson B, Hatcher D, Rathi S, Park J, Oh H. Condylar degeneration in anterior open bite patients: a cone bam computed tomography study. Oral Surg Oral Med Oral Pathol Oral Radiol. 2022;133:221–228.

Pirttiniemi P, Peltomaki T, Muller L, Luder H. Abnormal mandibular growth and condylar cartilage. Eur J Orthod. 2009;31:1–11.

Rathi S, Hatcher DC. Considerations for use of CBCT in orthodontics. Calif Dent Assoc J. 2019;47:111–120.

Shah LM, Hatcher DC. Juvenile idiopathic arthritis. In: Tamimi D, Hatcher DC, eds. Specialty Imaging: Temporomandibular Joint. Philadelphia: Amirsys – Elsevier, 2016:458–463.

Sommerfeldt DW, Rubin CT. Biology of bone and how it orchestrates the form and the function of the skeleton. Eur Spine J. 2001;10:S86–S95.

Tamimi D, Jalali E, Hatcher DC. Temporomandibular joint imaging. Radiol Clin N Am. 2017;65:157–175.

Trypkova B, Major P, Nebbe B, Prasad N. Craniofacial symmetry and temporomandibular joint internal derangement in female adolescents: a posteroanterior cephalometric study. Angle Orthod. 2000;70:81–88.

7

Cephalometric Radiographic Assessment of Facial Asymmetry

Guilherme Janson and Aron Aliaga-Del Castillo

Introduction

Several studies evaluating asymmetric malocclusions have been reported in orthodontics (Cheney 1961; Wertz 1975; Alavi et al. 1988; de Araujo et al. 1994; Rose et al. 1994; Burstone 1998; Janson et al. 2001; Azevedo et al. 2006; Janson et al. 2007a; Sanders et al. 2010; Minich et al. 2013). Systematic diagnosis and treatment planning have been proposed to achieve adequate and functional treatment results depending on the individual patient's characteristics (Wertz 1975; Lewis 1976; Forsberg et al. 1984; Shroff et al. 1997; Burstone 1998; Rebellato 1998; Shroff and Siegel 1998; Janson et al. 2003a, 2003b, 2004, 2007a; Turpin 2005; Cassidy et al. 2014). Class II subdivision malocclusion subjects have been compared with subjects with normal occlusion in order to evaluate intrinsic characteristics of the asymmetric malocclusion (Janson et al. 2001; Azevedo et al. 2006; Sanders et al. 2010).

These comparisons have been performed using clinical evaluation, photographs, dental models, 2D radiographs, and computed tomography (Wertz 1975; Lewis 1976; Ritucci and Burstone 1981; Forsberg et al. 1984; Alavi et al. 1988; Rose et al. 1994; Janson et al. 2001; Vitral et al. 2004). In the last years, the use of cone-beam computed tomography (CBCT) has become an important auxiliary tool for asymmetry diagnosis (Sanders et al. 2010; Minich et al. 2013; Cachecho et al. 2014; Cassidy et al. 2014; Huang et al. 2017). However, its use is limited to specific malocclusions depending on patient's requirements and ethical issues (American Academy of Oral and Maxillofacial Radiology 2013).

Although CBCT use has been increased, there are still clinicians that do not have access to this diagnostic tool and others that do not include it in their clinical practice as a routine exam. Therefore, the use of clinical parameters and 3D evaluations based on 2D radiograph methods are considered an adequate option for diagnosis, even with their limitations. In addition, they are easier to ask and be obtained by the patients. In this way, this chapter will focus on different 2D radiographic methods that explain the characteristics of asymmetric malocclusions and establish some clinical implications for their diagnosis and treatment planning.

Radiographic Methods for Diagnosis of Asymmetry

Different radiographic methods have been used to evaluate asymmetry. Among them, panoramic, posteroanterior, and submentovertex radiographs could be mentioned.

Panoramic radiographs could be used to detect mandibular asymmetry, differences in the shape and positions of the right and left condyles, differences in the height and width of the ramus, mandibular midline deviation, etc. (Peltola et al. 1995). However, distortion and magnification limit the accuracy of the obtained information.

The most frequent 2D method to evaluate asymmetry has been the posteroanterior radiograph. It allows frontal evaluation of the subjects. Although this projection could bring information about skeletal and dental asymmetries, it does not show the anteroposterior location of the dental components in relation to the skeletal structures.

To overcome these limitations, the submentovertex is also used to evaluate facial asymmetry (Ritucci and Burstone 1981; Forsberg et al. 1984; Arnold et al. 1994; Rose et al. 1994; Janson et al. 2001). The submentovertex radiograph is an option to evaluate skeletal and dental symmetry of the maxillary and mandibular components. It allows an analysis based on an axial projection.

In the next topics, the analyses of some of these radiographic projections will be described.

Posteroanterior Radiographs

The posteroanterior radiographs are most commonly used and they are obtained positioning the subject in the cephalostat, with the forehead and nose slightly touching the film cassette, according to Harvold's method (Harvold 1954). During exposure, the subjects should keep their teeth in centric occlusion.

Cephalometric structures, lines, planes, and measurements are obtained according to the method of Grummons and Kappeyne van de Coppello (1987). The tracings of the posteroanterior radiograph include orbits, contours of the nasal cavity, crista galli, zygomatic arches, mandibular contour from one condyle to the other, left and right maxillary contours, lateral aspects of the frontal bone, lateral aspects of the zygomatic bones, maxillary and mandibular central incisors, and maxillary and mandibular first molars (Figures 7.1 and 7.2). For paired structures, the distance to the reference midline is determined for both landmarks, and the difference between the distances is calculated. For unpaired points, the horizontal distance to the midline is determined.

Submentovertex Radiographs

The submentovertex projection allows the use of specific skeletal landmarks to determine the sagittal axis and to use specific coordinate systems. For the submentovertex radiograph, the patient should be positioned in the cephalostat and seated on a bench without backrest. The patient's head should be rotated posteriorly until the Frankfurt plane

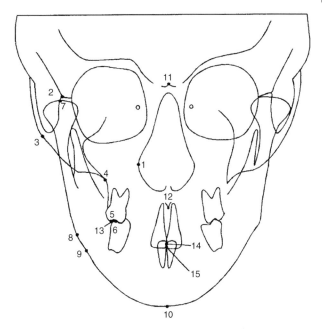

Figure 7.1 Structures and landmarks of the posteroanterior radiograph. 1, Most lateral point on outline of nasal orifice in region of each piriform aperture; 2, superolateral reference point, point located at lateral aspect of each frontozygomatic suture; 3, lateral aspect of each zygomatic arch centered vertically; 4, point located at depth of concavity of each lateral maxillary contour at junction of maxilla and zygomatic buttress; 5, buccal cusp tip of each maxillary first molar; 6, buccal cusp tip of each mandibular first molar; 7, point located on the superior surface of head of each condyle centered mediolaterally; 8, point located at each gonial angle of mandible; 9, point located at each antegonial notch; 10, menton, most inferior point on anterior border of mandible at symphysis; 11, most superior point of crista galli located ideally in skeletal midline; 12, tip of anterior nasal spine; 13, mean contact point between each maxillary and mandibular first molar; 14, midpoint between maxillary central incisors; 15, midpoint between mandibular central incisors. *Source:* Reproduced with permission from Janson et al. (2001)/Elsevier.

becomes parallel with the radiographic film cassette. In order to maintain this position, the patient should handle, with the two hands, an auxiliary support located in front of him/her (Janson et al. 2001).

During the exam, the subjects should maintain their teeth in centric occlusion, as they do not present functional mandibular deviation (Forsberg et al. 1984; Lew and Tay 1993; O'Byrn et al. 1995). One could argue that radiographs should be taken in centric relation to detect any functional mandibular deviation that might interfere with the evaluation of mandibular asymmetry in relation to the maxilla and the cranial base (Ritucci and Burstone 1981; Williamson 1981; Forsberg et al. 1984). Nevertheless, centric occlusion is preferred in patients without functional mandibular deviation.

Cephalometric structures, lines, planes, and measurements are obtained according to Ritucci and Burstone (1981), with some modifications (Forsberg et al. 1984; Janson

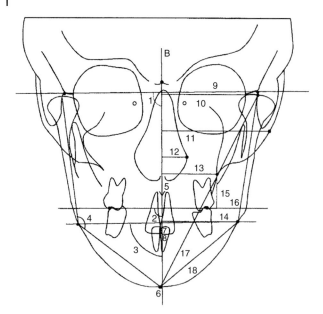

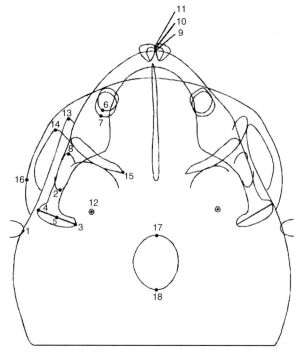

Figure 7.2 Angular and linear measurements from the posteroanterior radiograph. 1, Z plane angle, angle between Z plane and Cg–ANS line; 2, occlusal plane angle, angle between occlusal plane and Cg–ANS line; 3, antegonial plane angle, angle between antegonial plane and Cg–ANS line; 4, antegonial angle, angle between mandibular ramus and mandibular body; 5, anterior nasal spine deviation, horizontal distance between anterior nasal spine and X-line (vertical line representing medial plane drawn at right angle to Z plane through root of crista galli); 6, mandibular deviation, horizontal distance between menton and X-line; 7, maxillary dental midline deviation, horizontal distance between dental maxillary midline and X-line; 8, mandibular dental midline deviation, horizontal distance between dental mandibular midline and X-line; 9, frontozygomatic suture to X-line distance, horizontal distance between frontozygomatic suture and X-line; 10, condylion to X-line distance, horizontal distance between condylion and X-line; 11, zygoma distance, distance between zygomaxillary arch and X-line; 12, piriform aperture to X-line distance, horizontal distance between lateral wall of piriform aperture and X-line; 13, maxillary buttress to X-line distance, horizontal distance between maxillary buttress and X-line; 14, antegonial notch to X-line distance, horizontal distance between antegonial notch and X-line; 15, maxillary first molar height, vertical distance between maxillary buttress and buccal cusp tip of maxillary first molar; 16, condylion to antegonial notch distance, size of mandibular ramus from condylion to antegonialnotch; 17, condylion to menton distance, mandibular length from condylion to menton; 18, menton to antegonial notch distance, mandibular body size from menton to antegonial notch. *Source:* Reproduced with permission from Janson et al. (2001)/Elsevier.

Figure 7.3 Structures and landmarks of submentovertex radiograph. 1, Metallic ear rod point, medial center of each metallic ear rod; 2, gonion point, midpoint mediolaterally on posterior border of each gonial angle; 3, medial condylar point, tangent point to each medial condylar border of line drawn parallel to each mandibular body line; 4, lateral condylar point, tangent point to each lateral condylar border of line drawn parallel to each mandibular body line; 5, condylar midpoint, midpoint between lateral and medial condylar points on each condyle; 6, distal mandibular first molar point, most distal point in line with central groove on each mandibular first molar; 7, distal maxillary first molar point, most distal point in line with central groove on each maxillary first molar; 8, coronoid process point, most anterior point relative to transcondylar axis on each coronoid process; 9, mandibular midline, most anterior point of mandibular body (skeletal point); 10, mandibular dental midline, point contact between mesial surfaces of crowns of mandibular central incisors; 11, maxillary dental midline, point contact between mesial surfaces of crowns of maxillary central incisors; 12, foramina spinosa points, geometric center of each foramen spinosa; 13, angulare, most anterior point relative to transpterygomaxillary axis of triangular opacities present at external orbital angle where maxillary and mandibular orbital rims meet and zygomatic arch inserts; 14, buccale, point on internal surface of each zygomatic arch where arch turns medially and directly starts upon a backward sweep; 15, pterygomaxillary fissure, most medial and posterior point of each pterygomaxillary fissure; 16, zygion points, intersections of lateral borders of zygomatic arches with line parallel to transpterygomaxillary axis drawn across section of greatest bizygomatic width; 17, basion, most anterior point relative to transspinosum axis on border of foramen magnum; 18, opisthion, most posterior point relative to transspinosum axis on border of foramen magnum. *Source:* Reproduced with permission from Janson et al. (2001)/ Elsevier.

et al. 2001). The tracings of the submentovertex radiograph include foramen magnum, foramen spinosum, metallic ear rods, mandibular condyles, gonial angles, coronoid processes, posterior cranial vault, zygomatic arches, anterior cranial vault, pterygomaxillary fissures, vomer, maxillary and mandibular first molars, and maxillary and mandibular central incisors. The structures and landmarks used in this projection are illustrated in Figure 7.3 (Janson et al. 2001).

The method of Ritucci and Burstone (1981) evaluates the craniodental structures asymmetries in relation to different coordinate systems. The coordinate systems used are the mandibular, the cranial floor, and the zygomaxillary complex. In addition, the angular measurement between the abscissa of the coordinate systems can also be obtained (Janson et al. 2001).

The coordinate system consists of two axes perpendicular to each other. These axes allow evaluation of lateral and anteroposterior positions of structures of interest.

The transcondylar axis is established in the mandibular coordinate system, passing through the condylar points. This axis allows evaluation of symmetry of the anteroposterior positioning of the mandibular structures. Another axis, drawn perpendicular to the transcondylar axis from its midpoint, is used to assess symmetry of the transverse positioning of these structures (Figure 7.4).

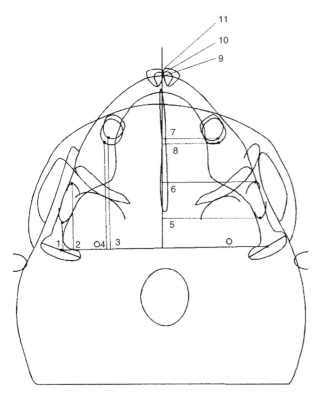

Figure 7.4 Measurements from the submentovertex radiograph. Mandibular coordinate system. Anteroposterior: 1, Gonion to transcondylar axis; 2, coronoid process point to transcondylar axis; 3, distal mandibular first molar point to transcondylar axis; 4, distal maxillary first molar point to transcondylar axis. Transverse: 5, gonion to intercondylar axis; 6, coronoid process point to intercondylar axis; 7, distal mandibular first molar point to intercondylar axis; 8, distal maxillary first molar point to intercondylar axis; 9, mandibular midline to intercondylar axis; 10, mandibular dental midline to intercondylar axis; 11, maxillary dental midline to intercondylar axis. *Source:* Reproduced with permission from Janson et al. (2001)/Elsevier.

Following this thinking, the transspinosum and interspinosum axes are constructed for the coordinate system of the cranial floor, and the transpterygomaxillary and interpterygomaxillary axes are constructed for the zygomaxillary coordinate system (Janson et al. 2001); and the transmaxillary molar, transmandibular molar, intermaxillary molar, and intermandibular molar axes are constructed for the maxillary and mandibular dental coordinate systems, respectively (Janson et al. 2007a).

For paired structures, the distance to the reference axis is determined for both landmarks, and the difference in the horizontal distance is calculated. For unpaired points, the horizontal distance to the midline is determined.

Evaluation of Asymmetries in Class II Subdivision Malocclusions using Radiographic Methods

These radiographic methods were used in investigating dentoskeletal asymmetries in Class II subdivision malocclusions and showed that they present the following characteristics (Alavi et al. 1988; de Araujo et al. 1994; Rose et al. 1994; Janson et al. 2001): (i) they are predominantly dentoalveolar; (ii) primarily characterized by distal positioning of the mandibular first molar on the Class II side and; (iii) secondarily by mesial positioning of the maxillary first molar on the Class II side and; (iv) consequently present a more frequent deviation of the mandibular dental midline to the Class II side; (v) the maxillary and mandibular dental arches have greater asymmetry than normal occlusion arches.

Based on these characteristics, a systematic approach for treatment of Class II subdivision malocclusions was developed which consists of classifying them in a clinical frontal analysis into two main types (Janson et al. 2001, 2003a, 2003b, 2007a): Type 1 – in which the maxillary dental midline will be coincident with the facial midline and the mandibular midline will be deviated and; Type 2 – in which the maxillary dental midline is deviated with the facial midline and the mandibular midline is coincident. Among Class II subdivision malocclusions, 61.36% has type 1, 18.18% has type 2 Class II subdivision malocclusion, and 20.45% has combined characteristics (Janson et al. 2007a).

Once the Class II malocclusion type has been diagnosed a treatment protocol has to be defined. For type 1, the following treatment alternatives can be used: removable or fixed functional appliances or; Class II elastics if the patient profile does not accept extractions or; 3-premolar extractions if extractions are accepted (Figure 7.5). For type 2, asymmetric headgear can be used in growing patients, or 1-premolar extraction (Figure 7.6).

The advantages of type 1 Class II subdivision malocclusion treatment with 3-premolar extraction over 4-premolar extraction protocols are that: (i) Treatment of Class II

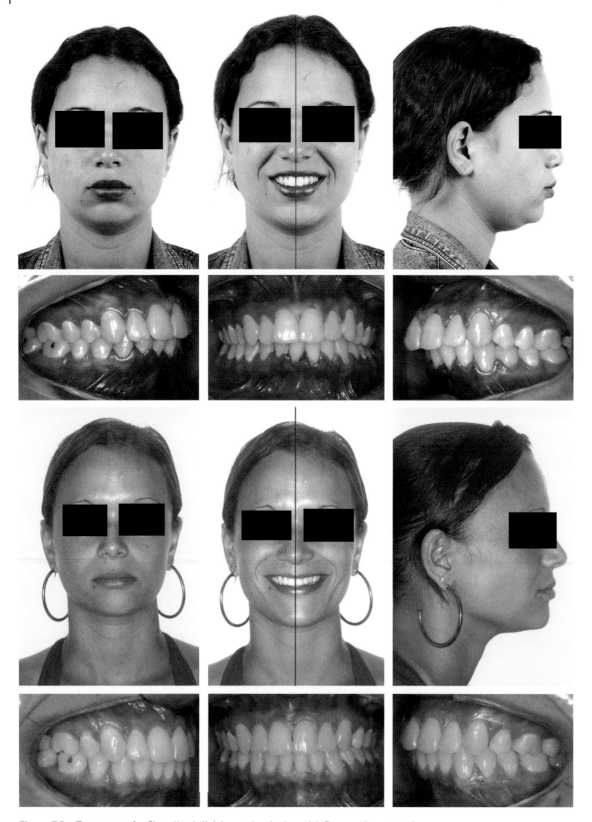

Figure 7.5   Treatment of a Class II subdivision malocclusion with 3-premolar extractions.

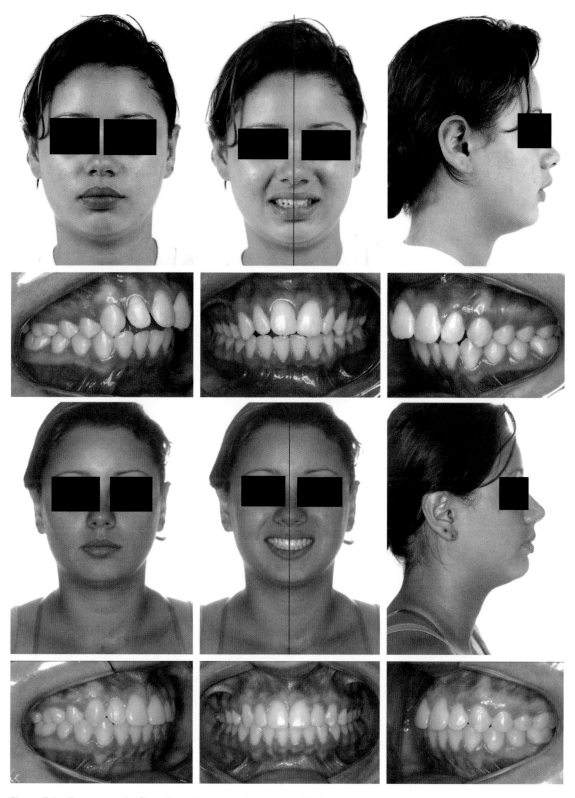

Figure 7.6 Treatment of a Class II subdivision malocclusion with 1-premolar extraction.

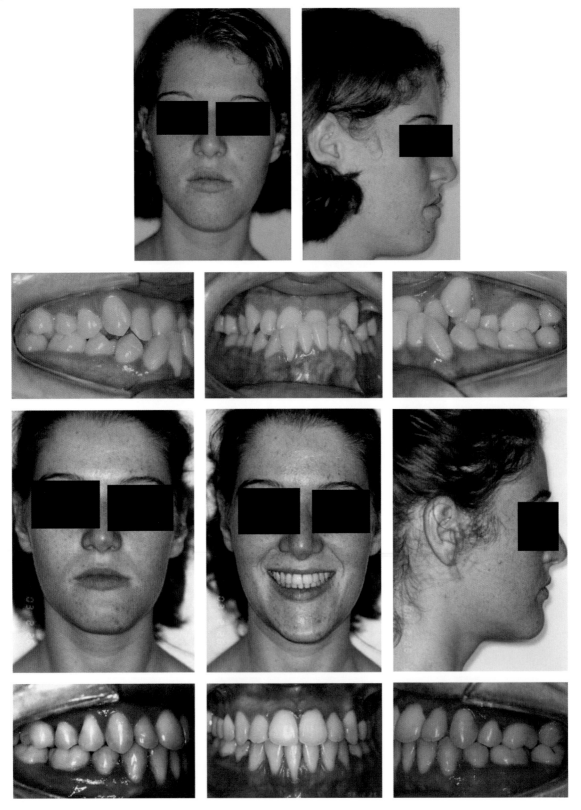

Figure 7.7 Treatment of a Class III subdivision malocclusion with 3-premolar extractions.

subdivision malocclusions with extraction of 3-premolar shows a better treatment success rate in correcting the maxillary-to-mandibular dental midline deviation and consequently a better correction of the anteroposterior discrepancy of the posterior segments, compared with 4-premolar-extraction treatment. It provides therefore, a simpler mechanics (Janson et al. 2003a); (ii) The 3-premolar asymmetric extraction protocol in Class II subdivision malocclusions produces significantly less mandibular incisor and soft-tissue retraction than the 4-premolar extraction protocol (Janson et al. 2007b); (iii) The treatment protocols with asymmetric extractions do not induce undesirable dentoskeletal effects in the frontal plane (Janson et al. 2004); (iv) Smile attractiveness with asymmetric extractions is similar to treatment with symmetric extractions (Janson et al. 2014).

One has to consider asymmetric third molar extractions in Class II subdivision cases treated with asymmetric premolar extractions (Janson et al. 2007c). The quadrants which had premolar extractions may have enough space for third molar eruption and function while the quadrant or quadrants which did not have premolar extractions may not have available space for third molar eruption, which will have to be extracted.

Although detailed studies have not been conducted on Class III subdivision malocclusions, a similar systematic approach can be applied in predominantly dentoalveolar malocclusions (Janson et al. 2003b). However, they should be inversely classified, as follows: they are classified as Type 1 when there is coincidence of the mandibular dental midline with the facial midline and deviation of the maxillary midline and; as Type 2 when there is deviation of the mandibular dental midline with the facial midline and coincidence of the maxillary midline. Consequently, their treatment is analogous to Class II subdivision malocclusions (Janson et al. 2009) (Figure 7.7).

Concluding Remarks

- The posteroanterior and submentovertex radiographs are useful and reliable to perform a correct diagnosis of asymmetry;
- They have been used in evaluation of dentoskeletal asymmetries in Class II subdivision malocclusions, allowing development of a systematic approach for diagnosis and treatment;
- Recognition of the characteristics of subdivision malocclusions is essential for more favorable treatment planning, which will simplify orthodontic mechanics and require less compliance from the patient and less chair time for the clinician.

References

Alavi DG, BeGole EA, Schneider BJ. Facial and dental arch asymmetries in Class II subdivision malocclusion. Am J Orthod Dentofac Orthop. 1988;93:38–46.

American Academy of Oral and Maxilofacial Radiology. Clinical recommendations regarding use of cone beam computed tomography in orthodontics. Position statement by the American Academy of Oral and Maxilofacial Radiology. Oral Surg Oral Med Oral Pathol Oral Radiol. 2013;116:238–257.

Arnold TG, Anderson GC, Liljemark WF. Cephalometric norms for craniofacial asymmetry using submental-vertical radiographs. Am J Orthod Dentofac Orthop. 1994;106:250–256.

Azevedo AR, Janson G, Henriques JF, Freitas MR. Evaluation of asymmetries between subjects with Class II subdivision and apparent facial asymmetry and those with normal occlusion. Am J Orthod Dentofac Orthop. 2006;129:376–383.

Burstone CJ. Diagnosis and treatment planning of patients with asymmetries. Semin Orthod. 1998;4:153–164.

Cachecho C, Hans MG, Palomo JM. A three-dimensional evaluation of Class II subdivision malocclusion correction using Cartesian coordinates. Semin Orthod. 2014;20:287–298.

Cassidy SE, Jackson SR, Turpin DL, Ramsay DS, Spiekerman C, Huang GJ. Classification and treatment of Class II subdivision malocclusions. Am J Orthod Dentofac Orthop. 2014;145:443–451.

Cheney EA. Dentofacial asymmetries and their clinical significance. Am J Orthod. 1961;47:814–829.

de Araujo TM, Wilhelm RS, Almeida MA. Skeletal and dental arch asymmetries in Class II division 1 subdivision malocclusions. J Clin Pediatr Dent. 1994;18:181–185.

Forsberg CT, Burstone CJ, Hanley KJ. Diagnosis and treatment planning of skeletal asymmetry with the submental-vertical radiograph. Am J Orthod. 1984;85:224–237.

Grummons DC, Kappeyne van de Coppello MA. A frontal asymmetry analysis. J Clin Orthod. 1987;21:448–465.

Harvold EP. A Roentgen Study of the Postnatal Morphogenesis of the Facial Skeleton in Cleft Palate. Oslo: University of Oslo, 1954.

Huang M, Hu Y, Yu J, Sun J, Ming Y, Zheng L. Cone-beam computed tomographic evaluation of the temporomandibular joint and dental characteristics of patients with Class II subdivision malocclusion and asymmetry. Korean J Orthod. 2017;47:277–288.

Janson G, Branco NC, Morais JF, Freitas MR. Smile attractiveness in patients with Class II division 1 subdivision malocclusions treated with different tooth extraction protocols. Eur J Orthod. 2014;36:1–8.

Janson G, Carvalho PE, Cancado RH, de Freitas MR, Henriques JF. Cephalometric evaluation of symmetric and asymmetric extraction treatment for patients with Class II subdivision malocclusions. Am J Orthod Dentofac Orthop. 2007b;132:28–35.

Janson G, Cruz KS, Barros SE, Woodside DG, Metaxas A, de Freitas MR, Henriques JF. Third molar availability in Class II subdivision malocclusion. Am J Orthod Dentofac Orthop. 2007c;132:e215–e221.

Janson G, Cruz KS, Woodside DG, Metaxas A, de Freitas MR, Henriques JF. Dentoskeletal treatment changes in Class II subdivision malocclusions in submentovertex and posteroanterior radiographs. Am J Orthod Dentofac Orthop. 2004;126:451–463.

Janson G, Dainesi EA, Henriques JF, de Freitas MR, de Lima KJ. Class II subdivision treatment success rate with symmetric and asymmetric extraction protocols. Am J Orthod Dentofac Orthop. 2003a;124:257–264. quiz 339.

Janson G, de Lima KJ, Woodside DG, Metaxas A, de Freitas MR, Henriques JF. Class II subdivision malocclusion types and evaluation of their asymmetries. Am J Orthod Dentofac Orthop. 2007a;131:57–66.

Janson G, De Souza JE, Barros SE, Andrade P Jr, Nakamura AY. Orthodontic treatment alternative to a Class III subdivision malocclusion. J Appl Oral Sci. 2009;17:354–363.

Janson GR, Metaxas A, Woodside DG, de Freitas MR, Pinzan A. Three-dimensional evaluation of skeletal and dental asymmetries in Class II subdivision malocclusions. Am J Orthod Dentofac Orthop. 2001;119:406–418.

Janson G, Woodside DG, Metaxas A, Henriques JF, de Freitas MR. Orthodontic treatment of subdivision cases. World J Orthod. 2003b;4:36–46.

Lew KK, Tay DK. Submentovertex cephalometric norms in male Chinese subjects. Am J Orthod Dentofac Orthop. 1993;103:247–252.

Lewis PD. The deviated midline. Am J Orthod. 1976;70:601–616.

Minich CM, Araujo EA, Behrents RG, Buschang PH, Tanaka OM, Kim KB. Evaluation of skeletal and dental asymmetries in Angle Class II subdivision malocclusions with cone-beam computed tomography. Am J Orthod Dentofac Orthop. 2013;144:57–66.

O'Byrn BL, Sadowsky C, Schneider B, BeGole EA. An evaluation of mandibular asymmetry in adults with unilateral posterior crossbite. Am J Orthod Dentofac Orthop. 1995;107:394–400.

Peltola JS, Kononen M, Nystrom M. Radiographic characteristics in mandibular condyles of orthodontic patients before treatment. Eur J Orthod. 1995;17:69–77.

Rebellato J. Asymmetric extractions used in the treatment of patients with asymmetries. Semin Orthod. 1998;4:180–188.

Ritucci R, Burstone CJ. Use of Submental Vertical Radiograph in the Assessment of Asymmetry. Farmington: University of Connecticut, 1981.

Rose JM, Sadowsky C, BeGole EA, Moles R. Mandibular skeletal and dental asymmetry in Class II subdivision malocclusions. Am J Orthod Dentofac Orthop. 1994;105:489–495.

Sanders DA, Rigali PH, Neace WP, Uribe F, Nanda R. Skeletal and dental asymmetries in Class II subdivision malocclusions using cone-beam computed tomography. Am J Orthod Dentofac Orthop. 2010;138:542.e1–542.e20. discussion 542–543.

Shroff B, Lindauer SJ, Burstone CJ. Class II subdivision treatment with tip-back moments. Eur J Orthod. 1997;19:93–101.

Shroff B, Siegel SM. Treatment of patients with asymmetries using asymmetric mechanics. Semin Orthod. 1998;4:165–179.

Turpin DL. Correcting the Class II subdivision malocclusion. Am J Orthod Dentofac Orthop. 2005;128:555–556.

Vitral RWF, de Souza Telles C, Fraga MR, de Oliveira RS, Tanaka OM. Computed tomography evaluation of temporomandibular joint alterations in patients with Class II division 1 subdivision malocclusions: condyle - fossa relationship. Am J Orthod Dentofac Orthop. 2004;126:48–52.

Wertz RA. Diagnosis and treatment planning of unilateral Class II malocclusions. Angle Orthod. 1975;45:85–94.

Williamson EH. Dr. Eugene H. Williamson on occlusion and TMJ dysfunction. Part 2. J Clin Orthod. 1981;15:393–404, 409–410.

8

EMG and Ultrasonography of Masticatory Muscles

Stavros Kiliaridis

Introduction

During the postnatal growth of bones, a continuous remodeling process takes place to maintain a form that is appropriate for its biomechanical environment. Masticatory muscle function has been considered to be a local environmental factor that plays an important role in influencing craniofacial growth, as has been shown in animal experiments and clinical studies. These investigations have shown that the elevator muscles of the mandible influence both the transverse and the vertical facial dimensions. It is possible that the loading of the jaws by masticatory muscles stimulates sutural growth, increases bone apposition, and results in greater transverse growth of the maxilla with broader bone bases for the dental arches. Furthermore, increased demands in masticatory muscle function are often associated with an anterior growth pattern and well-developed angular, coronoid, and condylar processes in the mandible (Kiliaridis 2006). Thus, certain facial asymmetries have been considered to be related to an asymmetric muscular balance, induced after an environmentally established unilateral malocclusion, as is the functional lateral crossbite (Pirttiniemi 1998).

Understanding the Functional Profile of the Muscle

The investigations which explored the interrelation between masticatory muscles and dentofacial morphology have relied on various characteristics of muscles that could be measured in order to define the level of the muscle capacity. In animal experimental studies, electrophysiologic methods and muscle biopsies could identify the characteristics of the functional profile of the muscle cells composing the muscle, i.e. the muscle fibers, that through their contraction create force and movement. Nevertheless, most of the clinical studies do not permit extensive use of such procedures, so other methods were implemented to identify the functional profile of the muscles of different individuals. In order to better understand the implementation of these methods, an effort will be done to present an overview of the basic function of the muscles.

The contraction of the muscle fiber is based on the size changes of sarcomers which are the basic functional elements of the striated fibers. Sarcomeres are organized so that their contractile proteins are situated in striated form; they function as a unit during development of active tension. Under physiologic and not experimental conditions, the contraction of a muscle fiber is initiated after a signal from the nervous system that reaches the motor endplate, situated on the fiber's sarcolemma, where an amount of acetylcholine is released from the nerve ending after the nerve stimulation. Due to this shower of acetylcholine at the motor endplate, the ion channels in the sarcolemma of the muscle fiber open and allow sodium ions to pass through. This induces a depolarization of the sarcolemma in a waveform that departs from the end plate and travels rapidly along the entire fiber and the internal of the fiber via the T-tubules, which are an organized network of channels. The initiation of this wave, called the *action potential,* releases calcium ions that then trigger almost simultaneous contraction of all the sarcomeres in the fiber (Franzini-Armstrong 2018).

In the center of the sarcomere thick filaments composed of myosin molecules are arranged in a hexagon with adjacent thin filaments. The thin filaments, *actin*, are attached to the Z-plate, which forms the borders between the sarcomeres (Luther 2009). The procedure of the muscle contraction is based on the sliding of the actin filaments along the thick *myosin* filaments, to bring the Z-plates closer to each other. The sliding process is achieved thanks to the "head" of the myosin molecules attached to an active site on an actin molecule, forming a cross-bridge between the thick and thin filaments. The transformation of the ATP to ADP releases energy that bends the myosin heads toward the center of the myosin filament, pulling also the attached actin filament to this direction and reducing the length of the sarcomere (Canepari et al. 2010).

Electrophysiologic methods of isolated muscle fibers after electric stimulation of the single fiber could distinguish them to *slow-twitch* and *fast twitch* and after repetition of the stimulation, the fibers were distinguished if they were reaching fatigue quickly, *fast fatigue*, or not, i.e. *fatigue resistant*. The electrophysiologic contractive profile of the fibers was related to an oxidative contraction for fibers that are slow twitch and resistant to fatigue, in contrast to glycolytic contraction of fibers which are fast twitch and fast fatigue. Thus, another way to characterize the muscle fibers is through the application of histochemical or immunohistochemical methods to differentiate them in *Type I* fibers which are those with oxidative contraction, slow twitch, and resistant to fatigue, and the *Type II* fibers which are those with glycolytic contraction and fast twitch. Two subcategories of the Type II fibers presented differentiation in fatigue, i.e. the *Type IIa* characterized by fast twitch and more fatigue resistant than the *Type IIb* fibers characterized by fast twitch and fast fatigue (Schiaffino and Reggiani 2011). The muscle fibers characteristics are decided by the motoneuron, and all the fibers innervated

by the same motoneuron, i.e. belong to the same motor unit and present the same functional profile. Analysis of the composition and size of the fibers provides a good insight in the functional profile of the muscle. Nevertheless, the analysis of biopsy samples of masticatory muscles in humans is a rare method used in the clinic.

The muscle strength of each of the elevator muscles cannot be measured independently under clinical conditions. Nevertheless, the result of their synergy is evaluated as bite force. The level of bite force is a complicated function, as it depends on the number of the activated motor units and their frequency of activation.

Thus, as it is explained beautifully by Astrand and Rodahl (1986) "in activities with low force demands, slowly contracting small motor units are recruited first, with relatively low frequency of contraction. With increasing demand for force, the 'old' motor units increase their discharge rate, and in addition, new motor units are recruited. The fast-contracting motor units gradually start their activity and then at a relatively high frequency. The gradation of a muscle contraction is brought about by varying the number of active motor units (recruitment) and their frequency of excitation (rate coding)." The number and size of the muscle fibers determine the muscle strength. Thus, an evaluation of the strength of a muscle can be based on the amount of the contractive elements producing the muscle force by measuring the cross-section or the thickness of a muscle.

Clinical Methods to Record Masticatory Muscles Functional Capacity

Bite Force

Bite force is the measured effect of the contraction of the jaw elevator muscles, mainly the masseter, temporalis, and medial pterygoid. Various levels of measurements of the bite force were recorded, the one mostly used, was the maximal bite force, while others as the chewing bite force, and the maximal bite force endurance have been also recorded but in less extent. Maximal bite force was used as an indirect measure of the functional capacity of all the elevator muscles of the mandible, relatively simple to perform (Kiliaridis et al.1993). The suggested site for recording the maximal bite force was the molar region where the highest recordings can be performed (Koc et al. 2010), while keeping the intermolar distance approximately 11 mm apart by adapting the thickness of the bite fork to this size. This distance was suggested as the optimal one, as the bite force levels increase when clenching is performed with gradual augmentation of the jaw opening until about 11 mm of intermolar distance, while there is a decrease of the level of maximal bite force with further opening of the mandible, probably reflecting the average result of the optimum sarcomere length of the jaw elevator muscles (Bakke 2006).

The recording of maximal molar bite force as a measure of the functional capacity of the masticatory muscles provides big advantages as it is relatively simple, inexpensive, and quick to perform, serving large epidemiologic purposes, and being well accepted by the subjects. Nevertheless, this method has a drawback as the maximum bite force is generated bilaterally from the synergy of all the elevator masticatory muscles, transferred on the mandible. The contribution of the contraction forces of both sides is the reason why the method is less sensitive to identify minor or moderate asymmetric functional differences between the elevator muscles of the two sides. Another disadvantage of the maximum bite force recordings is associated with a large method error as reported in different studies due to the motivation level of the subject to bite as hard as possible, the intellectual level of the subjects to understand this demand, the triggering of dental, periodontal, muscle or joint pain, as well as the fear of breaking a tooth or restoration, or the result of fatigue (Carlsson 1974; Hellsing and Hagberg 1990; Bakke 2006).

Electromyography

Electromyography (EMG) is a method available for imaging muscle function and efficiency, by identifying their electrical potentials. The EMG is recording the action potentials generated by muscle fibers when they are recruited by the motoneuron and trigger almost simultaneous contraction of all the sarcomeres in the fiber. This method can be implemented to assess the electrical activity on different levels: from a muscle fiber, a motor unit, a single muscle, or a group of muscles. Nevertheless, the recording of the activity of a single muscle fiber or a motor unit is performed by an intramuscular electromyography with bipolar needle electrodes inserted through the skin into the muscle tissue, most of the time being used to detect single motor unit action potential. Though the intramuscular EMG is a very useful diagnostic method in the neurology, its invasive approach is not practical for routine use in dental clinical settings and demands a thorough knowledge in neurophysiology and pathology for correct interpretation of the findings.

Surface electromyography (sEMG) has been a widely used method in the fields of Oral Physiology as well as in Orthodontics using surface electrodes located on the surface of the skin, and it detects superimposed motor unit action potentials from many muscle fibers (Dahlstrom 1989). The recordings depend on the location of the electrodes, where the voltage between two electrodes (with a standardized interelectrode distance) is measured. Nowadays, surface bipolar, self-adhesive, and pre-gelled electrodes are often used with an inter-electrode distance of 20 mm, decreasing a source of recording error.

Masseter and anterior temporalis muscles are the muscles most frequently assessed by sEMG. The EMG activity of these muscles can be evaluated during static tests (in rest position, maximum, or sub-maximum voluntary contraction during clenching) or during active tests, such as chewing, swallowing, opening, or closing the mouth, protrusion, retrusion, and lateral deviation of the mandible. The clinical rest position of the mandible, determined by freeway space, is an active muscle position because of the tone of the muscles involved in it (Suvinen et al. 2003). Maximum voluntary contraction (MVC) is another static test frequently analyzed. The recordings of the EMG activity during isometric contraction are usually performed while maximum clenching of the teeth for 3–5 seconds in an intercuspal position or biting on a control substance, i.e. with cotton rolls placed on the lower second premolar and molars (Ferrario et al. 2000; Tartaglia et al. 2008).

The recordings of sEMG were not found to be very reproducible, presenting a larger error in the method (Cecere et al. 1996). This may be because of different factors as the inaccuracy of electrode placement with respect to underlying structures, variation in impedance of the skin, the subcutaneous fat layer, and the depth of the muscle under study (Mohl et al. 1990; Ferrario et al. 1991; Lund et al. 1995; Nordander et al. 2003).

The impact of the large methodologic error may influence longitudinal recordings where the exact placement of the electrodes is crucial. This is more serious in growing individuals when recordings are performed some years later, and changes have occurred due to growth of the face, creating difficulties to localize exactly the site where the electrodes should be placed. Similar problems may appear when bilateral recordings are compared, as the bilateral position of the electrodes may not correspond perfectly to the position of the underneath muscles, thus creating problems when evaluating a symmetric or asymmetric function.

Cross-section Surface and Thickness of Masticatory Muscles: Imaging Techniques – Ultrasonography of the Masticatory Muscles

Another approach to evaluate the masticatory muscles functional capacity was based on the cross-sectional dimensions of the muscles as this is observed using imagine techniques, historically starting from anatomic dissections which later verified the imagined results of computer tomography, the implication of magnetic resonance imaging (MRI), as well as the use of ultrasonography. The measurements performed using computer tomography were well correlated with the dissected anatomic cross section of the muscles, where it was also found that the masseter muscle was a good representative muscle of all the elevator muscles, with a strong association between its size and the size of the other muscles (Weijs and Hillen 1984, 1985). Given the large disadvantage of exposing the patient to radiation, MRI has been used and it was found to correlate well with the findings of the cross-section measurements of masticatory muscles with computer tomography (van Spronsen et al. 1989). MRI could be the ideal method to visualize the cross section of the masticatory muscles, but the high cost to implement this method, the difficulty to access it easily, and the difficulties to apply it easily on children, created barriers for its widespread use.

In parallel to these attempts to use the MRI imaging of the masticatory muscles, another imaging method was introduced, to visualize the cross section of the masseter muscle by ultrasonography as this muscle was proven to represent well the other elevator jaw muscles (Kiliaridis and Kälebo 1991). The ultrasonographic measurement of the cross-sectional dimension of the masseter was validated with the findings of the MRI and it was found to display a high correlation with MRI (Raadsheer et al. 1994; Braun et al. 1996). Furthermore, a strong correlation has been found between muscle thickness measurements and electromyographic activity (Georgiakaki et al. 2007). Ultrasonography of the masseter muscle was proven to be both reliable and accurate (Kiliaridis and Kälebo 1991), easily accessible as method, simpler, cheaper, and quicker to be used than the other imagining techniques.

The creation of the ultrasound image is based on that the transducer is transmitting pulses of high-frequency sound waves and then receiving their echoes analyze their acoustic and temporal properties (Walker et al. 2004). The sonographic image of a muscle is quite clear, being fairly well distinguished from surrounding tissues such as bone, subcutaneous adipose tissue, and skin (Pillen et al. 2008). The image of a healthy muscle appears as a low echo intensity structure with dark appearance. The dark muscle mass is surrounded by the perimysium that is echogenic sheath of connective tissue and is divided from the perimysium that is the echogenic sheath of connective tissue grouping muscle fibers into fascicles. Ultrasonography can be easily used to examine superficial structures as the masseter and temporal muscles, while other muscle groups as medial pterygoideus are not accessible, as the mandibular ramus creates

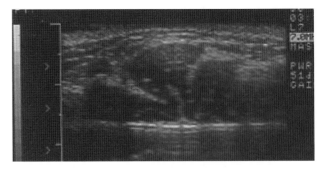

Figure 8.1 Transverse ultrasound scan of the masseter. The wide white shadow on the top depicts the skin echo; underneath, a narrow white line comes from the outer fascia of the muscle. During real-time scanning, the operator has a dynamic view of the examining area. For example, from relaxation to contraction and vice versa, it is easy to distinguish skin from fascia, although both are shown as white in the picture. The image of the masseter muscle is the dark area under the fascia. In the lower part, the echo from a bony structure is observed, which is the lateral surface of the ramus.

a bone barrier that is not penetrated by the ultrasound (Figure 8.1).

The ultrasonographic image of the masseter is obtained with a high-resolution linear-array transducer (e.g. 7–8.5 MHz) suitable for superficial structures, oriented perpendicularly to the ramus. The simplest use of ultrasonography in evaluating the masseter muscle is represented by the size assessment of the cross-section image of the muscle, by either measuring the thickness of the muscle or the surface of its cross section, two measures that are highly associated to each other. This procedure may quantify the extent of muscle hypertrophy or atrophy in respect to the age, growth phase, and gender of the subject. It is important when recording the muscle thickness to ensure that the transducer pressure on the skin is minimal, using rich amount of gel, as the muscle can easily be compressed, especially when the recording occurs in relaxed conditions, with excessive force on the transducer. This was clearly the case in the first publication on the thickness of the masseter muscle in adults, where the thickness of the muscle in relaxed conditions is substantially smaller than its thickness in contraction, something that was not the case in later studies (Kiliaridis et al. 2003; Charalampidou et al. 2008). Scanning the masseter obliquely would increase the thickness of the muscle. In order to avoid the distortion of the image, the angle of the transducer would be altered until the best echo of the mandibular ramus surface would be achieved. The site of measurement is aimed to be in the thickest part of the masseter, close to the level of the occlusal plane, approximately in the middle of the mediolateral distance of the ramus. The imaging and the measurements are performed bilaterally with the subject seated in an upright position, with the head in natural posture, under two different conditions: when the muscle is relaxed while the teeth are occluding gently, and when contracted during maximal clenching. The measurements are made directly from the image at the time of scanning, with a read-out of distance often to the nearest 0.1 mm. In a series of studies, it was found that ultrasonography was an accurate and reliable method, with a low error in measurement of the thickness of the masseter muscle (Reis Durão et al. 2017). The error of measurement was slightly larger in the measurements during the relaxed than during the contracted state, possibly due to the fact that the relaxed muscle was prone to more compression deformation than when in contraction.

Axial ultrasound images of the masseter enable to investigate not only the muscle cross-sectional area but also the muscle echo intensity that has been proposed as a clinically relevant noninvasive marker of muscle quality (Pillen et al. 2008; Fukumoto et al. 2012; Watanabe et al. 2013). In a series of recent studies, ultrasonography was proven a reliable method to evaluate structural alterations in the masseter muscles (Kiliaridis et al. 1995a; Egli et al. 2018), providing a qualitative estimation of neuromuscular and myopathic disorders because of the disease-related muscle replacement by fat and fibrous tissue (i.e. myosteatosis) (Pillen et al. 2008; Caresio et al. 2015; Minetto et al. 2019). The fibrous and adipose tissues have an acoustic impedance different from the echogenicity of healthy muscle tissue. This increases the number of reflecting interfaces in the muscle and turns the muscle mass to a whiter appearance due to increased echo intensity, like an image of the reflection of the car headlights in the fog.

While in the control subjects with healthy muscles, there is a clear visualization of bone and fascia and tendinous structures, being sharply visible without any interferences from the muscle tissue, in pathologic conditions, as is in Duchene Muscle Dystrophy, there is an increase intensity of echoes reflected from interfaces in the muscle mass, reducing the sharp bone echo. To evaluate qualitatively the severity of the muscle echogenicity we used criteria, based on a four-point scale from 0 to 3, as described in Kiliaridis et al. (1995a), according to Heckmatt et al. (1982).

Algorithms have been developed for other muscle groups to evaluate the degree of muscle tissue replacement and provide a clinically relevant noninvasive marker of muscle quality (Pillen et al. 2008; Fukumoto et al. 2012; Watanabe et al. 2013) linked to aberrations in the muscle tissue as could be the age-related, disuse-related, or disease-related loss of muscle mass. Such algorithms will be useful to be implemented in the masticatory muscles, adding substantial information on the thickness measures of the muscles.

Posterior Crossbite with Functional Shift. Effects on Masticatory Muscles?

An effort was made to evaluate the asymmetric function of the masticatory muscles mainly by sEMG, while differences in the cross-sectional area of the muscles were measured with implementation of imaging techniques, as ultrasonography. The malocclusion that was considered to be associated to an asymmetric muscle function was the posterior (or lateral) crossbite, and more specifically when functional mandibular shift occurs, as this requires an adaptation of the activity of the masticatory system to avoid the mediolateral cuspal interferences.

We approached this point by doing a systematic review of the literature (Tsanidis et al. 2016) trying to answer the questions if there is a cause and effect between the malocclusion and the functional asymmetry, whether a pre-existing functional muscular asymmetry leads to the development of a crossbite, or whether the creation of a crossbite due to problems such as bad habits leads to functional asymmetry. Our assumption was that a crossbite may lead to an orofacial functional asymmetry. Therefore, the correction of the functional unilateral posterior crossbite and elimination of the functional mandibular shift may normalize the orofacial functional asymmetry. We found four studies that fulfilled our eligibility criteria and evaluated masticatory muscle activity using absolute values obtained from sEMG (Kecik et al. 2007; De Rossi et al. 2009; Martín et al. 2012; Maffei et al. 2014). The treatment of the posterior crossbite was achieved by maxillary expansion, followed by retention. Two of the four studies included control groups in their study design. All four studies performed sEMG measurements in the rest position and found that the asymmetric activity of the masseter muscle was normalized following treatment, and three of them (Kecik et al. 2007; De Rossi et al. 2009; Martín et al. 2012), showed also normalization of the temporalis muscle. Similar results were also reported in these four studies regarding the sEMG measurements performed during maximal clenching. Following crossbite treatment, the masseter and temporalis muscles on the crossbite side showed a normalization of the initial asymmetric muscle activity.

Looking at the results of EMG studies, we should always bear in mind, as argued previously, that the EMG methodologic error is large and that EMG data can be affected by several artifacts, (Castroflorio et al. 2008). Furthermore, problems may appear when bilateral recordings are compared, as the bilateral position of the electrodes may not correspond perfectly to the position of the muscles underneath. This nonsystematic methodologic error in the placement of the electrodes may increase the normal biological variation of the sample, decreasing the possibility to reach statistically significant level, especially when the mean difference between samples is rather small. This may be an explanation for why some studies could not detect statistically significant differences in patients treated under similar conditions (Michelotti et al. 2019). The above-described issue related to the methodologic error of the EMG is the reason why sEMG was not used as diagnostic tool to detect functional aberrations of individuals and monitor possible small or moderate therapeutic improvements.

Based on the findings of the above-mentioned electromyographic studies, we expected that asymmetry would be revealed in the characteristics of the masticatory muscles, as for example in the ultrasonographic thickness of the masseter muscle. Therefore, we performed a cross-sectional study to measure if there are bilateral differences in the thickness of the masseter muscles in 38 untreated individuals with lateral crossbite, as well as in 18 subjects with successfully treated functional lateral crossbite, at least 3 years after the end of treatment, with all permanent teeth erupted (Kiliaridis et al. 2007). These findings were compared to the measures of a matched group of individuals created from a control group of 224 subjects without transversal malocclusions. We found that in the untreated group, the thickness of the masseter muscle on the crossbite side was 0.3 mm thinner than the one on the normal side, while no differences were found in the thickness of the masseter muscle between the left and the right side in the control subjects. Similarly, no differences were found in the thickness of the masseter muscle between the former crossbite side and the normal one in the treated group, 3 years after the end of their treatment.

It was argued that: "A possible explanation is that in the treated group the initially existing differences in the thickness of the masticatory muscles were reversible after orthodontic treatment, when the lateral crossbite and possible asymmetric muscle activity had been eliminated. In the functional crossbite subjects the prolonged bilateral difference in the activity level of the masticatory muscles may have worked as an asymmetric training stimulation, resulting in differences in the thickness of these muscles in the untreated group" (Kiliaridis et al. 2007). It is possible that this effect of asymmetric training stimulation on the masseter thickness is more obvious in children in late mixed dentition or permanent dentition, as was the case in our sample,

than in younger children in primary dentition or very early mixed dentition (Castelo et al. 2007). The decrease in the thickness of the masseter muscle at the crossbite side could be the consequence of the functional occlusal interferences that may cause reduction in the number of electromyographic activity periods of the masseter muscle per hour and their mean amplitude (Michelotti et al. 2005), which in its turn may cause thin muscle fibers (Kiliaridis et al. 1988; He et al. 2004). Such effects were found in biopsy material in subjects with posterior crossbite, where hypertrophic response of contralateral masseter and atrophic elements in ipsilateral masseter were found (Cutroneo et al. 2016).

The "rehabilitation" of the masseter muscle on the crossbite side that gradually occurred during the years after the crossbite treatment, is in line with the existing knowledge in work physiology that normal use of any skeletal muscle may increase the muscle size and strength (Sullivan et al. 1986; Abernethy et al. 1990). The capacity of the masticatory muscles to adapt in functional changes was observed after systematic chewing-gum training for a 4-week period, resulting in an average increase of the ultrasonographic thickness of the masseter muscle by 0.5 mm and 20% bigger maximal bite force values than their initial one (Kiliaridis et al. 1995b; Georgiakaki and Kiliaridis 1998).

The difference we found among the subjects of the sample between the cross-bite and the noncrossbite was rather small, almost as big as the methodologic error of the ultrasonographic measurements of the masseter. Thus, this method is not sufficiently reliable to be considered as diagnostic tool to detect asymmetric differences of a single individual, nor to measure small longitudinal changes on a subject, unless the expected differences are exceeding at least twice the error method.

Summarizing, unilateral functional posterior crossbite is associated with a habitual mandibular shift that leads to an asymmetric activity of the masticatory muscles and most possibly to an "asymmetric training effect" of these muscles. Orthodontic treatment of the unilateral posterior crossbite eliminates the need for the functional mandibular shift. This brings most probably a symmetrical functional charge of the muscles and gradually a symmetrical "training effect" of the muscles, given the appropriate length of time for the muscles to recover.

References

Abernethy PJ, Thayer R, Taylor AW. Acute and chronic responses of skeletal muscle to endurance and sprint exercise. A review. Sports Med. 1990;10:365–389.

Astrand P-O, Rodahl K. Textbook of Work Physiology. New York: McGraw-Hill, 1986:54–126.

Bakke M. Bite force and occlusion. Semin Orthod. 2006;12:120–126.

Braun S, Hnat WP, Freudenthaler JW, Marcotte MR, Honigle K, Johnson BE. A study of maximum bite force during growth and development. Angle Orthod. 1996;66:261–264.

Canepari M, Pellegrino MA, D'Antona G, Bottinelli R. Skeletal muscle fibre diversity and the underlying mechanisms. Acta Physiol (Oxford). 2010;199:465–476.

Caresio C, Molinari F, Emanuel G, Minetto MA. Muscle echo intensity: reliability and conditioning factors. Clin Physiol Funct Imaging. 2015;35:393–403.

Carlsson GE. Bite force and chewing efficiency. In: Kawamura Y, ed. Frontiers of Oral Physiology. Basel: Karger, 1974:265–292.

Castelo PM, Gavião MB, Pereira LJ, Bonjardim LR. Masticatory muscle thickness, bite force, and occlusal contacts in young children with unilateral posterior crossbite. Eur J Orthod. 2007;29:149–156.

Castroflorio T, Bracco P, Farina D. Surface electromyography in the assessment of jaw elevator muscles. J Oral Rehabil. 2008;35:638–645.

Cecere F, Ruf S, Pancherz H. Is quantitative electromyography reliable? J Orofac Pain. 1996;10:38–47.

Charalampidou M, Kjellberg H, Georgiakaki I, Kiliaridis S. Masseter muscle thickness and mechanical advantage in relation to vertical craniofacial morphology in children. Acta Odontol Scand. 2008;66:23–30.

Cutroneo G, Vermiglio G, Centofanti A, Rizzo G, Runci M, Favaloro A, Piancino MG, Bracco P, Ramieri G, Bianchi F, Speciale F, Arco A, Trimarchi F. Morphofunctional compensation of masseter muscles in unilateral posterior crossbite patients. Eur J Histochem. 2016;60:2605.

Dahlstrom L. Electromyographic studies of craniomandibular disorders: a review of the literature. J Oral Rehabil. 1989;16:1–20.

De Rossi M, De Rossi A, Hallak JE, Vitti M, Regalo SC. Electromyographic evaluation in children having rapid maxillary expansion. Am J Orthod Dentofac Orthop. 2009;136:355–360.

Egli F, Botteron S, Morel C, Kiliaridis S. Growing patients with Duchenne muscular dystrophy: longitudinal changes in their dentofacial morphology and orofacial functional capacities. Eur J Orthod. 2018;40:140–148.

Ferrario VF, Sforza C, D'Addona A, Miani A Jr. Reproducibility of electromyographic measures: a statistical analysis. J Oral Rehabil. 1991;18:513–521.

Ferrario VF, Sforza C, Colombo A, Ciusa V. An electromyographic investigation of masticatory muscles symmetry in normo-occlusion subjects. J Oral Rehabil. 2000;27:33–40.

Franzini-Armstrong C. The relationship between form and function throughout the history of excitation-contraction coupling. J Gen Physiol. 2018;150:189–210. [erratum: 2018;150:369].

Fukumoto Y, Ikezoe T, Yamada Y, Tsukagoshi R, Nakamura M, Mori N, Kimura M, Ichihashi N. Skeletal muscle quality assessed from echo intensity is associated with muscle strength of middle-aged and elderly persons. Eur J Appl Physiol. 2012;112:1519–1525.

Georgiakaki I, Kiliaridis S. Intensive chewing and chewing training on masseter muscle thickness. J Dent Res. 1998;77:1018. (Abstract).

Georgiakaki I, Tortopidis D, Garefis P, Kiliaridis S. Ultrasonographic thickness and electromyographic activity of masseter muscle of human females. J Oral Rehabil. 2007;34:121–128.

He T, Olsson S, Daugaard JR, Kiliaridis S. Functional influence of masticatory muscles on the fibre characteristics and capillary distribution in growing ferrets (*Mustela putonusfuro*) – a histochemical analysis. Arch Oral Biol. 2004;49:983–989.

Heckmatt JZ, Leeman S, Dubowitz V. Ultrasound imaging in the diagnosis of muscle disease. J Pediatr. 1982;101:656–660.

Hellsing E, Hagberg C. Changes in maximum bite force related to extension of the head. Eur J Orthod. 1990;12:148–153.

Kecik D, Kocadereli I, Saatci I. Evaluation of the treatment changes of functional posterior crossbite in the mixed dentition. Am J Orthod Dentofac Orthop. 2007;131:202–215.

Kiliaridis S. The importance of masticatory muscle function in dentofacial growth. Semin Orthod. 2006;12:110–119.

Kiliaridis S, Kälebo P. Masseter muscle thickness measured by ultrasonography and its relation to facial morphology. J Dent Res. 1991;70:1262–1265.

Kiliaridis S, Engström C, Thilander B. Histochemical analysis of masticatory muscle in the growing rat after prolonged alteration in the consistency of the diet. Arch Oral Biol. 1988;33:187–193.

Kiliaridis S, Kjellberg H, Wenneberg B, Engström C. The relationship between maximal bite force, bite force endurance, and facial morphology during growth. A cross-sectional study. Acta Odontol Scand. 1993;51:323–331.

Kiliaridis S, Engvall M, Tzakis MG. Ultrasound imaging of the masseter muscle in myotonic dystrophy patients. J Oral Rehabil. 1995a;22:619–625.

Kiliaridis S, Tzakis MG, Carlsson GE. Effect of fatigue and chewing training on maximal bite force and endurance. Am J Orthod Dentofac Orthop. 1995b;107:372–378.

Kiliaridis S, Georgiakaki I, Katsaros C. Masseter muscle thickness and maxillary dental arch width. Eur J Orthod. 2003;25:259–263.

Kiliaridis S, Mahboubi PH, Raadsheer MC, Katsaros C. Ultrasonographic thickness of the masseter muscle in growing individuals with unilateral crossbite. Angle Orthod. 2007;77:607–611.

Koc D, Dogan A, Bek B. Bite force and influential factors on bite force measurements: a literature review. Eur J Dent. 2010;4:223–232.

Lund JP, Widmer CG, Feine JS. Validity of diagnostic and monitoring tests used for temporomandibular disorders. J Dent Res. 1995;74:1133–1143.

Luther PK. The vertebrate muscle Z-disc: sarcomere anchor for structure and signalling. J Muscle Res Cell Motil. 2009;30:171–185.

Maffei C, Garcia P, de Biase NG, de Souza Camargo E, Vianna-Lara MS, Trindade Grégio AM, Reis Azevedo-Alanis L. Orthodontic intervention combined with myofunctional therapy increases electromyographic activity of masticatory muscles in patients with skeletal unilateral posterior crossbite. Acta Odontol Scand. 2014;72:298–303.

Martín C, Palma JC, Alamán JM, Lopez-Quiñones JM, Alarcón JA. Longitudinal evaluation of sEMG of masticatory muscles and kinematics of mandible changes in children treated for unilateral cross-bite. J Electromyogr Kinesiol. 2012;22:620–628.

Michelotti A, Farella M, Gallo LM, Veltri A, Palla S, Martina R. Effect of occlusal interference on habitual activity of human masseter. J Dent Res. 2005;84:644–648.

Michelotti A, Rongo R, Valentino R, D'Antò V, Bucci R, Danzi G, Cioffi I. Evaluation of masticatory muscle activity in patients with unilateral posterior crossbite before and after rapid maxillary expansion. Eur J Orthod. 2019;41:46–53.

Minetto MA, Caresio C, Salvi M, D'Angelo V, Gorji NE, Molinari F, Arnaldi G, Kesari S, Arvat E. Ultrasound-based detection of glucocorticoid-induced impairments of muscle mass and structure in Cushing's disease. J Endocrinol Investig. 2019;42:757–768.

Mohl ND, Lund JP, Widmer CG, McCall WD Jr. Devices for the diagnosis and treatment of temporomandibular disorders. Part II. Electromyography and sonography. J Prosthet Dent. 1990;63:332–336.

Nordander C, Willner J, Hansson GA, Larsson B, Unge J, Granquist L, Skerfving S. Influence of the subcutaneous fat layer, as measured by ultrasound, skinfold calipers and BMI, on the EMG amplitude. Eur J Appl Physiol. 2003;24:514–519.

Pillen S, Arts IM, Zwarts MJ. Muscle ultrasound in neuromuscular disorders. Muscle Nerve. 2008;37:679–693.

Pirttiniemi P. Normal and increased functional asymmetries in the craniofacial area. Acta Odontol Scand. 1998;56:342–345.

Raadsheer MC, van Eijden TM, van Spronsen PH, van Ginkel FC, Kiliaridis S, Prahl-Andersen B. A comparison of human masseter muscle thickness measured by ultrasonography and magnetic resonance imaging. Arch Oral Biol. 1994;39:1079–1084.

Reis Durão AP, Morosolli A, Brown J, Jacobs R. Masseter muscle measurement performed by ultrasound: a systematic review. Dentomaxillofac Radiol. 2017;46:20170052.

Schiaffino S, Reggiani C. Fiber types in mammalian skeletal muscles. Physiol Rev. 2011;91:1447–1531.

van Spronsen PH, Weijs WA, Valk J, Prahl-Andersen B, van Ginkel FC. Comparison of jaw-muscle bit-force cross-sections obtained by means of magnetic resonance imaging and high-resolution CT scanning. J Dent Res. 1989;68:1765–1770.

Sullivan JD, Olha AE, Rohan I, Schulz J. The properties of skeletal muscle. Orthop Rev. 1986;15:349–363.

Suvinen TI, Reade PC, Könönen M, Kemppainen P. Vertical jaw separation and masseter muscle electromyographic activity: a comparative study between asymptomatic controls and patients with temporomandibular pain and dysfunction. J Oral Rehabil. 2003;30:765–772.

Tartaglia GM, Moreira Rodrigues da Silva MA, Bottini S, Sforza C, Ferrario VF. Masticatory muscle activity during maximum voluntary clench in different research diagnostic criteria for temporomandibular disorders (RDC/TMD) groups. Man Ther. 2008;13:434–440.

Tsanidis N, Antonarakis GS, Kiliaridis S. Functional changes after early treatment of unilateral posterior cross-bite associated with mandibular shift: a systematic review. J Oral Rehabil. 2016;43:59–68.

Walker FO, Cartwright MS, Wiesler ER, Caress J. Ultrasound of nerve and muscle. Clin Neurophysiol. 2004;115:495–507.

Watanabe Y, Yamada Y, Fukumoto Y, Ishihara T, Yokoyama K, Yoshida T, Miyake M, Yamagata E, Kimura M. Echo intensity obtained from ultrasonography images reflecting muscle strength in elderly men. Clin Interv Aging. 2013;8:993–998.

Weijs WA, Hillen B. Relationship between the physiological cross-section of the human jaw muscles and their cross-sectional area in computer tomograms. Acta Anat (Basel). 1984;118:129–138.

Weijs WA, Hillen B. Physiological cross-section of the human jaw muscles. Acta Anat (Basel). 1985;121:31–35.

9

Localization and Problem List – 3-D Face Reconstruction

Karine Evangelista, Camila Massaro, Antonio Carlos de Oliveira Ruellas,
and Lucia H. Soares Cevidanes

Introduction

Facial asymmetry is a common find in orthodontics and comprises differences in morphology and/or position between right and left sides of the face using as a reference the midsagittal plane. Slight or subclinical asymmetries are present in most human faces and frequently are not noticed during a casual observation. Curiously, previous studies even demonstrated that perfect symmetric faces were perceived as less attractive than those with slight asymmetry (Swaddle and Cuthill 1995; Kowner 1996; Severt and Proffit 1997). However, when the asymmetry exceeds the acceptable degree and becomes noticeable, it may negatively affect occlusion, facial, and smile esthetics and should be carefully considered before initiating the orthodontic or surgical treatment.

In general, facial asymmetries can be clinically diagnosed in 12–44% of the patients (Severt and Proffit 1997; Sheats et al. 1998; Gribel et al. 2014). Considering a sample with patients seeking orthognathic surgery consultation, 34% demonstrated a clinically apparent facial asymmetry (Severt and Proffit 1997). In most of the cases (74%), asymmetry was identified in the lower third of the face. The upper face was asymmetric in only 5% of the patients, while the midface was not symmetrical in 36% of the cases (Severt and Proffit 1997). When affecting the middle and lower third of the face, the asymmetry was primarily explained by nose tip and chin deviation, respectively (Severt and Proffit 1997).

Dentofacial and Occlusal Asymmetries, First Edition. Edited by Birte Melsen and Athanasios E. Athanasiou.
© 2025 John Wiley & Sons Ltd. Published 2025 by John Wiley & Sons Ltd.

The facial asymmetry may involve one or more planes of space. Differences in the position, rotation, or a combination of both may occur. The adequate localization of the dental, skeletal, soft tissue, and functional asymmetry is highly important for the treatment plan. This chapter will present a review in three-dimensional (3D) face reconstruction for localization and listing of craniofacial regions of facial asymmetry problems.

Facial Asymmetry Diagnosis and Complementary Exams for Facial Asymmetry Localization

The identification of facial asymmetry is accomplished with patient interviews, clinical examination, and complementary imaging exams (Bishara et al. 1994; Burstone 1998; Legan 1998; Masuoka et al. 2007; Chia et al. 2008; Lee et al. 2010; Cheong and Lo 2011; Thiesen et al. 2015).

A careful intra and extraoral clinical examination is an essential tool to identify the asymmetry condition in vertical, anteroposterior, and transverse planes (Bishara et al. 1994; Burstone 1998; Legan 1998; Chia et al. 2008; Cheong and Lo 2011; Thiesen et al. 2015). During extraoral assessment, the patient should be in an upright position, looking forward, with teeth in occlusion and relaxed lips (Thiesen et al. 2015). Special attention should be given to the symmetry of the orbits and cheeks, chin deviations, leveling of lip commissures, mandibular lower border contour, gonial angle region, dental and facial midlines, inclination of the occlusal plane, gingival exposure, functional deviation of the mandible, and existing malocclusions (Bishara et al. 1994; Burstone 1998; Legan 1998; Chia et al. 2008; Lee et al. 2010; Cheong and Lo 2011; Thiesen et al. 2015). If the asymmetry is not properly localized, it may result in longer treatment time, delays related to changes in treatment direction, or eventually in unexpected or compromised outcomes (Lindauer 1998).

The presence of evident facial disproportion, midline deviation, inclination of the occlusal plane, and progressive and unilateral posterior open bite in the clinical evaluation suggests the presence of facial asymmetry and complementary diagnostic tools should be indicated to precisely locate the structures involved in the condition. Photographs, dental casts, radiographs, and tomography are examples of complementary exams indicated for asymmetry diagnostic and localization. Some specific cases, nuclear medicine tests are also recommended.

The conventional radiographs used in orthodontics, such as lateral and posteroanterior cephalometric and panoramic radiographs, provide limited information due to overlapping of the craniofacial structures, image magnification, and difficulty in standardizing the position of patient's head during image acquisition (Pirttiniemi et al. 1996; Legan 1998; Van Elslande et al. 2008; de Moraes et al. 2011; Damstra et al. 2013; Thiesen et al. 2015). A previous study compared posteroanterior cephalometric radiographs with cone-beam computed tomography (CBCT) exams to detect facial asymmetry in cases with chin deviation (Damstra et al. 2013). CBCT images were reliable and accurate while PA radiographs were not precise to assess asymmetries in the mandibular length (Damstra et al. 2013). Considering the limitations of a bidimensional assessment, the computed tomography, especially the full-face CBCT, is the complementary diagnostic tool of choice in cases with facial asymmetry.

The North American guidelines for CBCT use, proposed by the American Academy of Oral and Maxillofacial Radiology, recommends the use of CBCT scans to assess facial asymmetry (AAOMR 2013; Garib et al. 2014). According to the appendix of the proposed guidelines, facial asymmetry can be clinically presented as chin, mandibular, or midline deviations or occlusal cant discrepancies as well as other dental and craniofacial asymmetries. The European evidence-based recommendations for the use of CBCT, the SedentexCT guidelines, also propose the use of this exam for severe cases of skeletal discrepancies and orthognathic surgery planning (SEDENTEXCT 2012). In asymmetric cases with surgical indication, CBCT scan not only works as a valuable diagnostic tool but also allows the creation of 3D prototyped models to guide the surgery.

The CBCT exam provides a detailed 3D assessment of craniofacial asymmetries involving skeletal and soft tissue structures. Additionally, CBCT can better evaluate craniofacial morphology when compared with digital 2D images (de Moraes et al. 2011). The clinician should not expose the patient to multiple radiograph exams before taking a large field of view (FOV) CBCT to diagnose the asymmetry. The radiation dose of a large FOV CBCT exam is lower than the dose of multiple radiograph exams necessary to localize the asymmetry with better diagnostic information (Lorenzoni et al. 2012; Thiesen et al. 2015). In addition, the bidimensional images that clinician is familiar with can be easily generated from a CBCT exam taken with a large FOV.

For example, the coincidence between facial and dental midline can be assessed during clinical examination at smiling. The perpendicular line passing through the glabella, center of the interpupillary distance, or subnasal region can be used to determine the facial midline. The center of the chin and the tip of the nose frequently present variations and should not be used as reference (Bishara et al. 1994; Thiesen et al. 2015). If the clinical exam determines that a patient with 4mm midline deviation does not have functional shift, and that the etiology of the facial asymmetry is not dental, this is an indication to take a large FOV CBCT exam and it is important to know how to use this diagnostic record to localize the asymmetry properly. The CBCT exam will allow the localization of the asymmetry and the 3D quantification of the morphological error.

In 3D imaging analysis, patient's face can be assessed in all three planes of space. Clinicians are encouraged to use the 3D face reconstruction to evaluate vertical, anteroposterior, and transverse aspects as well as the rotation around the three axes (horizontal, axial, and vertical). The three aeronautical rotational descriptors known as pitch (vertical rotation), roll (lateral rotation), and yaw (horizontal rotation) are frequently used in imaging analysis (Ackerman et al. 2007; Yatabe et al. 2019), as shown in Figure 9.1. Face reconstruction for skeletal asymmetry analyses and the steps for a thorough 3D diagnosis using CBCT will be presented in the next topic. The identification of adequate references is important in evaluating asymmetry. The virtual preparation of the image data allows the correction of head tilts, through the head orientation step, and facilitates visual and quantitative evaluation of symmetry (Cevidanes et al. 2011). The appropriate operation of the CBCT exam will help the clinician to determine the correct location of the asymmetry and if the case diagnosis a nasomaxillary unilateral hypertrophy, sinus hypoplasia, hemimandibular hypertrophy, mandibular elongation/unilateral condylar hyperplasia, unilateral condylar resorption, or craniofacial microsomia. Each of this list of problems will also be discussed in this chapter later.

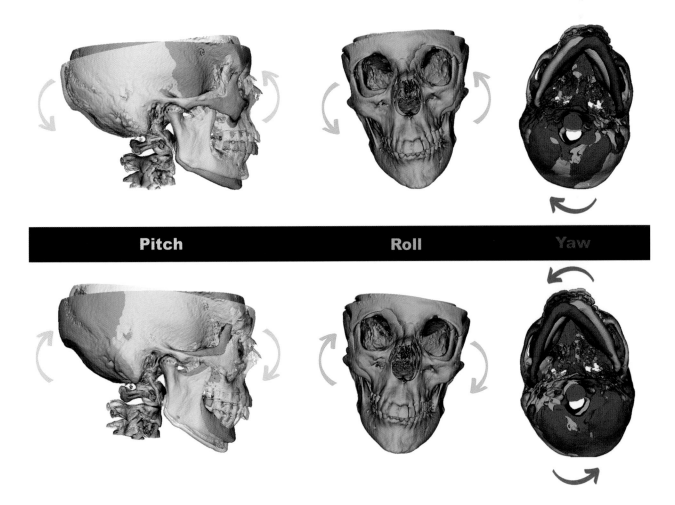

Figure 9.1 Schematic illustration of the rotational descriptors known as pitch (vertical rotation), roll (lateral rotation), and yaw (horizontal rotation).

Image Analysis in CBCT Scans for Skeletal Asymmetry

An important question to answer about patients with facial asymmetry is "Why do we want a thorough 3D diagnosis?". The craniofacial complex morphology is oriented by three planes of space: mediolateral, superoinferior, and anteroposterior. Asymmetric patients usually show more than one plane of space affected, such as cases of chin deviation in the horizontal plane and vertical asymmetry in mandibular ramus (Figure 9.2). However, the intrinsic interaction between all planes of space in the craniofacial complex may hide variations in planes of space affected with less severity. The interaction between all planes should always be considered in 3D diagnosis and consequently in the treatment planning. The 3D image analysis using linear and/or angular quantification will be able to identify the plane of space with more severe asymmetry features as well as if other planes are affected and how this combination is demonstrated.

Before 3D evaluation of CBCT scans, some steps are necessary to enhance the accuracy of asymmetry diagnosis. These steps will be discussed in the next topics.

Head Orientation

The patient's head position during tomographic acquisition can affect the diagnosis if head tilts occur (De Momi et al. 2006). Figure 9.3 shows a coronal view of CBCT scan and the rendering skull of the same patient before and after head orientation. Note that in the original image, the head shows a roll inclination. After the head orientation, the asymmetry in the mandible was properly revealed. The recommended position of the head for asymmetry diagnosis is with the horizontal plane of the head or Frankfurt plane perpendicular to the midsagittal plane. The components of the Frankfurt 3D plane consist of bilateral porion (Po) and bilateral infraorbitale (Or) (Ruellas et al. 2016). The midsagittal plane is determined through the alignment of glabella (G), crista galli (CG), and basio (Ba) (Ruellas et al. 2016). The position of the Frankfurt plane perpendicularly to midsagittal plane positions will automatically determine the coronal plane for each patient by software in image analysis. Figure 9.4 shows a 3D model obtained from a full-face CBCT scan with the Frankfurt plane perpendicular to the midsagittal plane after the head orientation step.

Scroll Through All Cross-Sectional Slices

Once the head is oriented with the Frankfurt plane perpendicular to the midsagittal plane, a navigation through all cross-sectional slices should be carefully performed. During the navigation, a search for anatomical structures in midline and bilateral regions of the skull brings information of symmetric and asymmetric regions of the skull in terms of morphology and/or position. The assessment of skull symmetry consisted in visualizing specific landmarks or regions of interest positions in all slices.

Landmarks placed in the midline of the skull are useful to detect horizontal asymmetry, by checking their positions in axial and coronal slices related to the midsagittal plane such as a vertical line fixed in the Nasion (Figure 9.5).

The assessment of bilateral regions is recommended to identify morphologic asymmetries between right and left sides, vertical rotation (roll), and horizontal rotation of the jaws (yaw). The image analysis of right and left

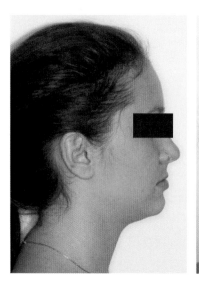 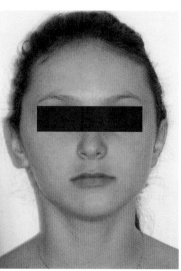

Figure 9.2 Facial photographs of a female patient with facial asymmetry. Note the lateral deviation of the chin to the left side and the asymmetry in the gonial angle region with the right side in a more inferior position.

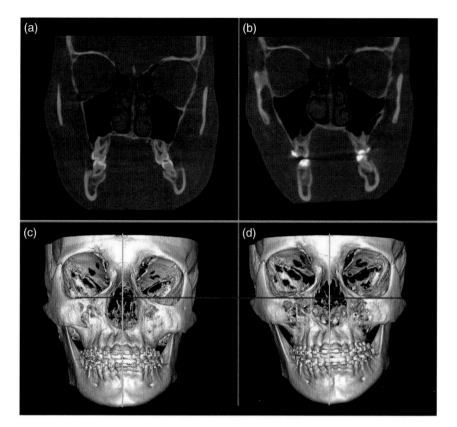

Figure 9.3 Head position in a coronal view of the scan and in the 3D model in original images (a and c), and after head orientation (b and d). In the original images, a roll inclination of the head is observed, and the left orbit is positioned inferiorly. The head orientation using as reference the Frankfurt plane perpendicular to the midsagittal plane, revealed a more evident asymmetry in the mandible. Note the horizontal position of the chin and the vertical position of the gonion.

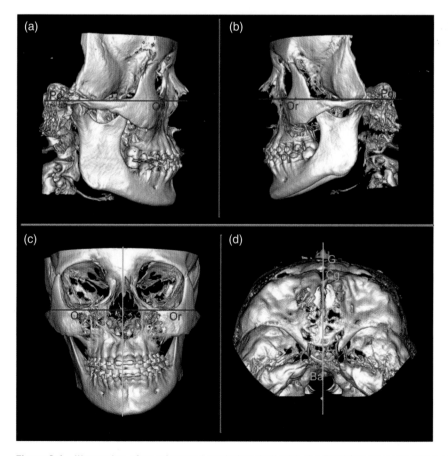

Figure 9.4 Illustration of an orientated rendering skull with the Frankfurt plane (red line) perpendicular to the midsagittal plane (yellow line).

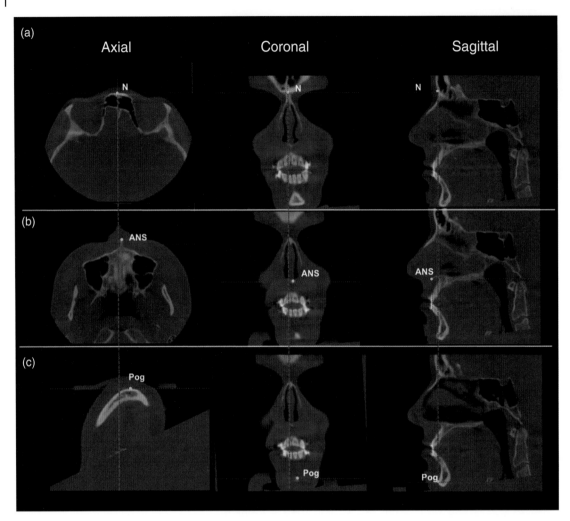

Figure 9.5 Axial, coronal, and sagittal slices with vertical red line fixed in midsagittal plane represented by Nasion (N) landmark (a). The horizontal position of anterior nasal spine (ANS) is seen in (b). The axial and coronal slices show a slight deviation of the ANS to the left side. The horizontal position of pogonion (Pog) is seen in (c). The axial and coronal slices show a marked asymmetry related to the midsagittal plane, with a deviation of the Pog landmark to the left side.

side consists into three approaches: (i) to check bilateral regions in axial and coronal slices relative to the horizontal line of reference, parallel to the Frankfurt plane, (ii) to check the latero-medial distance of bilateral regions relative to midsagittal plane, and (iii) to check the anteroposterior alignment of bilateral regions relative to a reference line parallel to coronal plane. Figure 9.6 shows the assessment of bilateral regions of maxilla and mandible.

Assessment of the 3D Rendering Viewing from Different Perspectives

In the 3D rendered view, it is possible to assess mandibular yaw rotation and lateral width of the zygomatic arches. From the frontal perspective, mandibular roll and yaw

rotations and the cant of the occlusal plane can be evaluated (Figure 9.7). Finally, from the lateral view, the assessment of the mandibular corpus, mandibular ramus, and condyle is performed.

List of Problems in Skeletal Craniofacial Asymmetries Through 3D Assessment

After a preliminary analysis of the CBCT scans, added by clinical signs observed in a clinical examination, the identification of a list of problems will enhance the asymmetry localization and guide further steps in image analysis by quantification of the problems detected. In this topic, a list of problems in skeletal craniofacial asymmetry will be presented through a 3D assessment. Later, asymmetry localization and quantification will be further discussed.

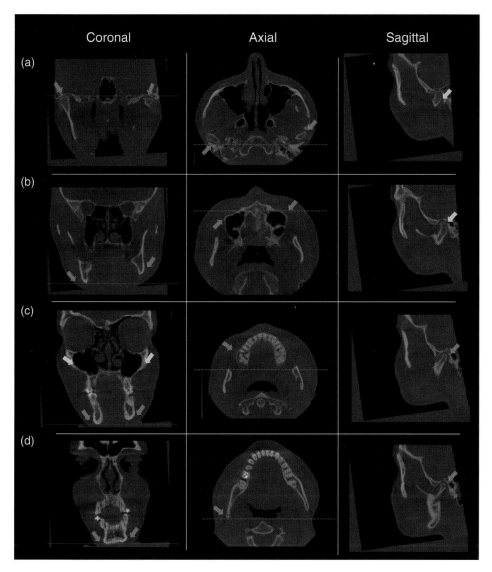

Figure 9.6 Coronal, axial, and sagittal views in different slices (a–d). Coronal views with a continuous reference line in blue parallel to Frankfurt plane revealed different condylar morphology (a), mandibular body with inferior position of the right side (b), different maxillary sinus morphology (c-yellow arrows) and mandibular body height (c- orange arrows) and mandibular symphysis with inferior position of the right side (d). Axial views with interrupted blue line parallel to coronal plane show condyles with posterior position of the right side (a), different sinus maxillary morphology with more anterior expansion on the left side (b), asymmetric maxillary morphology more expanded on the right side (c), and posterior position of the mandibular ramus on the right side (d). Sagittal views revealed different sizes in the middle region of right (a) and left (c) condyles, as well as in the slices aligned with the coronoid process in right (b-yellow arrows) and left (d-orange arrows) sides.

Zygomatic and Maxillary Unilateral Hypertrophy

Facial asymmetry can be secondary to a unilateral hypertrophy of the nasomaxillary complex. This condition occurs as a result of unilateral overgrowth of the zygomatic bone and maxillary structures on the affected side (Figure 9.8). Scrolling through all cross-sectional slices of the CBCT scan of a patient presenting with zygomatic and maxillary unilateral hypertrophy it is possible to note the sinuses differences in the coronal view, the zygomatic prominence in the axial views, as well as the thickness of the soft tissue in the right cheek region, and the mandibular deviation due to the elongated right zygomaticomaxillary hypertrophy (Figure 9.8).

Sinus and Maxillary Hypoplasia

Facial asymmetry may also be caused by maxillary sinus hypoplasia (MSH), which comprises an underdevelopment of the maxillary sinus (Erdem et al. 2002; Price and Friedman 2007; Khanduri et al. 2014). Etiology includes

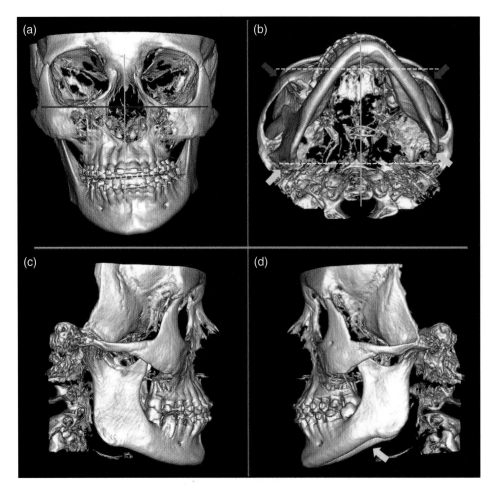

Figure 9.7 Rendered skull in different views. (a) Frontal view of the skull with orientation lines in continuous red (Frankfurt plane), continuous yellow (midsagittal plane), and interrupted red (occlusal plane) showing the occlusal cant with inferior position on the right side; (b) inferior view of the skull with orientation lines in continuous yellow (midsagittal plane) and interrupted yellow (parallels to coronal plane) showing the symmetric position and morphology of zygomatic arches (red arrows), and yaw rotation of the mandible to the left with anterior position of the mandibular ramus on the left side (yellow arrows); (c) right and (d) left views of the skull, showing the asymmetric position of the inferior border of the mandible and shorter mandibular ramus of the left side (yellow arrow).

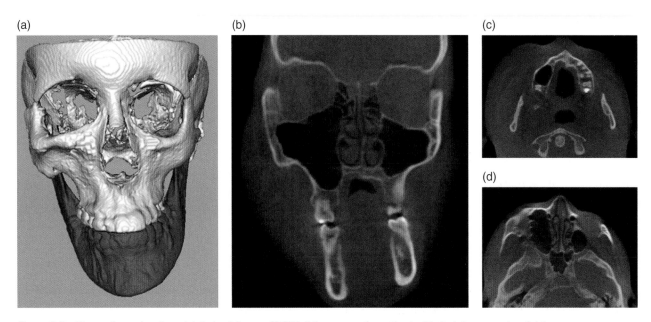

Figure 9.8 Three-dimensional model derived from a CBCT full face scan of a patient with facial asymmetry, right zygomaticomaxillary hypertrophy, and mandibular deviation to left side. (a) Note the sinuses difference and the zygomatic prominence in the coronal; (b) and axial (c and d) views, respectively, as well as the thickness of the soft tissue in the right cheek region (b and c), and the mandibular deviation due to the elongated right zygomaticomaxillary hypertrophy.

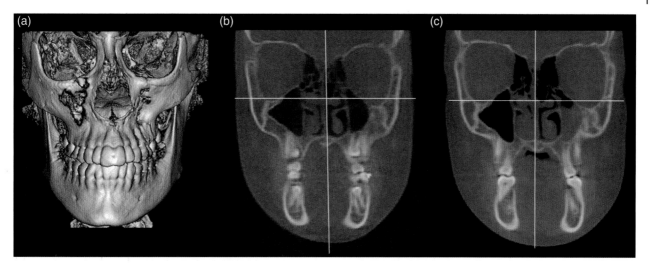

Figure 9.9 Patient presenting with sinus and maxillary hypoplasia in the left side. Note that the hypoplasia is not so evident in the 3D rendering skull at age 15. (a) Even after head orientation, note in the coronal view of the CBCT scans taken at 15; (b) and 16 (c) years of age that the sinus and maxillary hypoplasia on the left side as well as the facial asymmetry etiology is clear. Note the progressive difference in the orbital level and how the sinus is smaller and hypoplastic on the left side.

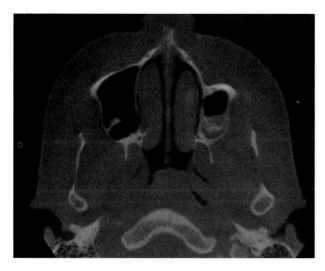

Figure 9.10 Axial slice of a CBCT scan from a patient with sinus and maxillary hypoplasia in the left side. Note that the left sinus is smaller than the right one.

an embryological underdevelopment or acquired causes such as trauma or infection (Price and Friedman 2007; Khanduri et al. 2014). Computed tomography facilitates the early diagnosis of MSH and should be included in the diagnosis process (Bindakhil and Mupparapu 2020). In the cross-sectional slices of a CBCT exam taken from a patient with MSH, differences in the orbital level and in the size of the right and left sinus can be noted (Figures 9.9 and 9.10).

Unilateral Condylar Hyperplasia

Unilateral condylar hyperplasia (UCH) is a morphological anomaly in mandibular condyles, expressed as two different conditions: hemimandibular hyperplasia and hemimandibular elongation. Hemimandibular hyperplasia or hemimandibular hypertrophy is defined as an excessive and unilateral mandibular growth resulting in vertical facial asymmetry and associated malocclusion (Obwegeser and Makek 1986). In severe cases, the increase in the mandibular height in the affected side results in a facial asymmetry characterized by a rotation of the mandible in the roll and yaw directions (Figure 9.11). Therefore, patients with this condition usually demonstrate a face with a "rotated appearance". The 3D models derived from CBCT scans are the most helpful tool for 3D diagnosis of hemimandibular hypertrophy (Figure 9.11).

Mandibular elongation is defined as a result of unilateral condylar hyperplasia with mild unilateral growth in condyle and related lengthening of the same side of mandible in horizontal plane (Obwegeser and Makek 1986). Consequently, chin deviation toward the healthy side and contralateral posterior crossbite are expressed as a clinical feature (Obwegeser and Makek 1986; Gateno et al. 2021). The affected condyle enlarges mildly, as well the condylar neck, with few changes in occlusal plane inclination (Figure 9.12).

While the hyperactivity of condylar growth causes hemimandibular hyperplasia with marked differences in ramus height, the gradual overactivity of condylar growth

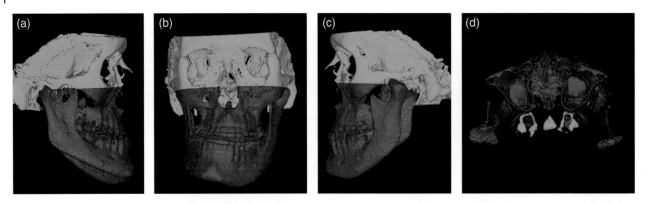

Figure 9.11 Patient presenting with facial asymmetry caused by left mandibular condyle, ramus, and body hypertrophy. 3D rendering solid views are helpful for diagnosis in this case and the cranial base and the clipped maxillomandibular structures are shown in different colors to facilitate visualization (a–d). Note the marked roll and yaw deviation of the mandible due to the hemimandibular hypertrophy in the left side.

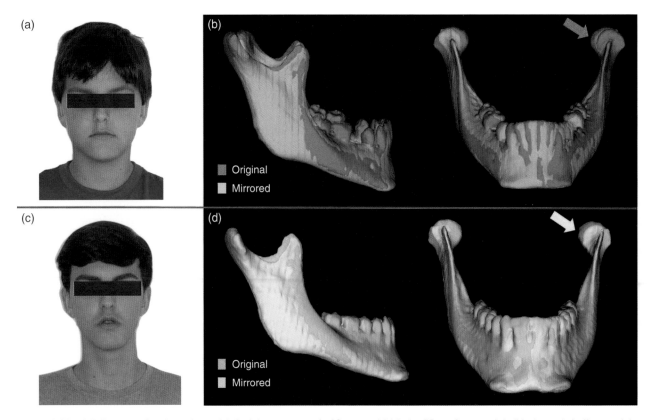

Figure 9.12 A follow-up of male patient with facial asymmetry. At 12 years old (a), the 3D surface models (b) showed similar condylar height (orange arrow). Extraoral frontal photograph (c) and 3D models (d) at 16 years old. Mandibular registration of the mirrored models shows a mildly condylar asymmetry at 16 years-old (yellow arrow), with greater condylar height in the right side not affecting the ramus height and occlusal plane inclination. Case report gently contributed by Dr. José Valladares-Neto.

brings about hemimandibular elongation (Obwegeser and Makek 1986). The diagnosis of UCH should be based on a thorough facial and intraoral examination, as well as tomographic images. Early diagnosis is a determining factor for the prognosis and treatment of this condition because approaches differ considerably according to the affected structures, patient's age, severity of the asymmetry, and whether the disease stage is active or passive. The 3D analysis is a valuable tool for differentiating the mandibular elongation from hemimandibular hyperplasia, through investigation of vertical asymmetry of ramus length as a result of disturbed condylar growth (Gateno et al. 2021). Additionally,

Figure 9.13 Planar scintigraphy image of the patient shown in Figure 9.12, presented with mandibular elongation and facial asymmetry. Sagittal sections of the right side (a) and left side (b) show the condylar uptake of radioisotope (yellow arrows). The planar scintigraphy ratio between right and left sides resulted in values under 10%.

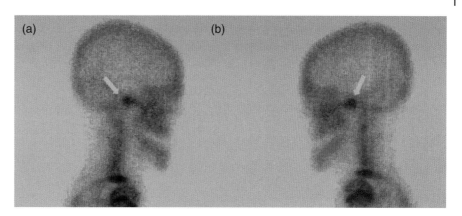

the treatment planning in cases of condylar hyperplasia is enhanced by 3D reconstruction through prototype creation for surgical planning. In both types of UCH, nuclear medicine tests, such as condylar scintigraphy and single-photon emission computed tomography (SPECT) scans have become a complementary exam for 3D diagnosis to confirm the type of asymmetric growth activity in the mandibular condyles (Figure 9.13). These tests are based on measuring the uptake of the radioisotope at the temporomandibular joint (TMJ) level to identify areas of increased osteoblastic activity (Hodder et al. 2000). Planar scintigraphy (PS) and SPECT with 99 mTc MDP radioisotope are the most frequently used, although the addition of SPECT to a CT scan (SPECT-CT) improves diagnostic precision.

Unilateral Condylar Resorption

Unilateral condylar resorption is characterized by a reduction in morphological remodeling in one side of the mandibular condyles resulted from a pathological process. The etiology comprises systemic disorders, such as osteoarthritis (OA) (Song et al. 2020), and local factors, such as mandibular trauma with condylar fracture (Baumann et al. 2004). The bone destruction of the TMJ can occur unilaterally causing malocclusion and facial asymmetry.

OA is a degenerative disorder caused by systemic inflammatory processes in osseous tissues of the joints (Pereira et al. 2011). The tissue damage of TMJ with OA leads to signs and symptoms of pain, movement limitations, clicking and crepitus sounds. Tomographic diagnosis can detect joint deformity, manifest as flattening, osteophyte formation, sclerosis, erosion, joint mice, and subchondral bone cysts (Song et al. 2020). The 3D face reconstruction is a valuable tool for image analysis to certify and quantify the morphology and asymmetry using as a reference the healthy side. Figure 9.14 shows a 3D mandibular model of

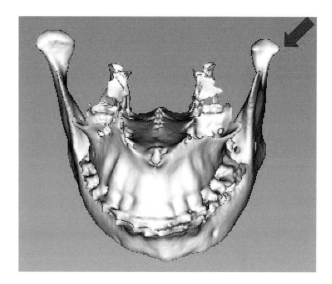

Figure 9.14 3D mandibular model of a patient with facial asymmetry and osteoarthritis (OA), showing the reduced morphology of left condyle (red arrow) as a result of unilateral condylar resorption.

a patient with facial asymmetry diagnosed with OA and unilateral condylar resorption in the left side.

Unilateral condylar resorption can also manifest after an episode of mandibular trauma. Mandibular trauma, especially during childhood involves the condylar region in 36 to 50% of subjects (Baumann et al. 2004). Due to under notification, mandibular fractures are estimated to be about twice as frequent as noticed or diagnosed, as many of them occur during early childhood and often pass with little discomfort (Pirttiniemi et al. 1996). In cases with fragments severely dislocated, there is an increased risk for ankylosis and/or resorption remodeling on the fracture side, particularly in children younger than 3 years of age (Baumann et al. 2004). The 3D mandibular reconstruction will identify condylar remodeling and asymmetries in patients with mandibular fractures. Figure 9.15 shows a PA

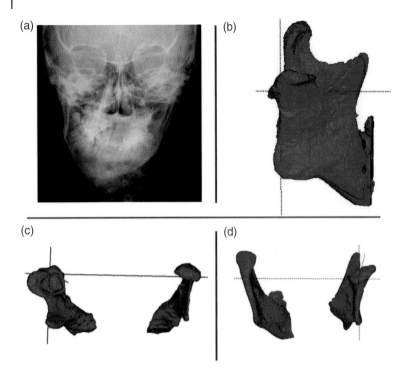

Figure 9.15 Patient with facial asymmetry and history of mandibular trauma at 3 months old. PA radiograph (a); right (b); superior (c); and posterior (d); views of the 3D surface models. The 3D mandibular reconstruction shows the deformity in the right TMJ, not visualized in the PA radiograph.

radiograph of a patient with history of mandibular trauma at 3 months old. At 16 years of age, she presented an evident asymmetry of TMJ morphology. In the PA radiograph, it is not possible to identify the condylar remodeling.

Patients with suspicion of OA and history of mandibular trauma must be follow-up with serial tomographic image analysis and 3D face reconstruction in order to establish early intervention, contributing to the facial asymmetry management.

Craniofacial Macrosomia

Craniofacial microsomia (CFM) is an anomaly caused by abnormal development of the first and second pharyngeal arches (Cohen et al. 1989). The jaws deformities occurring in CFM are commonly related to oculoauriculovertebral spectrum and Goldenhar syndrome (Gorlin et al. 1963). Variable underdevelopment of facial structures affects one side of the facial skeleton in 85% of the cases, resulting in facial asymmetry (Grabb 1965). The malformation is frequently seen in mandible, maxilla, zygoma and/or temporal bone, ear, and soft tissues (Cohen et al. 1989), as seen in Figure 9.16.

The deformities correction involves surgical procedures supported by current imaging techniques, such as tomographic analysis with 3D reconstruction (Maryanchik and Nair 2018). 3D face reconstruction is

important to recognize and document craniofacial osseous anomalies and soft tissue changes by the multidisciplinary team of clinicians, in light of the fact that any and all treatments instituted or planned must take into account all of the anomalies unique to the case of interest. The relevance of 3D diagnostic imaging and characterization of the syndromes involved will allow the planning and implementation of interdisciplinary intervention at an early stage. Additionally, the 3D assessment enhances the virtual surgical planning, modeling surgery, rapid prototyping techniques, and intraoperative navigation (Sun et al. 2020).

Asymmetry Localization and Quantification

After navigating through all slices of the CBCT scan and assessing the 3D rendering view, the comprehension of asymmetry localization and magnitude can be explored using computational tools in image analysis (Alhadidi et al. 2011; Bianchi et al. 2020; Evangelista et al. 2020). Figure 9.17 summarizes the steps for image analysis in asymmetry cases. The quantification of morphology and/or position asymmetries is crucial for determining which sites are the most affected and play the main role in facial asymmetry etiology, in order to guide the orthodontic treatment planning with or without surgical procedures.

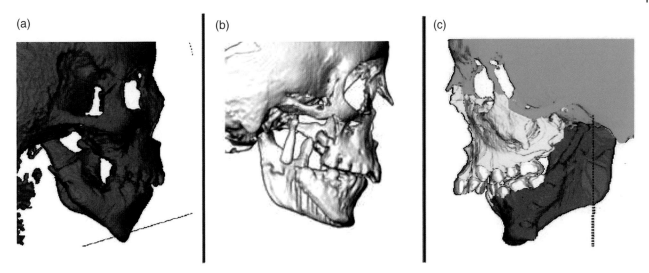

Figure 9.16 3D craniofacial reconstruction of three young patients with craniofacial microsomia (CFM), showing the lateral view of the affected side (a–c).

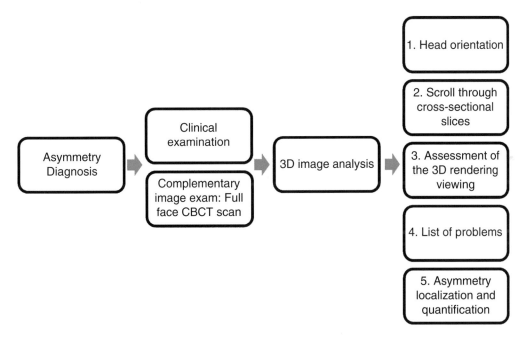

Figure 9.17 Flowchart for the image analysis steps in asymmetry cases.

Mirroring and Superimposition

The mirroring and superimposition are tools in image analysis of CBCT scans with great relevance in patients with asymmetry (Alhadidi et al. 2011, 2019; Cevidanes et al. 2011). The mirroring approach consists of inverting the position of right and left sides and then superimposing the inverted images. The superimposition can be performed using two different regions as reference in image registration: (i) cranial base superimposition and (ii)

mandibular regional superimposition (Evangelista et al. 2020). The cranial base registration is able to detect positional asymmetries of the middle and lower third of the face relative to the cranial base. The mandibular regional registration, using mandibular body and symphysis, is able to detect intrinsic morphological asymmetries in mandible (Cevidanes et al. 2011; Alhadidi et al. 2011, 2019; Solem et al. 2016). Figures 9.18 and 9.19 show 3D models with cranial base and mandibular superimposition, respectively.

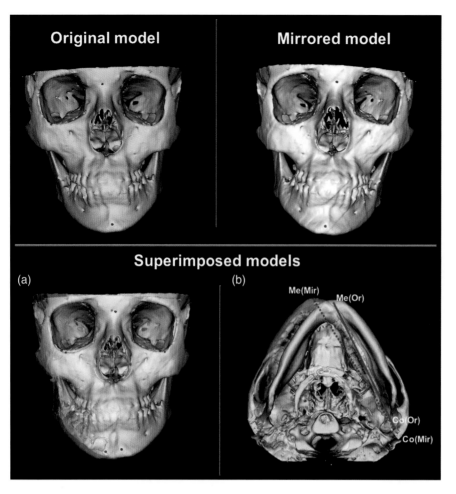

Figure 9.18 Original (yellow) and mirrored (white) 3D models. Superimposed models with semitransparency of mirrored models showing the larger asymmetry position in horizontal and vertical directions of the lower third of the face in frontal view. (a) Inferior view; (b) showing the mandibular yaw rotation evidenced by the angle between the red continuous (original) and interrupted (mirrored) lines.

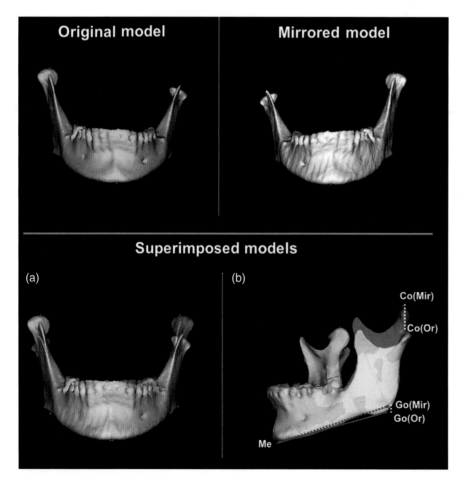

Figure 9.19 Original (Or, yellow) and mirrored (Mir, white) 3D models showing asymmetric morphology of the condyles, marked vertical asymmetry of mandibular ramus and condyles and, cant of the occlusal plane. The left condyle shows marked resorptive bone remodeling. Superimposed models with semitransparency of the mirrored models show regional asymmetry of mandibular ramus height in the frontal view. (a) Lateral view; (b) showing mandibular body length (Me-Go) in original left side (continuous red line) and in mirrored model (interrupted red line) and, the regional difference between right and left sides in condylion (Co) and gonion (Go) with interrupted white lines.

Quantification

The knowledge about the magnitude of asymmetries is a crucial step in the diagnosis process, in order to classify the severity and predominant directions of all irregularities. Traditionally, the asymmetries classification is based on the lower third of the face, in the presence of horizontal deviation of the chin. The calculation of the distance from central landmarks of the mandible to the facial midsagittal plane determines the classification system, divided into mild (<2 mm), moderate (2–4 mm), or severe (>4 mm) (Peck et al. 1991; Masuoka et al. 2005; Good et al. 2006; Thiesen et al. 2015). Unfortunately, other craniofacial regions are not yet explored in classification systems of asymmetries. The understanding of the asymmetry classification influences the treatment planning, establishing conservative approaches in orthodontics, or determining orthognathic surgical needs.

The quantification in reconstructed 3D faces is usually performed using automatic tools for linear and angular measurements in the image analysis software. Table 9.1 and Figures 9.18 and–9.20 show the linear and angular quantification of the mandibular asymmetry using as example the patient from Figures 9.2–9.7. The quantification showed a chin deviation of 7.00 mm to the left, and anterior nasal spine deviation of 1.49 mm to the left. These values confirmed a severe asymmetry located mainly in the mandible in the lower third of the face, with slight influence on horizontal position of the maxilla. The asymmetry in ramus height is expressed mainly by a more inferior

Table 9.1 Quantification values of positional and regional asymmetry of the patient presented in Figures 9.18 and 9.20.

Skull identification	Landmarks		
Reference planes			
Midsagittal plane (MSP)	Glabella (G), Crista galli (Cg), Basio (Ba)		
Frankfurt plane (FP)	Infraorbitale (Or), Porion (Po)		
Craniofacial regions			
Maxilla	Anterior nasal spine (ANS)		
Mandible	Condylion (Co), gonion (Go), menton (Me)		
Position related to reference planes		Values	Illustration
Maxilla deviation	ANS-MSP	1.49 mm	Figure 9.20a
Mandible deviation	Me-MSP	7.00 mm	Figure 9.20a
Condylion position (right)	Co(R)-FP	1.81 mm	Figure 9.20b
Condylion left position (left)	Co(L)- FP	1.35 mm	Figure 9.20c
Condylion position difference	Co(R)-FP – Co(L)- FP	0.46 mm	—
Gonion position (right)	Go(R)-FP	58.74 mm	Figure 9.20b
Gonion position (left)	Go(L)-FP	51.91 mm	Figure 9.20c
Gonion position difference	Go(R)-FP – Go(L)- FP	6.83 mm	—
Ramus roll (right)	CoGo(R).FP	81.01°	Figure 9.20a
Ramus roll (left)	CoGo(L).FP	94.30°	Figure 9.20a
Mandibular yaw	Co-Me(Or).CoMe(Mir)	6.10°	Figure 9.18b
Mandibular regional morphology			
Total ramus height (right)	Co-Go(R)	61.13 mm	Figure 9.20b
Total ramus height (left)	Co-Go(L)	49.96 mm	Figure 9.20c
Total ramus height difference	Co-Go(R)- Co-Go(L)	11.17 mm	—
Mandibular body length (right)	Go-Me(R)	83.77 mm	Figure 9.20b
Mandibular body length (left)	Go-Me(L)	82.34 mm	Figure 9.20c
Mandibular body length difference	Go-Me(L)- Go-Me(R)	1.43 mm	—
Condyle height difference	Co(R)-Co(L)	15.47 mm	Figure 9.19b
Gonion height difference	Go(R)-Go(L)	4.46 mm	Figure 9.19b

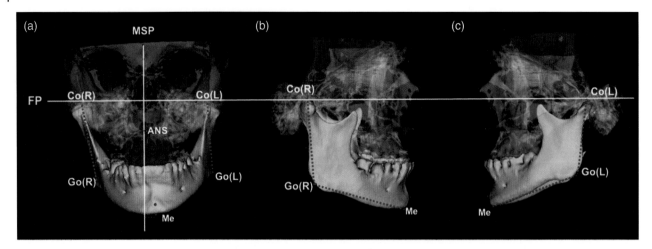

Figure 9.20 3D models showing the landmarks and reference planes for asymmetry quantification described in the Table 9.1.

position of the right gonion of 6.84 mm, with few differences in vertical position of the condyles (0.46 mm). The angular measurement (roll inclination) of mandibular ramus resulted in 81.01° on the right side and 94.30° on the left side. A mandibular yaw of 6.10° was identified.

Measurements after regional superimposition demonstrated larger distances of the right side in mandibular ramus height and mandibular body length of 11.17 and 1.43 mm, respectively. The difference in height between right and left condyle was 9.57 mm. For this case, the morphological asymmetry in condylar height caused the horizontal asymmetry of mandible position.

Determining the Asymmetry Directions

After quantification, the diagnostic process can be complemented though a critical analysis of the asymmetry directions, classified as:

1) Horizontal asymmetry: predominance of horizontal (right or left; anterior or posterior) deviation and subclinical asymmetry values in vertical direction.
2) Vertical asymmetry: predominance of vertical deviation with subclinical asymmetry values in horizontal direction.
3) Mixed (combined) asymmetry: a combination of evident horizontal and vertical asymmetries.

References

American Academy of Oral and Maxillofacial Radiology, AAOMR. Clinical recommendations regarding use of cone beam computed tomography in Orthodontics. Position statement by the American Academy of Oral and

Continuing the previous example, the measurements of the Table 9.1 revealed a patient with greater vertical asymmetry of the ramus height, and different size and height of the condyles due to left condyle remodeling. Although this vertical asymmetry was highlighted in the image analysis, the horizontal asymmetry was also markedly expressed by the chin deviation. Clinicians must be aware of these combined asymmetries in order to contemplate correction of both directions in the treatment plan.

Final Considerations

The 3D assessment of patients with facial asymmetry is one of the indications for a large field of view CBCT in orthodontics. A careful 3D image analysis is recommended to localize and quantify the facial asymmetry. This diagnostic tool will help the clinician to better treat the patient as a thorough diagnosis is needed for these cases.

Acknowledgments

- NIDCR R01 DE024450, for funding the image analysis tools developed for the asymmetry quantification.
- Dr. José Valladares-Neto for the gentle contribution of the images in Figure 9.12.

Maxillofacial Radiology. Oral Surg Oral Med Oral Pathol Oral Radiol. 2013;116:238–257.

Ackerman JL, Proffit WR, Sarver DM, Ackerman MB, Kean MR. Pitch, roll, and yaw: describing the spatial orientation of dentofacial traits. Am J Orthod Dentofac Orthop. 2007;131:305–310.

Alhadidi A, Cevidanes LH, Mol A, Ludlow J, Styner M. Comparison of two methods for quantitative assessment of mandibular asymmetry using cone beam computed tomography image volumes. Dentomaxillofac Radiol. 2011;40:351–357.

Alhadidi A, Paniagua B, Cook R, Tyndall D, Baqain Z, Cevidanes LH. The use of a custom-made virtual template for corrective surgeries of asymmetric patients: proof of principle and a multi-center end-user survey. Int J Comput Assist Radiol Surg. 2019;14:537–544.

Baumann A, Troulis MJ, Kaban LB. Facial trauma II: dentoalveolar injuries and mandibular fractures. In: Kaban LB, Troulis MJ, eds. *Pediatric Oral and Maxillofacial Surgery*. Philadelphia: Saunders, 2004.

Bianchi J, Paniagua B, Ruellas ACDO, Fillion-Robin JC, Prietro JC, Gonçalves JR, Hoctor J, Yatabe M, Styner M, Li T. *3D Slicer Craniomaxillofacial Modules Support Patient-Specific Decision-Making for Personalized Healthcare in Dental Research. Multimodal Learning for Clinical Decision Support and Clinical Image-Based Procedures*. New York: Springer, 2020.

Bindakhil M, Mupparapu M. CBCT evaluation of bilateral maxillary sinus hypoplasia with unilateral mandibular hypertrophy. J Orofacial Sci. 2020;12:61–63.

Bishara SE, Burkey PS, Kharouf JG. Dental and facial asymmetries: a review. Angle Orthod. 1994;64:89–98.

Burstone CJ. Diagnosis and treatment planning of patients with asymmetries. Semin Orthod. 1998;4:153–164.

Cevidanes LH, Alhadidi A, Paniagua B, Styner M, Ludlow J, Mol A, Turvey T, Proffit WR, Rossouw PE. Three-dimensional quantification of mandibular asymmetry through cone-beam computerized tomography. Oral Surg Oral Med Oral Pathol Oral Radiol Endod. 2011;111:757–770.

Cheong YW, Lo LJ. Facial asymmetry: etiology, evaluation, and management. Chang Gung Med J. 2011;34:341–351.

Chia MS, Naini FB, Gill DS. The aetiology, diagnosis and management of mandibular asymmetry. Orthod Update. 2008;1:44–52.

Cohen M Jr, Rollnick BR, Kaye CI. Oculoauriculovertebral spectrum: an updated critique. Cleft Palate J. 1989;26:276–286.

Damstra J, Fourie Z, Ren Y. Evaluation and comparison of postero-anterior cephalograms and cone-beam computed tomography images for the detection of mandibular asymmetry. Eur J Orthod. 2013;35:45–50.

De Momi E, Chapuis J, Pappas I, Ferrigno G, Hallermann W, Schramm A, Caversaccio M. Automatic extraction of the mid-facial plane for cranio-maxillofacial surgery planning. Int J Oral Maxillofac Surg. 2006;35:636–642.

De Moraes ME, Hollender LG, Chen CS, Moraes LC, Balducci I. Evaluating craniofacial asymmetry with digital cephalometric images and cone-beam computed tomography. Am J Orthod Dentofac Orthop. 2011;139:e523–e531.

Erdem T, Aktas D, Erdem G, Miman MC, Ozturan O. Maxillary sinus hypoplasia. Rhinology. 2002;40:150–153.

European Commission. CBCT for Dental and Maxillofacial Radiology: Evidence-Based Guidelines. Luxembourg: Publications Office, SEDENTEXCT,, 2012.

Evangelista K, Valladares-Neto J, Silva MAG, Cevidanes LHS, De Oliveira Ruellas AC. Three-dimensional assessment of mandibular asymmetry in skeletal Class I and unilateral crossbite malocclusion in 3 different age groups. Am J Orthod Dentofac Orthop. 2020;158:209–220.

Garib DG, Calil LR, Leal CR, Janson G. Is there a consensus for CBCT use in Orthodontics? Dental Press J Orthod. 2014;19:136–149.

Gateno J, Coppelson KB, Kuang T, Poliak CD, Xia JJ. A better understanding of unilateral condylar hyperplasia of the mandible. J Oral Maxillofac Surg. 2021;79:1122–1132.

Good S, Edler R, Wertheim D, Greenhill D. A computerized photographic assessment of the relationship between skeletal discrepancy and mandibular outline asymmetry. Eur J Orthod. 2006;28:97–102.

Gorlin RJ, Jue KL, Jacobsen U, Goldschmidt E. Oculoauriculovertebral dysplasia. J Pediatr. 1963;63:991–999.

Grabb WC. The first and second branchial arch syndrome. Plast Reconstr Surg. 1965;36:485–508.

Gribel BF, Thiesen G, Borges TS, Freitas MPM. Prevalence of mandibular asymmetry in skeletal Class I adult patients. J Res Dent. 2014;2:189–197.

Hodder S, Rees J, Oliver T, Facey P, Sugar A. SPECT bone scintigraphy in the diagnosis and management of mandibular condylar hyperplasia. Br J Oral Maxillofac Surg. 2000;38:87–93.

Khanduri S, Agrawal S, Chhabra S, Goyal S. Bilateral maxillary sinus hypoplasia. Case Rep Radiol. 2014;2014:148940.

Kowner R. Facial asymmetry and attractiveness judgement in developmental perspective. J Exp Psychol Hum Percept Perform. 1996;22:662–675.

Lee MS, Chung DH, Lee JW, Cha KS. Assessing soft-tissue characteristics of facial asymmetry with photographs. Am J Orthod Dentofac Orthop. 2010;138:23–31.

Legan HL. Surgical correction of patients with asymmetries. Semin Orthod. 1998;4:189–198.

Lindauer SJ. Asymmetries: diagnosis and treatment. Semin Orthod. 1998;4:133.

Lorenzoni DC, Bolognese AM, Garib DG, Guedes FR, Sant'anna EF. Cone-beam computed tomography and radiographs in dentistry: aspects related to radiation dose. Int J Dent. 2012;2012:813768.

Maryanchik I, Nair MK. Goldenhar syndrome (oculo-auriculo-vertebral spectrum): Findings on cone beam computed tomography – 3 case reports. Oral Surg Oral Med Oral Pathol Oral Radiol. 2018;126:e233–e239.

Masuoka N, Momoi Y, Ariji Y, Nawa H, Muramatsu A, Goto S, Ariji E. Can cephalometric indices and subjective evaluation be consistent for facial asymmetry? Angle Orthod. 2005;75:651–655.

Masuoka N, Muramatsu A, Ariji Y, Nawa H, Goto S, Ariji E. Discriminative thresholds of cephalometric indexes in the subjective evaluation of facial asymmetry. Am J Orthod Dentofac Orthop. 2007;131:609–613.

Obwegeser HL, Makek MS. Hemimandibular hyperplasia – hemimandibular elongation. J Maxillofac Surg. 1986;14:183–208.

Peck S, Peck L, Kataja M. Skeletal asymmetry in esthetically pleasing faces. Angle Orthod. 1991;61:43–48.

Pereira D, Peleteiro B, Araujo J, Branco J, Santos R, Ramos E. The effect of osteoarthritis definition on prevalence and incidence estimates: a systematic review. Osteoarthr Cartil. 2011;19:1270–1285.

Pirttiniemi P, Miettinen J, Kantomaa T. Combined effects of errors in frontal-view asymmetry diagnosis. Eur J Orthod. 1996;18:629–636.

Price DL, Friedman O. Facial asymmetry in maxillary sinus hypoplasia. Int J Pediatr Otorhinolaryngol. 2007;71:1627–1630.

Ruellas AC, Tonello C, Gomes LR, Yatabe MS, Macron L, Lopinto J, Goncalves JR, Carreira DGG, Alonso N, Souki BQ. Common 3-dimensional coordinate system for assessment of directional changes. Am J Orthod Dentofac Orthop. 2016;149:645–656.

Severt T, Proffit WR. The prevalence of facial asymmetry in the dentofacial deformities population at the University of North Carolina. Int J Adult Orthodon Orthognath Surg. 1997;12:171–176.

Sheats RD, McGorray SP, Musmar Q, Wheeler TT, King GJ. Prevalence of orthodontic asymmetries. Semin Orthod. 1998;4:138–145.

Solem RC, Ruellas A, Ricks-Oddie JL, Kelly K, Oberoi S, Lee J, Miller A, Cevidanes L. Congenital and acquired mandibular asymmetry: Mapping growth and remodeling in 3 dimensions. Am J Orthod Dentofac Orthop. 2016;150:238–251.

Song H, Lee JY, Huh KH, Park JW. Long-term changes of temporomandibular joint osteoarthritis on computed tomography. Sci Rep. 2020;10:1–10.

Sun Y, Du W, Xu C, Lin Y, Liu X, Luo E. Applications of computer-aided design/manufacturing technology in treatment of hemifacial microsomia. J Craniomaxillofac Surg. 2020;31:1133–1136.

Swaddle JP, Cuthill IC. Asymmetry and human facial attractiveness: symmetry may not always be beautiful. Proc R Soc Lond Ser B Biol Sci. 1995;261:111–116.

Thiesen G, Gribel BF, Freitas MPM. Facial asymmetry: a current review. Dental Press J Orthod. 2015;20:110–125.

Van Elslande DC, Russett SJ, Major PW, Flores-Mir C. Mandibular asymmetry diagnosis with panoramic imaging. Am J Orthod Dentofac Orthop. 2008;134:183–192.

Yatabe M, Gomes L, Ruellas AC, Lopinto J, Macron L, Paniagua B, Budin F, Prieto JC, Ioshida M, Cevidanes L. Challenges in measuring angles between craniofacial structures. J Appl Oral Sci. 2019;27:e20180380.

Part III

Management

10

Treatment Approaches

10.1

Very Early Treatment of Dentofacial Asymmetries: Why, When, and How?

Ute E.M. Schneider-Moser and Lorenz Moser

CHAPTER MENU

Introduction

Unilateral posterior crossbites (UPC) in the deciduous dentition are frequent findings, affecting between 8 and 22% of the children (Figure 10.1.1) (da Silva Filho et al. 2007; Shalish et al. 2013).

Studies have shown that the status of the primary occlusion affects the development of the permanent occlusion and that a UPC in the deciduous dentition will most likely be transferred to the mixed and permanent dentition (Kutin and Hawes 1969; Clifford 1971). Moreover, children with UPC have reduced bite force and asymmetrical muscle function leading to abnormal chewing or clenching which can negatively affect normal development of the orofacial system (Sever et al. 2011; Primožič et al. 2013).

Although research has shown that a spontaneous correction of a unilateral posterior crossbite can occur (Thilander et al. 1984; Kurol and Berglund 1992), the chances of its transfer from the primary to permanent dentition are by far higher, which can have long-term effects on the growth and development of the teeth, jaws, and the temporomandibular joint, leading ultimately to TMD and craniofacial asymmetry (Mohlin and Thilander 1984; Mongini and Schmid 1987; Riolo et al. 1987; O'Byrn et al. 1995; Piley et al. 1997; Egermark et al. 2001; Thilander et al. 2002; Kilic et al. 2008).

Early treatment is advised to normalize the occlusion and to create conditions for normal occlusal development, especially preventing the first molars to erupt in crossbite (Harrison and Ashby 2001; Lippold et al. 2013; Evangelista et al. 2020). Furthermore, postponement of treatment has been claimed to result in prolonged treatment of greater complexity (Lindner 1989; Bell and Kiebach 2014).

It seems, therefore, advisable not to delay orthodontic treatment to an older patient age, but to start treatment as soon as the crossbite is detected and the patient and the parents accept treatment (Viazis 1995; Bell and Kiebach 2014).

Dentofacial and Occlusal Asymmetries, First Edition. Edited by Birte Melsen and Athanasios E. Athanasiou.
© 2025 John Wiley & Sons Ltd. Published 2025 by John Wiley & Sons Ltd.

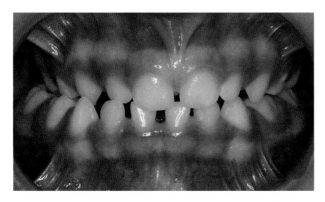

Figure 10.1.1 Unilateral posterior crossbite on the right with concomitant lower midline deviation.

Etiology

Fortunately, more than 80% of the early crossbites are only due to a transverse deficiency of the maxilla or of the upper dental arch, possibly associated with a low tongue posture, which causes a mandibular shift due to tooth interferences, and is not the result of underlying structural asymmetric mandibular growth (Shalish et al. 2013; Bell and Kiebach 2014). A thorough screening for associated factors, i.e. sucking habits, irregular tongue posture and function, impaired nasal breathing caused by enlarged tonsils and adenoids, or allergies involved in the etiology of the crossbite, besides heredity, is important for long-term stability of successful early orthodontic crossbite correction (Melsen et al. 1987; Oulis et al. 1994; Góis et al. 2008; Ovsenik 2009; Melink et al. 2010).

Diagnostic Evaluation

Clinical Examination

The most important part of the diagnostic process is the clinical examination. In presence of a UPC, children present a chin deviation to the affected side in maximum intercuspation. At a very young age, the asymmetry is limited to the lower facial third (Figure 10.1.2), without any repercussions on the midface or the maxillary arch in terms of a canted anterior occlusal plane (Primožič et al. 2013). Assessing maxillary constriction as the main causative factor can be performed by asking the children to close only until the first teeth contact (Figure 10.1.3). Spontaneous centering of the lower midlines during opening is a favorable sign for a mere functional asymmetry, while persistence of the mandibular midline deviation and tilting of the lower occlusal plane frequently indicate the development of a skeletal asymmetry (Figures 10.1.4 and 10.1.5).

Associated sagittal (Class II or III) and vertical (open or deep bite) dental and skeletal discrepancies should be clinically assessed and documented with standardized extraoral and intraoral photographs. It is advisable to add an intraoral frontal photograph upon opening to record any change in the lower midline. Alginate impressions or an intraoral scan are necessary for a thorough model analysis and for fabrication of the orthodontic appliance for crossbite correction.

In very young patients who present a UPC, it is very important to evaluate not only the maxillary transverse discrepancy and the resulting amount of upper dental crowding, but also the form of the lower dental arch. Thilander and Lennartsson (2002) have described that the combination of a narrow maxillary arch and a broad lower arch on the crossbite side, is a negative predictor for long-term stability of early crossbite correction by maxillary expansion, and hence an important diagnostic finding.

What About Radiographs?

In very young children who exhibit only a functional crossbite without any special redundant findings, taking radiographs on a regular basis is unnecessary and

Figure 10.1.2 (a) and (b) In very young children, a UPC causes only an asymmetry of the lower facial third.

(a)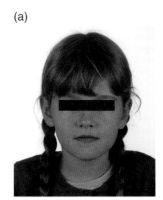

(b)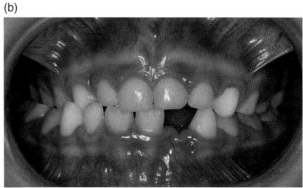

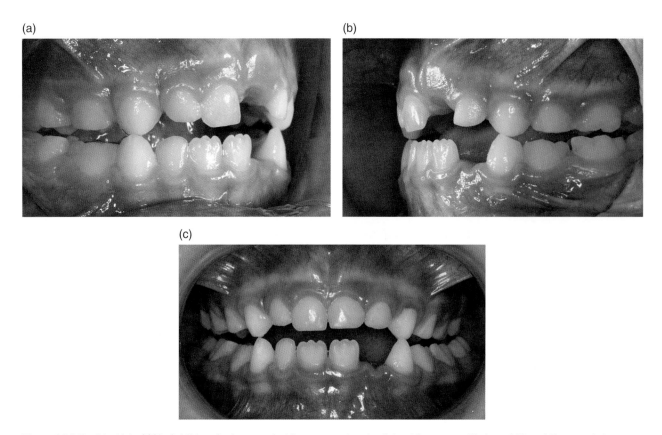

Figure 10.1.3 (a)–(c) In 80% of children in the pure deciduous or early mixed dentition, a mandibular midline shift toward the crossbite side from centric relation to centric occlusion is the main symptom.

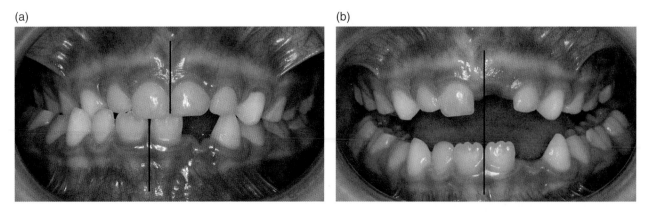

Figure 10.1.4 (a) and (b) If the midline deviation upon opening disappears, the crossbite is only functional in nature, while its persistence reveals an underlying skeletal asymmetry.

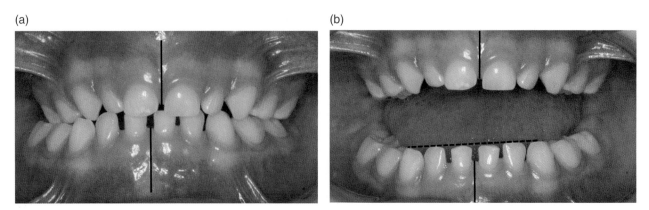

Figure 10.1.5 (a) and (b) In these patients, a cant of the lower anterior occlusal plane is a common finding, which is a second important criterion for a possible structural mandibular asymmetry.

should be avoided, as these records will not affect the primary treatment plan. Even in the presence of a non-centering mandibular midline upon opening, which might reveal an underlying skeletal asymmetrical component, taking radiographs is not mandatory at this stage, as the first orthodontic treatment approach will not differ from treatment of functional crossbites. However, should the first phase of treatment not lead to a complete correction of the crossbite or should cross-bite correction relapse during the later stage of growth, a thorough three-dimensional radiographic evaluation with cone beam computer tomography (CBCT) becomes necessary.

In very young patients with a history of congenital, developmental, or traumatic disturbances, additional sagittal or vertical discrepancies, or in the presence of congenitally missing deciduous teeth, taking additional pre-treatment radiographs can help the clinician to better estimate the complexity of the malocclusion and to inform the parents more reliably about the overall treatment needs.

Very Early Treatment for Unilateral Posterior Crossbite with Class I, II, III Malocclusion

Unilateral Posterior Crossbite and Class I Malocclusion

If the UPC is only caused by interferences of one or two single teeth. In this instance either grinding of these teeth or application of a simple criss-cross elastic can eliminate the problem in a very short time (6–12 weeks) (Figure 10.1.6).

As maxillary constriction is very often the main cause for a functional mandibular shift, early rapid palatal expansion in the deciduous dentition of around 4 or 5 years is the first treatment approach.

In the absence of any additional sagittal discrepancies, the gold-standard orthodontic appliance for UPC correction is the rapid palatal expander. With an activation of 1 turn per day, most maxillary transverse deficiencies can be resolved within 4–6 weeks. The maxilla should be over-expanded until the palatal cups of the maxillary

(a)

(b)

(c)

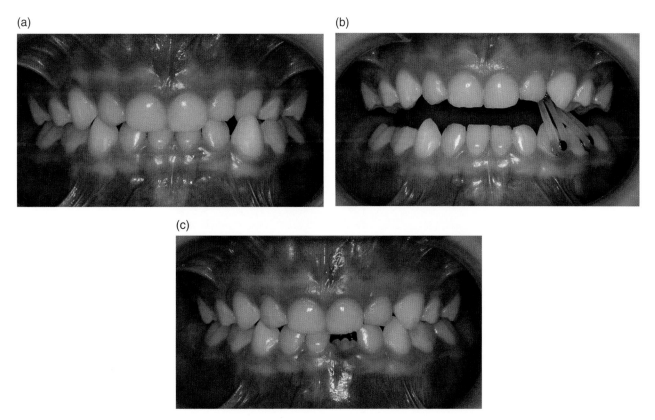

Figure 10.1.6 (a)–(c) Single tooth crossbite correction with 6 weeks of criss-cross elastic wear.

posterior teeth touch the buccal cusps of the lower posteriors, as some amount of relapse must be expected after removal of the appliance. After a stabilization period of 6–12 months, the appliance is removed and no further treatment is necessary, if the crossbite has been fully corrected and if no asymmetrical skeletal component is present (Figures 10.1.7–10.1.10).

Sometimes, the mandible does not center spontaneously after rapid palatal expansion. In this case, a buccal crossbite on the former well-occluding side, and insufficient correction of the former crossbite side will result. Crossbite elastics, either on one or on both sides, are very efficient accessories to reposition the mandible and to guide the attached muscles, which supports mandibular midline correction.

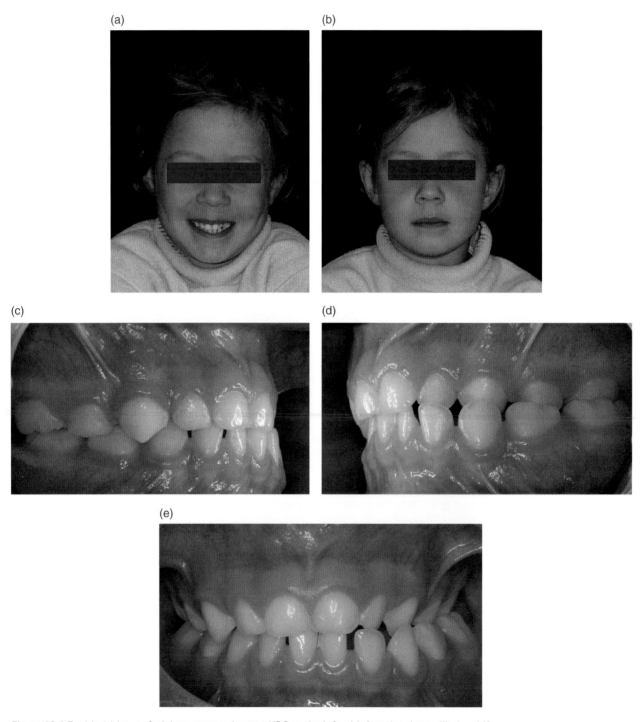

Figure 10.1.7   (a)–(e) Lower facial asymmetry due to a UPC on the left with functional mandibular shift.

(a) (b)

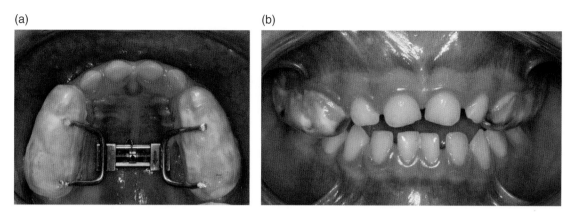

Figure 10.1.8 (a) and (b) One daily activation of the rapid maxillary expander's screw (0.25 mm/day) for 5 weeks has led to complete crossbite correction and spontaneous centering of the mandible and the lower midline.

(a) (b)

(c) (d)

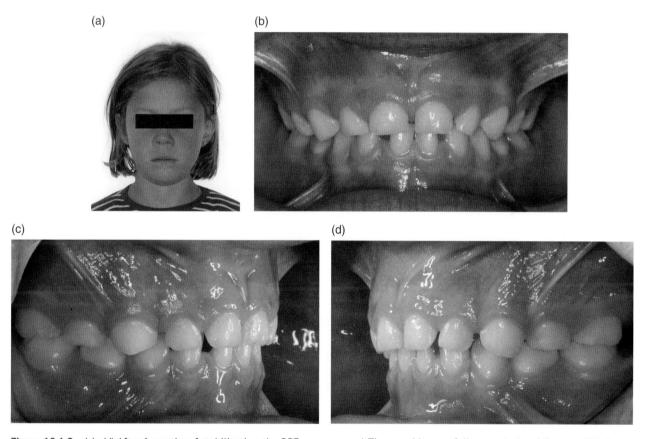

Figure 10.1.9 (a)–(d) After 6 months of stabilization, the RPE was removed. The crossbite was fully corrected and the mandible has centered spontaneously. No retention device was applied.

The 5-year-old little girl presented a unilateral crossbite on the right side due to a mandibular shift. Her mother was worried because of her asymmetric chewing pattern (Figure 10.1.11). After 6 weeks of maxillary expansion, incomplete crossbite correction on the right side and a buccal crossbite on the left were present (Figure 10.1.12).

Application of a criss-cross "box" elastic from the left upper and lower canines and first deciduous molars for 5 weeks has led to full correction of the transverse problem (Figure 10.1.13).

Four years later, at 9 years of age, the result of very early crossbite correction in the deciduous dentition has remained stable. Very likely, the patient will not require any further orthodontic treatment (Figure 10.1.14).

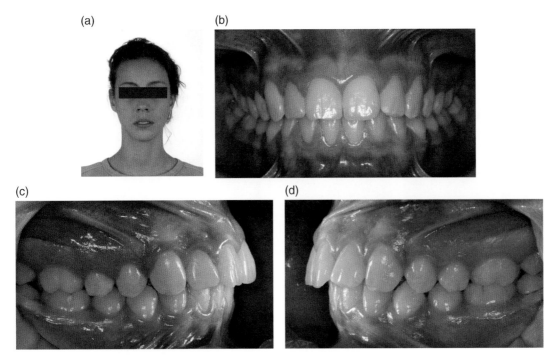

Figure 10.1.10 (a)–(d) Ten years later, very early crossbite correction has remained stable without any further treatment need.

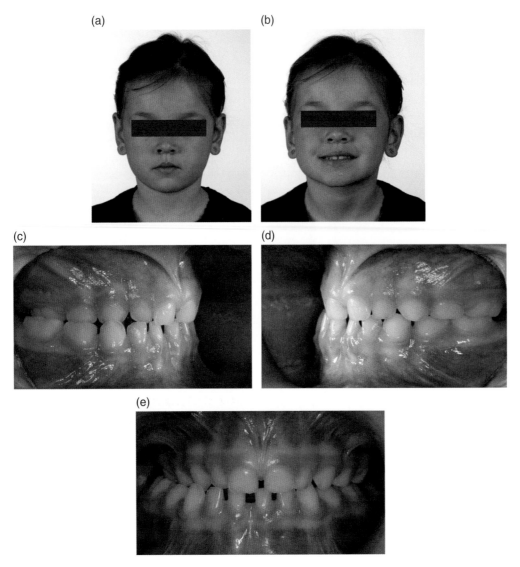

Figure 10.1.11 (a)–(e) The right UPC causes a chin deviation to the right side.

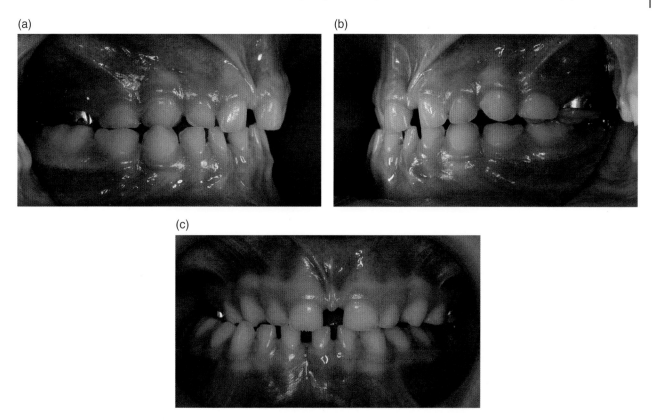

Figure 10.1.12 (a)–(c) Despite rapid maxillary expansion, the mandible did not center spontaneously.

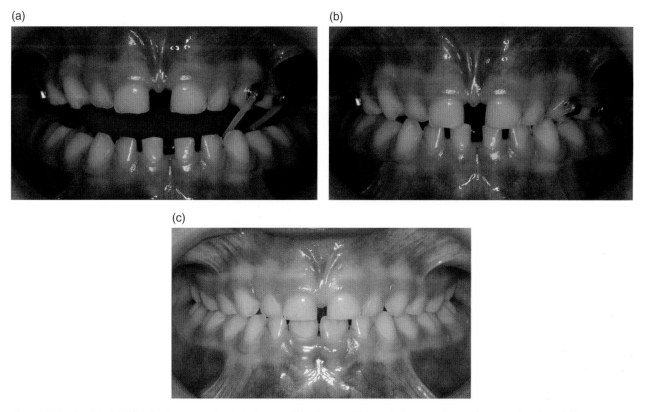

Figure 10.1.13 (a)–(c) A "box" criss-cross elastic helps to guide the mandible and the musculature for centering the midlines.

(a) (b)

(c) (d)

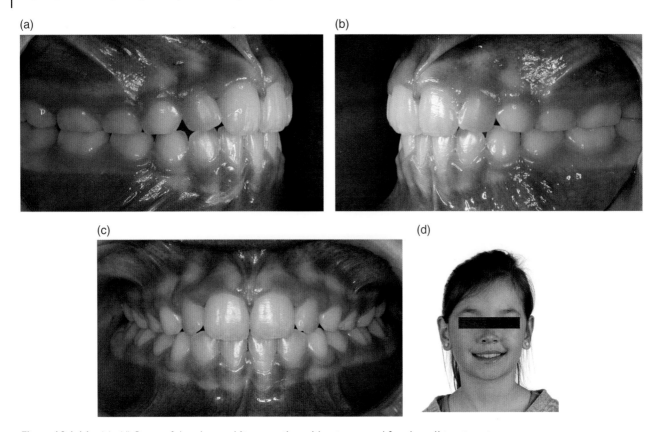

Figure 10.1.14 (a)–(d) Successful early crossbite correction without any need for phase II-treatment.

Unilateral Posterior Crossbite and Class III Malocclusion

Very young Class III patients with functional crossbites benefit from a concomitant correction of their transverse and sagittal discrepancies by very early treatment. Research has shown that more than 70% of early Class III treatments remain stable in the long term (>8.5 years posttreatment) and can therefore help to avoid the necessity of a later surgical intervention (Toffol et al. 2008; Masucci et al. 2011; Mandall et al. 2016).

Although Rosa et al. (2012) reported of a spontaneous correction of an associated anterior crossbite in 84% of patients around the age of 8 years previously treated with RPE alone, it is advisable to foresee the possibility to apply either Class III elastics (mild Class III) or a facemask to the RPE (moderate to severe) in very young patients with anterior crossbites.

At 6 years of age, the patient presented a maxillary constriction and a mild Class III malocclusion with a UPC on the left side, causing mandibular midline deviation was present (Figure 10.1.15). After 6 weeks of maxillary expansion, an additional Class III elastic was applied on the right side for another 6 weeks to overcorrect the deviated lower midline. Note the soldered hooks on the maxillary bands (Figure 10.1.16).

While monitoring the eruption of the permanent incisors, the Class III tendency worsened slightly. Bilateral Class III elastics for full-time wear were applied between bonded buttons on the lower canines and the hooks on the upper first molar bands (Figure 10.1.17). At age 8 years a bilateral Class I occlusion, normal transverse dimension, coinciding midlines, and an impressive normalization of both the preexisting facial asymmetry and the Class III traits can be evidenced (Figure 10.1.17).

When the Class III malocclusion is more severe, intermaxillary Class III elastics alone are not sufficient to correct the sagittal discrepancy; instead, a facemask at least for nighttime wear is indicated.

Especially in case of hereditary Class III malocclusion, a lateral cephalometric radiograph is mandatory to assess the Wits appraisal as an important diagnostic criterion for successful prognosis of interceptive Class III treatment, and for evaluation of the vertical skeletal dimension (Figure 10.1.18). In case of an increased Wits value associated with a hyperdivergent pattern, the parents should be informed about the looming risk of either a second phase of orthodontic treatment or, in the worst case of a combined orthodontic-orthognathic approach after the end of the growth period.

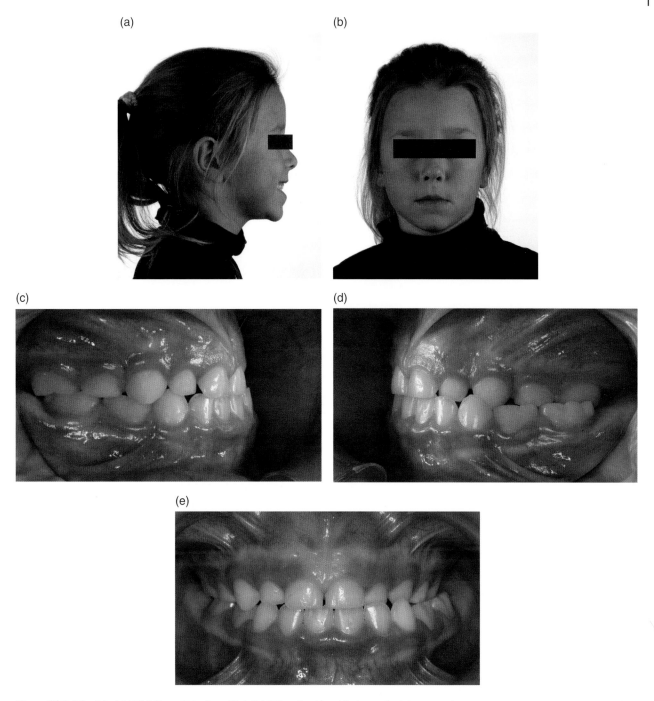

Figure 10.1.15   (a)–(e) Mild Class III traits with left UPC and noticeable lower facial asymmetry.

For the present patient, combined RPE and facemask therapy was performed. After 4 weeks of activation of the rapid palatal expander (1 turn daily), a facemask was applied for 10–12 hours. This wear time is usually enough to achieve adequate overcorrection of the anterior crossbite within 3–4 months (Figure 10.1.19). Without any retention or further orthodontic treatment, excellent maintenance of the achieved result can be assessed at age 14 years (Figure 10.1.20).

Unilateral Posterior Crossbite and Class II Malocclusion

Although the existing peer-reviewed literature suggests to postpone Class II treatment until the onset of the pubertal growth spurt in order to maximize the efficiency of the appliances (Tulloch et al. 1998; Thiruvenkatachari et al. 2013; Perinetti et al. 2015), the combination of a UPC with a

(a)

(b)

(c)

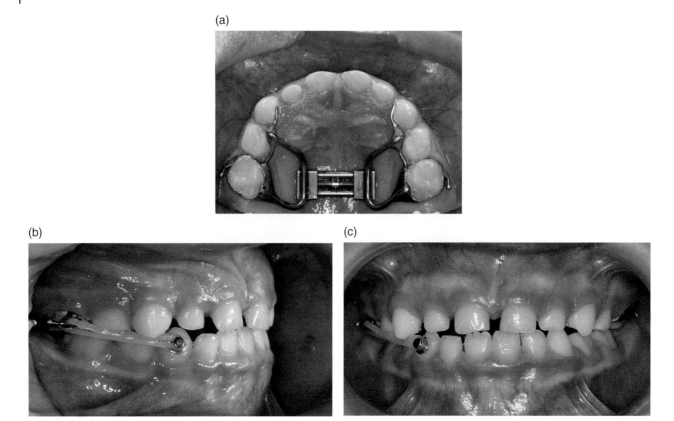

Figure 10.1.16 (a)–(c) Rapid maxillary expansion followed by application of a unilateral Class III elastic to center the midlines.

significant Class II malocclusion can justify to start orthodontic treatment as soon as the crossbite is diagnosed and the young patient is motivated to collaborate. Spontaneous improvement of the sagittal relationships after rapid maxillary expansion has been reported (McNamara 2002; Guest et al. 2010), but the evidence is controversial (Feres et al. 2015).

Very early correction of UPCs in Class II patients can be performed in two ways: rapid maxillary expansion or with a transpalatal arch for maxillary expansion and crossbite correction, followed by subsequent Class II correction with intermaxillary Class II elastics on the deciduous teeth. The great advantage of the Class II elastics is that they can be worn on a full-time basis as they cause much less discomfort than a bulky activator (Figure 10.1.21).

After intensive counseling for giving up the sucking habit, a rapid maxillary expander was inserted and activated once a day for 6 weeks (Figure 10.1.22). Immediately after crossbite correction, two buttons were bonded on the upper right deciduous canine and the lower right second deciduous molar for full-time application of a Class II elastic. On the left side, a criss-cross elastic was applied from the left upper first molar to both lower left deciduous molars to guide the mandible

toward the left side and to counteract the buccal crossbite tendency on the left side (Figure 10.1.23). Five months later, the UPC on the right side has been fully corrected and Class I dental relationships have been achieved. The patient gave up thumb-sucking (Figure 10.1.24). Facial symmetry and the lateral profile have been greatly improved by early intervention (Figure 10.1.25). Treatment success was maintained during the eruption of the anterior dentition (Figure 10.1.26).

An alternative to the application of Class II elastics – especially for UPC correction in dental open bite patients with tongue thrust or sucking habits (Figure 10.1.27) – is the insertion of a bonded rapid maxillary expander with acrylic occlusal coverage for maxillary expansion, followed by the application of an activator (Feres 2015). Six to nine months after correction of the crossbite, an activator with a high-pull headgear is prescribed for 12–14 hour/day. The average treatment time for this interceptive treatment is usually 15–18 months (Figure 10.1.28).

Good overall maintenance of the interceptive treatment success in all three dimensions was achieved. The eruption of the permanent dentition is monitored every 6 months. Very likely, the patient will not require a second phase of orthodontic therapy (Figure 10.1.29).

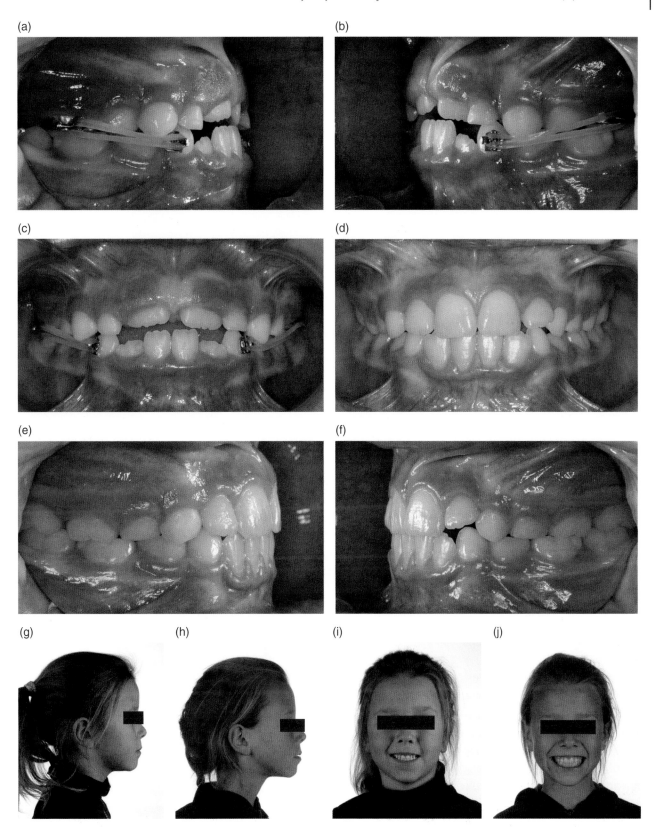

Figure 10.1.17 (a)–(j) Bilateral Class III elastics to counteract the Class II tendency.

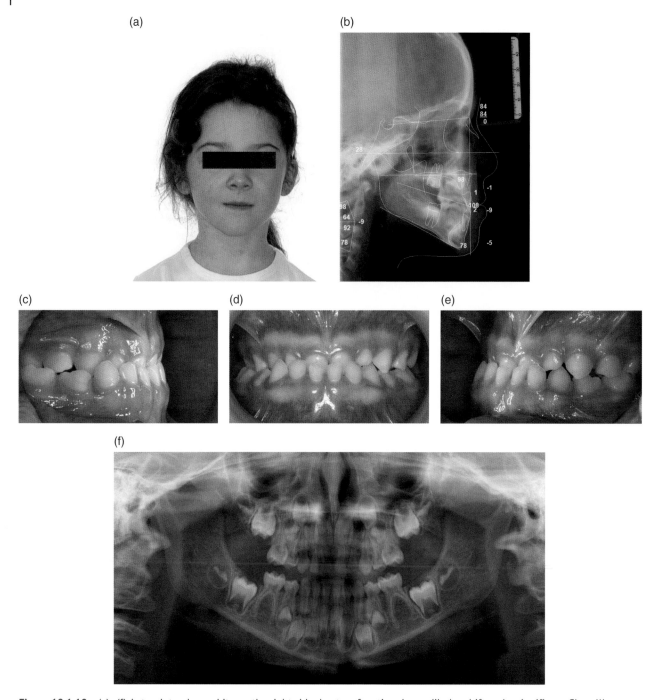

Figure 10.1.18 (a)–(f) Anterolateral crossbite on the right side due to a functional mandibular shift and a significant Class III hereditary growth pattern (Wits appraisal: −9 mm) are present at age 5 years. Note agenesis of all four second premolars.

What if a Class II Subdivision Develops After Early Crossbite Correction?

In 20% of young children with UPC, a true underlying skeletal asymmetry is present which may only be detected after a first attempt of crossbite correction has been undertaken. In these patients, either the corrected crossbite will relapse, or a unilateral Class II malocclusion will develop over time.

If the crossbite relapses within a short time, a second attempt of maxillary expansion with a RPE can be made, but the long-term prognosis is questionable.

(a)

(b)

(c)

(d)

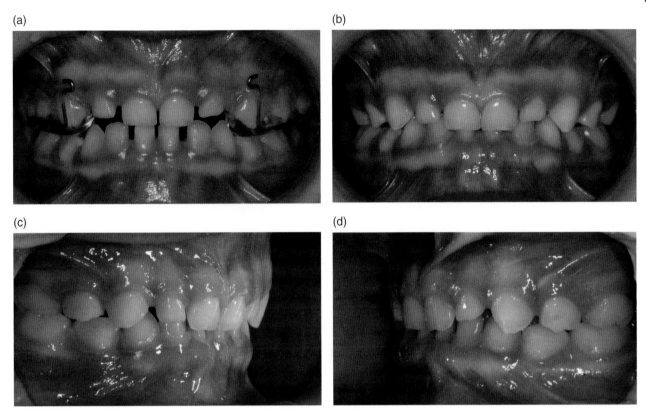

Figure 10.1.19   (a)–(d) Rapid maxillary expansion for 4 weeks followed by 6 months of facemask therapy have corrected the UPC and achieved bilateral Class I occlusion.

(a)

(b)

(c)

(d)

(e)

(f)

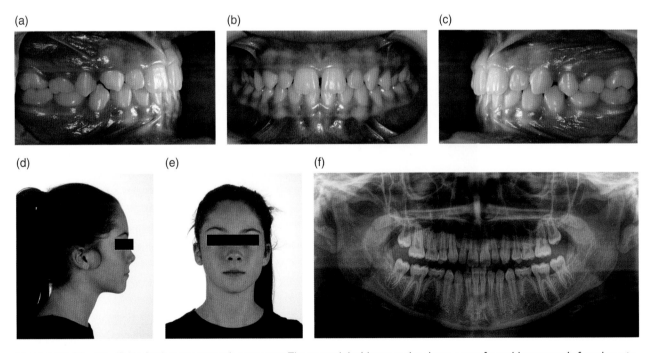

Figure 10.1.20   (a)–(f) No further treatment is necessary. The second deciduous molars have a very favorable prognosis for adequate long-term substitution of the congenitally missing second premolars due to their very long roots which do not exhibit any signs of root resorption.

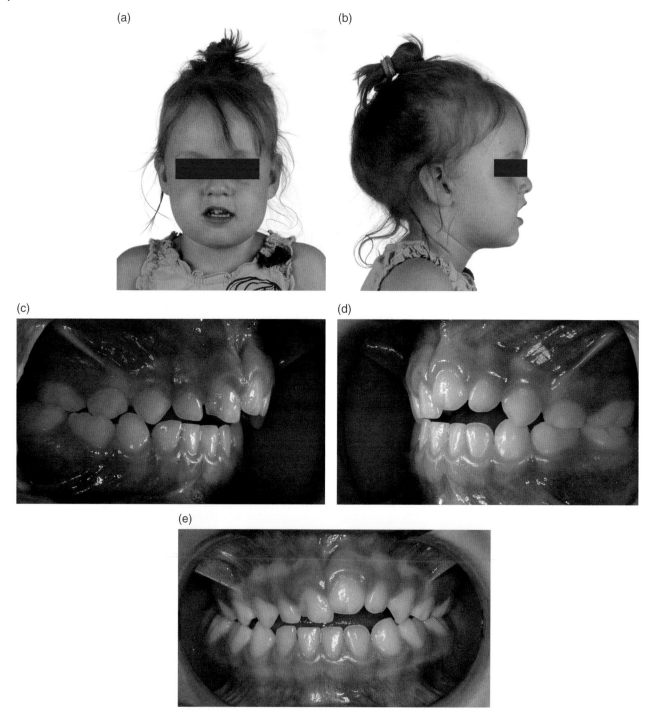

Figure 10.1.21 (a)–(e) A 4 1/2-year-old girl with UPC on the right in combination with severe Class II malocclusion and dental open bite due to thumb sucking.

If the crossbite remains stable, but a unilateral Class II malocclusion, a so-called "subdivision" develops, unilateral Class II elastics can be helpful to achieve a good posterior occlusion and centered dental midlines, as long as the subdivision malocclusion is mainly caused by an asymmetry of the lower dental arch and not by mandibular asymmetry (Azevedo et al. 2006; Janson et al. 2007; Lippold et al. 2013).

The 6-year-old girl was initially treated with a rapid maxillary expander for 9 months which corrected both the UPC on the right side and the concomitant midline deviation

(a)

(b)

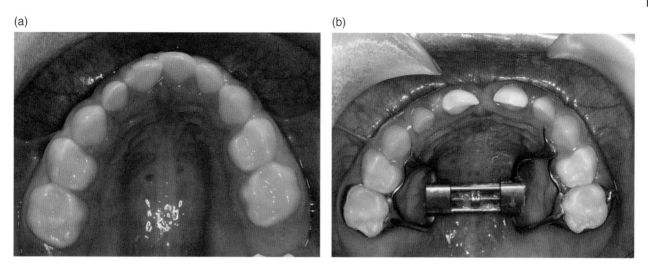

Figure 10.1.22 (a) and (b) Before and after 6 weeks of rapid maxillary expansion.

(a)

(b)

(c)

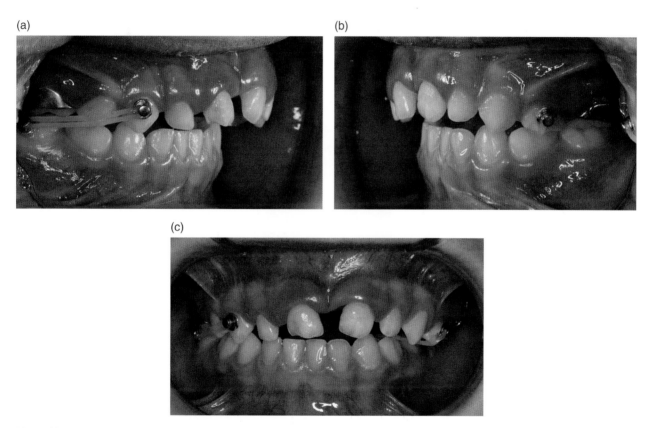

Figure 10.1.23 (a)–(c) Rapid maxillary expansion with Class II elastic on the right side and a criss-cross elastic on the left side.

(Figures 10.1.30 and 10.1.31). Already 1 year later, the patient returns with a Class II subdivision malocclusion on the right side. The maxillary midline coincides with the facial midline (Figure 10.1.32).

Two removable expansion plates and a unilateral Class II elastic on the right side are applied to counteract the subdivision. The great advantage of intermaxillary elastics is that they can be worn on a full-time basis in contrast to an activator with an incorporated midline correction. Eight months later, the Class II subdivision malocclusion has been corrected and midlines are coincident (Figure 10.1.33). Comparison of the patient's lateral

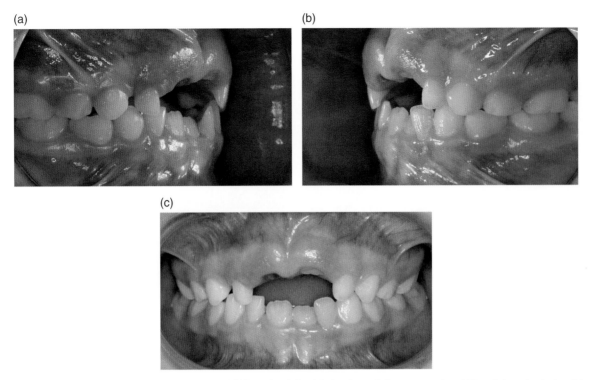

Figure 10.1.24 (a)–(c) Five months later, the UPC on the right side has been fully corrected and Class I dental relationships have been achieved. The patient gave up thumb-sucking.

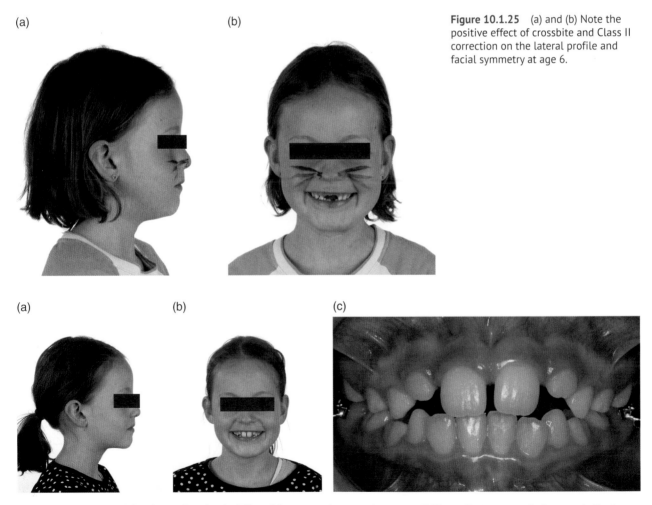

Figure 10.1.25 (a) and (b) Note the positive effect of crossbite and Class II correction on the lateral profile and facial symmetry at age 6.

Figure 10.1.26 (a)–(c) Good overall maintainability of the very early correction at age 8. The patient wears a lip bumper in the lower arch for space requirements.

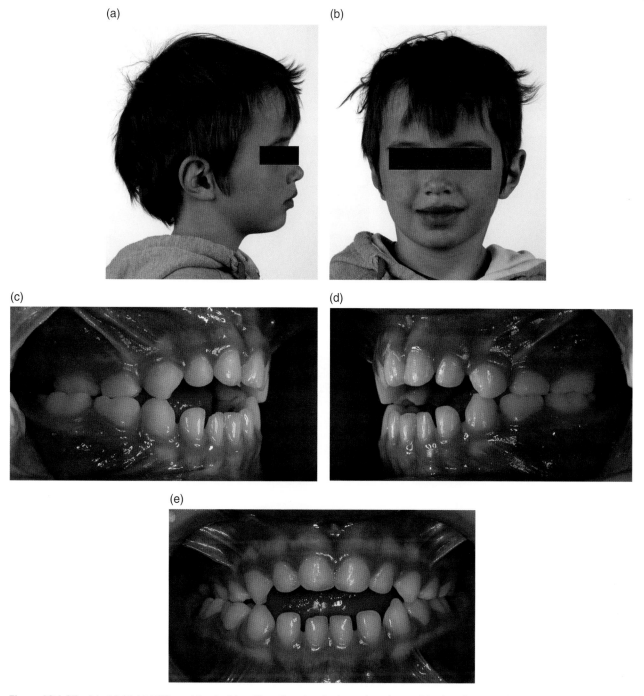

Figure 10.1.27 (a)–(e) Right UPC combined with a Class II malocclusion a dental open bite in a 6-year-old girl.

profile views and smiles pre- and posttreatment reveals the overall improvement of chin projection and facial symmetry (Figure 10.1.34).

Whether very early correction of Class II subdivision patients will remain stable in the long term cannot be guaranteed. According to the authors' expertise, very early rapid maxillary expansion coupled with Class II elastics on the affected side for achieving a solid Class I dental occlusion is a low-cost and efficient approach which might help to avoid a worsening of the mandibular dental arch asymmetry on the affected side. However, it will not be able to effectively counteract any Class II subdivision related to any true structural asymmetry like hemifacial microsomia.

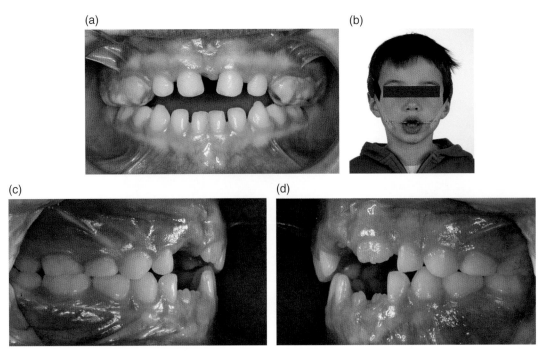

Figure 10.1.28 (a)–(d) Rapid maxillary expansion for 6 months followed by 9 months of van Beek-activator therapy.

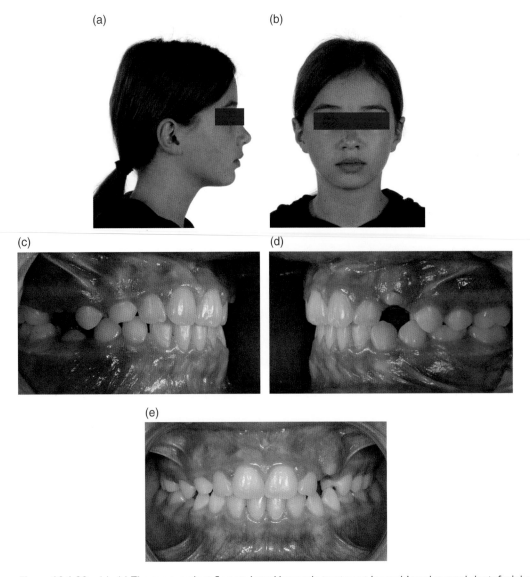

Figure 10.1.29 (a)–(e) The same patient 5 years later. Very early treatment has achieved normal dentofacial relationships. Very likely, the patient will not need to undergo a second phase of orthodontic treatment.

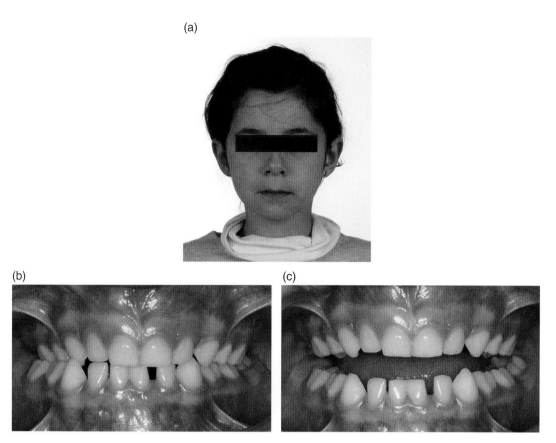

Figure 10.1.30 (a)–(c) At 6 years of age, a UPC on the right side with a lower midline deviation which persists during opening is evident. This can be a symptom of a skeletal asymmetry or a developing Class II subdivision.

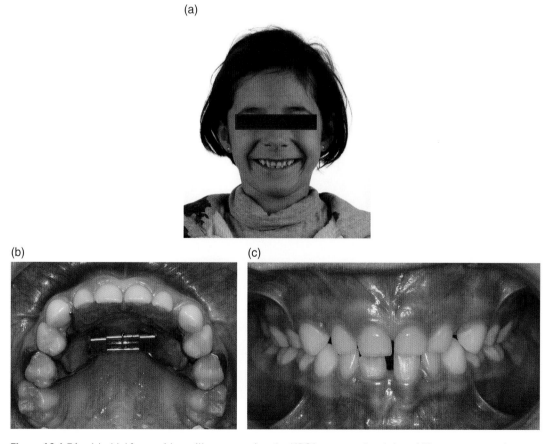

Figure 10.1.31 (a)–(c) After rapid maxillary expansion the UPC is corrected and the midlines are centered.

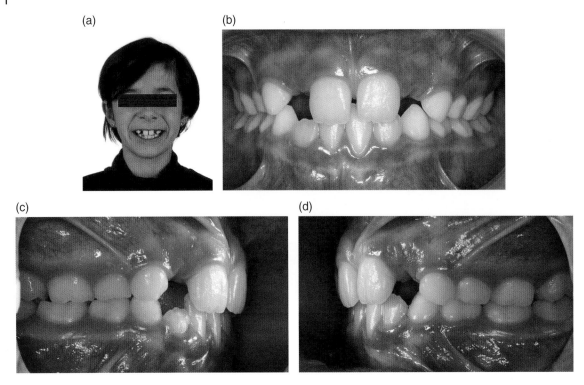

Figure 10.1.32 (a)–(d) One year later, a Class II subdivision malocclusion on the right side has developed. Note that the maxillary midline coincides with the facial midline.

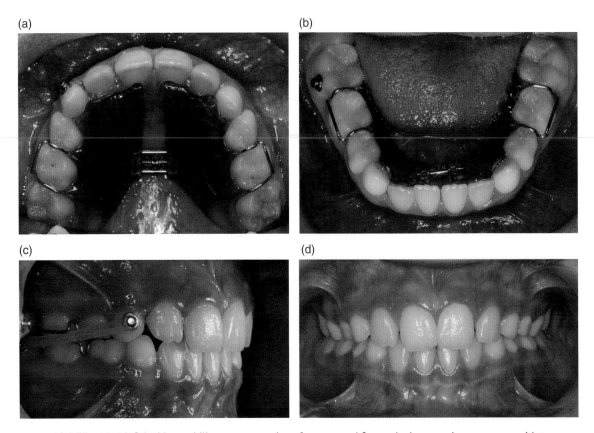

Figure 10.1.33 (a)–(d) Coincident midlines upon opening after a second 8-months interceptive treatment with two expansion plates and a unilateral Class II elastic for full-time wear.

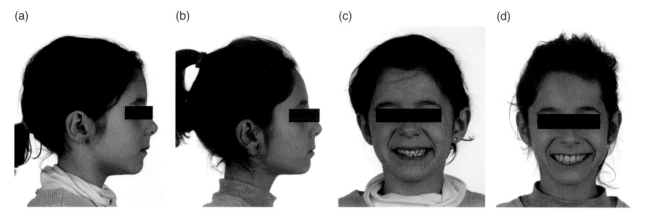

(a) (b) (c) (d)

Figure 10.1.34 (a)–(d) Apart from the positive effect on the lower facial asymmetry, Class II correction has also improved the patient's profile.

What About Stability of Very Early Crossbite Correction?

It has been reported in the literature that very early crossbite correction in the pure deciduous dentition yields a 30–40% relapse potential and cannot prevent eruption of the maxillary first permanent molars in crossbite in all patients, which implies that retreatment in the mixed dentition phase becomes necessary (Schroder and Schroder 1984; Thilander et al. 1984; Kantomaa 1986; Kurol and Berglund 1992; Primožič et al. 2013).

However, other studies have shown excellent long-term stability in 80–100% of the treated patients after early maxillary expansion, with permanent molars in normal transversal relation both in centric occlusion and in centric relation (Harrison and Ashby 2001; Cozzani et al. 2003; Malandris and Mahoney 2004; Mutinelli et al. 2008; Masucci et al. 2017; Tepedino et al. 2018). This controversy may depend on the presence or absence of an underlying skeletal asymmetry, the severity of the initial malocclusion, appliance and treatment management, and on retention time.

It is important to acknowledge, that when UPC correction is postponed until the mixed dentition or early permanent dentition, the concomitant pretreatment asymmetric muscle activity is not improved by maxillary expansion (Brin et al. 1996; Primožič et al. 2009). One could speculate that very early crossbite correction in the pure deciduous dentition may be helpful to overcome the problem of the persistent asymmetric postural and chewing pattern into adulthood with possible negative impact on the temporomandibular joint (Michelotti et al. 2019). An interesting study by Primožič et al. (2009) has shown that while very young children with UPC exhibit only lower facial asymmetry older children present also asymmetrical midface structures. Therefore, treating small children with UPCs very early might also be beneficial for avoiding a developmental structural midfacial asymmetry.

Early crossbite correction in the pure deciduous dentition is a relatively short (between 6 and 12 months) treatment utilizing simple and low-cost appliances. Above all, it causes only minimal discomfort to the little patients.

In a systematic review, Costa et al. (2017) revealed that an average retention time of 6 months in growing individuals is sufficient to guarantee satisfactory transverse stability of maxillary expansion, independent from the use of fixed (acrylic plate, Haas, Hyrax, and quad-helix) or removable (Hawley and Hawley expander) appliances.

If the functional posterior crossbite is the only problem, a second phase of orthodontic treatment can either be completely avoided or at least significantly reduced in complexity and in duration.

Summary

Considering the favorable effects of early crossbite correction, this opportunity should not be missed. Many children in their last year of kindergarten have adequate understanding and patience to cope with taking records, inserting an expansion appliance, and tolerating such a device for 6–12 months. They can then enjoy their first school year without the burden of major intraoral and extraoral changes during the delicate period of finding their place in a new environment.

References

Azevedo AR, Janson G, Henriques JF, Freitas MR. Evaluation of asymmetries between subjects with Class II subdivision and apparent facial asymmetry and those with normal occlusion. Am J Orthod Dentofac Orthop. 2006;129:376–383.

Bell RA, Kiebach TJ. Posterior crossbites in children: developmental-based diagnosis and implications to normative growth patterns. Semin Orthod. 2014;20:77–113.

Brin I, Ben-Bassat Y, Blustein Y, Ehrlich J, Hochman N, Marmary Y, Yaffe A. Skeletal and functional effects of treatment for unilateral posterior crossbite. Am J Orthod Dentofac Orthop. 1996;109:173–179.

Clifford FO. Cross-bite correction in the deciduous dentition: principles and procedures. Am J Orthod. 1971;59:343–349.

Costa JG, Galindo TM, Mattos CT, Cury-Saramago AA. Retention period after treatment of posterior crossbite with maxillary expansion: a systematic review. Dental Press J Orthod. 2017;22:35–44.

Cozzani M, Rosa M, Cozzani P, Siciliani G. Deciduous dentition-anchored rapid maxillary expansion in crossbite and non-crossbite mixed dentition patients: reaction of the permanent first molar. Prog Orthod. 2003;4:15–22.

Egermark I, Carlsson GE, Magnusson T. A 20-year longitudinal study of subjective symptoms of temporomandibular disorders from childhood to adulthood. Acta Odontol Scand. 2001;59:40–48.

Evangelista K, Valladares-Neto J, Garcia Silva MA, Soares Cevidanes LH. Three-dimensional assessment of mandibular asymmetry in skeletal Class I and unilateral crossbite malocclusion in 3 different age groups. Am J Orthod Dentofac Orthop. 2020;158:209–220.

Feres MF, Raza H, Alhadlaq A, El-Bialy T. Rapid maxillary expansion effects in Class II malocclusion: a systematic review. Angle Orthod. 2015;85:1070–1079.

Góis EG, Ribeiro-Júnior HC, Vale MP, Paiva SM, Serra-Negra JM, Ramos-Jorge ML, Pordeus IA. Influence of nonnutritive sucking habits, breathing pattern and adenoid size on the development of malocclusion. Angle Orthod. 2008;78:647–654.

Guest SS, McNamara JA Jr, Baccetti T, Franchi L. Improving Class II malocclusion as a side-effect of rapid maxillary expansion: a prospective clinical study. Am J Orthod Dentofac Orthop. 2010;138:582–591.

Harrison JE, Ashby D. Orthodontic treatment for posterior crossbites. Cochrane Database Syst Rev. 2001;1:CD000979.

Janson G, de Lima KJ, Woodside DG, Metaxas A, de Freitas MR, Henriques JF. Class II subdivision malocclusion types and evaluation of their asymmetries. Am J Orthod Dentofac Orthop. 2007;131:57–66.

Kantomaa T. Correction of unilateral crossbite in the deciduous dentition. Eur J Orthod. 1986;8:80–83.

Kilic N, Kiki A, Oktay H. Condylar asymmetry in unilateral posterior crossbite patients. Am J Orthod Dentofac Orthop. 2008;133:382–387.

Kurol J, Berglund L. Longitudinal study and cost-benefit analysis of the effect of early treatment of posterior cross-bites in the primary dentition. Eur J Orthod. 1992;14:173–179.

Kutin G, Hawes RR. Posterior cross-bites in the deciduous and mixed dentitions. Am J Orthod. 1969;56:491–504.

Lindner A. Longitudinal study of the effect of early interceptive treatment in 4-year-old children with unilateral cross-bite. Scand J Dent Res. 1989;97:432–438.

Lippold C, Stamm T, Meyer U, Végh A, Moiseenko T, Danesh G. Early treatment of posterior crossbite – a randomised clinical trial. Trials. 2013;14:20.

Malandris M, Mahoney EK. Aetiology, diagnosis and treatment of posterior cross-bites in the primary dentition. Int J Paediatr Dent. 2004;14:155–166.

Mandall N, Cousley R, DiBiase A, Dyer F, Littlewood S, Mattick R, Nute SJ, Doherty B, Stivaros N, McDowall R, Shargill I, Worthington HV. Early class III protraction facemask treatment reduces the need for orthognathic surgery: a multi-centre, two-arm parallel randomized, controlled trial. J Orthod. 2016;43:164–175.

Masucci C, Franchi L, Defraia E, Mucedero M, Cozza P, Baccetti T. Stability of rapid maxillary expansion and facemask therapy: a long-term controlled study. Am J Orthod Dentofac Orthop. 2011;140:493–500.

Masucci C, Cipriani L, Defraia E, Franchi L. Transverse relationship of permanent molars after crossbite correction in deciduous dentition. Eur J Orthod. 2017;39:560–566.

McNamara JA Jr. Early intervention in the transverse dimension: is it worth the effort? Am J Orthod Dentofac Orthop. 2002;121:572–574.

Melink S, Vagner MV, Hocevar-Boltezar I, Ovsenik M. Posterior crossbite in the deciduous dentition period, its relation with sucking habits, irregular orofacial functions, and otolaryngological findings. Am J Orthod Dentofac Orthop. 2010;138:32–40.

Melsen B, Attina L, Santuari M, Attina A. Relationships between swallowing pattern, mode of respiration, and development of malocclusion. Angle Orthod. 1987;57:113–120.

Michelotti A, Rongo R, Valentino R, D'Antò V, Bucci R, Danzi G, Cioffi I. Evaluation of masticatory muscle activity in patients with unilateral posterior crossbite before and after rapid maxillary expansion. Eur J Orthod. 2019;23(41):46–53.

Mohlin B, Thilander B. The importance of the relationship between malocclusion and mandibular dysfunction and some clinical applications in adults. Eur J Orthod. 1984;6:192–204.

Mongini F, Schmid W. Treatment of mandibular asymmetries during growth. A longitudinal study. Eur J Orthod. 1987;9:51–67.

Mutinelli S, Cozzani M, Manfredi M, Bee M, Siciliani G. Dental arch changes following rapid maxillary expansion. Eur J Orthod. 2008;30:469–476.

O'Byrn BL, Sadowsky C, Schneider B, BeGole EA. An evaluation of mandibular asymmetry in adults with unilateral posterior crossbite. Am J Orthod Dentofac Orthop. 1995;107:394–400.

Oulis CJ, Vadiakas GP, Ekonomides J, Dratsa J. The effect of hypertrophic adenoids and tonsils on the development of posterior crossbite and oral habits. J Clin Pediatr Dent. 1994;18:197–201.

Ovsenik M. Incorrect orofacial functions until 5 years of age and their association with posterior crossbite. Am J Orthod Dentofac Orthop. 2009;136:375–381.

Perinetti G, PrimozicJ FL, Contardo L. Treatment effects of removable functional appliances in pre-pubertal and pubertal Class II patients: a systematic review and meta-analysis of controlled studies. PLoS One. 2015;10(10):e0141198.

Piley J, Mohlin B, Shaw W, Kingdon A. A survey of craniomandibular disorders in 500 19-year-olds. Eur J Orthod. 1997;19:57–70.

Primožič J, Ovsenik M, Richmond S, Kau CH, Zhurov A. Early crossbite correction: a three-dimensional evaluation. Eur J Orthod. 2009;31:352–356.

Primožič J, Richmond S, Kau CH, Zhurov A, Ovsenik M. Three-dimensional evaluation of early crossbite correction: a longitudinal study. Eur J Orthod. 2013;35:7–13.

Riolo ML, Brandt D, Ten Have TR. Associations between occlusal characteristics and signs and symptoms of TMJ dysfunction in children and young adults. Am J Orthod Dentofac Orthop. 1987;92:467–477.

Rosa M, Lucchi P, Mariani L, Caprioglio A. Spontaneous correction of anterior crossbite by RPE anchored on deciduous teeth in the early mixed dentition. Eur J Paediatr Dent. 2012;13:176–180.

Schroder V, Schroder I. Early treatment of unilateral posterior crossbite in children with bilaterally contracted maxillae. Eur J Orthod. 1984;6:65–69.

Sever E, Marion L, Ovsenik M. Relationship between masticatory cycle morphology and unilateral crossbite in the primary dentition. Eur J Orthod. 2011;33:620–627.

Shalish M, Gal A, Brin I, Zini A, Ben-Bassat Y. Prevalence of dental features that indicate a need for early orthodontic treatment. Eur J Orthod. 2013;35:454–459.

da Silva Filho OG, Santamaria M Jr, Capelozza FL. Epidemiology of posterior crossbite in the primary dentition. J Clin Pediatr Dent. 2007;32:73–78.

Tepedino M, Iancu-Potrubacz M, Ciavarella D, Masedu F, Marchione L, Chimenti C. Expansion of permanent first molars with rapid maxillary expansion appliance anchored on primary second molars. J Clin Exp Dent. 2018;10:e241–e247.

Thilander B, Lennartsson B. A study of children with unilateral posterior crossbite, treated and untreated, in the deciduous dentition. Occlusal and skeletal characteristics of significance in predicting the long-term outcome. J Orofac Orthop. 2002;63:371–383.

Thilander B, Wahlund S, Lennartsson B. The effect of early interceptive treatment in children with posterior cross-bite. Eur J Orthod. 1984;6:25–34.

Thilander B, Rubio G, Pena L, de Mayorga C. Prevalence of temporomandibular dysfunction and its association with malocclusion in children and adolescents: an epidemiologic study related to specific stages of dental development. Angle Orthod. 2002;72:146–154.

Thiruvenkatachari B, Harrison JE, Worthington HV, O'Brien KD. Orthodontic treatment for prominent upper front teeth (Class II malocclusion) in children. Cochrane Database Syst Rev. 2013; (11):CD003452.

Toffol LD, Pavoni C, Baccetti T, Franchi L, Cozza P. Orthopedic treatment outcomes in Class III malocclusion. Angle Orthod. 2008;78:561–573.

Tulloch JF, Phillips C, Proffit WR. Benefit of early Class II treatment: progress report of a two-phase randomized clinical trial. Am J Orthod Dentofac Orthop. 1998;113:62–72.

Viazis AD. Efficient orthodontic treatment timing. Am J Orthod Dentofac Orthop. 1995;108:560–561.

10.2

Tooth Movement and Goal-oriented Mechanics in the Treatment of Patients Exhibiting Asymmetry

Bhavna Shroff, Steven M. Siegel, Steven J. Lindauer, and Birte Melsen

---

CHAPTER MENU

Introduction

Asymmetric malocclusions are common orthodontic problems that are challenging to correct successfully. The early recognition of the asymmetry, the proper localization (skeletal or dental), and treatment planning of the malocclusion, whether compensation or correction will insure the attainment of optimal treatment outcomes. The orthodontic management of a malocclusion presenting with some degree of asymmetry is challenging because of the necessity of asymmetric mechanics on the right and left quadrants of a dental arch to achieve an acceptable correction. Significant undesirable side effects may be associated with the correction of an asymmetric malocclusion and the analysis of the force system in the three dimensions is necessary step of goal-oriented treatment planning prior to the initiation of orthodontic therapy.

A critical step of planning treatment is to establish precise goals of treatment so the correction of identified problems can be achieved. A goal-oriented treatment approach allows the analysis of the ideal force system necessary to achieve the treatment objectives and the design of an appliance consistent with these goals. The careful analysis of the desired force system, its equilibrium, and the potential side effects that may arise will improve outcomes and the speed of treatment. The proper assessment of the force system is central to successful outcomes of treatment and clinicians can develop the appropriate biomechanics to achieve their treatment goals. If the nature of the asymmetry is misdiagnosed, the prognosis of successful treatment outcomes is greatly compromised and the results of treatment may be less than optimal.

In this chapter, different treatment strategies for the successful treatment of dental asymmetries are described. Key elements in the differential diagnosis and the analysis of force systems of a number of different orthodontic appliances used in contemporary clinical practice are discussed.

Dentofacial and Occlusal Asymmetries, First Edition. Edited by Birte Melsen and Athanasios E. Athanasiou.
© 2025 John Wiley & Sons Ltd. Published 2025 by John Wiley & Sons Ltd.

Diagnosis – Problem List

It is extremely important to establish the underlying cause of an occlusal asymmetry so that an appropriate treatment plan can be efficiently implemented. Asymmetric malocclusions may be caused by an underlying skeletal asymmetry, mandibular shifts from initial tooth contact to maximum intercuspal position, or dental asymmetry of purely dental origin (Pirttiniemi 1994; Bishara et al. 1994; Cohen 1995).

Skeletal asymmetries may be due to congenital anomalies such as hemifacial microsomia. Affected individuals have underdevelopment of the condylar-ramal complex on the involved side along with ear malformations (Figures 10.2.1a–c). Hemifacial microsomia has a variety of clinical presentations with varying degrees of deformation of the mandible on the affected side. A number of classification systems have been described as having various treatment protocols. The type and timing of treatment may depend on the degree of deformation and on the philosophy of treatment. Early treatment may involve the use of an asymmetric functional activator, distraction osteogenesis, or the placement of a costochondral rib graft (Mulliken et al. 1989; Kaplan 1989). Definitive orthognathic surgery may be required (Kaban et al. 1988). Treatment goals include optimizing facial growth and minimizing secondary asymmetric development of the maxilla and canting of the occlusal plane.

Progressive asymmetries may be seen in patients with Parry–Romberg syndrome in which there is a progressive hemifacial atrophy. There is evidence that this disease is of central nervous system origin. There is generally an active, progressive atrophic period followed by relative stability (Cory et al. 1997; Mazzeo et al. 1995).

Unilateral coronal synostosis (plagiocephaly) is associated with a progressive, growth-related skeleto-facial deformity involving the frontal bone and orbital rim and secondarily affecting the maxilla and mandible (Loomis et al. 1990; Arvystas et al. 1985). Condylar fracture during childhood has been associated with growth arrest and subsequent asymmetry. As normal facial growth continues, the mandible may progressively deviate toward the affected side. In many cases of early condylar fracture, normal mandibular growth will still occur. Stabilization of the occlusion during initial healing through intermaxillary fixation may be needed. In some cases, compensatory overgrowth of the fracture site occurs, producing an asymmetry with mandibular deviation away from the affected side.

Temporomandibular injury may produce an intracapsular hemarthroses which has the potential to cause joint ankyloses (Skolnick et al. 1994; Proffit et al. 1980). Along with asymmetry, a marked limitation upon opening due to the lack of translation of the condyle on the affected side may be seen clinically. Unilateral condylar or mandibular hyperplasia may result in an asymmetry in which the mandible deviates away from the affected side (Figure 10.2.2a–d). Condylar hypoplasia may also result in a skeletal asymmetry in which the mandible deviates toward the affected side. Compensatory maxillary asymmetry and canting of the occlusal plane may be associated with these skeletal asymmetries (Figure 10.2.3a–d). Temporomandibular disorders, particularly those involving unilateral degenerative joint disease, may be associated

Figure 10.2.1 (a) Frontal facial view of patient with hemifacial macrosomia. (b) Frontal cephalogram showing extent of underlying skeletal asymmetry.

(a)

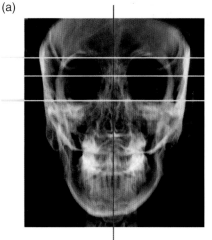

(b)

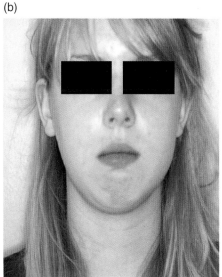

(a)

(b)

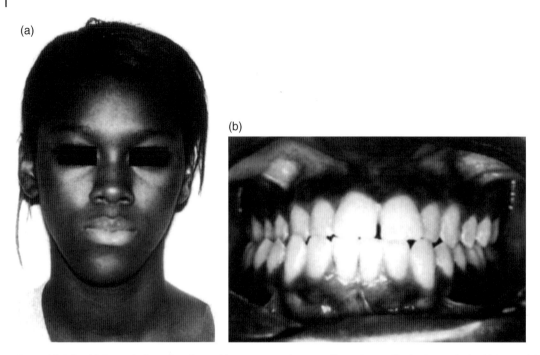

Figure 10.2.2 (a) Frontal view of patient with asymmetry due to unilateral mandibular hyperplasia. (b) Frontal intraoral view showing midline deviation away from the affected side.

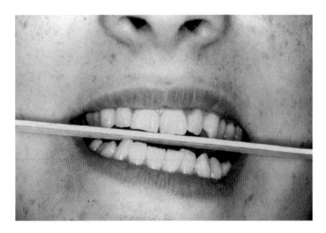

Figure 10.2.3 Bite stick in place to demonstrate canting of the occlusal plane.

with skeletal asymmetry (Figure 10.2.4a and b). Progressive condylar resorption, if occurring bilaterally, is associated with a progressive anterior open bite and increasing mandibular retrognathia (Huang et al. 1997). If the condylar resorption occurs unilaterally, it will be associated with a progressive asymmetry with the affected side becoming more Class II (Figure 10.2.5a and b). Neoplasia and fibrous dysplasia may cause facial and mandibular asymmetry (Arendt et al. 1990) (Figure 10.2.6a and b).

Radionuclide metabolic bone scans with 99-m-technetium phosphate may be useful in assessing the metabolic activity of the condyle in cases of hyperplasia, resorption, arthritis, fibrous dysplasia, and neoplasia. While not specific, the bone scan is more sensitive than conventional radiography and may be useful in diagnosis and treatment planning (Bohuslavizki et al. 1996; Matteson et al. 1985).

Asymmetries due to functional mandibular shifts are most often due to centric prematurities on cusp tips and inclines causing a lateral mandibular displacement upon full closure. A common example is seen in young patients with unilateral posterior crossbite (Figure 10.2.7a and b). At rest position, the mandible is symmetric but upon closure deviates to the side in crossbite. This is usually an indication of a maxillary transverse deficiency. It is important to distinguish a functional shift from true skeletal asymmetry. In the case of an asymmetry associated with a unilateral posterior crossbite with a functional shift, maxillary expansion is expected to correct the crossbite and reestablish symmetry of the occlusion. In the case of a unilateral posterior crossbite due to a true mandibular asymmetry, the need for surgical correction is more likely (O'Byrn et al. 1995).

Asymmetric malocclusions can also result from the malposition of a tooth or a group of teeth in the occlusal plane (first order), in the sagittal plane (second order) or the frontal plane (third order), or a combination of these. For example, the presence of a unilateral rotation of a molar can result in a dental asymmetry in the sagittal plane. Also, a difference in molar axial inclination in the

(a)   (b)

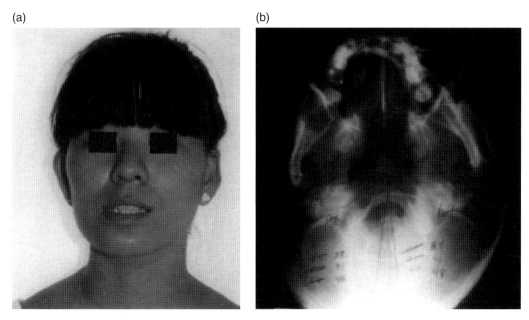

Figure 10.2.4 (a) Frontal view of patient with asymmetry associated with right temporomandibular joint disc displacement without reduction. (b) Submental vertex radiograph revealing the extent of the mandibular asymmetry.

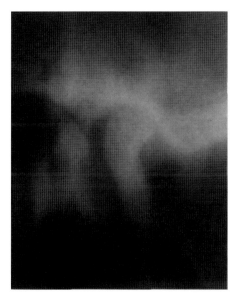

Figure 10.2.5 Corrected axis tomogram of left condyle revealing obliteration of normal joint space.

Molar Rotation (First Order)

Rotations of the maxillary permanent first molar are usually the result of premature loss of the deciduous molar. A mesial migration with forward tipping of the permanent molar accompanies rotation of the tooth resulting in a significant space loss in the posterior part of the dental arch. This rotation can also be due to ectopic mesial eruption of the molar. During normal development, the crowns of the maxillary molars are facing distally and as the maxilla moves downward and forward. The maxillary molars then upright and their crowns face occlusally (Burstone 1964; Andrews 1972).

The maxillary and mandibular arches must be carefully studied to recognize the presence of a molar rotation. A mesial-in rotation of a maxillary molar will result in a more Class II molar relationship on that side of the arch (Figure 10.2.8a–d). The malocclusion is evaluated in centric relation and the amount of overjet and overbite is recorded. Any discrepancy between centric relation and centric occlusion is also documented. The buccal occlusion on the right and left side are classified using the Angle classification and, if a dental asymmetry is diagnosed, specific steps will be taken during treatment planning to obtain a symmetric occlusion during the initial stages of orthodontic treatment.

From the occlusal view, the arches are evaluated for symmetry with respect to the median raphe and its projection on the mandibular arch. It is possible to superimpose a grid over the occlusal surface of the dental arch

sagittal plane will create an asymmetry of the occlusion between the right and left buccal segment of teeth. Similarly, the presence of a unilateral crossbite creates an asymmetric occlusion which will need asymmetric mechanics to be corrected. In this paper, the primary focus will be on the management of dental asymmetries resulting from abnormal molar rotation or incorrect axial inclination of the molars.

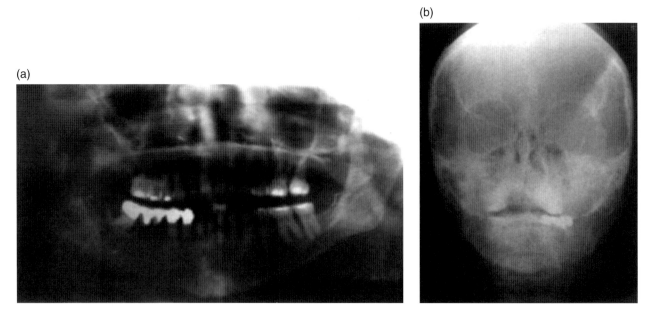

Figure 10.2.6 (a, b) Panoramic radiograph (a) and frontal cephalogram (b) of a patient with an acquired asymmetry secondary to the growth of a neurofibroma requiring resection of the left condylar-ramal complex.

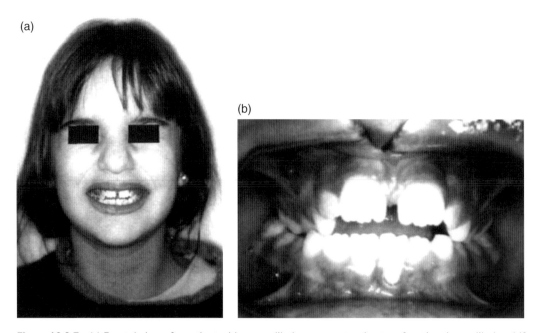

Figure 10.2.7 (a) Frontal view of a patient with a mandibular asymmetry due to a functional mandibular shift to the right in centric occlusion. (b) Frontal intraoral view of same patient demonstrating right side unilateral crossbite and lower midline shift to the right.

and evaluate the symmetry of the dental arch with respect to the median raphe (Proffit 1993). An easier and more efficient way to evaluate rotation of the molars is to draw a line along the mesial surface of the molar on each side of the arch and observe the point of intersection of these two lines (Figure 10.2.9a). If the right and left molars have the same amount of rotation, these lines will intersect at the median raphe (Figure 10.2.9b). If the right molar is more rotated than the left molar, the lines will intersect on the right side of the arch (Figure 10.2.9c). Once the diagnosis is established and the rotated tooth is identified, orthodontic treatment can be initiated with specific goals designed to correct the asymmetry early during treatment.

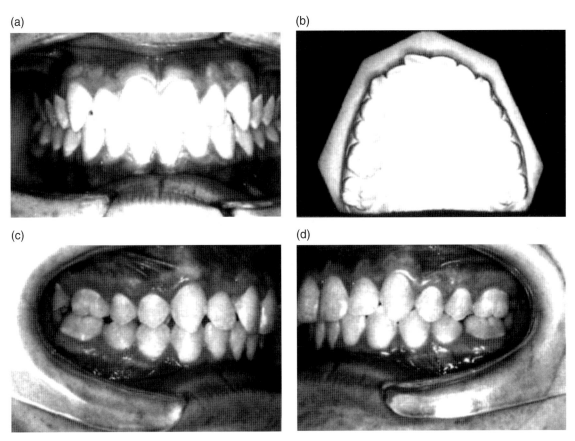

Figure 10.2.8 (a) Frontal view of a Class II subdivision malocclusion in the permanent dentition. (b) Observation of the occlusal aspect of the maxillary arch reveals a mesial-in rotation of the maxillary first permanent molar. As a result of this unilateral molar rotation, the right (c) and left (d) buccal occlusions are asymmetric. The right buccal occlusion is more Class II than the left buccal occlusion.

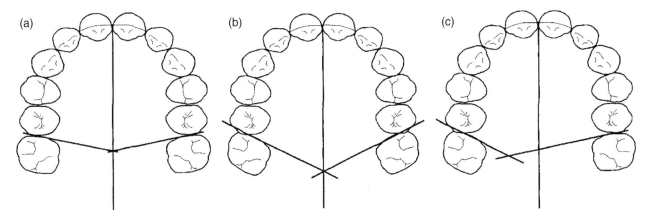

Figure 10.2.9 (a) An efficient way to assess molar rotation by tracing a line along the mesial surface of the molars on each side of the arch. (b) If the molar rotation is bilateral and of equal amount, these two lines will intersect at the median raphe. (c) If the molar rotation is on one side only, these two lines will intersect on the side of the rotated molar.

Molar Tipping (Second Order)

The presence of a dental asymmetry in the buccal occlusion may also be due to an abnormal axial inclination of the first permanent molar. Abnormal axial inclination of the molar in the second order results from an ectopic eruption pattern or from the early loss of a deciduous molar. During normal development, the maxillary molars have a distal axial inclination. With favorable growth of the facial complex, the molar will erupt with a more mesial axial

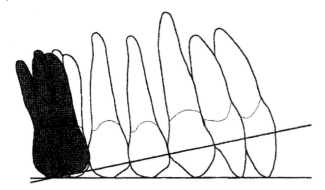

Figure 10.2.10 Assessment of the mesio-distal axial inclination of the molar can be easily done by tracing a horizontal antero-posterior line connecting the tip of the buccal cusps of the molar. If the molar is tipped forward, this horizontal line will intersect the incisors more gingivally.

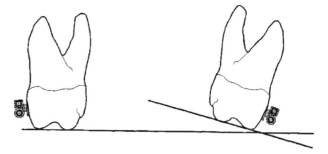

Figure 10.2.11 Evaluation of the bucco-lingual axial inclination of the molars is done with respect to a horizontal line in the frontal plane connecting the right and left molar.

inclination (Burstone 1964). In cases where the first permanent molar undergoes ectopic eruption, the mesial tipping of the permanent molar as it erupts accounts for a buccal occlusion that is more Class II on that side and a loss of space in the posterior part of the dental arch.

The diagnosis of such a discrepancy in axial inclination between the right and left buccal occlusion can be established by comparing the cant of the right and left posterior occlusal planes on a lateral cephalometric radiographic film taken at 45°. Orthodontic models can also be useful in this evaluation. A line drawn through the cusps of the molar and extended anteriorly will help visualization of the difference in axial inclination between the right and left permanent molars (Burstone 1962) (Figure 10.2.10). Panoramic or periapical radiographs can also be used, but they provide a less precise and reliable method as the two sides are magnified differently in the case of a skeletal asymmetry. Evaluation of the axial inclination of the molars than a cephalometric film taken at 45° or model evaluation may be better by using a cone-beam computed tomography (CBCT). However, these radiographs are valuable for assessing the distal space available to tip back the molar.

Posterior Crossbite (Third Order)

Dental asymmetries can also be observed in the frontal plane, and it is critical to differentiate between a dental or a skeletal crossbite. A thorough evaluation of the occlusion is necessary including the Angle classification, the amount of overjet, and overbite. Observation of the occlusion is made in centric relation and centric occlusion and any discrepancy is carefully noted. This is a very important step in diagnosing an asymmetric malocclusion because some

malocclusions presenting with a centric relation-centric occlusion discrepancy may appear to be asymmetric in centric occlusion when they are symmetric in centric relation (Faber 1981). The number of teeth involved in the crossbite should be recorded and their axial inclination in the frontal plane should also be evaluated.

Frontal cephalometric radiographs are useful in the evaluation of a posterior crossbite and they may help to differentiate a skeletal crossbite due to a narrow palate from a dental crossbite due to an abnormal axial inclination (third order) of the molar. Study models, plaster, or scanned virtual models can also bring important elements to the problem. To visualize the axial inclination of the molars in the frontal plane, a line is drawn through the cusps of the molars connecting the right and left molars of one arch and the axial inclinations of the two molars are compared (Figure 10.2.11).

Early Loss of Mandibular Deciduous Canines

Dental asymmetries are frequently due to the premature loss of deciduous teeth. Arch length deficiency will sometimes manifest with the unilateral resorption and loss of a deciduous canine which might result in the development of an asymmetric posterior occlusion. The loss of a mandibular deciduous canine in the mixed dentition results in a migration of the dental midline to the side of the missing canine as well as a mesial migration with or without forward tipping of the deciduous molars and permanent first molar on that side. This clinical situation needs to be addressed very early using a space maintainer such as a lingual arch to avoid the eruption of the premolars in a mesial position, thus creating a dental asymmetry more challenging to correct later. In the patient shown in Figure 10.2.12, a 9 years, 6-month-old patient presented regarding her dental midline discrepancy. The patient displayed a bilateral Class I molar relationship in the mixed

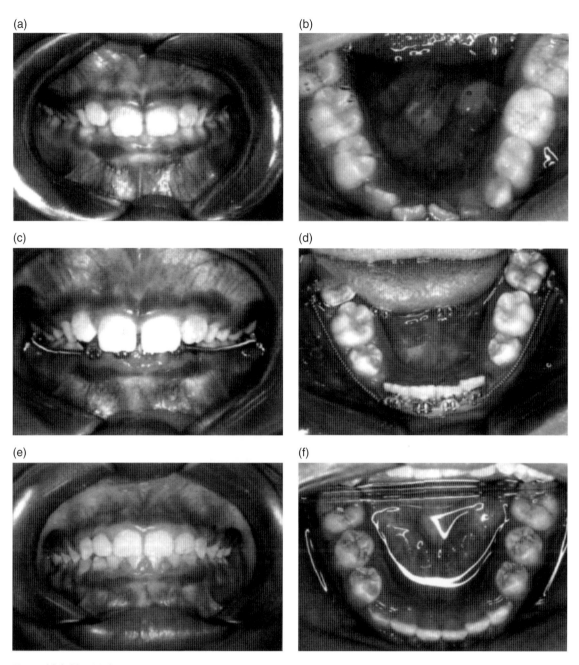

Figure 10.2.12 (a) Clinical example showing a dental midline discrepancy due to the premature loss of a mandibular canine. (b) Occlusal view of the mandibular arch shows the mandibular dental midline displaced to the right. (c) Early correction of this midline discrepancy included the opening of space for the right permanent canine using coil springs on a continuous 0.016″ stainless steel archwire (d). (e, f) At the end of this first phase of treatment, the midline was significantly corrected and space opened for the right mandibular canine.

dentition, an increased overjet and overbite relationship, and a significant midline discrepancy between the maxillary and mandibular arches. After the clinical examination, the nature of the midline discrepancy became apparent and was attributed to the early loss of the mandibular right canine (Figure 10.2.12a and b). The primary goals of the first phase of treatment were to correct the midline discrepancy and open the space for the right

mandibular permanent canine by bringing the mandibular incisors forward. This was achieved by using a continuous 0.016″ stainless steel archwire extending from right to left mandibular permanent first molars and open coiled springs extending from the first molars to the lateral incisors (Figure 10.2.12c and d). The results of the first phase of treatment were satisfactory and are shown in Figure 10.2.12e–h. Early orthodontic intervention allowed the patient to maintain a symmetric buccal occlusion. The premature loss of a second deciduous molar may cause a mesial tipping and mesio-lingual rotation of the permanent first molar which may result in an asymmetric posterior occlusion.

Treatment

Once the course of dental asymmetry is established, specific goals of treatments are determined and a mechanics plan is developed. It is important to correct an asymmetry in the buccal occlusion during the early stages of treatment. This allows the orthodontist to use symmetric mechanics during the rest of the orthodontic treatment and gives the practitioner more flexibility in the appliance design he or she chooses. The use of continuous archwire techniques makes it very challenging to efficiently correct dental asymmetry without significant undesirable side effects. It is advantageous to adopt a segmented approach during the initial phases of treatment to maximize the correction of such asymmetric malocclusions (Burstone 1962, 1966, 1985). The segmented arch technique allows the treatment of these asymmetries with excellent control of the side effects (Van Steenbergen and Nanda 1995).

Correction of dental asymmetries in clinical situations requiring extraction may be addressed through asymmetric extraction patterns including unilateral extraction, differential anchorage requirements, and the use of asymmetric space closure mechanics. In cases where non-extraction treatment is desired, maintenance and use of leeway space may help to reestablish arch symmetry. In cases involving asymmetric molar tipping and rotation, a variety of fixed or removable appliances may be considered to derotate, upright, and distalize the molar to a symmetric position within the arch.

Correction of Unilateral Molar Rotation

When the diagnosis of a molar rotation is established, the first step in the correction of the malocclusion is to determine the desirable force system (Smith and Burstone 1984; Burstone 1989, 1994). For example, if the right maxillary first molar is rotated mesial-in, a counterclockwise moment is necessary to correct the rotation of the molar. The equilibrium diagram shows that mesio-distal forces are produced on the right and left side of the dental arch (Figure 10.2.13). The molar which rotates will also be tipped forward and the molar on the opposite side of the arch will be tipped back (Figure 10.2.14).

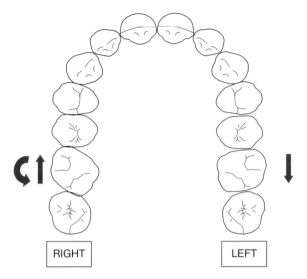

Figure 10.2.13 Equilibrium diagram generated when a molar is rotated unilaterally. In addition to the counterclockwise moment necessary for the rotation of the molar, mesio-distal forces are created on each side of the dental arch.

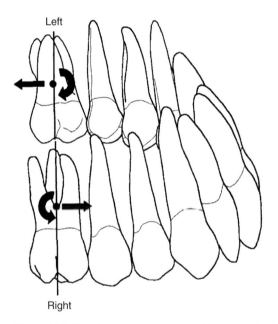

Figure 10.2.14 Force system generated in the sagittal plane. As the right molar is rotated mesial out, it will tip forward while the molar on the left side of the arch will simultaneously tip back.

When a continuous archwire is used to achieve correction of the molar rotation with a toe-in bend for example, the molar will move buccally and the premolars will move lingually creating an abnormal buccal overjet in the premolar and the molar areas. The presence of an abnormal overjet in the molar premolar area will need further correction and this can be a lengthy process using continuous archwires of increasing cross sections. The correction of a unilateral molar rotation can be efficiently achieved using a transpalatal arch which will help to obtain a statically determinate force system (Burstone 1989; Burstone and Manhartsberger 1988).

Clinically, after the alignment of the teeth using light flexible archwires, a rigid segment of wire (0.017×0.025 stainless steel) is placed from the premolar area on the right side of the dental arch extending to the left molar. A transpalatal arch (0.032×0.032 TMA or 0.030 stainless steel) is then placed with the unilateral first-order activation. The side effects discussed above are not expressed clinically because of the occlusion of a large number of teeth included in the anchorage unit. As the molar rotation is corrected, the occlusion will improve and become more Class I. In the sagittal plane, the axial inclination of the left molar will be maintained because of the rigid segment of wire placed as anchorage. On the right side, the molar will feel a mesial force but the amount of forward tipping of the tooth clinically visible will be minimized by the presence of adjacent teeth.

Current Mechanics Used to Correct a Class II Subdivision Malocclusion

A number of different treatment modalities are available to the clinician to correct an asymmetric buccal occlusion resulting from an abnormal axial inclination of the molar on one side of the arch only. For example, unilateral Class II elastics can be used in association with a continuous archwire but this approach may cause a number of undesirable side effects (Figure 10.2.15). These side effects will depend on the amount and point of application of the force as well as the length of elastic wear. Significant canting of the maxillary anterior occlusal plane due to the vertical

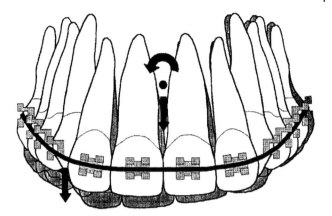

Figure 10.2.16 Frontal view. Unilateral Class II elastic wear creates a cant of the anterior occlusal plane because of the extrusive component of Class II elastics.

component of the Class II elastic is observed extruding the side of the arch where the elastic is worn (Figure 10.2.16). The occlusal plane on the side of the correction will also steepen as a result of the vertical forces applied to the anterior portion of the maxillary and mandibular arches. This will make the stability of the treatment questionable especially if adequate growth does not occur. Skewing of the arches with possible maxillo-mandibular midline discrepancy can develop along with flaring of the mandibular incisors. The development of an asymmetric overjet is usually the initial sign of the development of these side effects.

Unilateral Class II elastic correction has also been achieved with the use of open coil springs or sliding jigs to tip back the molar unilaterally thus correcting its mesio-distal axial inclination. Unilateral molar distalization in the maxillary arch is more predictable prior to the eruption of the second molar (Gianelly et al. 1991). The coil spring delivers a distal force to the crown of the molar and a tip-back moment and a mesial force to the premolars and canine, tipping these teeth forward. Nance buttons have been sometimes recommended to enhance anchorage in the maxillary arch but with varying degrees of success as soft tissue can rarely be anticipated to deliver valid anchorage. Unilateral Class II elastics can be used in this situation to counteract the mesial force delivered by the coil spring (Figure 10.2.17). Undesirable side effects due to the extrusive component of the Class II elastics include canting of the anterior occlusal plane and lower molar extrusion. Skewing of the dental arches as well as flaring of the lower incisors are common side effects experienced with the use of these mechanisms. Sliding jigs have also been advocated to correct the mesio-distal axial inclination of the molar (Thurow 1966; Tweed 1966). These jigs are sliding on continuous archwires and although the Class II elastic is not directly attached to the archwire, most of the undesirable

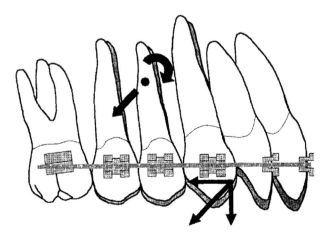

Figure 10.2.15 Force system generated by Class II elastics on a continuous archwire.

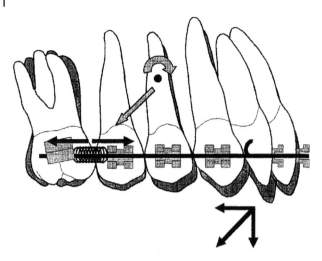

Figure 10.2.17 When unilateral Class II elastic is used with coil springs as shown, undesirable side effects associated with the extrusive component of the Class II elastic are still expressed.

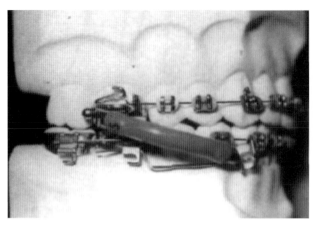

Figure 10.2.19 Jasper Jumper in place for Class II correction. Points of attachment at headgear tube of maxillary molar band and lower rectangular sectional archwire.

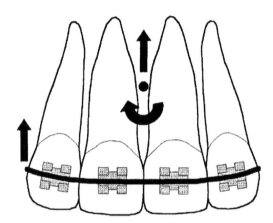

Figure 10.2.18 Application of an intrusive force unilaterally will result in canting of the anterior occlusal plane.

side effects described above can be observed with this appliance system.

Unilateral tip-back bends incorporated in 2×4 appliances or continuous archwires have also been advocated for the unilateral correction of a tipped molar. The force system includes a unilateral tip-back moment at the molar on the side of the tip-back bend but also a unilateral intrusive force on the anterior portion of the arch on the same side. This results in a cant of the anterior occlusal plane which is difficult to correct (Figure 10.2.18a and b).

The Jasper Jumper appliance (American Orthodontics, Sheboygan, Wisconsin, USA) and more of this type of appliance when used unilaterally have also been advocated for the correction of a unilateral Class II occlusion. This appliance is usually associated with a continuous round wire in the maxillary arch and a heavy rectangular archwire in the mandibular arch (Blackwood 1991; Cope

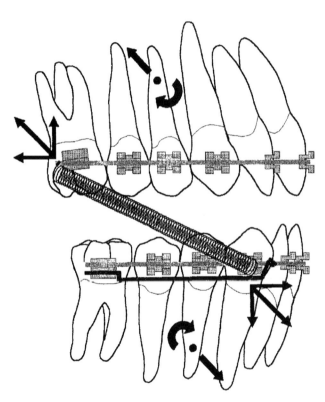

Figure 10.2.20 Force system delivered by the Jasper Jumper. The molar will not only feel a distal force and tip back but also feel an intrusive force.

et al. 1994) (Figure 10.2.19). The maxillary molar will not only tip back but will also feel an intrusive force (Figure 10.2.20). As a result of the buccal point of application of the intrusive force, the maxillary molar might also tip buccally thus increasing the buccal overjet. In the mandibular arch, the anterior section of the arch will feel a mesial force and an intrusive force. This may result in a cant of the lower anterior occlusal plane intruding the

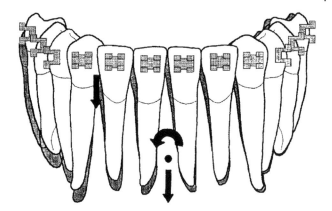

Figure 10.2.22 Frontal view of the mandibular arch. The effect of the unilateral intrusive force results in canting of the anterior occlusal plane.

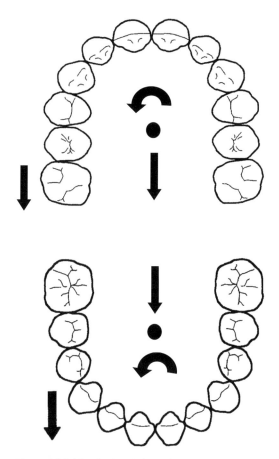

Figure 10.2.21 Occlusal view of both the maxillary and mandibular dental arches shows the mesial movement of the mandibular arch on the side of the Jasper Jumper and the skewing of the mandibular arch.

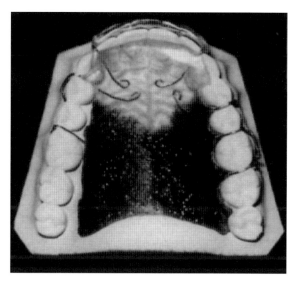

Figure 10.2.23 Shamy appliance with a unilateral tip-back spring on the right side of the maxillary arch.

anterior teeth on the side where the Class II correction is needed and flaring of the lower incisors (Figure 10.2.21). Skewing of the mandibular and maxillary arches may also occur as a result of the unilateral application of such a force system creating an asymmetric overjet and a potentially significant midline discrepancy (Figure 10.2.22). Some cases of Class II subdivision malocclusion have mandibular arch asymmetries with a lower midline shift toward the Class II side (de Araujo et al. 1994; Rose et al. 1994).

The use of a unilateral Jasper Jumper may be advantageous in these clinical situations to aid the midline correction. Control of lower incisor position and lower arch anchorage may be enhanced by incorporating the second molars in a rigid archwire and by the addition of anterior lingual crown torque.

Treatment strategies using the Pendulum appliance in the correction of unilateral Class II malocclusion may present some advantages but also some drawbacks as a distal force on the lingual surface will augment the mesial rotation that is a part of the problem. Removable appliances as well as Class II elastics rely on patient compliance for successful treatment outcomes but may have an unfortunate influence to the inclination of the occlusal plane. A typical Shamy appliance uses the entire arch as anchorage and a unilateral tip-back spring is used to correct the unilateral Class II relationship (Cetlin and Ten Hoeve 1990) (Figure 10.2.23). One of the side effects of this treatment is the potential loss of anterior anchorage and the subsequent forward movement of the maxillary anterior teeth which may or may not be a desirable side effect. The Pendulum appliance uses anchorage from the palate and TMA springs are designed to tip back the molars unilaterally or bilaterally (Figure 10.2.24). Control of anchorage, especially in the anterior portion of the arch, may limit the use of this appliance to very specific situations.

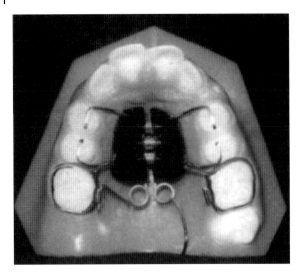

Figure 10.2.24 Pendulum appliance which can be used for unilateral or bilateral tip-back. The springs are made of TMA.

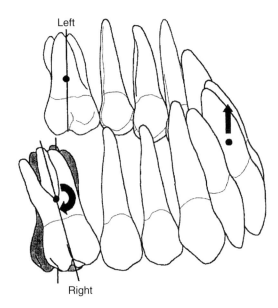

Figure 10.2.25 The desired force system necessary to achieve a unilateral molar tip-back and intrude the anterior teeth simultaneously.

Asymmetric headgear (unilateral face bow) use has also been advocated for the correction of a unilateral Class II occlusion (Haack and Weinstein 1958). Although this appliance system is effective at delivering a unilateral distal force (Hershey et al. 1981), a net lateral force is also felt at the inner bow and has a tendency to create a lingual cross-bite on the side which receives the greater distal force. Headgear use may also be limited because of patient compliance.

Unilateral Tip-back Mechanics

The correction of an asymmetric buccal occlusion due to an abnormal axial inclination (second order) of one molar can be achieved by using unilateral tip-back moments. Often these malocclusions are associated with a deep overbite and simultaneous treatment of the posterior asymmetry and the overbite is advantageous during orthodontic therapy. The initial step of treatment includes determination of the desired force system to tip back the molar unilaterally without significant side effects on the rest of the dental arch. In the example that will be discussed in this chapter, the right buccal occlusion is Class II and the left buccal occlusion is Class I with a significant anterior deep bite. The asymmetry present between the right and left buccal occlusion is due to the forward tipping of the maxillary right first molar. The force system necessary to correct this buccal asymmetry includes a tip-back moment on the right maxillary first molar to correct its axial inclination and intrusive forces on the anterior segment of teeth to correct the deep overbite (Figure 10.2.25). It is possible to use a distal force applied at the bracket of the molar to produce a tip-back moment but

this usually results in significant undesirable side effects in the anterior portion of the arch. The use of couples is more desirable and such a force system can be delivered by a transpalatal arch. The right and left molars can be connected by a transpalatal arch and a tip-back moment can be delivered to the right molar to correct its axial inclination. At equilibrium, the left molar will feel a tip-forward moment that can be easily counteracted by using a rigid continuous archwire connecting teeth in the rest of the arch (Figure 10.2.26). This approach to treatment is only used in the permanent dentition.

Another approach is available to the clinician when simultaneous correction of the dental asymmetry and the deep overbite are desirable (Shroff et al. 1995, 1997). The use of a three piece base arch produces bilateral tip-back moments which are necessary to correct the axial inclinations of the molar on the right side of the dental arch (Figure 10.2.27). Tip-back springs are hooked bilaterally to the distal extensions of a rigid anterior segment of wire connecting the four anterior teeth. The point of force application on the anterior segment of wire is through the estimated center of resistance of the anterior teeth and the four incisors are intruded with control of their axial inclination. The molars will tip back and extrude bilaterally. As the molars tip-back, the hooks of the tip-back springs slide back along the distal extension of the anterior wire, changing the anterior point of force application. It is therefore necessary to monitor the position of the hooks during treatment.

In clinical situations where the axial inclination of a molar needs to be corrected unilaterally, it is possible to use

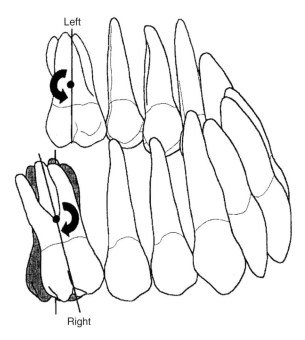

Figure 10.2.26 Force system generated when a unilateral tip-back moment is applied using a transpalatal arch.

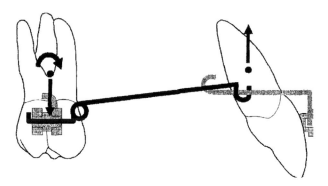

Figure 10.2.27 Schematic representation of a three piece base arch.

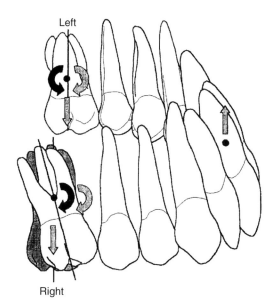

Figure 10.2.28 Force system developed when a transpalatal arch with a second-order activation is used simultaneously with a three piece base arch. The right molar will feel a tip-back moment and the left molar will maintain its axial inclination as the incisors are intruded.

a palatal arch combined with a three piece base arch. A unilateral activation is incorporated in the palatal arch on the side that needs the molar to be uprighted and the three piece base arch will deliver bilateral tip-back moments and simultaneously intrude the anterior teeth. As a result of simultaneously using a palatal arch with unilateral activation and a three piece base arch, the molar on the opposite side of the arch will experience a tip forward moment from the palatal arch and a tip-back moment from the three piece base arch (Figure 10.2.28). The molar on that side of the arch will therefore maintain its axial inclination.

The three piece base arch includes an anterior segment of wire passively positioned into the brackets of the four incisors and fabricated of $0.021'' \times 0.025''$ stainless steel. This rigid anterior segment extends distally to the position of the canines. Bilateral tip-back springs fabricated of $0.017' \times 0.025$ TMA are engaged into the auxiliary tubes of the molar bands and extend mesially to be hooked on the distal extension of the anterior segment of wire. The anterior portion of the tip-back springs has a hook that is free to slide distally along the extension of the anterior segment of wire as the crown of the molar tips back. The intrusive force applied on the anterior segment of teeth is 70 g on the right and left sides and the tip-back moments are approximately 2100 g-mm if a distance of 30 mm separates the anterior and posterior segments. A transpalatal arch fabricated of $0.032'' \times 0.032''$ TMA or $0.030''$ stainless steel is used simultaneously with the three piece base arch and activated unilaterally delivering equal and opposite moments to each side of the arch. A tip-back bend is incorporated in the transpalatal arch and the entire arch is twisted by incorporating a bend at its apex. The resulting force system includes an intrusive force on the anterior segment of teeth and an increased tip-back moment on the molar that needs to be corrected. The molar on the opposite side of the dental arch will maintain its axial inclination because the moment from the palatal arch will cancel the moment from the three piece base arch. Buccal segments of wires are not used with the three piece base arch to encourage the distal drifting of the premolars and canines as the molar uprights on that side of the arch. Figure 10.2.29a–c show the pretreatment views of the buccal right and left occlusion of a patient presenting with a Class II division 2

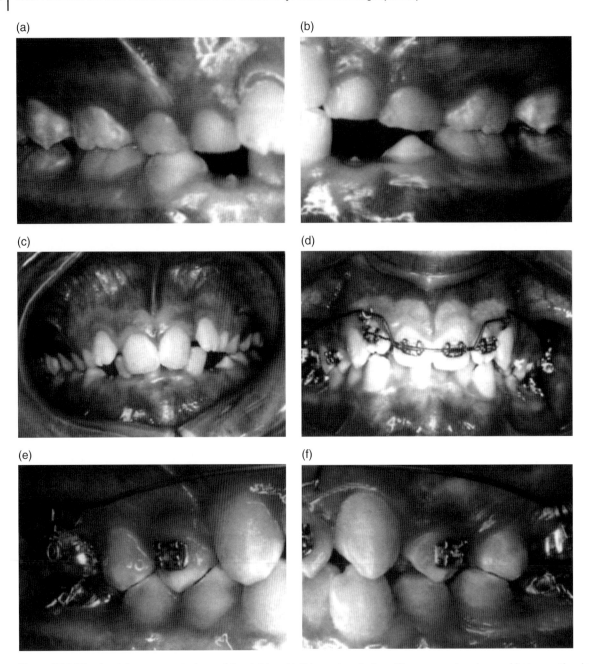

Figure 10.2.29 (a–c) Pretreatment views of the right and left buccal occlusions. The asymmetry observed between the right and left buccal occlusion is primarily due to the axial inclination of the left molar which is tipped forward. (d) The anterior segment of the three piece base arch observed in the frontal view. (e, f) Right and left buccal occlusion after correction of the asymmetry.

subdivision malocclusion. The left molar is tipped forward and needs to be uprighted to achieve a symmetric buccal occlusion. In Figure 10.2.29d–f the anterior segment of the three piece base arch is observed in the frontal view (d) as well as the right and left buccal occlusion (e, f). The extrusive forces experienced by the molar are usually counteracted by the forces of occlusion.

Once the axial inclination of the molar is corrected unilaterally and the buccal occlusion on the right and left sides are

symmetrical, the second step of orthodontic treatment can be initiated using symmetric mechanics in all four quadrants.

Conclusion

Patients presenting with significant clinical asymmetry pose special problems and treatment challenges to the orthodontist. Determination of the underlying cause of the asymmetry is an important first step in the formulation of an appropriate goal-oriented treatment plan. Meticulous clinical and radiographic evaluation, related dental cast analysis in centric relation and centric occlusion as well as a thorough review of the past medical and dental history are necessary to evaluate the asymmetry in three planes of space. Asymmetries may be solely of skeletal, dental, or functional origin or may express combination of these factors. When possible, the etiology of the asymmetry should be determined. This is particularly important when evaluating skeletal asymmetry. It is essential to determine whether the asymmetry is stable or progressive in nature secondary to abnormal growth or pathology. Progressive asymmetries which may be present in conditions such as condylar hyperplasia or condylar resorption may require deferring definitive orthognathic surgery until active metabolic activity stabilizes. In some cases, condylectomy with the placement of a costochondral rib graft may be indicated.

In the case of dental arch asymmetries, the treatment plan not only helps to identify the appropriate force system and the appropriate appliance design necessary to address the asymmetry but also minimizes undesirable side effects such as inadvertent tipping of the anterior occlusal plane. In this chapter, treatment strategies that can prove useful in fulfilling these objectives have been presented. Unilateral molar rotation, uprighting, and Class II correction using a variety of fixed and removable appliances have been reviewed. The best appliance to use in a given clinical situation is dependent on proper diagnosis and the clinician's thorough knowledge of the desired force system to achieve optimum treatment results.

References

Andrews LF. The six keys to normal occlusion. Am J Orthod. 1972;62:296–309.

de Araujo TM, Wilhelm RS, Almeida MA. Skeletal and dental arch asymmetries in Class II division I subdivision malocclusions. J Clin Pediatr Dent. 1994;18:181–185.

Arendt DM, Whitt JC, Hon CB, Curran TJ, Bate WS. Facial asymmetry. J Am Dent Assoc. 1990;120:688–690.

Arvystas MG, Antonellis P, Justin A. Progressive facial asymmetry as a result of early closure of the left coronal suture. Am J Orthod. 1985;87:240–246.

Bishara SE, Burkey PS, Kharouf JG. Dental and facial asymmetries: a review. Angle Orthod. 1994;64:89–98.

Blackwood HO. Clinical management of the Jasper Jumper. J Clin Orthod. 1991;25:755–760.

Bohuslavizki KH, Brenner W, Kerscher A, Fleiner B, Tinnemeyer S, Sippel C, Wolf H, Clausen M, Henze E. The value of bone scanning in pre-operative decision-making in patients with progressive facial asymmetry. Nucl Med Commun. 1996;17:562–567.

Burstone CJ. The rationale of the segmented arch. Am J Orthod. 1962;48:805–821.

Burstone CJ. Distinguishing developing malocclusion from normal occlusion. Dent Clin North Am. 1964;2:479–491.

Burstone CJ. Mechanics of the segmented arch technique. Angle Orthod. 1966;36:99–120.

Burstone CJ. Applications of bioengineering to clinical orthodontics. In: Graber TM, ed. Current Orthodontic Concepts and Techniques. Philadelphia: WB Saunders, 1985:154.

Burstone CJ. Precision lingual arches: active applications. J Clin Orthod. 1989;23:101–109.

Burstone CJ. The precision lingual arch: hinge cup attachments. J Clin Orthod. 1994;23:151–158.

Burstone CJ, Manhartsberger C. Precision lingual arches: passive applications. J Clin Orthod. 1988;22:444–451.

Cetlin NM, Ten Hoeve A. Non extraction treatment. J Clin Orthod. 1990;17:396–404.

Cohen MM Jr. Perspectives on craniofacial asymmetry. III. Common and/or well-known causes of asymmetry. Int J Oral Maxillofac Surg. 1995;24:127–133.

Cope JB, Buschang PM, Cope DD, Parker J, Blackwood HO. Quantitative evaluation of craniofacial changes with Jasper Jumper therapy. Angle Orthod. 1994;64:113–122.

Cory RC, Clayman DA, Faillace WJ, McKee SW, Gama CH. Clinical and radiographic findings in progressive facial hemiatrophy (Parry-Romberg syndrome). Am J Neuroradiol. 1997;18:751–757.

Faber RD. The differential diagnosis and treatment of crossbites. Dent Clin North Amer. 1981;25:53–68.

Gianelly AA, Bednar J, Dietz VS. Japanese NiTi coils used to move molars distally. Am J Orthod Dentofac Orthop. 1991;99:546–566.

Haack DC, Weinstein S. The mechanics of centric and eccentric cervical traction. Am J Orthod. 1958;44:346–357.

Hershey HG, Houghton CW, Burstone CJ. Unilateral face-bows: a theoretical and laboratory analysis. Am J Orthod. 1981;79:229–249.

Huang YL, Pogrel MA, Kaban LB. Diagnosis and management of condylar resorption. J Oral Maxillofac Surg. 1997;55:114–119.

Kaban LB, Moses MH, Mulliken JB. Surgical correction of hemifacial microsomia in the growing child. Plast Reconstr Surg. 1988;82:9–19.

Kaplan RG. Induced condylar growth in a patient with hemifacial microsomia. Angle Orthod. 1989;59:85–90.

Loomis MG, Radkowski MA, Pensler JM. Maxillary deformation in unilateral coronal synostosis. J Craniofac Surg. 1990;1:73–76.

Matteson SR, Proffit WR, Terry BC, Staab EV, Burkes EJ Jr. Bone scanning with^{99m}technetium phosphate to assess condylar hyperplasia. Report of two cases. Oral Surg Oral Med Oral Pathol. 1985;60:356–367.

Mazzeo N, Fisher JG, Mayer MH, Mathieu GP. Progressive hemifacial atrophy (Parry-Romberg syndrome). Case report. Oral Surg Oral Med Oral Pathol Oral Radiol Endod. 1995;79:30–35.

Mulliken JB, Ferraro NF, Vento AR. A retrospective analysis of growth of the constructed condyle-ramus in children with hemifacial microsomia. Cleft Palate J. 1989;26:312–317.

O'Byrn BL, Sadowsky C, Schneider B, BeGole EA. An evaluation of mandibular asymmetry in adults with unilateral posterior crossbite. Am J Orthod Dentofac Orthop. 1995;107:394–400.

Pirttiniemi PM. Associations of mandibular and facial asymmetries - a review. Am J Orthod Dentofac Orthop. 1994;106:191–200.

Proffit WR. Contemporary Orthodontics. St. Louis: Mosby-Year Book, 1993.

Proffit WR, Vig KW, Turvey TA. Early fracture of the mandibular condyles: frequently an unsuspected cause of growth disturbances. Am J Orthod. 1980;78:1–24.

Rose JM, Sadowsky C, BeGole EA, Moles R. Mandibular skeletal and dental asymmetry in Class II subdivision malocclusions. Am J Orthod Dentofac Orthop. 1994;105:489–495.

Shroff B, Lindauer SJ, Burstone CJ, Leiss JB. Segmented approach to simultaneous intrusion and space closure: biomechanics of the three-piece base arch appliance. Am J Orthod Dentofac Orthop. 1995;107:136–143.

Shroff B, Lindauer SJ, Burstone CJ. Class II subdivision treatment with tip back moments. Eur J Orthod. 1997;19:93–101.

Skolnick J, Iranpour B, Westesson PL, Adair S. Prepubertal trauma and mandibular asymmetry in orthognathic surgery and orthodontic patients. Am J Orthod Dentofac Orthop. 1994;105:73–77.

Smith RJ, Burstone CJ. Mechanics of tooth movement. Am J Orthod. 1984;85:294–307.

Thurow R. Edgewise Orthodontics. St. Louis: CV Mosby, 1966.

Tweed C. Clinical Orthodontics. St. Louis: CV Mosby, 1966.

Van Steenbergen E, Nanda R. Biomechanics of orthodontic correction of dental asymmetries. Am J Orthod Dentofac Orthop. 1995;107:618–624.

11

Treatment Principles

11.1

Dentofacial Orthopedics in the Management of Hemifacial Microsomia and Nager Syndrome Cases

Birte Melsen and Athanasios E. Athanasiou

CHAPTER MENU

Introduction

Hemifacial microsomia is a congenital disorder of the craniofacial region that affects the development of the lower half of the face and commonly also the ears, facial skin, and mouth. It is called as such because it occurs mainly on one side of the face as the small jaw, but it can be also manifested at both sides of the face simultaneously in 10–15% of patients. Its main etiopathogenic units are the condyle and gonial angle, mostly unilaterally, and the ear abnormalities vary greatly in its external and middle parts (Choi et al. 2015). It presents similar manifestations with the Goldenhar syndrome (additionally, vertebral defects and epibular dermoids) but its etiology is heterogeneous (Tuin et al. 2015). Hemifacial microsomia results from the malformation of the first and second branchial arches (Poswillo 1973). It is considered the second in prevalence syndrome after cleft lip and palatal; it occurs in 1/3500–1/5600 births, and it is not inherited (Tuin et al. 2015). Hemifacial microsomia can present variable signs and symptoms, ranging from the slight asymmetry of face to the complete absence of one ear, small ipsilateral face, facial nerve palsy, and the cleft of the mouth corner (Tuin et al. 2015).

The extent that characterizes the involvement of the temporomandibular joint (TMJ) determines timing and type of treatment that has focused on the possibilities of influencing the growth of the different determinants of mandibular form and size by controlling the quantity and quality of the condylar cartilaginous proliferation. McNamara (1980) reviewed the results of studies on functional appliances performed on animals or based on clinical observations of young children. Also the similar effect of condylar growth by bringing the mandible forward was described many years ago (Weinmann and Sicher 1955) and experiments performed on rats underlined the importance of the treatment timing when trying to generate longer mandibles in these animals (Stutzmann and Petrovic 1979). The influence on growth of the human mandible with a functional appliance was shown to be dependent on the turnover rate meaning the growth potential of the child (Petrovic et al. 1991). The influence of the occlusion and function was the focus of several of the Moyer's symposia held in Ann Arbor, Michigan, United States, and monograph no. 4 focused specifically on determinants of mandibular form and growth (McNamara et al. 1975), where the influence of function was discussed and demonstrated by Harvold (1975). Later Harvold (1983) published the concept on which the treatment of hemifacial microsomia was based. The treatment principles of hemifacial microsomia have been chosen according to the age. In reference to the use of functional appliances at an early age, there are two benefits. First, depending on the amount that a favorable growth response takes place, the outcome of surgical treatment, if necessary, would be better. Second, any necessary surgical reconstruction would be focused mainly on the osseous components (Proffit and Turvey 1991).

The present chapter will present examples of slow distraction in young children by means of functional appliances (Harvold activator), splints, and pivot appliances, respectively. These case reports illustrate how the relation muscle-bone interaction will be able to influence the condylar growth in patients with insufficient height of the mandible unilaterally.

Case Reports

Case Report 1

The patient was diagnosed as a hemifacial microsomia without any dental anomalies and affection of ears and tags (Figure 11.1.1a–d). The patient at the age of 4 years referred from the pedodontist who had noted the asymmetric opening pattern. The asymmetry of the face had not been noted until then. The careful clinical examination performed at the Orthodontic Clinic verified a marked deviation of the mandible to the left side, which was significantly exaggerated during maximal opening. The profile evaluation gave the impression of a relative mandibular retrognathism with a rather convex profile. The patient exhibited a complete deciduous dentition with neutral molar relationship on the right side and distal molar relationship on the left side. Both arches were asymmetrical and there was a midline discrepancy of 4 mm.

Evaluation of both the frontal and the panoramic radiographs revealed a pronounced asymmetry of the mandible with the chin deviation to the left (Figure 11.1.1f). Measuring the maximal length from the muscle attachment, the dimension of the right side was 26 mm longer than the left side. Left condyle and ramus were underdeveloped. According to Chierici (1983), the patient presented with a Type II mandibular deformity with missing condylar head and neck. A pronounced pre-angular notch was also present on both sides (Figure 11.1.1f).

The extraoral photograph of the sagittal view demonstrated a mandibular retrognathism and a convex profile obviously caused by the increased sagittal jaw relationship related to the short-left side of the mandible. Labial inclination of the lower incisors and lingual inclination of the upper incisors compensated for the increased sagittal jaw relationship resulting in 3 mm overjet. The posterior margins of the ramus deviated 13 mm horizontally at the level of the external cranial base.

The frontal cephalometric radiograph confirmed the marked asymmetry and showed a compensatory inclination of the lower incisors to the right and of the upper incisors to the left. The spina mentalis of the mandible deviated 15 mm from the midline constructed as a perpendicular to the orbital roof through Crista Galli.

When the patient's parents were informed about the mandibular malformation, they were provided with different approaches to the treatment of their daughter's problem. They could wait until the end of growth and then perform a surgical-orthodontic treatment (Kaban et al. 1981), treat during pre-pubertal and pubertal growth, and finish with surgery, if necessary (Ousterhout and Owsley 1983; Vargervik 1985), or start as soon as possible with the use of functional appliances and still possibly have the need for surgery when reaching adulthood.

The parents selected the third option with the use of a functional appliance (Harvold activator) with a construction bite above the rest position. The principle of this treatment approach is illustrated in Figure 11.1.2 and has been previously described in detail (Melsen et al. 1986).

In this approach, the activator with a construction bite that lowered the condyle on the affected side over the freeway space forcing the mandible into the correct midline by rotating the mandible around the healthy condyle was fabricated and used. The acrylic was removed from occlusal contact which allowed the maxillary teeth in the underdeveloped side to erupt. In the unaffected side, the acrylic was maintained with full coverage. The patient was instructed to wear the activator each night and 1–2 hours a day (Figure 11.1.1e).

After 6 months, the activator was replaced with a new one to stay above the freeway space (Figure 11.1.1g). This was repeated every 6 month, after 4 years a new set of radiographs and photographs were produced (Figure 11.1.1h–l), and the treatment continued. Two years later, the treatment was terminated and at the age of 12 years a new set of diagnostic records was produced (Figure 11.1.1m–q).

At the age of 12 years, the face appeared symmetric and when opening the mouth, the patient performed a symmetric movement of the mandible. The occlusion was normal in all three planes of space and the midlines coincided. Radiographic analysis confirmed that the asymmetry was significantly reduced although the panoramic radiograph demonstrated that the condylar process of the affected side was still underdeveloped and had maintained the Type II deformity classification (Chierici 1983). However, the difference in ramus height between affected and non-affected sides had been reduced significantly. The spontaneous uprighting of the incisors in the frontal view was obvious. The frontal cephalometric radiograph confirmed the reduction of the asymmetry in all planes of space. The extraoral photograph of the sagittal view demonstrated significant decrease in both the mandibular retrognathism and the convexity of the profile that characterized the patient pre-treatment.

The conclusion of this treatment confirmed the studies by Harvold (1983).

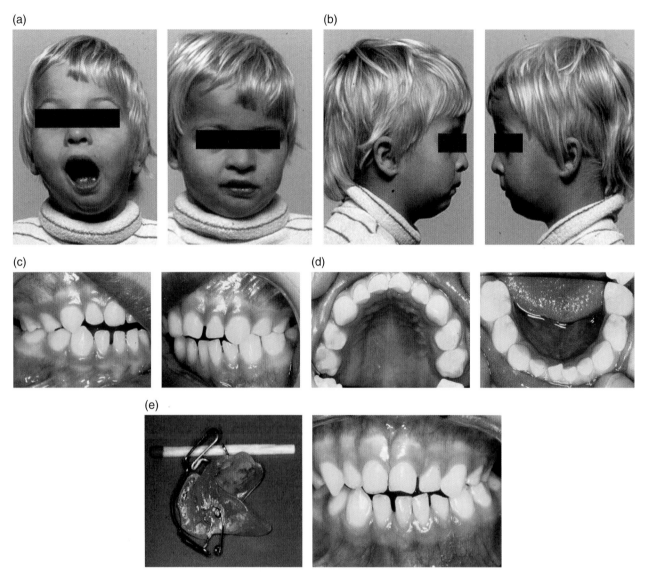

Figure 11.1.1 (a–d) A 4-year-old female patient diagnosed with a hemifacial microsomia without any dental anomalies and affection of ears and tags. The careful clinical examination verified a marked deviation of the mandible to the left side, which was significantly exaggerated during maximal opening. The profile evaluation gave the impression of a relative mandibular retrognathism with a rather convex profile. The patient exhibited a complete deciduous dentition with neutral molar relationship on the right side and distal molar relationship on the left side. (e) The Harvold activator was made with a construction bite that lowered the condyle on the affected side over the freeway space forcing the mandible into the correct midline by rotating the mandible around the healthy condyle was fabricated and used. (f) Evaluation of both the frontal and the panoramic radiographs revealed a pronounced asymmetry of the mandible with the chin deviation to the left. (g) After 6 months the activator was replaced with a new one to stay above the freeway space. (h–l) After 4 years a new set of radiographs and photographs were produced and the treatment continued. (m–q) Two years later the treatment was terminated and at the age of 12 years a new set of diagnostic records was produced. Assessment of the panoramic and frontal radiographs showed that the difference in ramus height between affected and non-affected side had been reduced significantly, the extraoral photograph of the sagittal view demonstrated significant decrease of both the mandibular retrognathism and the convexity of the profile that characterized the patient pre-treatment.

(f)

(g)

(h)

(i)

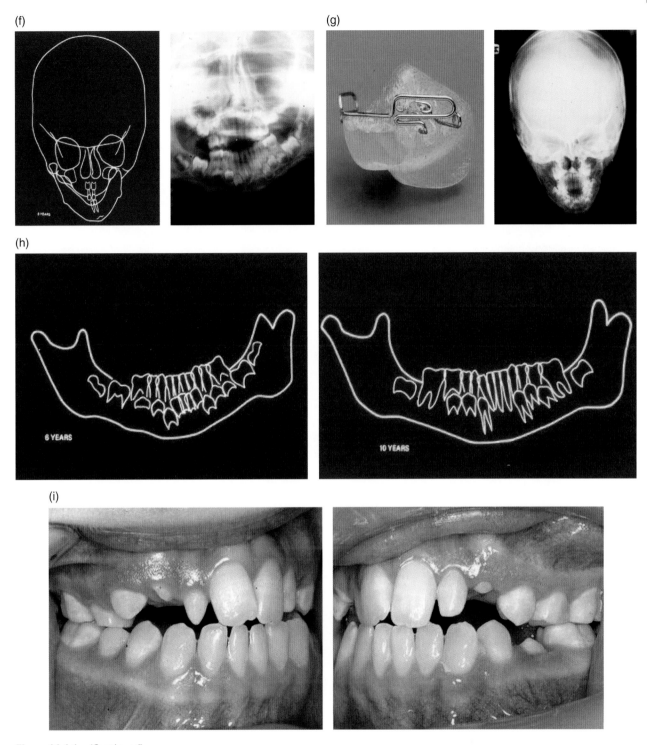

Figure 11.1.1 (Continued)

(j)

(k)

(l)

(m)

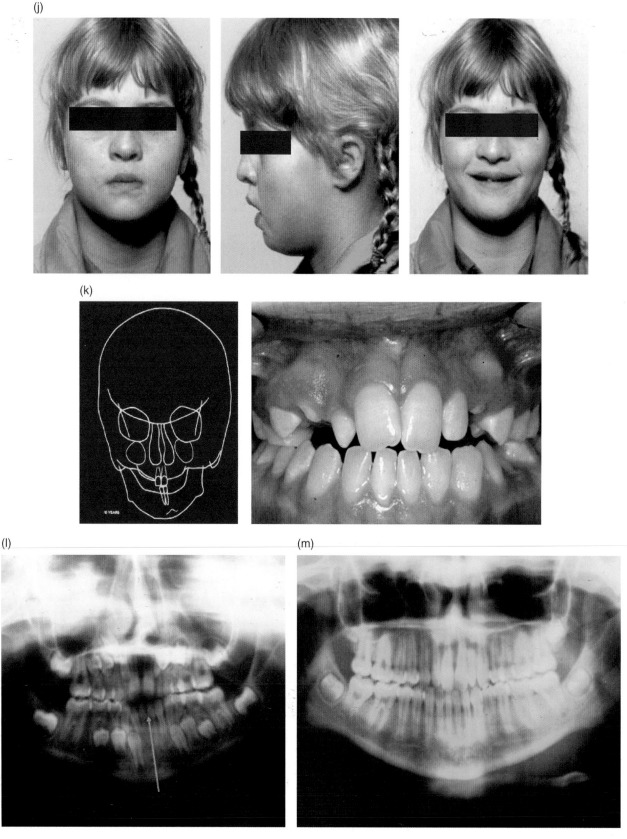

Figure 11.1.1 (Continued)

(n)

(q)

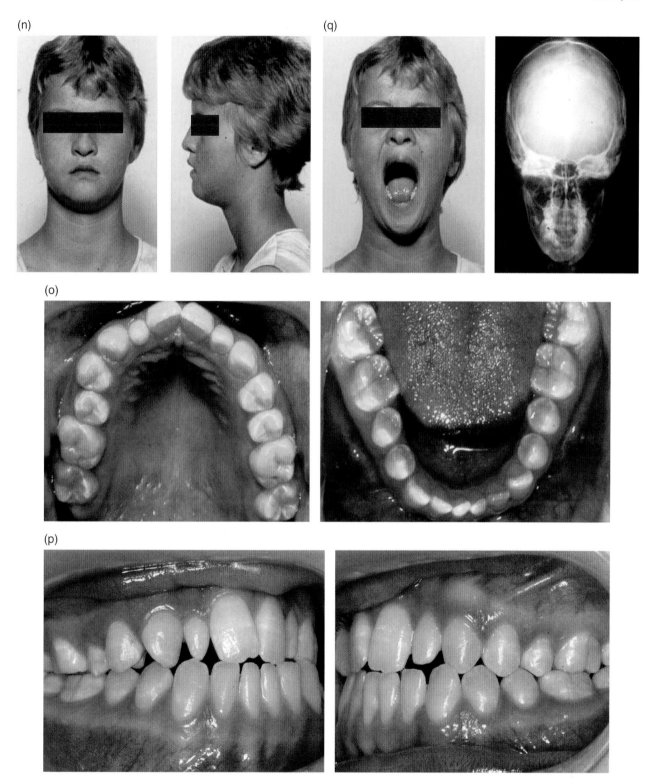

(o)

(p)

Figure 11.1.1 (Continued)

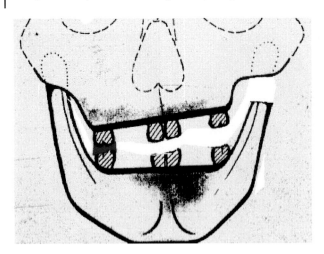

Figure 11.1.2 The principle with the use of a functional appliance with a construction bite above the rest position.

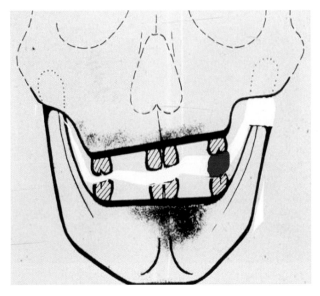

Figure 11.1.3 The approach applied in the treatment by means of a splint that could be used 24 hours per day in order to generate an open bite on the affected side. The idea was to use the patient's muscle force to maintain the deformed mandibular ramus lowered by the masticatory force.

Case Report 2

The patient was a 12-year-old boy suffering from hemifacial microsomia that was reflected mainly by a tilted occlusal plane. At that age, a major part of the growth had taken place and it was concluded that the condylar distraction as applied in the case report 1 would not be sufficient to generate the desired effect. Therefore, a splint therapy that could be used 24 hours per day was planned and executed. The approach applied in this treatment is illustrated in Figure 11.1.3.

The clinical examination revealed a boy with an asymmetric face with the mandible deviating toward the left side and an occlusal plane tilted downward on the right side (Figure 11.1.4a). He also exhibited skin tags and ear deformity on the affected side.

The principle in his treatment was, opposite of the patient of case report 1, namely to generate an open bite on the affected side with a splint that was used almost full-time (as close to 24 hours a day). The idea was to use the patient's muscle force to maintain the deformed mandibular ramus lowered by the masticatory force.

The first step of this treatment was to perform the resilience test in order to measure how much the patient could distract the affected condyle and still generate contact on the healthy side. The test was done by adding layers of aluminum foil with a thickness of 0.2 mm on the affected side of the mouth and ask the patient to occlude on the healthy side. When occluding on the healthy side, the patient would rotate the mandible around the healthy condyle. Once the resilience test had verified how much the patient could distract the condyle, a set of study casts were produced and mounted in an adjustable activator, a vacuum-pulled 1 mm splint was produced and a selective grinding was so that the splint did not rise the bite as it would be perforated in single places (Figure 11.1.4b and c). The aluminum foil used to demonstrate the resilience was then placed in the housing of the condyle (Figure 11.1.4d).

Afterward, an acrylic splint with occlusal contact on the affected side and an opening corresponding to the resilience was produced. Patient was instructed to wear the splint full time. After 1 year, an open bite was generated on the affected side and the splint was activated to be above the freeway space (Figure 11.1.4e). After 2 years, the face appeared symmetrical and the splint was adjusted so that the upper left molars were free to erupt. When looking at the posttreatment panoramic radiograph (Figure 11.1.4h) the characteristics and comparison of the mandibular condyles in the non-affected and affected sides at the final stage of treatment can be noted and fixed appliances are visible in the upper dental arch for alignment and leveling. Although the patient's mandibular position at the chin point shows to be symmetric, the skin tags and ear deformity on the affected side remained present (Figure 11.1.4i).

Case Report 3

This patient was a 4-year-old boy treated with a pivot appliance. The boy was suffering from a Nager syndrome first described in the medical literature by Nager and de Reynier (1948). Nager syndrome belongs to a group of disorders collectively known as acrofacial dysostoses (AFDs). These disorders are characterized by craniofacial and limb abnormalities.

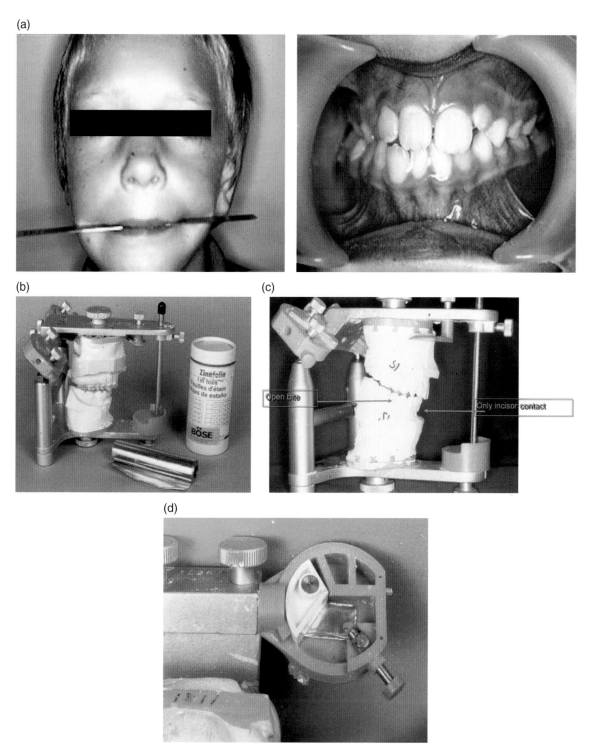

Figure 11.1.4 (a) The clinical examination revealed a boy with an asymmetric face with the mandible deviating toward the left side and an occlusal plane tilted downward on the right side. He also exhibited skin tags and ear deformity on the affected side. (b–d) The resilience test in order to measure how much the patient could distract the affected condyle and still generate contact on the healthy side was done by adding layers of aluminum foil with a thickness of 0.2 mm on the affected side of the mouth and ask the patient to occlude on the healthy side. Once the resilience test had verified how much the patient could distract the condyle, a set of study casts was produced and mounted in an adjustable activator, a vacuum-pulled 1 mm splint was produced and a selective grinding was so that the splint did not rise the bite as it would be perforated in single places. (d) The aluminum foil used to demonstrate the resilience was then placed in the housing of the condyle. (e) An acrylic splint with occlusal contact on the affected side and an opening corresponding to the resilience was produced. (f, g) After 2 years, the face appeared symmetrical and the splint was adjusted so that the upper left molars were free to erupt. (h) When looking at the posttreatment panoramic radiograph the characteristics and comparison of the mandibular condyles in the non-affected and affected sides at the final stage of treatment can be noted and fixed appliances are visible in the upper dental arch for alignment and leveling. (i) The patient's mandibular position at the chin point shows to be symmetric but the skin tags and ear deformity on the affected side remained present.

(e)

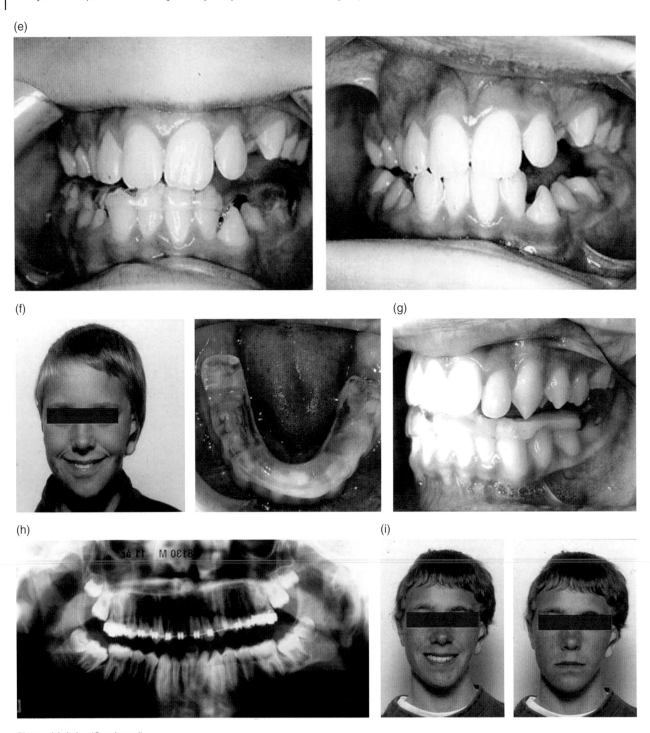

(f)

(g)

(h)

(i)

Figure 11.1.4 (Continued)

The family of the patient did not want clinical images published, but the panoramic radiograph revealed that there was no condyle on the left side of the mandible (Figure 11.1.5a). To stress, the boy of a minimum pivot resting the deciduous molars were build up on the affected side. This generated an open bite on the healthy side. A panoramic radiograph taken 3 years later demonstrated almost 1 cm of extra growth and a shape which simulated a condyle (Figure 11.1.5b). Two images of the condylar area illustrate that a condyle-like structure had developed. The yellow line indicates the increased length from the last tooth bud to the distal contour of the mandible (Figure 11.1.5c).

(a)

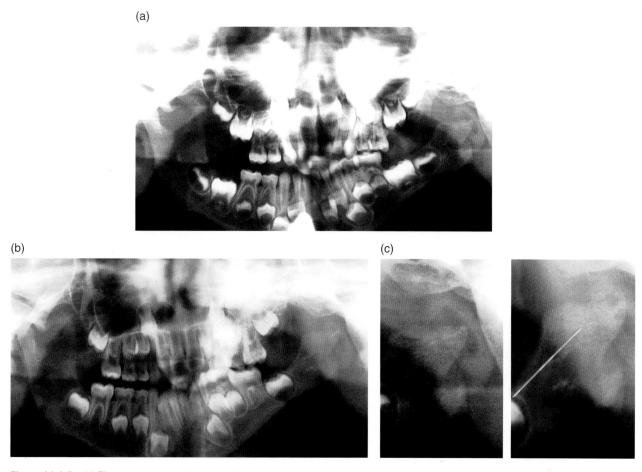

(b)   (c)

Figure 11.1.5 (a) The panoramic radiograph of the male patient with Nager syndrome at the age of 4-years revealed the absence of condyle on the left side of the mandible. (b) The panoramic radiograph taken after 3 years of treatment by the pivot appliance demonstrated almost 1 cm of extra growth and a shape which simulated a condyle. (c) The two images of the condylar area illustrate that its structure had developed. The yellow line indicates the increased length from the last tooth bud to the distal contour of the mandible (Figure c).

Discussion

The advantage of the non-surgical methods with slow distraction was clearly the good effect on both hard and soft tissue and with a limited need for finishing orthodontic treatment. The big disadvantage was obviously the long treatment times and the need for collaboration by the patient. To overcome the need for the long treatment and to offer a treatment to the patients who did not receive slow distraction treatment when they were young, based on CT scanning and production of stereometric models, Harvold (1975) demonstrated distraction elongation of the ramus in adult patients (Figure 11.1.6a). In this approach, a comprehensive and lengthy orthodontic treatment was needed to obtain a satisfactory occlusion. Although the midline and the occlusion were corrected, the disadvantage of the distraction of this approach was that the function and thereby the soft tissues were not part of the treatment. The clear disadvantage was that when observing the changes occurring during the remaining growth period, they comprised only the hard tissues and not the muscles (Figure 11.1.6b–f). Although the occlusion was corrected surgically the face remained asymmetrically as the function was not influenced.

A different combination with slow distraction followed by surgical distraction may allow for the muscle function to follow the improved occlusion and the remaining skeletal deviation can be corrected with a surgical distraction focusing on the correction of the asymmetric occlusion.

Studies concerning the long-term efficiency of distraction osteogenesis in correcting face asymmetry in hemifacial macrosomia patients have expressed reservation regarding the use of this method at an early age because its results may not hold up in the long term (Marquez et al. 2000; Polley and Figueroa 1997).

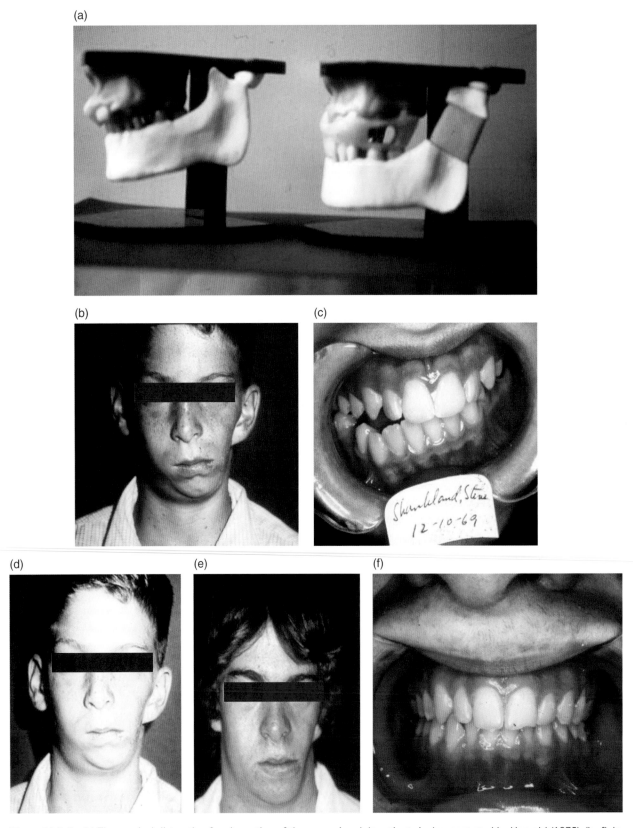

Figure 11.1.6 (a) The surgical distraction for elongation of the ramus in adult patients is demonstrated by Harvold (1975). (b–f). In this case of hemifacial microsomia, a comprehensive and lengthy orthodontic treatment was needed to obtain a satisfactory occlusion. Although the midline and the occlusion were corrected, the disadvantage of the distraction of this approach was that the function and thereby the soft tissues were not part of the treatment thus with the face to remain asymmetric.

The patients described in this chapter were treated for the asymmetry being part of a hemifacial microsomia. In cases characterized as hemifacial microsomia and with the condylar head missing, the asymmetry is reported to increase in severity with age (Caldarelli and Valvassori 1979; Rune et al. 1981). Cases of hemifacial microsomia of mild severity and without missing condylar cartilage may remain asymmetric but without further deterioration. In these cases, the skeletal mandibular asymmetry is not progressive in nature and growth of the affected side in these patients parallels that of the non-affected side (Polley et al. 1997).

In the cases presented in this chapter, the patients did not exhibit a normal condylar cartilage. However, in spite of this doubtful prognosis, all patients responded positively to the slow distraction applied. The general principle followed in the three cases was to generate a change in muscle activity which was deviating from normal (Harvold 1983). The aim of the treatment was to establish a new stress system that led to bone apposition in the region of the condylar region.

The problem that the cases presented was a ramus that was too short unilaterally to support the mandible in a correct relation to the skull. The first case suffered from a facial asymmetry and a pronounced convexity of the face. The means by which the necessary stress system could be established was an activator with the construction bite above the freeway space. Thereby the sensory input from the periodontium was maximized as a result of the slow distraction. The multiplane analysis proposed by Grayson et al. (1983) has demonstrated that the correction of the asymmetry was normally more pronounced anteriorly than in the posterior planes. The cases described in this paper demonstrated that with slow distraction the corrections were clearly more in the posterior planes including the glenoid fossa region. This finding also corroborates with a report on activator treatment using implants as growth markers (Birkebæk et al. 1984; Bjørk 1963).

The three cases clearly demonstrated that generation of a normal muscle balance is possible even in absence of a condyle. Although similar case reports suggest that treatment of hemifacial microsomia should be initiated early enough so that the stimulus could to some degree normalize the deficient tissues and induce bone apposition (Sidiropoulou et al. 2003), the small number of cases published and the long treatment time that is necessary for this kind of management could be considered as drawbacks for this concept of management.

Since a study of large populations has been missing, Lópes et al. (2022) performed a systematic review of the literature on treatment of hemifacial microsomia. A total number of 1137 papers were collected that satisfied the search criteria, but only 27 strictly fulfilled all the criteria. Of these, 21 were only case reports. In most of these reports, applied vertical correction and stabilization of the occlusal plane were performed. This systematic literature review further demonstrated that the evidence derived from the available literature was of poor quality and the authors concluded that well-designed prospective studies of homogenous samples with long-term follow-up should be performed.

Realistically speaking, this requirement has no chance to be fulfilled. As the prevalence of hemifacial microsomia is small and the variation in the severity big, not even multi-center collaboration would fulfill minimum requirements for prospective clinical trials. The only solution would be if the requirements for registrations would be standardized and assembled in a common databank which after 10–15 years would improve the basis on which patients with hemifacial microsomia can be treated. A similar approach has been attempted regarding cleft palate management protocols without reaching a final solution.

Conclusion

The cases described in this chapter demonstrated that treatments of mandibular asymmetries, if started early, can be done with slow distraction thus avoiding surgery.

It is, however, imperative that the patients accept long treatment times and in addition, the risk that surgery at the end of growth might be necessary.

There is no doubt that the response to treatments is varying between patients and that the severity, but also the genetics, play a role in the success. The slow distraction will always contribute to a better final result.

References

Birkebæk L, Melsen B, Terp S. A laminografic study of the tempero-mandibular joint following activator treatment. Eur J Orhod. 1984;6:257–266.

Bjørk A. Variations in the growth pattern of the human mandible: longitudinal radiographic study by the implant method. J Dent Res. 1963;42:400–411.

Caldarelli DD, Valvassori GE. A radiographic analysis of first and second branchial arch anomalies. In: Converse JM, McCarthy JG, Wood-Smith D, eds. Symposium on Diagnosis and Treatment of Craniofacial Anomalies. St. Louis: The CV Mosby Company, 1979.

Chierici G. Radiologic assessment of facial asymmetry. In: Harvold EP, ed. Treatment of Hemifacial Mircrosomia. New York: Alan R Liss, 1983.

Choi JW, Kim BH, Kim HS, Yu TH, Kim BC, Lee SH. Three-dimensional functional unit analysis of hemifacial macrosomia mandible – a preliminary report. Maxillofac Plast Reconstr Surg. 2015;37:28.

Grayson BH, Boral S, Eisig S, Kolber A, McCarthy JG. Unilateral craniofacial microsomia. Part 1. Mandibular analysis. Am J Orthod. 1983;84:225–230.

Harvold EP. Centric relation. A study of pressure and tension systems in bone modeling and mandibular positioning. Dent Clin N Am. 1975;19:473–484.

Harvold EP. The theoretical basis for the treatment of hemifacial microsomia. In: Harvold EP, Vagervik K, Chierici G, eds. Treatment of Hemifacial Microsomia. New York: Alan R Liss Inc, 1983.

Kaban LB, Mulliken JB, Murray JE. Three-dimensional approach to analysis and treatment of hemifacial microsomia. Cleft Palate J. 1981;18:90–99.

Lópes DF, Acosta DM, Rivera DA, Mejia CM. Hemifacial micosomia: treatment alternatives – a systematic review of literature. J Clin Pediatr Dent. 2022; 46:15–30.

Marquez IM, Fish LC, Stella JP. Two-year follow-up of distraction osteogenesis: its effect on mandibular ramus height in hemifacial microsomia. Am J Orthod Dentofac Orthop. 2000;117:130–139.

McNamara JA. Functional determinants of craniofacial size and shape. Eur J Orthod. 1980;2:131–159.

McNamara JA, Connelly TG, McBride MC. Histological studies of temporomandibular joint adaptations. In: McNamara JA, ed. Determinant of Mandibular Form and Growth. Monograph 4, Cranial Growth Series, Center for Human Growth and Development. Ann Arbor: University of Michigan, 1975:209–227.

Melsen B, Bjerregård J, Bundgård M. The effect of treatment with functional appliance on a pathologic growth pattern

of the condyle. Am J Orthod Dentofac Orthop. 1986; 90:503–512.

Nager FR, de Reynier JP. Das Gehörorgan bei den angeborene Kopfmissbildungen. Basel: S Karger, 1948.

Ousterhout DK, Owsley JK Jr. Skeletal surgery in hemifacial microsomia. In: Harvold EP, ed. Treatment of Hemifacial Microsomia. New York: Alan R Liss Inc, 1983.

Petrovic A, Stutzmann J, Lavergne J, Shaye R. Is it possible to modulate the growth of the human mandible with a functional appliance? Int J Orthod. 1991;29(1–2):3–8.

Polley JW, Figueroa AA. Distraction osteogenesis: its application in severe mandibular deformities in hemifacial microsomia. J Craniofac Surg. 1997;8:422–430.

Polley JW, Figueroa AA, Liou EJ, Cohen M. Longitudinal analysis of mandibular asymmetry in hemifacial microsomia. Plast Reconstr Surg. 1997;99:328–339.

Poswillo D. The pathogenesis of the first and second branchial arch syndrome. Oral Surg Oral Med Oral Pathol. 1973;35:302–328.

Proffit WR, Turvey TA. Dentofacial asymmetry. In: Proffit WR, White RP Jr, eds. Surgical – Orthodontic Treatment. St. Louis: Mosby Year Book, 1991:483–549.

Rune B, Selvik G, Sarnäs KV, Jacobsson S. Growth in hemifacial macrosomia studied with the aid of roentgen stereophotogrammetry and metallic implants. Cleft Palate J. 1981;18:128–146.

Sidiropoulou S, Antoniades K, Kolokithas G. Orthopedically induced condylar growth in a patient with hemifacial microsomia. Cleft Palate Craniofac J. 2003;40:645–650.

Stutzmann J, Petrovic A. Intrinsic regulation of the condylar cartilage growth rate. Eur J Orthod. 1979;1:41–54.

Tuin J, Tahiri Y, Paliga JT, Taylor JA, Bartlett SP. Distinguishing Goldenhar syndrome from craniofacial microsomia. J Craniofac Surg. 2015;26:1887–1892.

Vargervik K. Muscle activity and bone formation. Prog Clin Biol Res. 1985;187:269–279.

Weinmann JP, Sicher A. Bone and Bones. St. Louis: The C.V. Mosby, 1955: 108.

11.2

Rational Diagnosis and Treatment of Dental Asymmetries

Joseph Bouserhal, Nikhillesh Vaiid, Ismaeel Hansa, Zakaria Bentahar, Lea J. Bouserhal, and Philippe J. Bouserhal

Introduction

Dental asymmetries are considered as one of the most difficult scenarios to manage in orthodontics. A correct differential diagnosis constitutes the cornerstone for any biomechanical application. These asymmetries could be classified by their location as either posterior or anterior, by their orientation in the occlusal, the sagittal, or the frontal plane, and by their etiology which could be dental, functional, or skeletal. Anterior asymmetries are generally more difficult to treat due to their interaction with smile esthetics. Posterior asymmetries, which are more discrete, have to be also considered for a better occlusal intermaxillary relationship and in the pursuit of excellence in orthodontics. The aim of this chapter is to identify different types of dental asymmetries, to develop a differential diagnosis, and to apply individualized treatment mechanics depending on each case.

The objectives of orthodontic treatment encompass dentofacial esthetics, functional occlusion, periodontal health, and stability. As Peck et al. (1990) mentioned, symmetry plays an important role in dentofacial esthetics. Asymmetry may be expressed as mandibular deviations, occlusal cants, dental midline shifts, or simple gingival height discrepancies (Sarver and Ackerman 2003). Perfect symmetry seldom occurs in nature, however, and the development of the human face and dentition is no different (Lundstrom 1961).

Some degree of facial and dental asymmetry occurs in virtually all individuals (Bishara et al. 1994; Ferrario et al. 1993; Ming 2006; Sheats et al. 1998; Smith and Bailit 1979; Yoon et al. 2013). Facial asymmetry can have dental, functional, or skeletal causes or a combination of the three (Bishara et al. 1994; Joondeph 2000). An asymmetry in a single dimension has the potential to cause other asymmetries in other dimensions within the craniofacial complex. The question then arises: What is a clinically acceptable asymmetry for the various dentofacial features? Beyer and Lindauer (1998) suggest midline asymmetry greater than 2.2 mm is discernible. Choi (2015) suggested that facial asymmetries within 3–4% and 3–4 mm are not clinically detectable.

According to Sheats et al. (1998), the most common asymmetries in patients presenting for orthodontic treatment were mandibular midline deviation from the facial midline, occurring in 62% of patients, followed by lack of dental midline coincidence (46%), maxillary midline deviation from the facial midline (39%), molar classification asymmetry (22%), maxillary occlusal asymmetry, (20%) and mandibular occlusal asymmetry (18%). Facial asymmetry (6%), chin deviation (4%), and nasal deviation (3%) made up the remainder.

Dental deviations should be treated as far as possible with intra-arch mechanics, functional deviations with inter-arch mechanics, and skeletal deviations with orthognathic surgery. While some degree of asymmetry is definitely part of natural appearance, symmetry is the ideal that we should treat toward (Pinho et al. 2007).

Classification of Dental Asymmetries

Facial asymmetry can be classified into skeletal, functional, or dental. Dental asymmetries, although somewhat associated with skeletal asymmetry, can be categorized into posterior and anterior depending on their location.

The posterior asymmetries can then be further classified into occlusal, sagittal, and frontal plane asymmetries, while anterior asymmetries can be divided into asymmetries of dental, functional, or skeletal origin.

Diagnosis of Dental Asymmetries

The diagnosis of asymmetry follows the traditional comprehensive orthodontic clinical examination including photographs, study models, occlusograms, and cone beam computed tomography (CBCT) (or panoramic radiograph, lateral cephalometric radiography, submental cephalometric radiography, and frontal cephalometric radiography, if a CBCT is unavailable).

The extra-oral clinical examination of asymmetry is performed with the patient in the natural head position and involves utilizing some specific facial planes and landmarks, i.e. the interpupillary line, and a vertical line

through the glabella perpendicular to the inter-pupillary line, tip of the nose, and center of the philtrum and chin (Figure 11.2.1). The clinical examination for asymmetry can be performed by looking from a frontal view. In addition, looking from inferior view of the mandible can aid in determining the extent of deviation (Cheney 1961) (Figure 11.2.2). Alternatively, a straight instrument or piece of floss placed in line with the facial midline can aid in visualization of asymmetry (Figure 11.2.3).

A frontal facial photo is ideal to investigate asymmetry, where the anatomical landmarks and constructed lines can be drawn digitally and compared, which may be awkward when done in-person. The presence of an occlusal cant should also be assessed at this stage. This can be done by asking the patient to bite on a tongue blade which is positioned in the canine area, and comparing it to the interpupillary line (Arnett and Bergman 1993) (Figure 11.2.4). Furthermore, a frontal examination of the patient smiling, with their mouth closed and then slightly opened, will also aid in observing any asymmetry of the smile or cant of the occlusal plane, respectively.

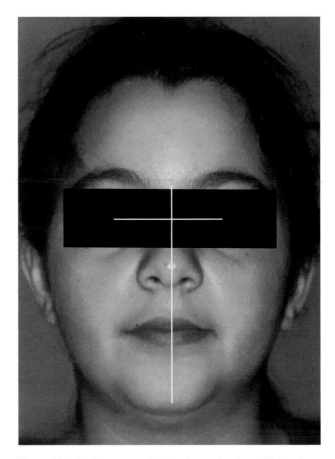

Figure 11.2.1 An extra-oral clinical examination utilizing the interpupillary line, and a vertical line through the glabella perpendicular to the interpupillary line.

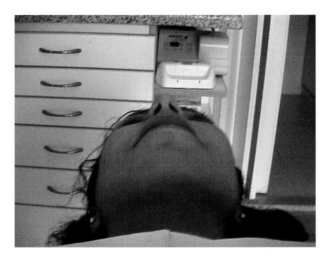

Figure 11.2.2 A clinical examination can be performed by looking from inferior view of the mandible.

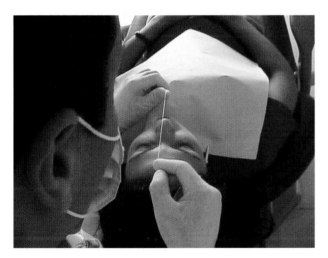

Figure 11.2.3 A straight instrument or piece of floss placed in line with the facial midline can aid in visualization of asymmetry.

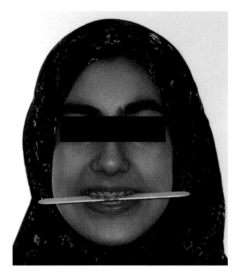

Figure 11.2.4 The presence of an occlusal cant assessed by asking the patient to bite on a tongue blade and comparing it to the inter-pupillary line.

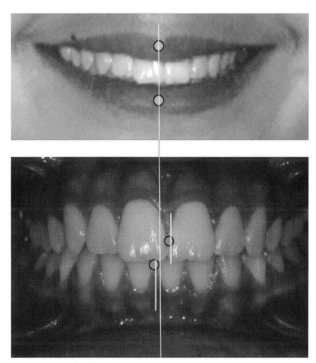

Figure 11.2.5 Examination of dental midline asymmetry.

A clinical examination should involve screening for functional asymmetries such as mandibular dental midline deviations during opening, centric relationship, first contact of the occlusion, and in occlusion (Bishara et al. 1994). True dental or skeletal asymmetries will exhibit similar midline discrepancy in both centric relation and centric occlusion. Conversely, functional asymmetries due to occlusal interferences will show a midline discrepancy between centric relation and centric occlusion as the mandible shifts laterally.

Moving intra-orally, the facial midline is coincident with the upper lip philtrum and the midpalatal suture, and these landmarks should be used when measuring the upper dental midline deviation. In both the upper and lower arches, the labial or lingual frena should not be used

as a reference landmark, due to their alveolar insertion which adapts and alters based on tooth position (Figure 11.2.5).

Dental arch asymmetry should also be investigated at this point and can be further inspected using a dental cast. The dental cast can also be investigated for asymmetry via an occlusogram, which involves the use of a grid to aid in measurement of dental arch asymmetries (Faber 1992;

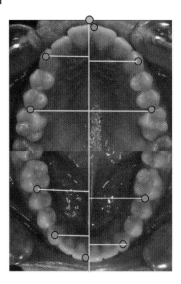
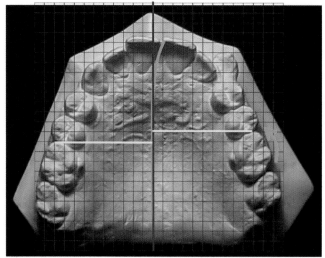

Figure 11.2.6 Asymmetry of dental arches evaluation.

Fiorelli and Melsen 1999; White 1982). This allows for discrete measurements of the left and right differences and asymmetries in different planes (Figure 11.2.6).

Dental arch asymmetries can be caused by skeletal factors, such as the rotation of the entire dental arch and the maxillary base, or by local factors such as the premature loss of primary teeth. Asymmetry of the buccolingual inclination of the posterior teeth, especially in cases with a unilateral crossbite, should be assessed to determine if an asymmetry is of dental, functional, or skeletal origin.

In certain cases, where the cause of asymmetry is unclear, a therapeutic diagnosis can be attempted. An outwardly apparent asymmetric occlusion may become symmetric after leveling and aligning of the arches or via the use of an occlusal splint. This usually manifests itself when there is an initial premature contact that causes a functional mandibular deviation.

The radiographic examination for asymmetry should start with conventional panoramic and cephalometric radiographs. The panoramic radiograph enables the clinician to view the condyles for size and shape discrepancies, as well as irregular cortical borders (Figure 11.2.7). While the condylar length and ramus length may be measured as well, positioning errors of the patient tends to make these measurements unreliable and is better evaluated using CBCT.

A lateral cephalometric radiograph can be used to identify mandibular asymmetry by observing the two borders of the mandible (Figure 11.2.8). This also has some reliability issues, however, as the patient's head positioning may lead to small discrepancies between the borders of the mandible (Bishara et al. 1994). Hence only gross and obvious asymmetry can be reliably identified. Frontal and submental cephalometry has been the traditional go-to method for evaluating skeletal asymmetry due to the right and left

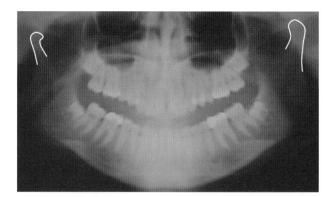

Figure 11.2.7 Panoramic radiographic examination.

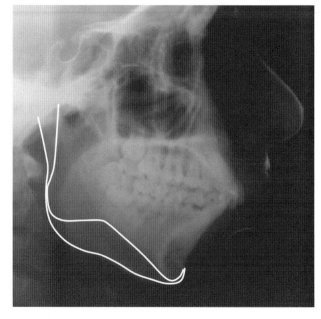

Figure 11.2.8 Identification of mandibular asymmetry on a lateral cephalometric radiograph.

Figure 11.2.9 Frontal cephalometric evaluation.

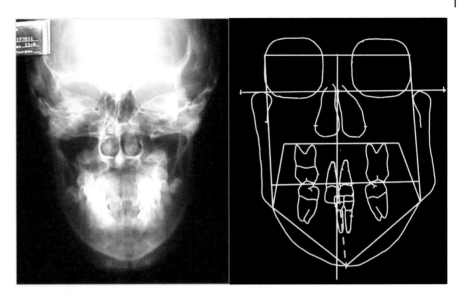

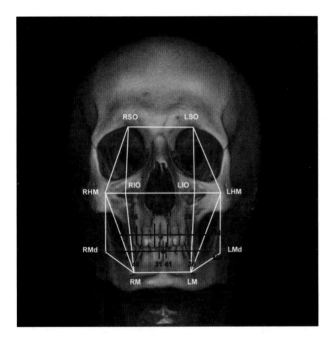

Figure 11.2.10 3D cephalometric analysis.

structures being equidistant from the film and X-ray source. Hence, landmarks on either side of the midline can be measured and contrasted with greater accuracy (Figure 11.2.9).

With the development and subsequent popularization of CBCT, 2D radiographs, especially when facial asymmetry is involved, have largely become redundant. Faure et al. (2013) have conceived a useful analysis when investigating and measuring asymmetry using CBCT volumes (Figure 11.2.10). While the hard tissue analysis is important and requires a comprehensive work-up, the soft tissue is actually of greater importance. Even if the hard tissue is significantly asymmetric, if the soft tissue is favorable and camouflages the

asymmetry, then skeletal correction may not be required, and dental compensation could be performed.

Management of Posterior Dental Asymmetries

Occlusal Plane

One of the most common sources of occlusal asymmetry is the mesial-in rotation of the maxillary first molars (Figure 11.2.11). When this is present, the most effective method of dealing with the asymmetry is the transpalatal arch (TPA), which is activated to derotate the offending tooth, and hence also has a distalizing reaction force on the contralateral molar (Nanda and Margolis 1996). Figure 11.2.12

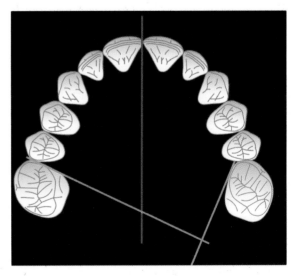

Figure 11.2.11 Occlusal asymmetry with mesial-in rotation of the maxillary first molar.

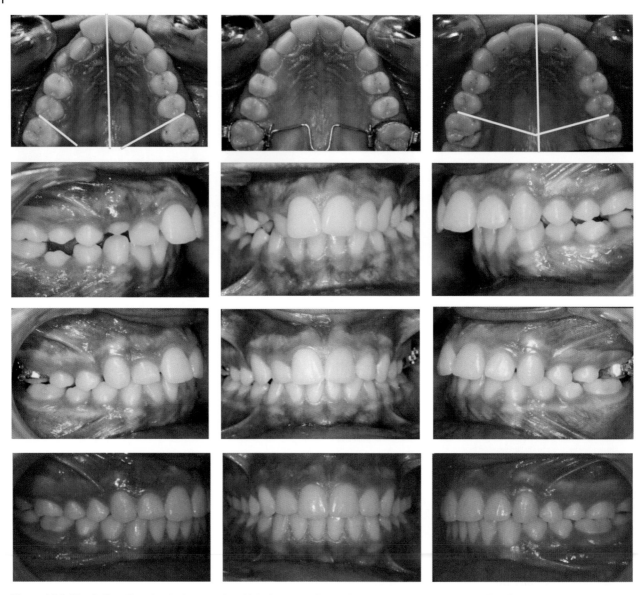

Figure 11.2.12 A Class II malocclusion case in which the upper first molars were rotated mesially in. The first molars were derotated using a TPA and headgear.

shows a Class II malocclusion case in which the upper first molars were rotated mesially in. The first molars were then derotated using a TPA and headgear, thus also aiding Class II correction.

Sagittal Plane

Molar Tipping

Tipping of the maxillary molar is another common problem associated with the early exfoliation of the primary second molar (Figure 11.2.13). In the mixed dentition, both fixed and removable appliances can be used to tip back the molar and regain space (Figure 11.2.14). Extra-oral anchorage is

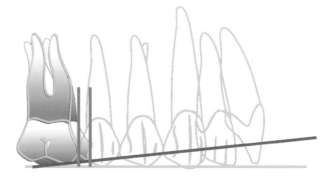

Figure 11.2.13 Tipping of the maxillary first molar is a common problem associated with the early exfoliation of the primary second molar.

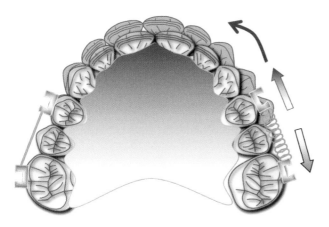

Figure 11.2.14 Orthodontic appliances are used to tip back the molar and regain space.

particularly useful to prevent unwanted proclination due to the side effects caused by the appliances. Figures 11.2.15 and 11.2.16 display a case in which an upper removable appliance was used in conjunction with a J-hook headgear to distalize the molars and correct the Class II malocclusion while maintaining the anterior anchorage.

Asymmetrical Class II

A Class II subdivision malocclusion occurs in about 3% of Class II malocclusion patients and can be particularly challenging to treat (Kula et al. 1998). In non-extraction cases, unilateral forces are often applied, which leads to inadvertent side effects. In the case of unilateral Class II elastics, this leads to extrusion of the canine area on the Class II side and canting of the occlusal plane (Figure 11.2.17). To mitigate this effect, an opposite force is required. This can be done using a traditional J-hook or TADs (Figure 11.2.18). Figure 11.2.19 exhibits the use of a J-hook headgear in addition to a unilateral Class II elastics on the right side in order to treat the Class II, division 2, subdivision right malocclusion. To avoid the use of Class II elastics entirely, and prevent unwanted deleterious effects of proclining the lower incisors (Balut et al. 2019), en-masse distalization can be performed using TADs or a cervical headgear if indicated (Figure 11.2.20).

Asymmetrical Space Closure

Often times differential space closure is required during treatment in order to center the midline (Figure 11.2.21). Using closing loops and tiebacks, differential anchorage, or through increasing or decreasing the number of anchoraged teeth, can all be utilized to obtain the desired midline correction. Figure 11.2.22 shows a case in which extractions were performed, and the lower space closed asymmetrically in order to align the midlines.

Frontal Plane

The most common asymmetry viewed frontally is unilateral crossbites. Skeletal and dental crossbites can be distinguished based on the inclination of the affected teeth (Figure 11.2.23). If the maxillary teeth are palatally inclined, then the crossbite is usually due to a dental origin. In this case, correction can be done in a variety of ways, including via archwire, elastics, removable appliances, quadhelix, or a combination of thereof.

When the affected maxillary teeth are inclined labially and are in crossbite, then this points toward a skeletal problem, which can be confirmed by an examination of the palatal vault anatomy. If the patient is young enough, a regular rapid palatal expansion (RPE) can be utilized to expand and split the suture. Thereafter, extra labial root torque will be required to correct the inclination of the teeth (Figure 11.2.24). Figure 11.2.25 exhibits a case of maxillary constriction which was treated using an RME followed by conventional fixed appliances. Extra labial root torque was placed during treatment to prevent flaring of the posterior dentition and prevent hanging cusps. If the patient is an adolescent or a young adult, expansion may be performed using miniscrew-assisted rapid palatal expansion (MARPE).

Management of Anterior Dental Asymmetries

Axial Inclination

When a midline deviation is recognized, the face should be assessed for symmetry. If the face is symmetrical, then the midline discrepancy will be of dental origin, and hence treated orthodontically. If the face too is asymmetrical, then orthodontic-surgical correction may be required.

Dental midline deviations may present in a few ways: (i) only the upper midline may be deviated, (ii) only the lower midline is deviated, (iii) upper and lower midlines deviate in opposite directions, and (iv) both upper and lower midlines are deviated in the same direction (Jerrold et al. 1990) (Figure 11.2.26).

The axial inclination of the anterior teeth may also be a cause of midline discrepancy. In order to assess this, the interdental papilla and contact point should be perpendicular to the horizontal plane. If the line between the papilla and contact point is not perpendicular to the horizontal plane, then the incisors are inclined (Figure 11.2.27). Figure 11.2.28 displays the use of extractions and proper bracket positioning to correct the axial inclination of the upper incisors.

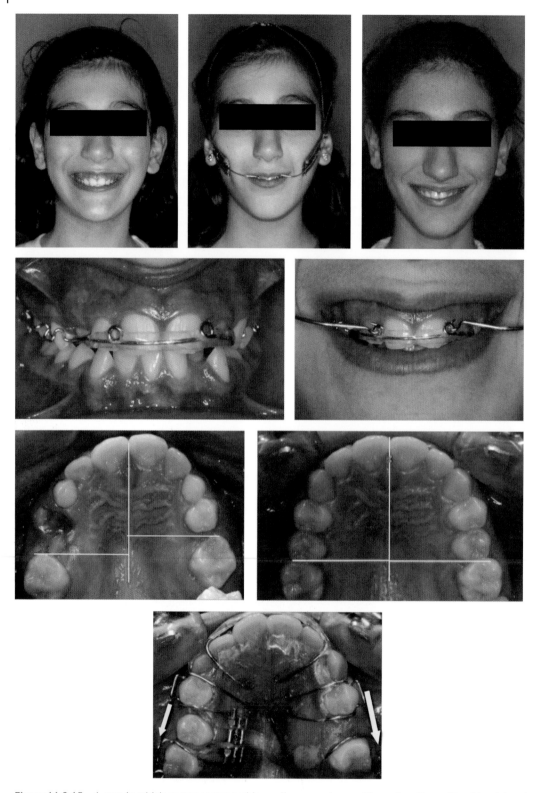

Figure 11.2.15 A case in which an upper removable appliance can be used in conjunction with a J-hook headgear to distalize the molars while maintaining the anterior anchorage.

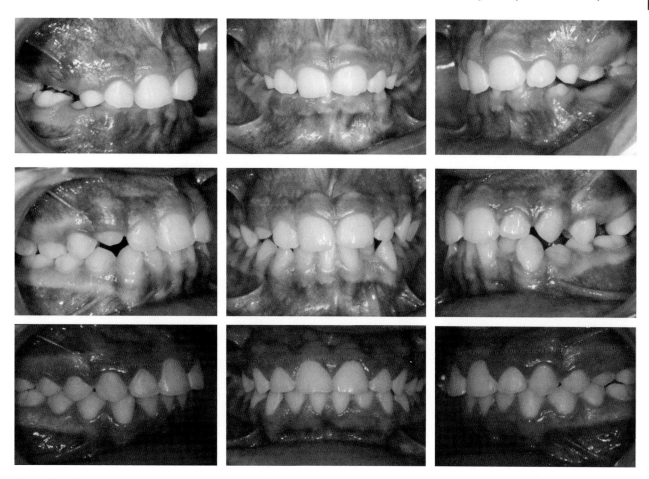

Figure 11.2.16 Asymmetry management and malocclusion correction.

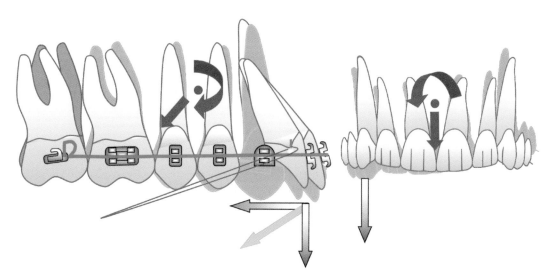

Figure 11.2.17 The use of unilateral Class II elastics may lead to extrusion of the canine area on the Class II side and canting of the occlusal plane.

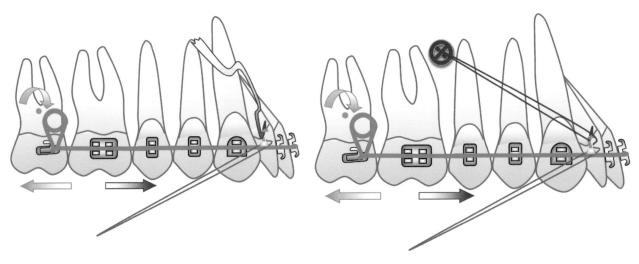

Figure 11.2.18 A traditional J-hook or TAD can be used to mitigate this effect.

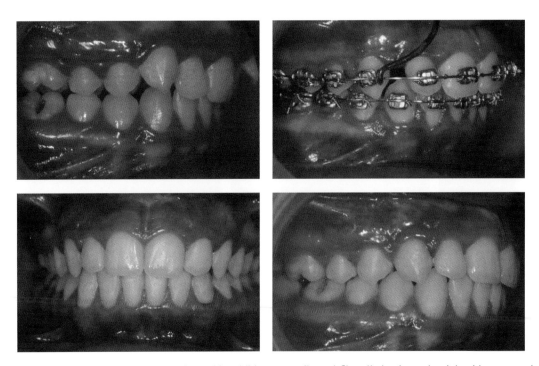

Figure 11.2.19 A J-hook headgear is used in addition to a unilateral Class II elastic on the right side to treat the Class II, division 2, subdivision right malocclusion.

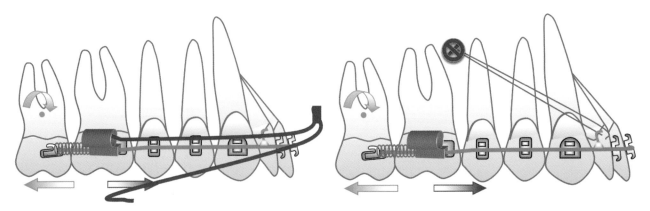

Figure 11.2.20 To avoid Class II elastics use, and prevent proclining the lower incisors, en-masse distalization can be performed using TADs or a cervical headgear if indicated.

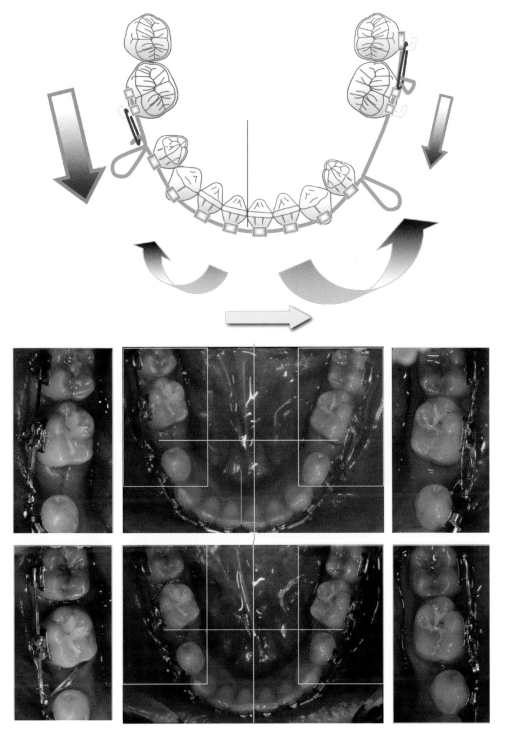

Figure 11.2.21 Space closure management using closing loops, tiebacks, and differential anchorage to obtain the desired midline correction.

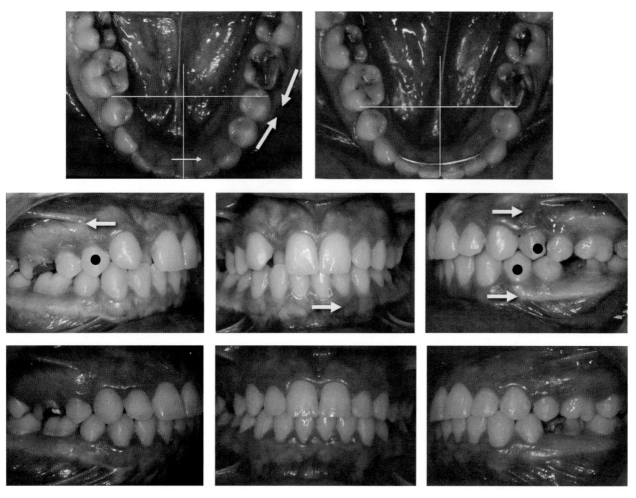

Figure 11.2.22   A case in which extractions were performed, and the lower space closed asymmetrically in order to align the midlines.

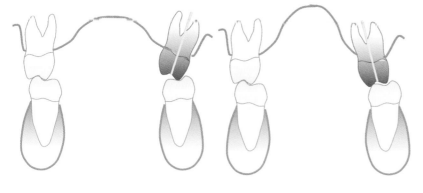

Figure 11.2.23   Skeletal and dental crossbites can be distinguished based on the inclination of the affected teeth.

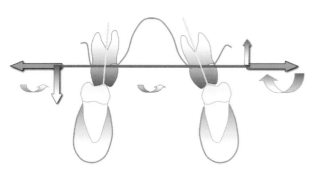

Figure 11.2.24   Rapid palatal expansion can be utilized to expand and split the suture. Extra labial root torque will be required to correct the inclination of the teeth.

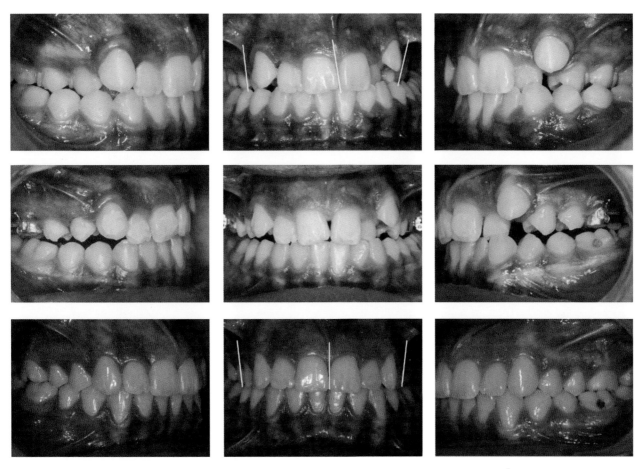

Figure 11.2.25 A case of maxillary constriction treated using rapid palatal expansion followed by conventional fixed appliances: Extra labial root torque was placed on the upper lateral segments to prevent flaring and hanging cusps.

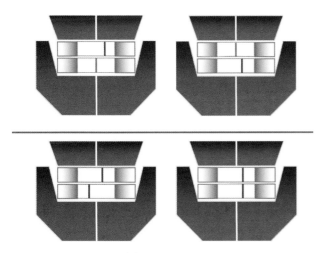

Figure 11.2.26 Dental midline deviations may present in a few ways: (1) only the upper midline may be deviated, (2) only the lower midline is deviated, (3) upper and lower midlines deviate in opposite directions, and (4) both upper and lower midlines are deviated in the same direction.

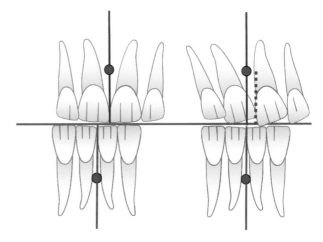

Figure 11.2.27 The axial inclination of the anterior teeth may also be a cause of midline discrepancy. The interdental papilla and contact point should be perpendicular to the horizontal plane.

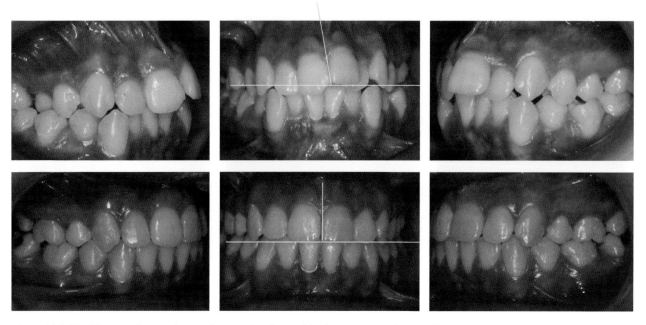

Figure 11.2.28 The use of extractions and proper bracket positioning to correct the axial inclination of the upper incisors is shown.

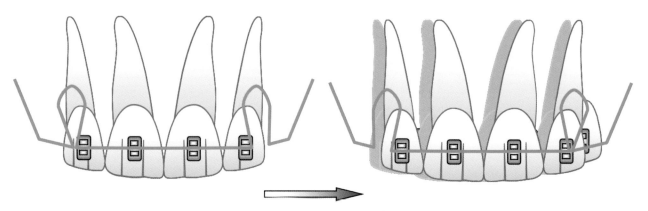

Figure 11.2.29 Asymmetrical space closure using closing loops is an excellent way of correcting midline discrepancies.

Closing Loops on a Continuous Archwire

Asymmetrical space closure using closing loops is an excellent way of correcting midline discrepancies (Jerrold et al. 1990). The loops should be close to the lateral incisor bracket, and the unilateral activation should be gentle (Figure 11.2.29). Figure 11.2.30 shows a patient in which asymmetrical space closure was used to center the upper midline after extraction of four premolars.

Asymmetrical Directional Forces

Asymmetric mechanics are required to treat asymmetrical problems, such as midline deviations and occlusal plane cants (Figure 11.2.31). These mechanics should not utilize the dentition for anchorage, as the reaction forces may cause

undesired side effects. Hence, extra-oral anchorage such as J-hooks and headgears, or bone-borne anchorage such as TADs are preferable (Figure 11.2.32). Figure 11.2.33 shows the asymmetrical use of J-hooks in the first and third quadrants. The J-hook attached to the first quadrant was used for distalizing the dentition and correcting the Class II malocclusion and upper midline deviation. The J-hook in the third quadrant was used to extrude the lower left anterior segment, thus correcting the lower anterior cant.

Tooth-by-Tooth Movement

When correcting midline deviations, it is prudent to close the space strategically in order to make the treatment efficient. Uncontrolled space closure can cause anchorage loss

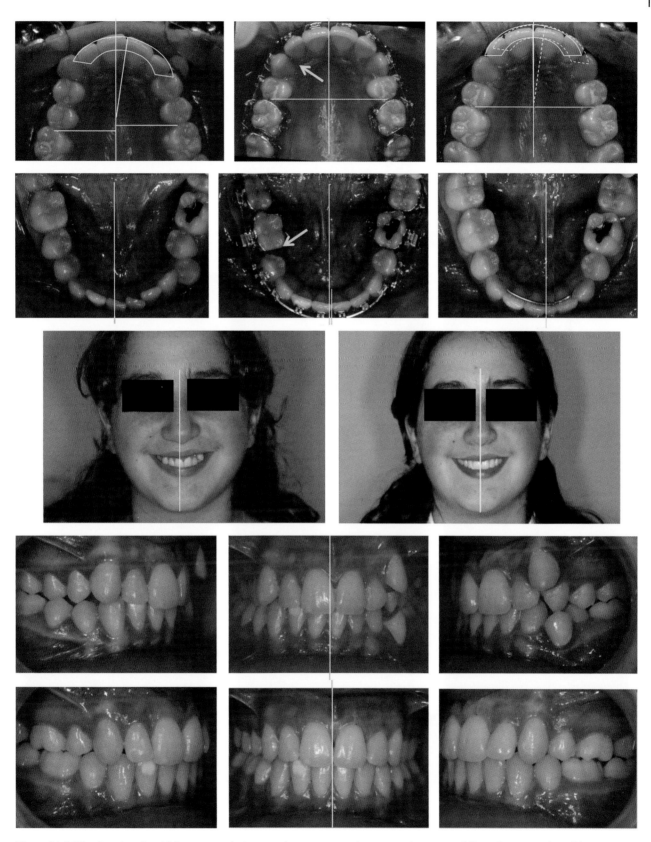

Figure 11.2.30 A patient in which asymmetrical space closure was used to center the upper midline after extraction of four premolars.

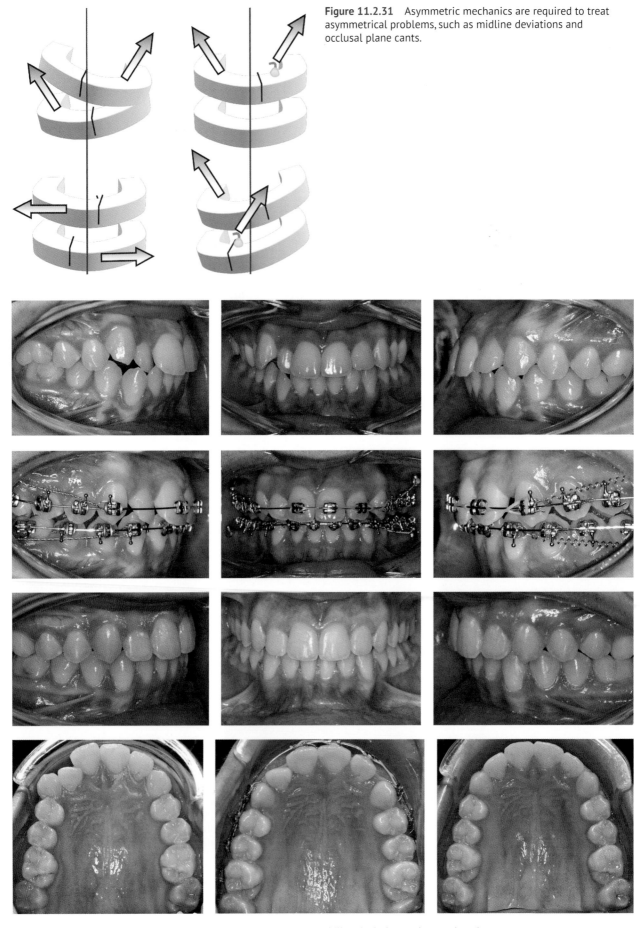

Figure 11.2.31 Asymmetric mechanics are required to treat asymmetrical problems, such as midline deviations and occlusal plane cants.

Figure 11.2.32 A case in which TADs were used to correct upper midline deviation and control anchorage.

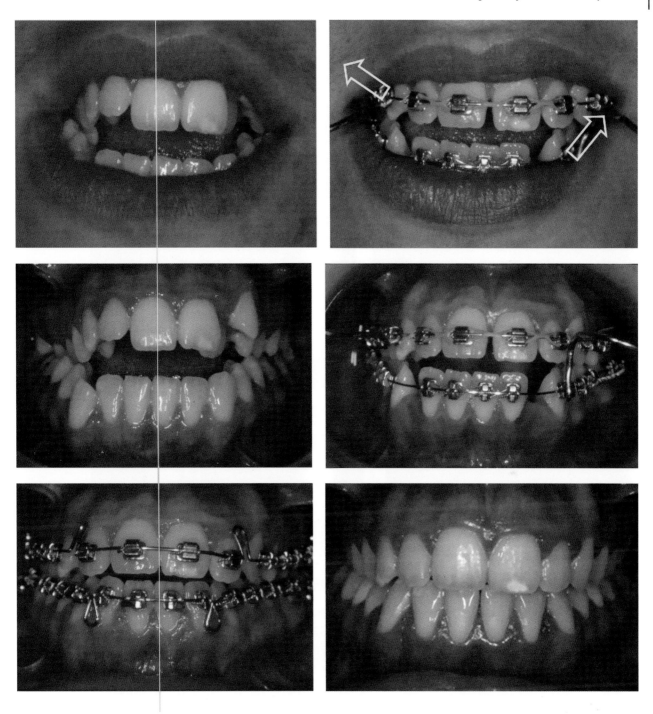

Figure 11.2.33 Asymmetrical use of J-hooks for malocclusion management, midline deviation, and occlusal plane cant correction.

and the extraction spaces may close without resolving the problem. Thus use of oblique anterior intermaxillary elastics may be required, which may produce side effects such as an anterior occlusal plane cant and asymmetric smile. Moving each tooth separately using sequentially activated open coil springs and powerchains, and using figure 8's on the anchor units, is an effective way to center the midlines during space closure (Figure 11.2.34).

Anterior Rotational Control

A canted occlusal plane is a complicated orthodontic problem. Traditionally treated with orthognathic surgery, occlusal cants have more recently been corrected using TADs for less invasive treatment. Appliances such as J-hooks, asymmetric auxiliary arches, or cantilevers with sectional mechanics can also be utilized

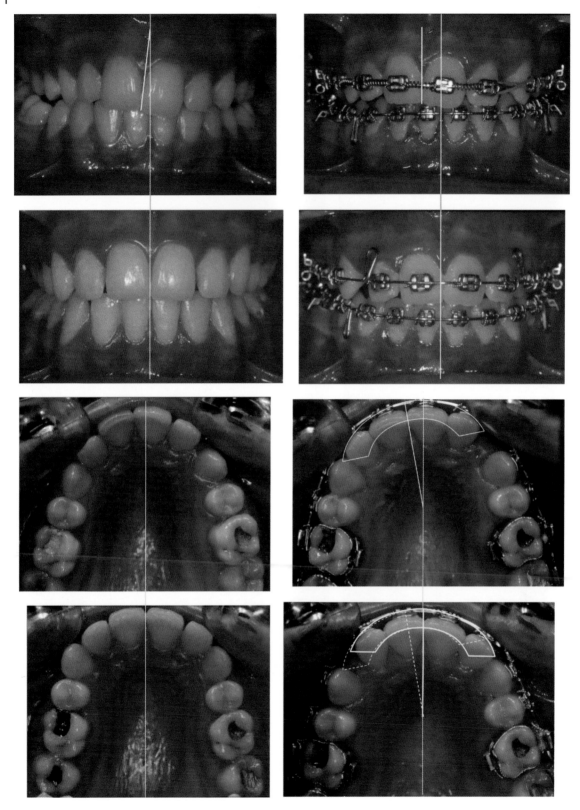

Figure 11.2.34 Moving each tooth separately, using sequentially activated open coil springs and powerchains, to center the midlines.

(van Steenbergen and Nanda 1995). These asymmetric mechanics allow for the intrusion of one side and extrusion of the other. The reaction forces are mitigated by using a TPA (Figure 11.2.35).

A novel method is the "Yin-Yang" archwire, described by Liou et al. (2019), which is a continuous archwire that is ligated conventionally to each bracket. It essentially consists of a curve of Spee (CoS) on one side of the archwire and reverse CoS (RCoS) on the other using a rectangular TMA archwire (Hansa et al. 2020) (Figure 11.2.36).

Asymmetrical Extractions

When a patient presents with a symmetric face but with deviated midlines and extractions are warranted, asymmetric extraction patterns are a great way to facilitate mechanics, make treatment more efficient, and decrease treatment duration (Nanda and Margolis 1996).

Depending on the molar and canine relationship and the distribution of crowding, asymmetric extraction patterns could include unilateral extractions or dissimilar teeth

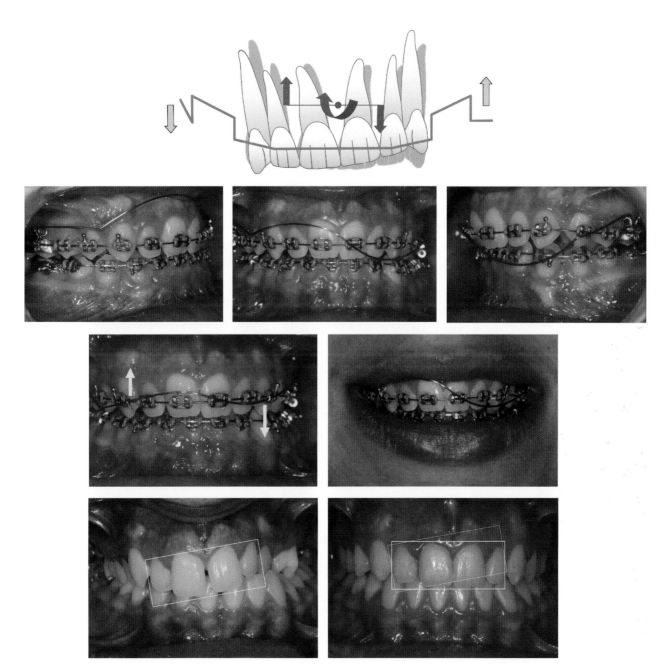

Figure 11.2.35 A case where asymmetrical rotational control is applied to correct the cant of the anterior occlusal plane.

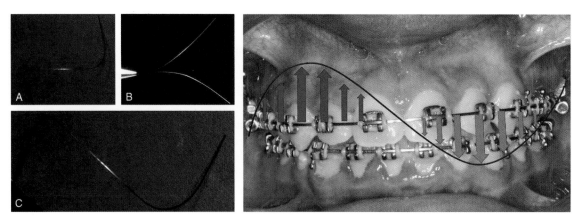

Figure 11.2.36 The "Yin-Yang" archwire consists of a curve of Spee on one side of the archwire and reverse curve of Spee on the other, using a rectangular TMA archwire.

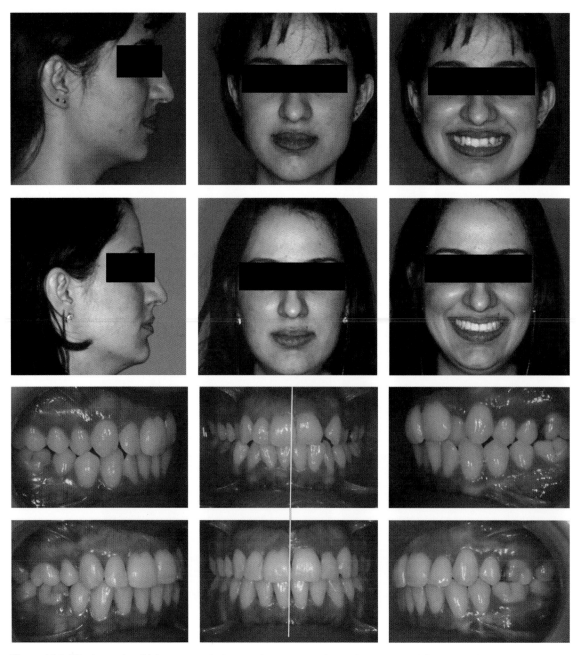

Figure 11.2.37 A case in which asymmetrical extractions were performed to correct midline deviation.

being extracted in the four quadrants (Janson et al. 2003). Figure 11.2.37 shows such a case in which the upper midline was deviated to the left. As extractions were warranted, the decision was made to extract the upper right first premolar and the upper left second premolar, in addition to the lower second premolars in order to aid midline correction.

accurate diagnosis. Once the diagnosis is determined, treatment planning in all three dimensions should be performed and individualized. Dental asymmetries should ideally be treated using dental movements, functional asymmetries addressed with interarch controlled mechanics, and skeletal asymmetries resolved with orthognathic surgery.

Conclusions

In summary, the treatment of dental asymmetries requires a comprehensive 3D investigation in order to obtain an

Acknowledgment

The authors would like to thank Dr. Elie El Amm for the graphic illustrations.

References

Arnett GW, Bergman RT. Facial keys to orthodontic diagnosis and treatment planning. Part I. Am J Orthod Dentofac Orthop. 1993;103:299–312.

Balut N, Hansa I, González E, Ferguson DJ. Bone regeneration after alveolar dehiscence due to orthodontic tooth movement – a case report. APOS Trends Orthod. 2019;9:117.

Beyer JW, Lindauer SJ. Evaluation of dental midline position. Semin Orthod. 1998;4:146–152.

Bishara SE, Burkey PS, Kharouf JG. Dental and facial asymmetries: a review. Angle Orthod. 1994;64:89–98.

Cheney EA. Dentofacial asymmetries and their clinical significance. Am J Orthod. 1961;47:814–829.

Choi KY. Analysis of facial asymmetry. Arch Craniofacial Surg. 2015;16:1.

Faber RD. Occlusograms in orthodontic treatment planning. J Clin Orthod. 1992;26:396–401.

Faure J, Oueiss A, Treil J, Braga J. The use of geometric morphometry to study facial asymmetries: relationship between basicranial shape and maxillofacial and occlusal pathologies. J Dentofac Anomalies Orthod. 2013;16:303.

Ferrario VF, Sforza C, Miani A, Tartaglia G. Craniofacial morphometry by photographic evaluations. Am J Orthod Dentofac Orthop. 1993;103:327–337.

Fiorelli G, Melsen B. The "3-D occlusogram" software. Am J Orthod Dentofac Orthop. 1999;116:363–368.

Hansa I, Ismail A, Vaid NR. Abordagem não invasiva para correção do plano oclusal inclinado: relato de caso. Rev Clínica Ortod Dent Press. 2020;19:145–152.

Janson G, Dainesi A, Henriques C, de Freitas R, Jero K. Class II subdivision treatment success rate with symmetric and asymmetric extraction protocols. Am J Orthod Dentofac Orthop. 2003;124:257–264.

Jerrold L, Lowenstein LJ, York N. The midline: diagnosis and treatment. Am J Orthod Dentofac Orthop. 1990;97:453–462.

Joondeph DR. Mysteries of asymmetries. Am J Orthod Dentofac Orthop. 2000;117:577–579.

Kula K, Esmailnejad A, Hass A. Dental arch asymmetry in children with large overjets. Angle Orthod. 1998;68.45–52.

Liou EJ-W, Mehta K, Lin JC-Y. An archwire for non-invasive improvement of occlusal cant and soft tissue chin deviation. APOS Trends Orthod. 2019;9:19–25.

Lundstrom A. Some asymmetries of the dental arches, jaws, and skull, and their etiological significance. Am J Orthod. 1961;47:81–106.

Ming TC. Spectrum and management of dentofacial deformities in a multiethnic Asian population. Angle Orthod. 2006;76:806–809.

Nanda R, Margolis MJ. Treatment strategies for midline discrepancies. Semin Orthod. 1996;2:84–89.

Peck S, Peck L, Kataja M. Skeletal asymmetry in esthetically pleasing faces. Angle Orthod. 1990;61:43–48.

Pinho S, Ciriaco C, Faber J, Lenza MA. Impact of dental asymmetries on the perception of smile esthetics. Am J Orthod Dentofac Orthop. 2007;132:748–753.

Sarver DM, Ackerman MB. Dynamic smile visualization and quantification: part 2. Smile analysis and treatment strategies. Am J Orthod Dentofac Orthop. 2003;124:116–127.

Sheats RD, McGorray SP, Musmar Q, Wheeler TT, King GJ. Prevalence of orthodontic asymmetries. Semin Orthod. 1998;4:138–145.

Smith RJ, Bailit HL. Prevalence and etiology of asymmetries in occlusion. Angle Orthod. 1979;49:199–204.

van Steenbergen E, Nanda R. Biomechanics of orthodontic correction of dental asymmetries. Am J Orthod Dentofac Orthop. 1995;107:618–624.

White L. The clinical use of occlusograms. J Clin Orthod. 1982;16:92–103.

Yoon SJ, Wang RF, Na HJ, Palomo JM. Normal range of facial asymmetry in spherical coordinates: a CBCT study. Imaging Sci Dent. 2013;43:31–36.

12

Orthodontics, Maxillofacial Surgery, and Asymmetries

12.1

Dental Arch Shape in Relation to Class II Subdivision Malocclusion

Birte Melsen and Padhraig S. Fleming

Introduction

Class II subdivision malocclusion is a common orthodontic presentation characterized by the presence of asymmetric molar relationships. The etiology of Class II subdivision is varied involving asymmetric dental positions, a skeletal asymmetry, or a combination of these (Cassidy et al. 2014). The majority of subdivisions, however, appear to have posterior positioning of the mandibular molar being contributory often reflecting an underlying skeletal issue (Alavi et al. 1988; Rose et al. 1994; Janson et al. 2001; Azevedo et al. 2006). Moreover, aberrant positioning of the glenoid fossa allied to the presence of a functional displacement may also be contributory (Li et al. 2015).

Dental Arch Form

Dental arch form asymmetry may involve the presence of asymmetric crowding or spacing due to underlying dentoalveolar disproportion. This may also be aggravated by the presence of hypodontia, or the premature loss of primary teeth. Asymmetric crowding in the maxillary arch may, for example, introduce associated space loss with mesial movement of the contralateral maxillary molar and deviation of the maxillary midline to the same side. Correction may therefore necessitate space creation on the contralateral (Class II) side in order to address the maxillary midline shift.

Up to 60% of subdivisions involve mandibular midline shift, in isolation, with 20% having upper midline deviation alone and the remaining 20% mixed characteristics (Janson et al. 2007). Mandibular midline shift may present due to uneven mandibular space conditions with the midline deviating to the crowded quadrant. As such, space creation in the side away from which the midline has shifted (Class I) may be considered. Bilateral removal of maxillary bicuspids may be considered in order to preserve the pre-existing molar relationships (Janson et al. 2017).

Mandibular asymmetry is a common finding in cases with asymmetric molar relationships and predisposes to the deviation of the lower dental midline to the side to which the chin-point is deviated. While more severe skeletal asymmetry may be associated with vertical elements and may necessitate a combined orthodontic-surgical approach, the occlusion can be corrected by tooth movement in the presence of milder skeletal asymmetry. Extractions may be required in both arches in order to provide sufficient space for lower midline correction while also permitting molar correction and the achievement of Class I incisor relationship. Non-extraction approaches may also be used particularly in the presence of limited lower arch crowding (Akın et al. 2019).

It is important to appreciate that Class II subdivision may present a complex array of features not limited to midline shift and/or molar asymmetry. In particular, vertical issues and asymmetric positioning of the canines are to be expected. Moreover, arch form changes including transverse mismatch are common findings. During orthodontic treatment in symmetric situations, increases in arch dimensions may be planned to alleviate crowding, to address transverse discrepancies, and to a lesser extent alter smile esthetics (Fleming et al. 2008). In the presence of subdivisions, the transverse dimension may require careful management in order to maintain optimal arch coordination, particularly in the canine region.

In this chapter, case reports of two patients with Class II subdivision are presented and compared. Neither of the cases presented with a facial asymmetry that might indicate a combined orthodontic-surgical approach. The malocclusions were both Class II subdivision and allied goals of maintaining a Class II molar relationship on the subdivision side, neutral canine relationship, and coincident dental midlines. Both cases were treated with one premolar extraction on the Class II side. The influence of the arch form and the canine position on the appropriate planning of patients exhibiting Class II subdivision will be emphasized.

Case 1

An adult male presented with a Class II subdivision on a mild skeletal Class II pattern with mandibular retrognathia. There was no obvious mandibular asymmetry.

Lips were competent with normal soft tissue protrusion. Both upper and lower arches were crowded with palatal displacement of the maxillary left lateral incisor. The maxillary canines were both buccally positioned. The upper midline was displaced to the Class I (neutral) side and the lower midline coincided with the facial midline (Figures 12.1.1–12.1.3).

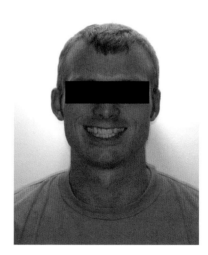

Figure 12.1.1 Patient presenting with a Class II subdivision malocclusion with upper midline shift to the left side, dual-arch crowding and a chief complaint relating to the maxillary arch crowding and the prominence of the maxillary canines.

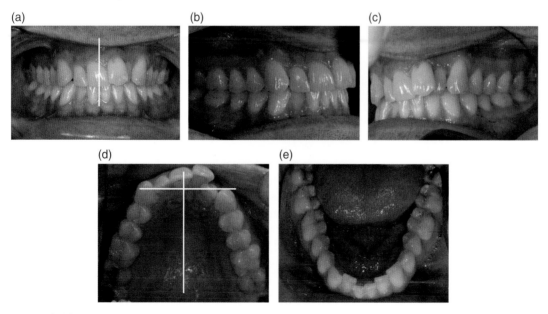

Figure 12.1.2 (a–e) Intra-oral images illustrating the presence of a maxillary midline shift to the left side. The posterior occlusion is Class I on the left side and Class II on the right. The maxillary occlusal view highlights that the canine on the right side is placed anterior in relation to the canines on the left side.

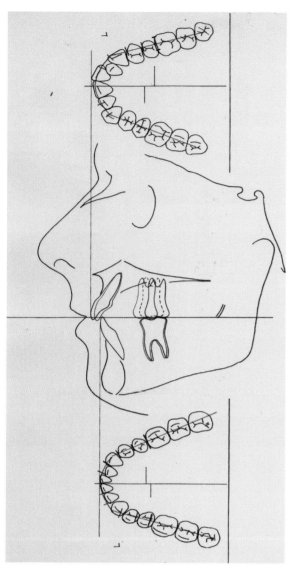

Figure 12.1.3 Combined tracing of the lateral cephalogram and the occlusogram highlighting planned tooth movements.

One upper premolar (#14) was extracted on the Class II side in order to provide space to address the maxillary midline deviation while correcting the Class II canine relationship on the right side. The Class II molar relationship on the right side was to be preserved (Figure 12.1.4). Following canine retraction, the maxillary midline was corrected and space generated for the correction of the palatally-displaced lateral incisor (Figure 12.1.5). Alignment of the upper left lateral incisor was accomplished with an overlay arch (0.016-inch NiTi) (Figure 12.1.6) prior to torque expression, finishing, and detailing (Figure 12.1.7). The maxillary midline was corrected relative to the midfacial axis and was coincident with the lower dental midline (Figure 12.1.8).

The outcome was retained with a bonded retainer from first premolar to first premolar with and a removable retainer in the upper arch. The upper retainer was discarded after 12 months leading to minor change in the position of the maxillary left lateral incisor at 5-year follow-up (Figure 12.1.9).

Case 2

The second case was also treated with premolar extraction of the Class II side. There was, however, a significant difference from the first case as the canines on the distal side were placed further distally compared to the neutral side (Figures 12.1.10–12.1.13). This situation was mirrored in the lower arch. The distal movement of the upper canine following the extraction of the first premolars was done with power arms both labially and lingually (Figure 12.1.14). This movement resulted in a pronounced flattening of the arch. This change was replicated in the lower arch as a result of the occlusion. Consequently, while a neutral occlusion was achieved, the arch form was distorted in both arches. In order to restore optimal arch shape and symmetry, extension arms originating from the Class I side were inserted to rotate the anterior segments around the canine (Figure 12.1.15). These arches generated space anterior to the right canine. An anterior movement was generated using an asymmetrically activated transpalatal arch in the maxillary arch with a vertical tube on the right side to improve maxillary arch symmetry (Figure 12.1.16). The lower arch was corrected using an expansion spring extending from the left first molar to the anterior segment. At the end of the treatment, the patient exhibited a smile characterized by a symmetrical position of canines (Figure 12.1.17).

Discussion

Both cases presented highlight the complex nature of Class II subdivision malocclusion. While the definition refers to asymmetric molar relationships, the management is dictated by the etiology, the location, and extent of any associated midline shifts and space conditions. Furthermore, the impact of arch asymmetry in relation to the antero-posterior and transverse positioning of the canines is critical (Figures 12.1.18 and 12.1.19).

In Case 1, the antero-posterior position of the maxillary canines faithfully reflected the midline shift and asymmetric molar relationships. As such, asymmetric extraction allied to careful anchorage management produced relatively simple correction of the malocclusion without

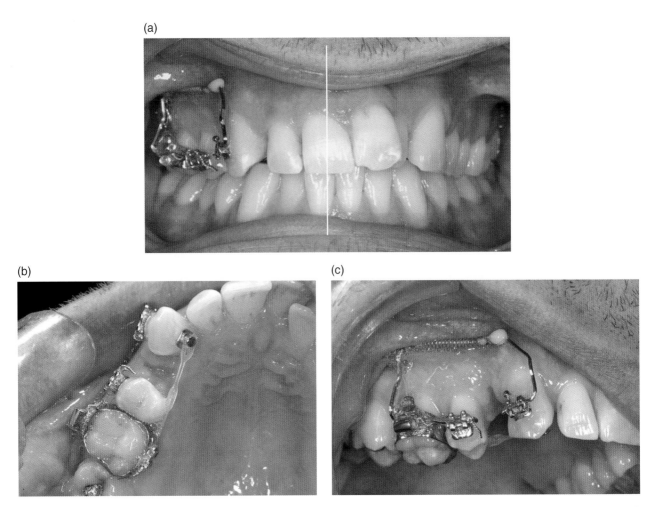

Figure 12.1.4 (a–c) Distal movement of the right upper canine being performed with power arms on the buccal side and elastomeric chain on the lingual aspect.

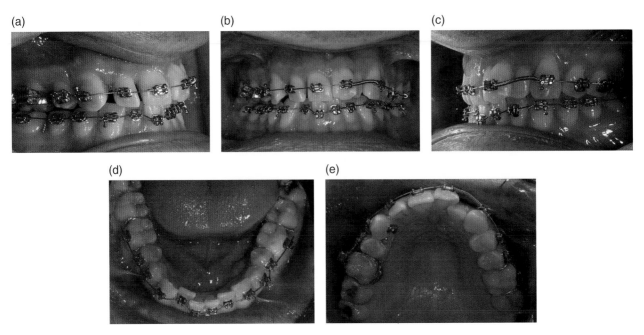

Figure 12.1.5 (a–e) The retraction of the maxillary right canine into a Class I position has resulted in passive drifting of the incisors allowing levelling of the upper incisors. Additional space, however, was required in the region of the lingually displaced maxillary left lateral incisor.

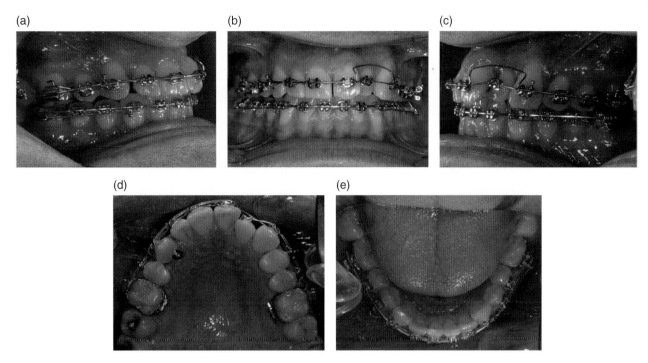

Figure 12.1.6 (a–e) A step was introduced to a 0.017 × 0.025-inch stainless base archwire to increase the space for the alignment of lingually displaced maxillary left lateral incisor. An overlay 0.016-inch NiTi wire was applied to correct the position of #22.

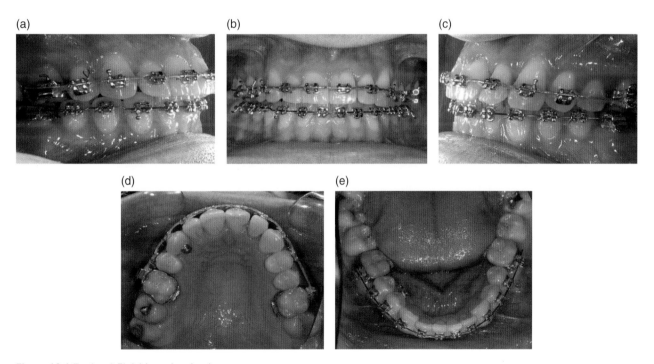

Figure 12.1.7 (a–e) Finishing wires in place.

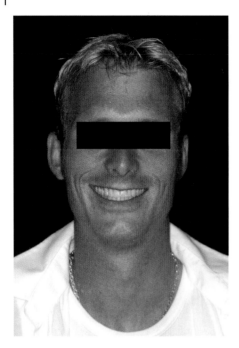

Figure 12.1.8 Smiling photograph illustrating coincidence of the maxillary and mandibular midlines.

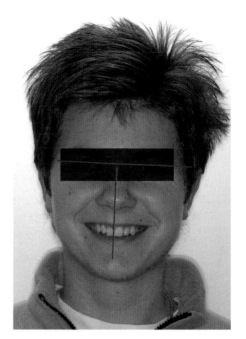

Figure 12.1.10 Patient presenting with a Class II subdivision malocclusion with an upper midline shift to the right side. There was crowding of both arches with a chief complaint involving upper arch irregularity.

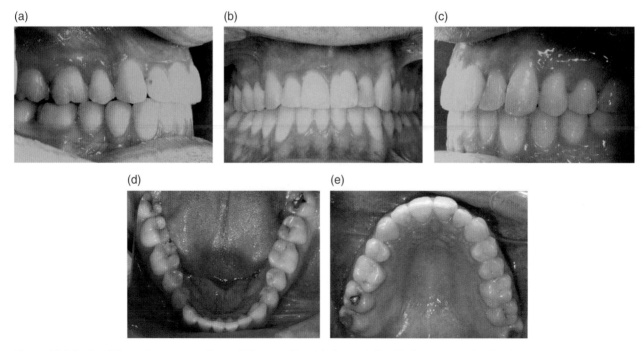

(a) (b) (c)

(d) (e)

Figure 12.1.9 (a–e) Treated outcome at 5-year follow-up. Class I incisor relationship has been maintained with a well-interdigitated posterior occlusion. Minor relapse in the position of the lingually placed #22 occurred as no retainer was used in the upper arch.

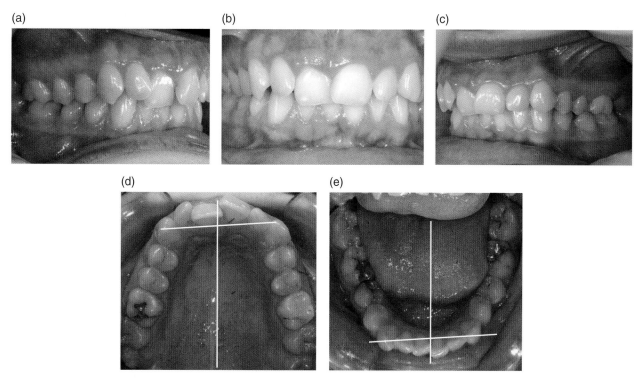

Figure 12.1.11 (a–e) Intra-oral photographs highlighting crowding of the anterior maxillary region and a Class II subdivision with a distal occlusion on the right side. The maxillary canine on the Class II side was more posteriorly located than on the left side.

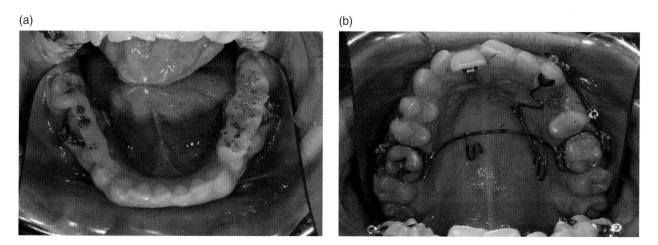

Figure 12.1.12 (a) As in Case 1, asymmetric extraction of a maxillary first premolar was performed on the Class II side. The maxillary left canine was subsequently displaced distally with power arms both lingually and buccally. (b) The bite was opened with a lingual attachment on the lingually inclined maxillary right central incisor and a transpalatal arch with a vertical tube on the Class I side served as anchorage and allowed for a light forward movement of the distally-positioned molar on the right side.

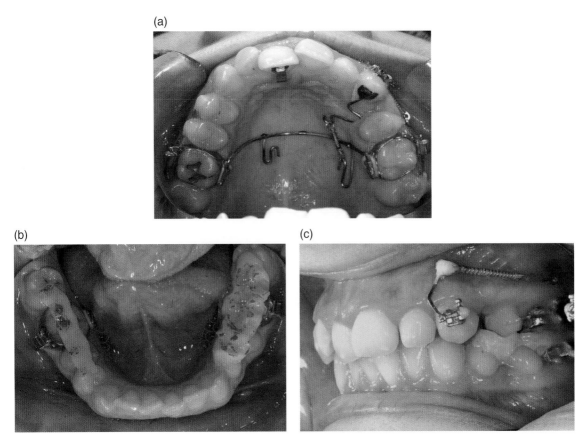

Figure 12.1.13 (a–c) The maxillary left canine was retracted to a Class I position. A fixed posterior bite plane was added to facilitate correction.

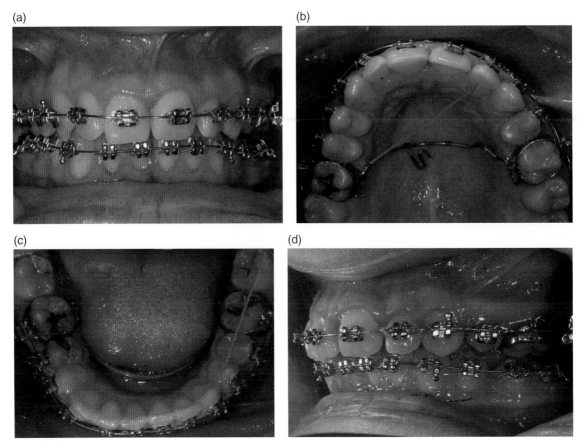

Figure 12.1.14 (a–d) Following space closure, both upper and lower arch were significantly flattened on the left side with associated rotation of the anterior segments.

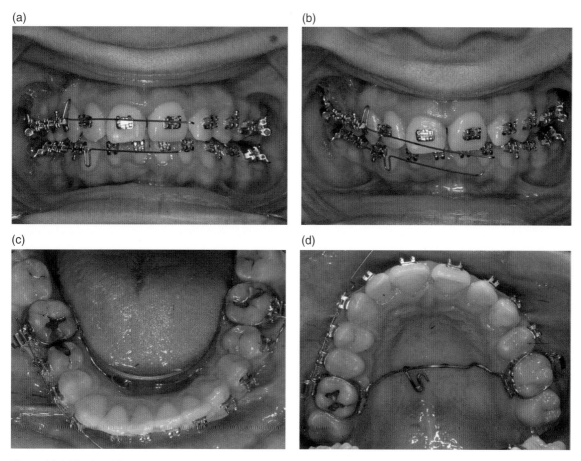

Figure 12.1.15 (a–d) Power arms extending from the right side were applied to move the left incisors anteriorly.

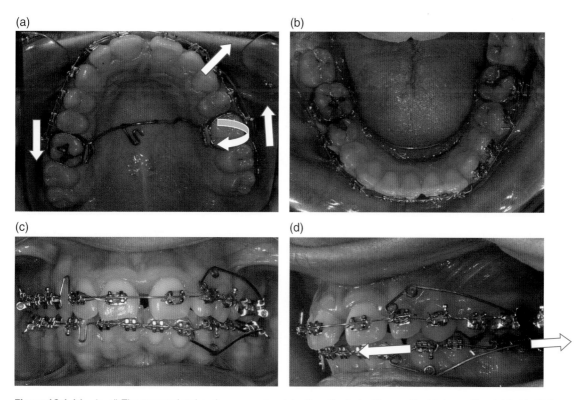

Figure 12.1.16 (a–d) The transpalatal arch was asymmetrically activated with a vertical tube on the right side. This was geared at rotating the molar on the left side distally, moving the canine buccally, the left molar distally and the right molar mesial. Segments extending from the molars to the canines in the upper and the lower arches supported the forward movement of the lateral incisors and canines.

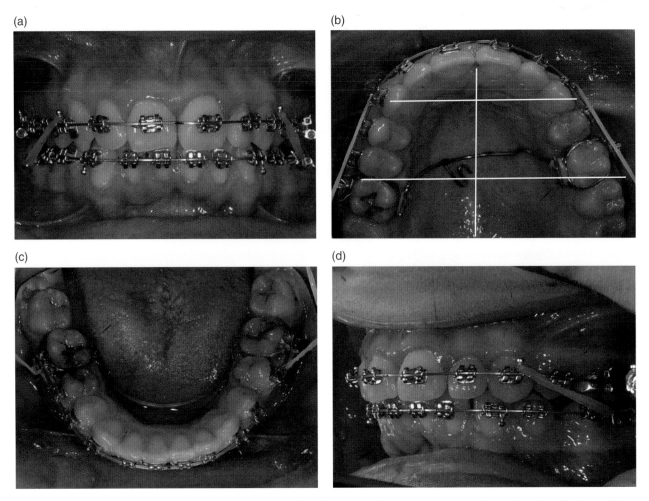

Figure 12.1.17 (a–d) Regeneration of arch symmetry with Class I canines and correct antero-posterior positioning of both maxillary canines.

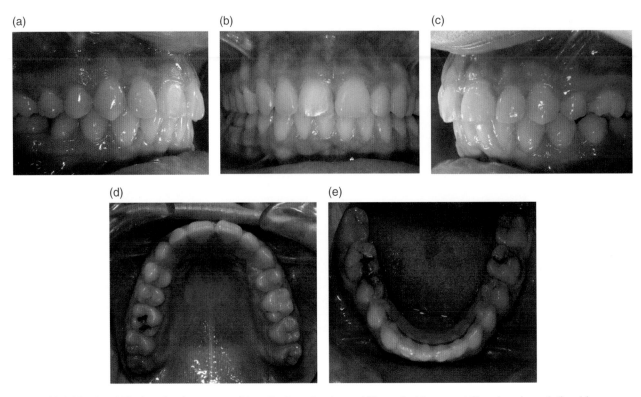

Figure 12.1.18 (a–e) Final occlusal outcome with well-aligned arches, midline coincidence and Class I canine relationships. A lower fixed retainer was placed from first premolar to first premolar.

Figure 12.1.19 Smiling photograph illustrating midline coincidence and symmetrical positioning of the canines.

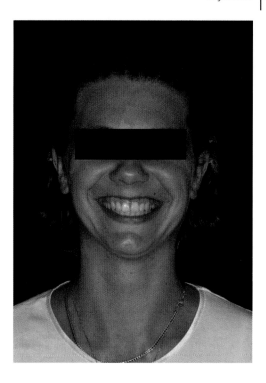

introducing arch asymmetry. Conversely, the second case was complicated by the aberrant positioning of the canines (Uysal et al. 2009). The latter dictated the use of differential moments and mechanics in order to restore arch symmetry.

The achievement of optimal outcomes in the presence of Class II subdivision hinges on careful evaluation of the skeletal and dental features with particular attention to the presence of arch form issues. Moreover, the characteristics of the arches in three spatial planes should be considered, rather than focusing purely on the antero-posterior inter-arch relationships and space conditions in orthodontic camouflage of Class II subdivision.

References

Alavi DG, BeGole EA, Schneider BJ. Facial and dental arch asymmetries in Class II subdivision malocclusion. Am J Orthod Dentofac Orthop. 1988;93:38–46.

Akın M, Erdur EA, Öztürk O. Asymmetric dental arch treatment with Forsus fatigue appliances: long-term results. Angle Orthod. 2019;89:688–696.

Azevedo AR, Janson G, Henriques JF, Freitas MR. Evaluation of asymmetries between subjects with Class II subdivision and apparent facial asymmetry and those with normal occlusion. Am J Orthod Dentofac Orthop. 2006;129:376–383.

Cassidy SE, Jackson SR, Turpin DL, Ramsay DS, Spiekerman C, Huang GJ. Classification and treatment of Class II subdivision malocclusions. Am J Orthod Dentofac Orthop. 2014;145:443–451.

Fleming PS, Dibiase AT, Lee RT. Arch form and dimensional changes in orthodontics. Prog Orthod. 2008;9:58–64.

Janson GR, Metaxas A, Woodside DG, de Freitas MR, Pinzan A. Three-dimensional evaluation of skeletal and dental asymmetries in Class II subdivision malocclusions. Am J Orthod Dentofac Orthop. 2001;119:406–418.

Janson G, de Lima KJ, Woodside DG, Metaxas A, de Freitas MR, Henriques JF. Class II subdivision malocclusion types and evaluation of their asymmetries. Am J Orthod Dentofac Orthop. 2007;131:57–66.

Janson G, Lenza EB, Francisco R, Aliaga-Del Castillo A, Garib D, Lenza MA. Dentoskeletal and soft tissue changes in Class II subdivision treatment with asymmetric extraction protocols. Prog Orthod. 2017;18:39.

Li J, He Y, Wang Y, Chen T, Xu Y, Zeng H, Feng J, Xiang Z, Xue C, Han X, Bai D. Dental, skeletal asymmetries and functional characteristics in Class II subdivision malocclusions. J Oral Rehabil. 2015;42:588–599.

Rose JM, Sadowsky C, BeGole EA, Moles R. Mandibular skeletal and dental asymmetry in Class II subdivision malocclusions. Am J Orthod Dentofac Orthop. 1994;105:489–495.

Uysal T, Kurt G, Ramoglu SI. Dental and alveolar arch asymmetries in normal occlusion and Class II division 1 and Class II subdivision malocclusions. World J Orthod. 2009;10:7–15.

12.2

Asymmetric Application of Lingual Arches

Kwangchul Choy

Introduction

Asymmetric occlusions are very common in the typical orthodontic patient. A unilateral crossbite can result in improper coordination of upper and lower arches. Subdivision patients present a asymmetric sagittal molar relationships in which the patient exhibits Class II on one side and Class III on the other, or Class I on one side and Class II or III on the other. Correction of these asymmetric occlusions is one of the most challenging subjects in the field of orthodontics, particularly in subdivision patients that we commonly see. There are many possibilities in correction of asymmetries, such as functional appliances in growing patients, asymmetric extraction or asymmetric mechanics in adult patients, or orthognathic surgery for severe skeletal asymmetries. In recent years, TADs have been used as the new treatment modality for asymmetry correction. However, some patients opt out of such demanding procedures, or discrepancies are relatively small or dental origin so that problems of asymmetric occlusion could be solved by orthodontics means only. Differential diagnosis regarding the nature and amount of asymmetry is the most important criteria in deciding the treatment modality; however, it is beyond the scope of this chapter.

In the case that the dental origin is identified as the cause of asymmetry, asymmetric activation of lingual arch can produce a unique force system that can correct the asymmetries that labial arches cannot. With continuous archwire in the labial brackets, all the teeth are connected from the most posterior end on one side to the other end. This makes it seem as though every tooth would be under the control of a continuous full archwire; this begs the question of why one would need to connect the bilateral molars directly across the dental arch by a lingual arch. The continuous full archwire can hardly control the posterior molar position of the dental arch due to inherent limitations that are distal flexibility and adjacent anchorage problem, necessitating the bilateral molars to be connected directly across the dental arch by a lingual arch (Burstone and Choy 2015).

Asymmetric tooth movement is very difficult. Suppose there are some ideas suggested for asymmetric movement of posterior teeth. The lingual archwire is fabricated so that it is passively fitted to the final position of a tooth. For

(a)
(b)

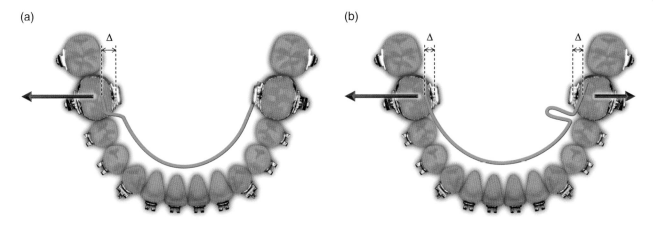

Figure 12.2.1 Lingual arch designs for unilateral expansion based on shape-driven concept. This is not a valid force diagram because it does not follow Newton's first law. (a) A step-out bend (Δ) for producing unilateral expansive force; (b) a loop was incorporated to reduce the force/deflection rate so that lower force is produced on left side.

example, to expand lower right first molar the lingual arch is made with step out bend (Δ) on the right side only for unilateral expansion (Figure 12.2.1a), or the lingual arch is bilaterally activated with same amount (Δ); however, the left side loop was incorporated in order to reduce the force/deflection rate so that lower force is produced on left side (Figure 12.2.1b). These efforts of so-called "shape-driven concept" or "differential force system" are in fact in vain because it does not obey the Newton's first law; in other words, there are always equal and opposite forces, so that magnitude of left and right expansive forces should be equal and opposite to each other. No matter how cleverly we design the appliances we cannot overcome the Law of nature and this is why asymmetric tooth movement is very difficult to produce. Asymmetric application of lingual arch is no exception because it should also follow Newton's law. However, distribution of stress in the PDL is modified so that asymmetric tooth movement is produced.

Color Code of the Wire and Force System

When the wire, or especially the lingual arch, is engaged into the attachments, it is not possible to tell if the wire is passive or active unless the lingual arch is removed from the attachments. For better understanding the state of the wires in the figure, the wires are depicted in two colors. The green-colored wire means there is no internal stress in the wire so that the wire is passive and thus, no force system is produced. The orange-colored wire means internal stress exists in the wire. The wire is elastically bent, which produces a certain force system that therefore entails some kind of tooth movement.

The force system is depicted in different colors in the figure. The red-colored arrows represent the force system acting on the tooth. It is the deactivation force system because, as it is in the name, it is the force system produced during deactivation of the appliance. The blue-colored arrows are the force system acting on the appliance. It is called the activation force system because it is the force system applied to activate the appliance by orthodontist's hand. The gray-colored arrows are undefined or incorrect force system. The yellow colored arrows are replaced equivalent force system (Burstone and Choy 2015).

Shape-driven Concept

There are two basic concepts used in application of active lingual arches – a shape driven, and a force-driven concept. The shape-driven concept of an appliance means the wire is permanently deformed into certain shape so that it is passive to the final position of the teeth. The wire is elastically bent during the insertion of the wire into the attachments and it moves the teeth as the wire deactivates. One of the most typical appliances made from shape shape-driven concept is the ideal archwire and a wire with reversed shape. The ideal-shaped archwire made from super elastic wire is elastically bent and engaged into crowded tooth. As the wire deactivates, and sequential changing of the wire by increasing stiffness, misaligned teeth eventually follow the shape of an ideal archwire. Perhaps you will end up with ideally aligned dentition by this procedure. A mandibular arch showing deep curve of Spee is treated with a wire with reverse curve of Spee, so-called compensation curve with an anticipation of a reverse shape of the wire will flatten the occlusal plane in a straight line. The appliance designed based on this shape-driven concept may work properly in some cases; however, it does not always produce the correct force system – especially in asymmetric applications as we have discussed in Figure 12.2.1. This chapter will focus on delineating active application of lingual arch particularly in asymmetric applications for posterior crossbite and sagittal asymmetric molar relationship (Burstone 1989).

Force-driven Concept and Definition of Shapes

As a response to the shape-driven concept, the force-driven concept is developed to deliver correct force system. In the force-driven concept only the force system is considered, rather than the shape of the appliance. The appliance designed by force-driven concept has two characteristics. First, the initial force system including magnitude and Moment/Force (M/F) ratio is correct. Second, the Force/Deflection (F/D) rate is reduced and the appliance is over activated to maintain initial correct force system hence, it moves the teeth rapidly without round tripping; therefore, a force-driven appliance eliminates unnecessary tooth movement.

To obtain the correct shape, computers with beam theory and iterative method is required, but we will use the same principle to obtain the correct shape at clinically acceptable level (Burstone and Koenig 1981).

Unilateral Expansion

Designing Valid Force System

Suppose that we would like to expand the lower right molar only. The first step is to design a valid force diagram that is in equilibrium. Being in equilibrium means all the forces and moments acting on an object sum to zero. At first glance, a single force only acting on the right molar by differential forces would be the best choice, but in fact is an invalid choice because it is not in equilibrium, as seen in Figure 12.2.2a. Only force diagrams that satisfy the equilibrium are valid and any others are not applicable. Some valid possibilities are using differential moments between left and right molar.

First method is applying bilateral equal and opposite forces obliquely so that the line of action passes near the crown on the right side and the center of resistance on the left side (red arrows in Figure 12.2.2b). It is valid force diagram because equal and opposite forces cancel each other out and the lingual arch is in equilibrium. On the right molar, the force is acting on a bracket (crown level) hence, the molar tips to the buccal side. The location of the center of rotation is slightly apical yet very close to the center of resistance of the molar. On the left molar, the line of action of the force passing through the center of resistance and the left molar translates. Uniform stress distribution on the reactive unit (left molar) is less likely to move or more resistant to tooth movement. However, the same expansive force is applied, only the right side expands, because a single force at the crown on the right side produces high stress in the alveolar crest and the apex of the root, which causes a system that is prone to tipping. Side effects would be vertical component of forces, but extrusive force would be neutralized by occlusal forces.

The single force acting at the center of resistance of the left molar is clinically impossible due to anatomic limitation. Hence, it is replaced with equivalent force system at the bracket which is depicted in yellow colored force system (Figure 12.2.2b). The yellow replaced equivalent force system acting at the bracket is identical force system with the red single force acting directly at the center of resistance. It can be seen that an expansive horizontal force with counterclockwise moment is needed at the bracket for translation of the left molar. The M/F ratio required would

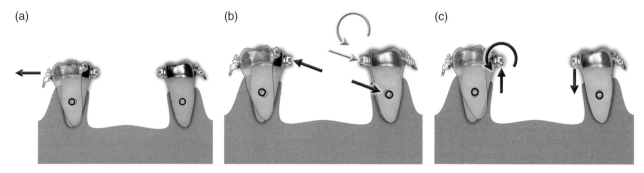

(a)   (b)   (c)

Figure 12.2.2 Various force systems for unilateral expansion. (a) Single force is acting on the right molar only. This are not a valid force diagram; (b) equal and opposite force (red arrows) are in equilibrium. The yellow arrows are replaced equivalent force system at the bracket (method 1); (c) a moment is applied at the right molar with accompanied vertical forces on each side (method 2).

be the distance between the bracket and the center of resistance. Suppose the distance between the lingual bracket and the center of resistance is 8 mm and the expansive force is 100 g, required moment is counterclockwise 800 gmm (M/F = 8 mm). Theoretically, this method is valid; however, it is problematic. Translating a tooth by delivering a force with line of action passing through the center of resistance is practically very difficult for many reasons. The identification of location of the center of resistance is very difficult because it is influenced by many factors such as length and shape of the root, amount of periodontal support around the root, and angulation of a tooth itself. Even if the exact location of center of resistance is identified, small deviation of the line of action of force from the center of resistance could result in significant rotation of a tooth. It is analogous to standing an egg on end on flat table. Even if center of mass of the egg is known it is very difficult.

A better possibility is method 2. The moment is applied at the right molar with accompanied vertical forces on each side (Figure 12.2.2c). It is also a valid force diagram because the moment on the right side is canceled by equal and opposite couple produced by two vertical forces. Notice that there are no horizontal expansive forces. Then how does it produce unilateral expansion without any horizontal force? A couple applied at a tooth rotates around the center of resistance. In other words, the center of rotation is identical with center of resistance. The force system acting on the right molar is totally different from the method 1. However, the effect of the tooth by a single horizontal force acting at the bracket by method 1 and the effect of the tooth by a couple by method 2 are clinically indistinguishable because center of rotation is very close to each other. The side effects of method 2 are vertical forces. The distance between two lingual attachments of the molar would

be one of the largest inter bracket distances provided in the oral cavity and hence the vertical force can be kept minimum because the distance between two bracket-times the vertical force is the magnitude of counteracting moment to cancel the couple acting on the right molar. The occlusal forces can minimize the extrusion of the right molar. The intrusive force on the left molar may tip the molar lingually because the force is passing lingual to the center of resistance, but the magnitude is very low so that the effect would be negligible or additional slight expansion of the lingual arch can compensate it. The major advantage of method 2 is that the force system is not so sensitive to position of the moment or vertical forces and frequent adjustment of the lingual arch may not be necessary.

Simulation of Force System

First, a passive shape of the lingual arch is fabricated with minimal clearance between the soft tissues. Anatomic structures like mandibular or maxillary torus are bypassed for patient comfort (Figure 12.2.3a,b) (Burstone and Manhartsberger 1988). Next, apply the deactivation force system that was predetermined previously on the passive shape. Hold tightly the right end of the lingual arch by plier and a single force is applied on the left side downwards. It is better to use finger than a plier to avoid unnecessary moments to the left side. The wire (lingual arch) is elastically bent and twisted in three dimensions to reach a certain shape. This shape is called a simulated shape and this procedure is called simulation (Figure 12.2.4a). If specific magnitude of couple is required, a ruler to measure the distance between two lingual brackets and a force gauge is necessary. For example, suppose 1000 gmm of moment is required on the right molar and measured inter bracket distance is 30 mm, then 33 g (= 1000 gmm/30 mm) of force

(a)

(b)

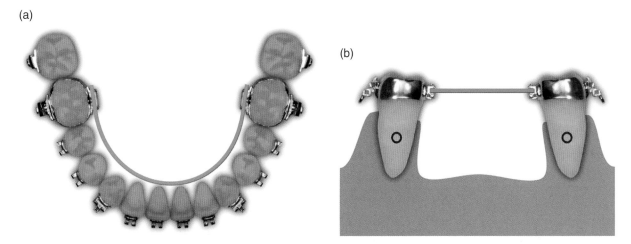

Figure 12.2.3 The passive shape of a lingual arch. (a) Occlusal view; (b) frontal view.

(a)　　　　　　　　　　　　　　　　　　　　(b)

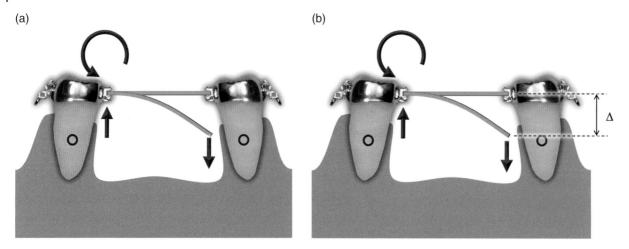

Figure 12.2.4 Simulation of deactivation force system. Passive shape (green color), Simulated shape (orange color). (a) The left side of the wire is push downward while right side is fixed; (b) amount of deviation is recorded.

is applied on the left free end during simulation. The amount of deviation is recorded (Figure 12.2.4b).

Next step is to permanently bend the wire in exactly the same way as the simulated shape; this shape is called a deactivated shape, which represents the final shape of the wire before activation (Figure 12.2.5a). The lingual arch undergoes bending and twisting during simulation. Looking from the lingual perspective, the free end on the left side is not parallel with the bracket (Figure 12.2.5b). However, once it is activated by an upward single force on the free end on the left side, it will be parallel with the lingual bracket and there would be no moment necessary to engage the wire into the bracket (Figure 12.2.6a). This activated shape would be identical to the passive shape we made at the first step hence, there will be no interference between the lingual arch and the soft tissue. From the occlusal perspective, only the right molar shows buccal movement while the left molar stand still at the original position (Figure 12.2.6b). It is not possible to distinguish if it is passive or active unless the lingual arch is removed from the bracket. Obtaining the accurate shape using computer using iteration method follows the same procedure (Burstone and Koenig 1981).

A patient who presented with severe lingual inclination of the lower second molar was treated by unilateral expansion (Figure 12.2.7a,b). A pontic connecting between the second molar and second premolar was removed and unilateral expansion lingual arch by method 2 was activated and inserted. Buccal crown and lingual root moment were applied on the left second molar accompanied with minimal vertical forces. Note that the left second molar rotated to buccal side while right second molar maintained its original position without any horizontal expansive forces (Figure 12.2.7c).

(a)

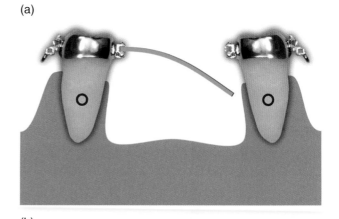

(b)

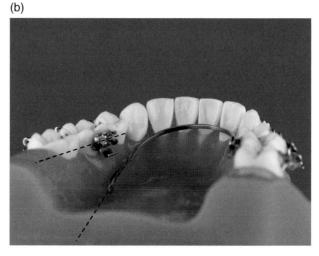

Figure 12.2.5 Deactivated shape. (a) Deactivated shape is fabricated exactly same as the simulated shape; (b) looking from the lingual perspective, the free end on the left side is not parallel with the bracket.

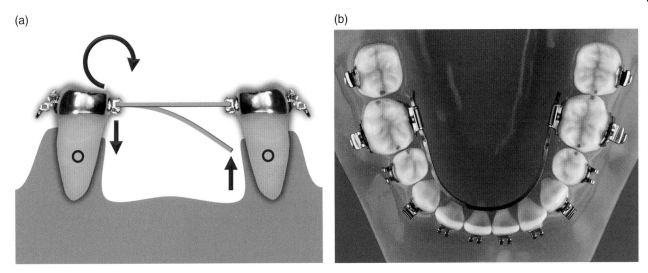

Figure 12.2.6 Activated shape. (a) Before activation (green color), After activation (orange color). Activated shape is identical with the original passive shape; (b) The red dots on the tooth show buccal movement of the right molar while the left molar keeps the original position.

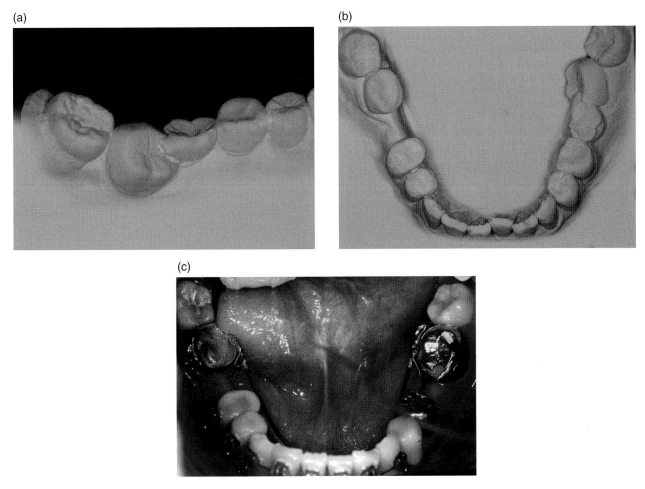

Figure 12.2.7 (a) and (b) A patient with a severely lingually tipped mandibular left second molar that needs unilateral expansion; (c) the left second molar moved buccally while the position of the right second molar has been preserved.

Unilateral Tip-back and Unilateral Tip-forward

In a case with asymmetric sagittal molar relationship, unilateral or asymmetric bilateral intermaxillary elastics in continuous full arch is commonly used but it needs patient cooperation and have three-dimensional adverse side effects such as occlusal plane canting or result in lack of arch coordination. The unilateral tip-back and tip-forward force system caused by a very unique activation of the lingual arch can be used in these cases. It is very difficult to produce this kind of force system in continuous labial archwire (systems).

First, design the valid force system. The simplest force system you may think could be equal and opposite forces on each molar such as a distal force on the right side and a mesial force on the left side (Figure 12.2.8a). However, this force diagram is not valid because the force is not in equilibrium. The forces are equal and opposite but as they are

not in the same line of action which produces a clockwise couple. If counterclockwise couple is added on left and/or right molars, then the force diagram is valid. Some examples of valid force diagrams with mesio distal forces are depicted in Figure 12.2.8b,c. In addition to correction of asymmetric sagittal molar relationship, when bilateral counterclockwise rotation (Figure 12.2.8b) or unilateral counterclockwise rotation of the right (or left) molar is required (Figure 12.2.8c) these force systems would be desirable. However, mesio distal forces are not successful because the magnitude of force is very low due to large inter bracket distance. Therefore, mesio distal single force is replaced with equal and opposite couples (Figure 12.2.8d). The force system is valid and the clinical manifestation from couple is very similar to mesio distal single force at the bracket as described above.

Let's suppose you would like to tip back the upper left molar and tip forward the upper right molar. The first step is to determine valid and desired force system that is equal

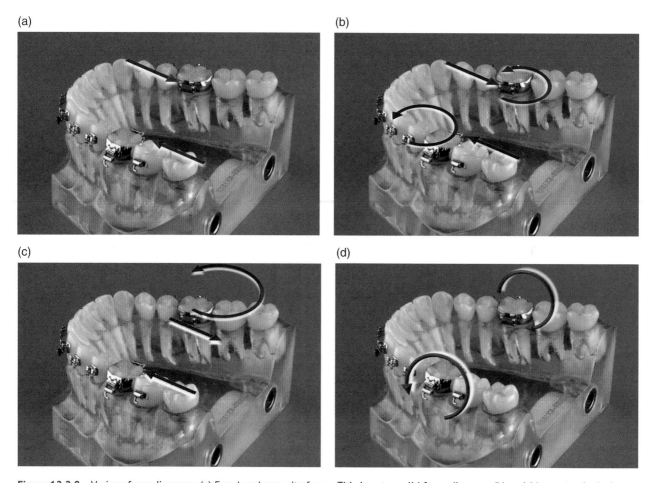

Figure 12.2.8 Various force diagrams. (a) Equal and opposite forces. This is not a valid force diagram; (b) and (c) counterclockwise couple is added on left and/or right molars to satisfy the equilibrium; theses are valid force diagrams but have irrelevant clinical effects; (d) mesio distal single forces are replaced with equal and opposite couples. This is valid force diagram.

Figure 12.2.9 Unilateral tip back and tip forward lingual arch. (a) Passive shape; (b) Simulation. The deactivation force system is applied and the lingual arch is elastically twisted at apex (a area) and bend (b area). (c) Scan the QR code or visit the URL. 3D movie file shows the distortion of the lingual arch in three dimensions (Illustration by Dr. N. Rinaldi with permission).

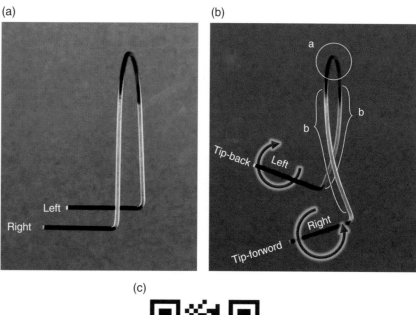

(a)   (b)   (c)

https://youtu.be/YxUd4X8CLGA

and opposite couple in this case. The second step is fabrication of passive shape that is contoured with minimal clearance between the soft tissue (Figure 12.2.9a). The third step is simulation of the deactivation force system on the passive shape which is predetermined in the first step. Each free end is gripped with plier and equal and opposite couple is applied. The lingual arch will be twisted and bent to reach simulated shape by elastic deformation. The apex of the lingual arch is twisted and straight parts between the free end and the apex are bent and gentle curvature is produced bilaterally in opposite direction (Figure 12.2.9b). Next step is to permanently deform the wire to fabricate the lingual arch into deactivation shape that is exactly same as simulated shape. The wire is twisted and bent in three dimensions so that it is better depicted in movie file. Scan the QR code to access it (Figure 12.2.9c). During this procedure, over bending of the wire and bending in opposite direction to reach the final deactivated shape is required to prevent permanent deformation. Before it is activated in the mouth of the patient, "trial activation" is performed to apply activation force system on the lingual arch to check if the activated shape is same as passive shape. If the deactivated shape is correctly fabricated, once it is engaged into

the brackets the activated shape would follow the passive shape that we make in the first step (Figure 12.2.10).

The patient in Figure 12.2.11 has asymmetric occlusion with class I molar relationship on the right side and class II molar relationship on the left side (Figure 12.2.11a,b). The panoramic radiograph clearly shows that the upper left buccal segment has been tipped forward. The perpendicular projection of the center of resistance to occlusal plane of the right molar lies on the central pit, but on the left side, it lies distal to the central pit (Figure 12.2.11c). Mentally uprighting the upper left molar can correct the class II molar relationship. The objective of treatment is to rotate the upper left molar around the center of resistance and hence, applying couple on the upper left molar is the required force system. The unavoidable accompanying tip-forward moment on the right side is unnecessary. With the unilateral tip back and tip forward lingual arch inserted, the force system would look like the figure depicted on the labial side (Figure 12.2.11d,e). In order to cancel the unwanted tip-forward moment on the right side, cantilever tipback spring is inserted bilaterally on the labial side. The force system from the tip back spring is the tipback moment on

(a)

(b)

(c)

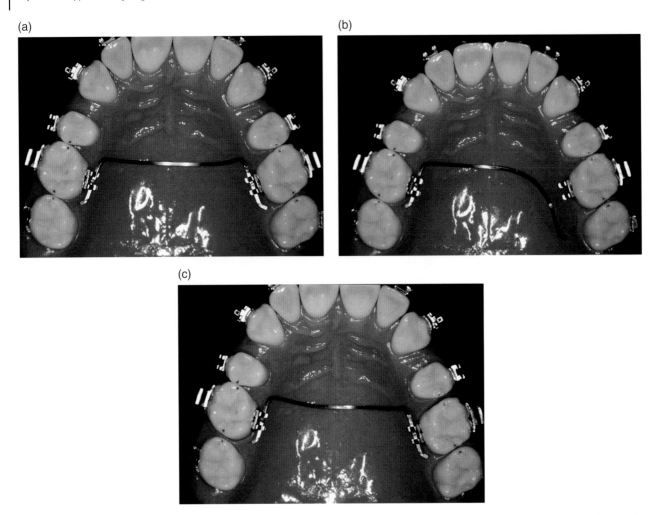

Figure 12.2.10 (a) Passive shape; (b) deactivated shape; (c) activated shape. Upper left molar tipped backward, and upper right molar tipped forward.

the bilateral molar, intrusive force on anterior free end, and extrusive force on the posterior teeth (Figure 12.2.11f,g). In the upper right molar tip forward moment from the lingual arch and tip-back moment from the tip back spring cancel each other out while in the upper left molar, there would be tip back moment from both lingual arch and labial tip-back spring. The remaining unnecessary vertical forces are eliminated by a small piece of wire engaged into upper first bicuspid. It is activated so that it produces extrusive force on the anterior teeth and intrusive force on the posterior teeth to cancel the vertical forces from the tip back springs (Figure 12.2.11h,i). In this patient, the first premolar was later extracted. Summing of the force system from several appliances there is a couple produced on the upper left first molar and all other unnecessary adverse side effects are concentrated on the first bicuspid. After asymmetric applications of lingual arch treatment shows tip

back on the upper left molar only and the upper right molar maintained its original position (Figure 12.2.11j,k).

Summary

Lingual archwire connecting molars across the arch can produce very unique force systems that continuous labial archwires cannot. To the extent possible, the specific amount of bend in "mm", amount of angle of twist in "degrees" for proper activation of an appliance were not used, as those numbers can vary in accordance with size and shape of the cross section of the wire, material and overall configuration of the lingual arch. Rather, emphasis was put on principle over the technique in this chapter, aiming to explain the "why" and not the "how." Once the valid force system is designed, start with the passive shape and simulation of the predetermined force system will

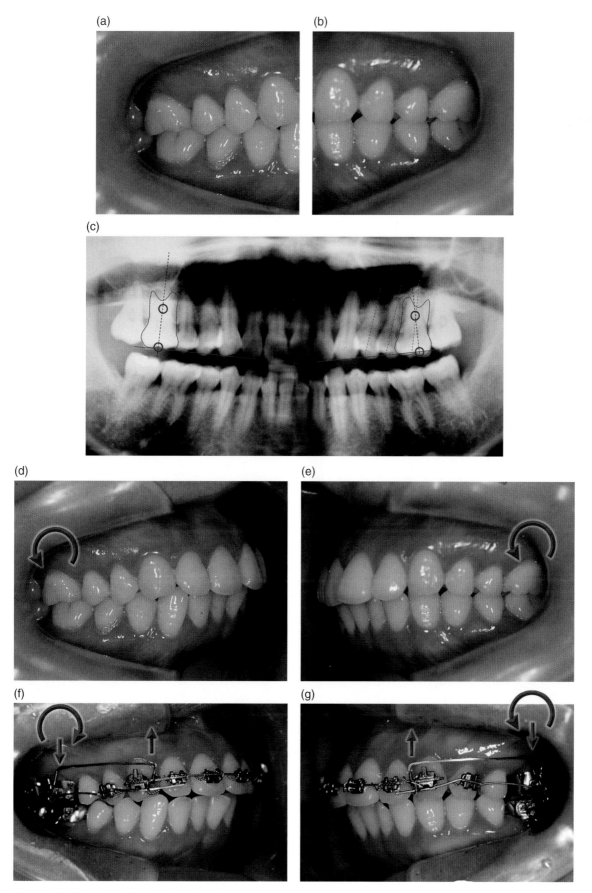

Figure 12.2.11 (a) and (b) A patient with Class I molar relationship on the right and Class II molar relationship on the left side; (c) Panoramic view shows that upper left buccal teeth tipped forward (red dotted line); (d) and (e) the force system from the lingual arch; (f) and (g) the force system from bilateral tip back springs; (h) and (i) force system from the wire pitted against the first premolar; (j) Before treatment; (k) After application of active lingual arch.

(h)

(i)

(j)

(k)

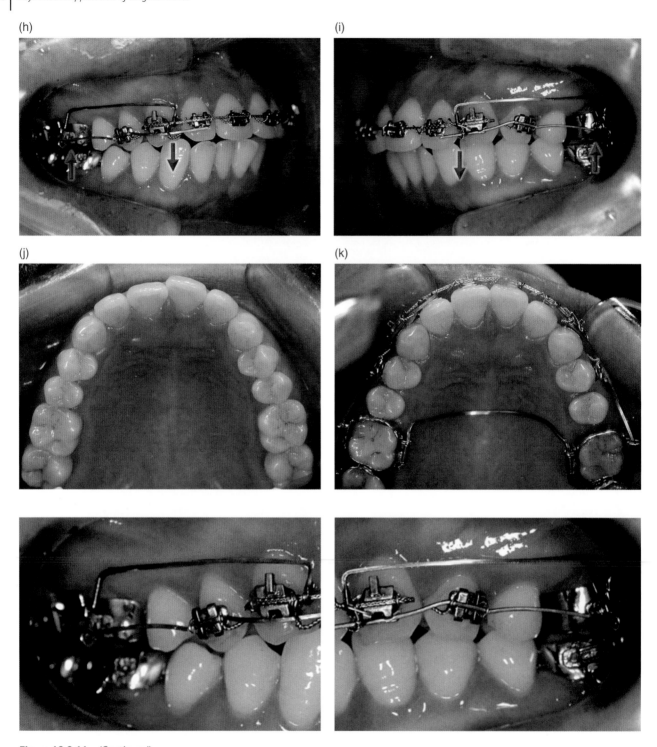

Figure 12.2.11 (Continued)

show you the correct shape. The simulation method to obtain the correct shape is applied to any other asymmetric applications such as unilateral rotation, unilateral constriction of the lingual arch and of course any other symmetric application as well. Only unilateral expansion and unilateral tip back and tip-forward mechanic were covered in this chapter, nevertheless, the simulation method to obtain the correct deactivated shape is universal and its application is limited only by law of nature and your imagination. There is no doubt that the application of sound biomechanical principle may give rise to development of asymmetric application.

References

Burstone CJ. Precision lingual arches. Active applications. J Clin Orthod. 1989;23:101–109.

Burstone CJ, Choy K. The Biomechanical Foundation of Clinical Orthodontics. Chicago: Quintessence Publishing Company Inc., 2015:229–274.

Burstone CJ, Koenig HA. Precision adjustment of the transpalatal lingual arch: computer arch form predetermination. Am J Orthod. 1981;79:115–133.

Burstone CJ, Manhartsberger C. Precision lingual arches. Passive applications. J Clin Orthod. 1988;22:444–451.

12.3

Skeletal Anchorage for the Correction of the Canted Occlusal Plane

George Anka and Athanasios E. Athanasiou

Treatment of the Canted Occlusal Plane

The canted occlusal plane problem has not being addressed as a real issue in the clinical orthodontics. In the past, its clinical consideration was minimal, if any, and doing correction in this area was often associated with complications. One reason is that the clinical technique was complex and required complete cooperation from the patient's side. Orthodontists seldom integrated the correction of the occlusal plane, especially the canted one, into the actual treatment plan. If it was considered a significant issue within the therapy and part of the chief complaint, such as face asymmetry, facial esthetic, jaw function, and temporomandibular dysfunction (TMD) problems, the procedure of choice most of the time was orthognathic surgery treatment. In the first author' practice, by conducting "orthodontics and dentofacial orthopedics", an attempt to minimize the need of surgery by using temporary anchorage devices (TADs) is routinely utilized. The term "orthodontics and dentofacial orthopedics" refers to the movement of teeth together with their supporting alveolar bone so that by camouflage surgery is avoided. A good number of patients would decline treatment when surgical intervention is the only option.

The use of TADs is presented in this chapter as a possible alternative in doing orthodontic treatment without or limited surgical intervention in problems involved the canted occlusal plane. By using this concept, a new dimension in orthodontics for treating the canted occlusal plane is presented according to the limitations of camouflage therapy based on the envelope of discrepancy (Graber et al. 2011) (Figure 12.3.1). The concept presented in this chapter focuses on the middle range of motion using TADs for producing the orthopedic effect (Anka and Grummons 2009). By using this concept, a deviated mandible can be corrected to a certain degree thus, minimizing the asymmetry of the face and the jaws as well as by rehabilitating the oral function. The challenge is great especially if considering that form follows function (Kondo 2007). On the other hand, the question remains whether the function will follow if a change of the structure will be attempted. Unfortunately, the answer is negative unless the deviated function is corrected by efficient oral rehabilitation which is necessary for stability. Therefore, with all treatments of asymmetries with a canted occlusal plane primarily involved, the practice of myofunctional therapy is recommended to be part of the overall treatment plan.

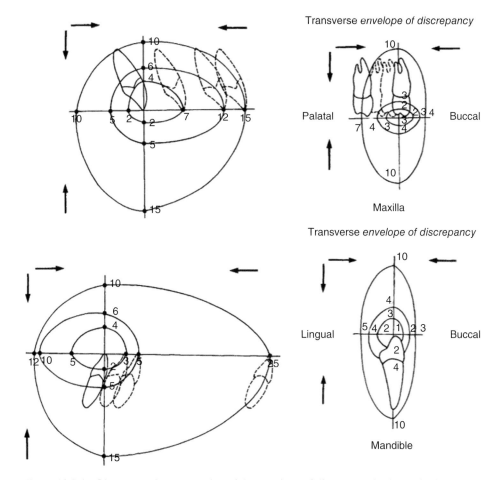

Figure 12.3.1 Diagrammatic presentation of the envelope of discrepancy in the sagittal and transverse planes. The inner envelope shows the range of orthodontic tooth movement alone, the middle envelope explains the range of combined orthodontic tooth movement with growth modification and orthopedic effect, and the outer shell illustrates the range of orthognathic surgery range. *Source:* Reprinted from Graber et al. (2011) with permission.

By performing orthodontic procedures for the correction of an occlusal problem often the skeletal problem becomes less apparent (Raghuraj et al. 2015). Since it is not possible to change the underlying structures, a camouflage treatment could be used to manage the problem. In such cases, search and assessment regarding etiology becomes the first priority based on a detailed classification of the malocclusion and the skeletal relationships (Moyers et al. 1980; White et al. 1976; Proffit 1986; Graber 1963). Making identification of the cause of malocclusion simple, it can be divided into three main categories in which treatment should be directed to the tissues involved.

Firstly, diseases and syndromes: Crouzon syndrome, Apert syndrome, hemangioma, plexiform neurofibromas, torticollis, premature closure of cranial sutures, craniosynostosis, scoliosis, etc.

Secondly, posture: Respiratory problems that affect posture, tongue trust related to swallowing and sucking, sitting and/or sleeping on one side, etc.

Thirdly, growth: Hypoplasia, hyperplasia, cleft lip and palate, skeletal heredity, etc.

It seems that is feasible to deal mostly with the malocclusions related to the second category only, namely posture. Sometimes it can be difficult to correct this kind of problem, as patients are reluctant to change their habits. As an example, when it comes to their appearance, they like their hairstyle, which they prefer to let the hair dropped on the side of the head that may or may not cover one of the eyes. This habit will first affect the symmetry of the left and right eyes; then the maxilla bone might tilt to one side, effect the occlusal plane, and head posture can sometimes be severely affected (Chihiro et al. 2015). However, when this problem is explained by the doctor to the patient, his/her reaction can vary, and the treatment outcome will differ as well. The problem of the canted occlusal plane mostly begins with asymmetry of the mandible, which will force the maxilla to adapt and will result in a deviation of both jaws (Kheir and Kau 2016). In the etiological category of disease, it can sometimes involve more complex problems such as scoliosis (Saccucci et al. 2011). Scoliosis can trigger one-sided chewing thus causing unilateral posterior crossbite. Adolescent idiopathic scoliosis is defined as a spinal curve or curves of 10° or more in about 2.5% of most populations. However, in only about 0.25%, the curve does progress to the point that treatment is justified (Visscher et al. 2001). It is recommended to treat patients with scoliosis during a young age so that the problem can be identified early and be treated efficiently. After orthodontic treatment for deep overbite has finished and an excellent posterior occlusal relationship has been achieved, posttreatment radiographic evaluation revealed a normal-appearing spine (Saccucci et al. 2011). Physical exercises have been described as giving the patient significantly improved posture. Abnormal scoliotic and kyphotic curves in the spine have been also associated with general health problems such as headaches, backaches, and limited range of back motion. Following various types of rehabilitation dental treatments, all these symptoms disappeared, and the spine on posttreatment radiographic examination appeared normal (Saccucci et al. 2011).

It is quite understandable that many of the cases with canted occlusal plane will involve a multidisciplinary approach of dental and medical disciplines due to their complex nature and three-dimensional manifestations of malocclusion. The deviated direction of the maxillary and mandibular bones that affects the occlusal plane of the upper and lower dentition can be of *Roll*, *Yaw*, and *Pitch* movement and combinations (Figure 12.3.2). The role of orthodontist in correcting or camouflaging the asymmetry can be limited depending on the *Roll*, *Yaw*, and *Pitch* characteristics and severity of the problem.

The *Yaw* movement is probably the biggest obstacle in dealing with the camouflage treatment at the contemporary clinical approach of dentoalveolar orthopedics. The problem involves the skeletal deformation or asymmetry of the maxilla and mandible expressed between two or more maxillary or mandibular movements. Camouflage treatment depends on the impact of the combined action of the treatment of the maxilla and mandible toward the cranial base. Among the mentioned three movements, the *Yaw* movement will make the configuration of the two jaws so that deformity can be beyond the ability of correction with conventional orthodontics and even with the assistance of TADs. In these cases, observation of the three-dimensional CT images show that the landmarks Porion are not located in the exact mesialdistal location thus, directly influencing the left and right part of the maxilla as well as the molar location.

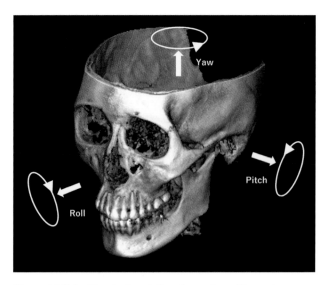

Figure 12.3.2 The deviated directions of maxilla and mandible that affect both upper and lower occlusal planes can be of *Roll*, *Yaw*, and *Pitch* movements and combinations. *Roll* describes when the vertical position of the teeth is different on the right and left sides – viewed as up-down deviations around the transverse axes. *Pitch* is when the vertical relation of the teeth to the lips and cheeks can be conventionally described as up-down deviations around the anteroposterior axes. *Yaw* is a rotation of the jaw or dentition to one side or the other, around a vertical axis, produces a skeletal or dental midline discrepancy.

The limitation of *Roll* motion correction may vary depending on the case, but the most common modification is up to 3° (Kheir and Kau 2016). However, the absence of a good number of cases and statistical data prevents from determining how much influence can take place occlusally. The correction of the *Roll* will affect the TMJ region and the adaptation ability of the joint toward the changes of the position of the occlusal plane. Precautions should be taken in correcting the cant of the occlusal plane by extruding and intruding the four quadrants of the posterior occlusal planes involved which are the main causes of the canted problems (Figure 12.3.3). Many cases with canted occlusal plane already present symptoms of TMD and joint adaptation may not be expected. In these cases, treatment should be designed in such a way to improve TMD symptoms and conditions as well as to correct the canted occlusal plane.

Assessment of the canted occlusal plane by means of CBCT has been recommended (Kheir and Kau 2016), but it seems that at present the standardization of the method is not easily achievable. Since the occlusal plane is projected in the three dimensions of space its superimposition before and after treatment to show the differences of the correction is not feasible yet. The necessity of easing superimposing

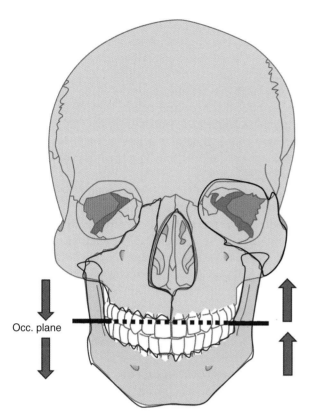

Figure 12.3.3 To correct the canted occlusal plane all four quadrants of posterior teeth should be considered for intrusion or extrusion.

Occ. plane

the plane of two periods (before and after treatment) to the cranial base of the skull will be appropriate to understand the effect of orthopedic outcome. The three-dimensional evaluation will also assist to follow the direction and how the occlusal plane has moved and corrected.

The next problem is knowing the adaptive ability of the TMJ structure to endure a compression or distraction, which happens when the canted occlusal plane is altered. For the movement of the correction of the canted occlusal plane, it is wise to consider all four quadrants of posterior teeth (Figure 12.3.3).

Sometimes, it is possible to intrude or extrude one quadrant for the correction of the canted occlusal plane that may help decreasing the asymmetry. Still, the maneuver will be depending on the condyle adaptation ability of the new environment. The spaces and structures between the condyle and fossa namely mandibular fossa anatomical configuration, disc, and the bilaminar zone are the structures that might influence the success of the treatment. Therefore, the treatment plan should be adapted to each case according to their temporal articular mandibular condition. In doing the correction of the canted occlusal plane, it is also recommended to do a functional analysis of the TMJ by using axiograph or other jaw tracking devices, and

combine its findings with the radiographic findings regarding the articular structures of the TMJs. Clinical evaluation of the position of the mandible in rest and in maximum intercuspation is also required. These clinical findings are significant in determining whether there is a functional change due to occlusal interferences. The functional shift caused by occlusal interferences may be contralateral to the side of the problem, and care should be taken if any change due to treatment may worsen the situation. Any occlusal interference must be detected and related to the actual asymmetrical condition (Bishara et al. 1994). The TMJ problem will affect the mandibular position toward the maxilla, and the joint condition must first be addressed to avoid a wrong or incomplete diagnosis. Management of TMD symptoms must come first before starting the camouflage treatment. The treatment of the canted occlusal plane is needed not only for esthetic reasons but also for restoring function and associated problems such as TMD. An association between craniofacial asymmetry and unilateral TMJ sounds in adult patients has been documented (Yáñez-Vico et al. 2013).

Interestingly, the laypersons' perception toward the canted occlusal plane is not to the degree of the actual tilting as orthodontists assess on the frontal cephalometric radiographs. However, people do accept canted occlusal planes up to 3–4° (Olivares et al. 2013).

Correction of the camouflage treatment takes place in the dentoalveolar region and not in the basal bone itself since dentoalveolar bone changes are relatively straightforward and predictable. However, correction of the deviated basal bone that caused the canted occlusal plane may not be easy, but still can be done if the volume of the alveolar bone allows the dental movement in such a way to camouflage and to restore oral masticatory function. When tilting of the occlusal plane is severe, for example 3° or more, distraction osteogenesis of the condylar neck area is also a choice to correct the asymmetric mandible, if indicated (Grayson and Santiago 1999).

Clinical analysis of the face is essential because asymmetry needs to be documented and reviewed all times, and with the aim to change the structures, if possible. After a thorough overall analysis of the face takes place, personalization of the treatment can be done using all the data collected (Meneghini and Biondi 2012).

In the frontal cephalometric radiograph, the Mid-Sagittal Reference Line is the first variable to primarily identify the deviation between the left and right sides of the face, and afterward to assess and measure the asymmetry in detail (Figure 12.3.4). It should be noted that this variable is primarily a two-dimensional measurement, and it will be challenging to interpret a three-dimensional problem especially when the interpupillary line is not perpendicular to

The measurement

Grummons   Frontal   Analysis
(simplified)

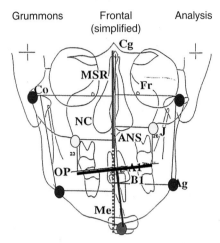

With the courtesy from Dr. Duane Grummons

Figure 12.3.4 Landmarks of the Grummons frontal cephalometric analysis: Ag, antegonial notch; ANS, anterior nasal spine; Cg, cristal galli; Co, condylion (most superior aspect); Fr, foramen rotundum; J, jugal process; Me, menton; MSR, mid-sagittal reference line at cristal galli drawn toward ANS; NC, nasal cavity at the widest point; Z, zygomatic frontal suture, median aspect; ZA, zygomatic arch; A1, upper central incisor edge; and B1, lower central incisor edge.

the upper median line of the head because the left and right eyes are not symmetrical toward the median line. It should be noted that in prosthodontic work, the interpupillary line guides the arrangement of upper anterior teeth. The occlusal plane of the upper anterior teeth must be parallel to the interpupillary line. However, in orthodontic patients, these two lines are not necessarily parallel to each other (Bhuvaneswaran 2010). This finding has been presented in several reports (Kokich et al. 1999; Rifkin 2000; Kavitha 2019; Revilla-León et al. 2019) and for this reason the midline of the face (maxilla) should be selected when the interpupillary line is not parallel (Figure 12.3.5).

The use of the line N-ANS as orientation baseline is preferable and by drawing a line from the left orbital rim perpendicular to the N-ANS an interpupillary line can be formed. The search for an orientation baseline in studying head asymmetry presents great difficulty in cases with a deviated nasal septum (Figure 12.3.6). The maxillary bone differences of left and right side will make the case a complex one and the deviation of the maxilla to one side and the asymmetrical structure of the temporal bones will affect the location of Porion (Figure 12.3.7).

Dealing with asymmetry cases, an aim should be to avoid further deterioration thus, giving to the patient a better quality of life rather than correcting the entire entity, which may be related to hereditary or acquired etiological factors. The challenge is what orthodontic and dentoalveolar orthopedic procedures should be used in dealing with this kind of asymmetry, which often is mainly characterized by the canted occlusal plane.

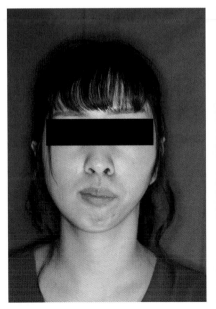
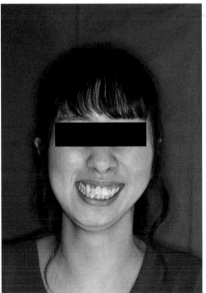
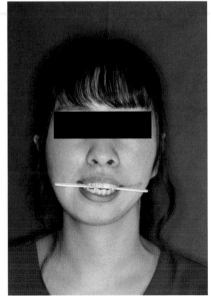

Figure 12.3.5 Un-face assessment of face asymmetry and evaluation of the canted occlusal plane with the use of a wooden tongue depressor.

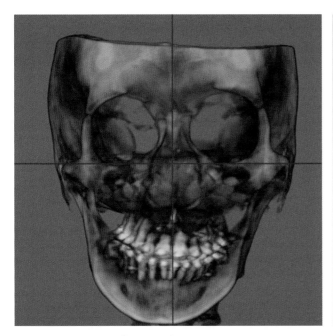
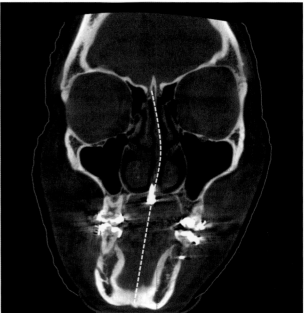

Figure 12.3.6 The 3-D reconstruction and CBCT sections show the deviated nasal septum, the asymmetry of the left and right mandibular rami and body that resulted to a shift of the maxilla and the mandible to the right.

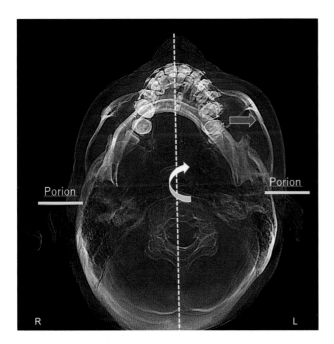

Figure 12.3.7 When the temporal bones are asymmetrical then, as a result, the left and right Porion will not be located on the same line.

Biomechanics for the Correction of the Canted Occlusal Plane

The introduction of TADs in clinical practice almost 20 years ago has significantly contributed to the development of camouflage treatment for the management of face asymmetries, especially in the correction of the canted occlusal plane. The use of TADs provides a semi-fixed anchorage that can be placed in strategic locations that might be difficult or impossible in the past, resulting in a predictable and reliable way of bone-borne anchorage. TADs' use and design can be of various types, varying from single-standing TADs to extended bone-borne plates, so that the technique and the biomechanics have provided many options in correcting the occlusal plane.

The Trans-Palatal Arch (TPA) Plus Hooks

This device is a modification of the trans-palatal arch (TPA) with hooks. The following case is an example of understanding its function and how it works to correct the canted occlusal in combination with TADs.

The patient is a 16Y2M female with TMD symptoms, including reciprocal clicking on her right TMJ, mandibular deviation to her right side upon opening and closing the mandible, limited opening to 30 mm, and masticatory muscles painful to palpation, especially on the left and right lateral and medial pterygoid muscles. MRI reveals an anterior disc displacement of the right TMJ (Figure 12.3.8).

Patient underwent TMD splint therapy for 1 month, with fair-to-good response resulting in relief of the dysfunction symptoms. The patient's lower right first molar presented poor prognosis and its preservation was problematic. Her dentist asked if the second molar could move

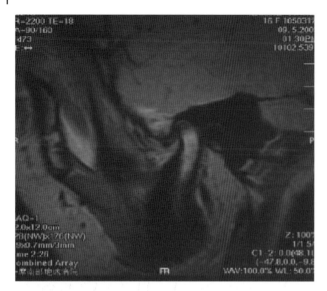

Figure 12.3.8 MRI examination reveals an anterior disc displacement of the right TMJ.

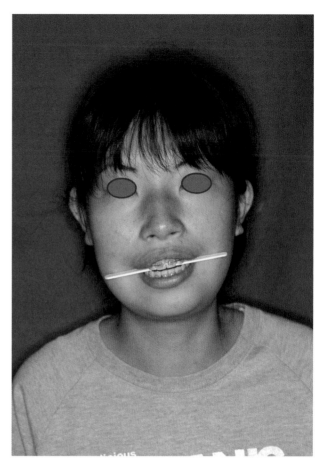

Figure 12.3.9 Un-face facial photograph.

orthodontically in such a way as to replace it. Un-face extraoral and intraoral photographs of the patient appear in Figure 12.3.9. Patient presented with a Class III molar relationship in both sides. The upper second molar lingual cusps caused occlusal interferences during lateral excursions. Treatment began with the extraction of upper second premolars, the lower right first molar, and the lower left second premolar. Resin was placed on the upper first molars to reduce occlusal interferences and ease the alignment of the second molars (Figure 12.3.10). The course of treatment and the result of the use of TPA with hooks is presented in Figure 12.3.11. The method has successfully corrected the canted occlusal plane as seen in the frontal cephalometric radiographs (Figure 12.3.12), the un-face photographs (Figure 12.3.13) and the intraoral photographs (Figure 12.3.14). This case finished using fixed appliances. Although every case has different characteristics and treatment outcomes, the 3° of correction of the inclination of the occlusal plane should be noted. Perhaps the limit of correction of the canted occlusal plane lies significantly on the condyle adaptation coping with the drastic changes induced by the therapy. In this case, the opening and closing movements of the mandible were improved and showed no limitation. Temporomandibular functional evaluation after orthodontic treatment reveals that clicking was still present, without pain, and no ongoing muscle tenderness anymore.

The TPA plus hooks has been successfully used after the Benefit plate (PSM Medical Solutions, Gunningen, Germany) was integrated into the system. The arms provide maneuvering of the force in different directions using coil springs or elastics (Figure 12.3.15). This maneuverability

adds flexibility in moving and guiding the occlusal plane in an oral environment involving deviated oral function and TMD problems. However, when increasing the vertical height of the bite, the masticatory force encountered will be difficult to predict and measure. Therefore, adjustment of force direction during the treatment, when necessary, may be required.

The placement of single-standing screw-type TADs was the standard procedure before the Benefit system was available. The location chosen as the implantation area is the alveolar bone between the first molars and the second premolars, about 5–10 mm below the cervical region of the palatal alveolar bone. The selection of the site for placement depends on the quality and quantity of the alveolar bone in this area. This location is considered a safe site for the implantation with regards to the distance from the lingual root of the first molar and the root of the second premolar since there is enough length that the clinician can reassure the safety of the procedure, even without a surgical guide. The anatomical limitations of tooth movement also need to be taken into account in the treatment plan. The lateral side of palatal alveolar bone placement provides ample distance

(a)

(b)

(c)

(d)

(e)

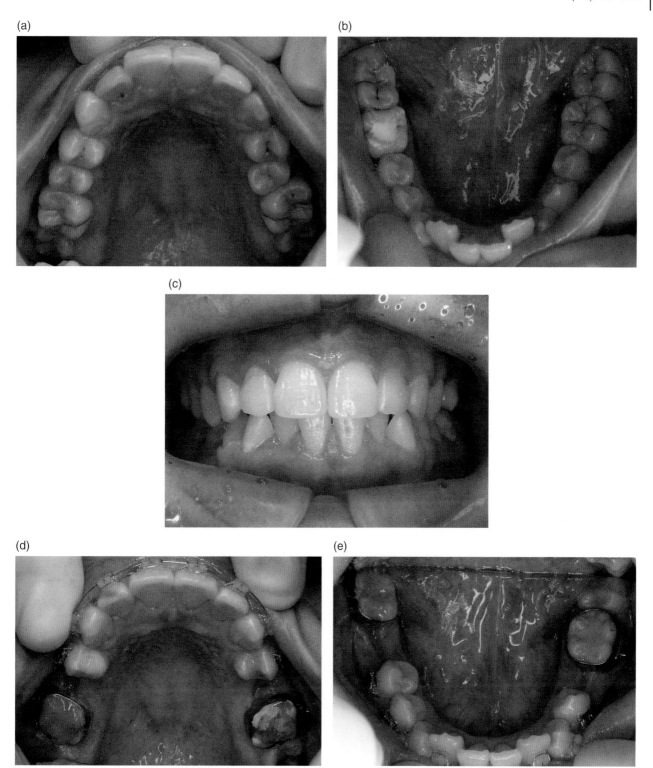

Figure 12.3.10 (a)–(e) The upper second molar lingual cusps caused occlusal interferences during lateral excursions. Treatment began with the extraction of upper second premolars, the lower right first molar, and the lower left second premolar. Resin was placed on the upper first molars to reduce occlusal interference and ease the alignment of the second molars.

(a)

(b)

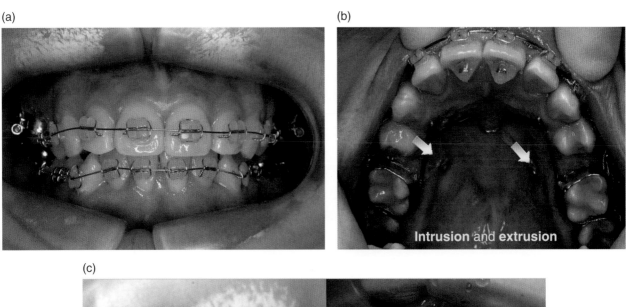

(c)

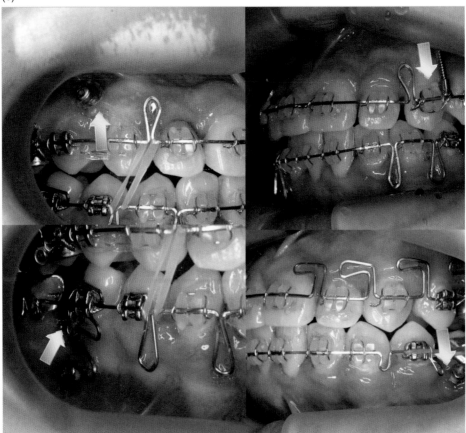

Figure 12.3.11 (a)–(c) Intraoral photographs taken during the course of treatment and the result of the use of TPA plus hooks.

between the implanted TAD's screw since it is far away from the roots. There will be minimum or no risk for any collusion between the screws and the roots as the dentition moves mesially or distally. Therefore, it is essential to calculate and observe the distance of the en-masse movement of the treatment plan before the therapy commences. The range of limitation for the en-masse movement depends on the anatomy

of the occlusal view available in the posterior area distally to the upper second molars, as seen in Figure 12.3.16. The third molars should be removed to provide enough space when there is a need to distalize the dentition. Although theoretically, the upper dentition could move at a considerable distance, the anatomical configuration of the most backward cortical wall of the maxilla will prevent this movement since

(a) (b) (c)

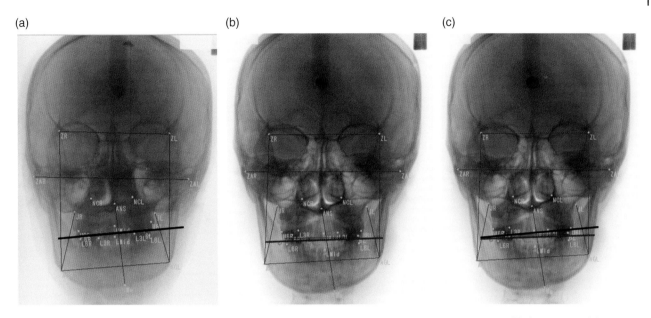

Figure 12.3.12 Frontal cephalometric radiographs taken before the start (a) and at the end of treatment (b) show successful correction of the canted occlusal plane as much as 3° (c).

Figure 12.3.13 Comparison of the initial occlusal plane with the one after treatment.

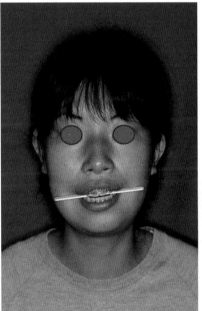 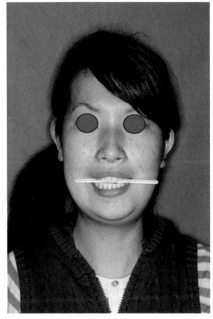

the outer cortical bone will run in a curve inward. Therefore, the maxillary intermolar width will constrict with further posterior movement. The lateral aspect of a radiograph repeatedly shows that the nasal floor is stacking between the roots of the molars (Figure 12.3.17). If there is a desire to further move the tooth or teeth distally the risk of perforating the sinus floor or blunting the apexes is high. The need for distalizing the molars will vary significantly between individuals. Therefore it is essential to thoroughly assess the

CBCT or panoramic radiographic images of the patient before making the final treatment plan. It should be noted that in the mandible the situation is opposite with the intermolar width to increase with distal movement and, on the other hand, the cortical bone of the lingual side not to permit the mesialization of the posterior teeth (Figure 12.3.18). The differences of the intermolar widths in the maxilla and the mandible during distalization of the dentition are apparent.

(a)

(b)

(c)

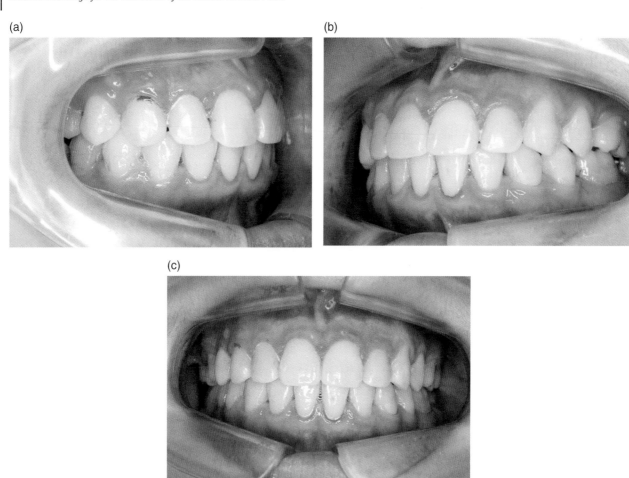

Figure 12.3.14 (a)–(c) Intraoral photographs taken after the treatment.

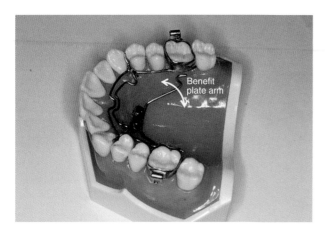

Figure 12.3.15 The TPA plus hooks with the Benefit plate integrated into the system.

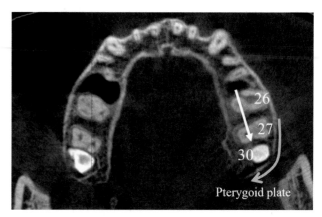

Figure 12.3.16 By observing the maxillary wall from the occlusal view, the outer cortical bone will run in a curve inward so that the intermolar width will constrict as teeth move posteriorly.

When upper and lower teeth move distally, at one point, the relationship between upper and lower posterior molars will gradually become end-to-end thus leading to crossbite. When a Class III molar relationship of skeletal etiology is corrected by moving the lower molars distally, this crossbite phenomenon frequently happens. Depending on the age and maturity of the palatal bone, the Alt-RAMEC protocol to expand and advance forward the maxillary bone

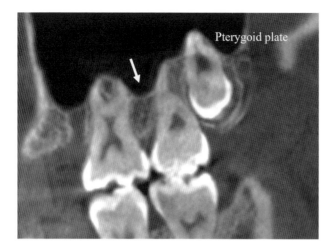

Figure 12.3.17 The lateral aspect of the radiograph shows that the nasal floor is stacking between the roots of the molars. Attempts to move the molars distally may risk perforation of the sinus floor or blunting the apexes of the roots.

orthopedically may be used (Liou and Tsai 2005). This procedure might help avoid the crossbite of the posterior teeth and keep the correct relation of the molars as expansion of the maxilla and distalization of the lower dentition take place to compensate each other. Therefore, it becomes obvious that calculation of the space in need is necessary for the treatment plan of the mesial and distal movements related to the widths of the maxilla and mandible to maintain proper molar relations and good interdigitation. Each anatomical structure should be understood when moving teeth mesial or distally, as it will change the intermolar width and may cause a disturbance in occlusion.

Details of TPA Plus Hooks

The TPA plus hooks is one of the few devices intended to control en-masse the entire dentition within the dental arch in the three-dimensional space and correct the canted occlusal plane. Therefore, it is essential to provide information about its details. After the TADs became available for clinical use (Kanomi 1997), there were several attempts to move more than one tooth at a time, known as the en-masse movement (McGuire et al. 2006; Vibhute 2011; Tan et al. 2017; Becker et al. 2018; Barthélemi et al. 2019; Khlef et al. 2019). In addition, when the cooperation of young patients in using headgear is problematic distalization of posterior teeth becomes a challenge and the jumping-the-bite type of appliances have been effectively used. With the popularity of adults seeking orthodontic treatment nowadays, a better way of moving the molars was necessary and the TADs came into the clinical practice just in time.

The fabrication of the TPA plus hooks includes the following (Figure 12.3.19):

1) Placement bands on the molars.
2) A lingual arch connects the two bands and a TPA reinforcement behind the lingual arch increases the rigidity of the complex.
3) Hooks are soldered to the lingual side behind the first premolars. The length of the hook depends on the type, extrusion, or intrusion of the en-mass movement. The position of the TADs is also related to the planed movement.
4) Finger wire is soldered on the anterior part of the medial side of the premolars. The finger wire will

(a) 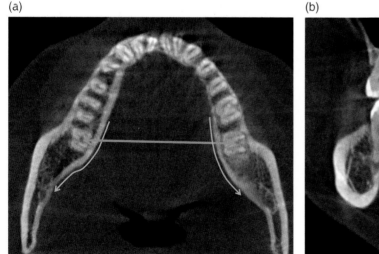 (b)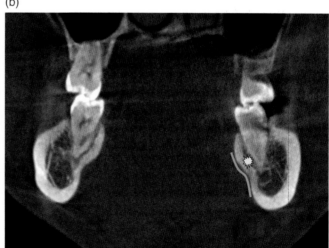

Figure 12.3.18 (a) and (b) In the mandible, the intermolar width will increase as teeth move distally and the cortical bone of the lingual side will not permit to move them medially.

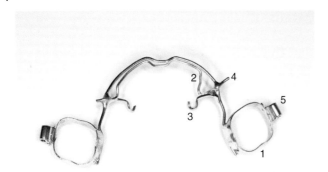

TPA plus hooks

Figure 12.3.19   The TPA plus hooks appliance.

hold the entire posterior dentition during the en-mass movement.

5) Bonding of labial brackets and insertion of wire will engage all teeth together as the entire dentition moves distally or mesially.

6) The above design aims to make a rigid construction that can hold all posterior teeth in one group with or without the anterior teeth together to make the en-masse movement of the entire dentition possible.

This construction becomes more effective when the Benefit plate is added as the range of maneuverability increases significantly (Figures 12.3.20 and 12.3.21). The forces are delivered by using an elastic chain of as much as 300 g per side. The forces will decline rapidly within less than a few days and drop down to 200 g, giving a rest period for bone remodeling. It is anticipated that generation of continuous excessive force might not be necessary, as the value of the ultimate power needed for the en-masse movement is not precisely known. Therefore a range of force will

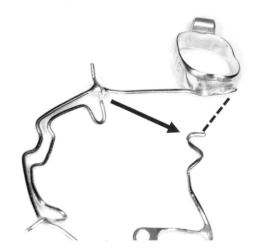

Figure 12.3.21   Configuration of the TPA plus hooks system for distalization and intrusion during the en-masse movement.

be appropriate. Nevertheless, the intermittent force works well and the en-masse movement can change position of the entire group of teeth in a predictable direction.

The TPA plus hooks system is intended to assist in correcting the canted occlusal plane which is dominated by *Roll* and *Pitch* motions, respectively. Especially when doing the *Roll* movement in the correction of the canted occlusal plane, it should be noted that the center of resistance of the maxilla is different from the one of the mandible. Therefore, in correcting one problem, it should be expected to deal with the consequences of fixing another one that will occur. In this case, a *Yaw* problem may occur when correcting the canted occlusal plane by using *Roll* movement and having a deviated midline (Figure 12.3.22).

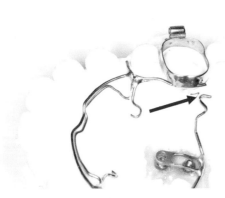

Figure 12.3.20   Configuration of the TPA plus hooks system combined with the Benefit plate for distalization and extrusion during the en-masse movement.

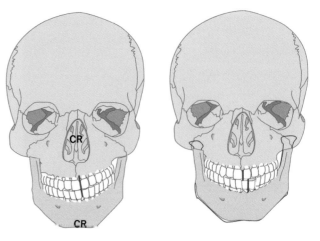

Figure 12.3.22   The Center of Resistance of the maxilla is different from the one of the mandible. Therefore, in correcting one problem, the clinician should be aware of the consequences of fixing another one that may develop.

Figure 12.3.23 (a) and (b) Female patient with canted occlusal plane before and after orthodontic treatment.

(a)

(b)

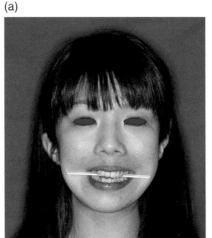
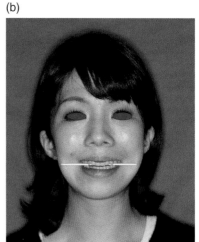

To revise the canted occlusal plane, the clinician should be ready to do all the three-dimensional movements, namely *Pitch*, *Roll*, and *Yaw*. No device can make all three-dimensional actions at once, and a combination of all TADs is recommended.

The application of the TPA plus hooks will be able to correct different types of canted occlusal planes, and the other accessories can be of benefit in case an irregular position of the occlusal plane calls for individual attention and care. The occlusal plane can be corrected easily when the treatment involves extraction in the molar region, but using TADs and TPA plus hooks has helped even nonextraction cases to benefit from the method.

The use of the TPA plus hooks is presented in the following nonextraction treatment of a case with a canted occlusal plane (Figure 12.3.23). Correction in the range of 2–3° of the canted occlusal plane using TPA plus hooks is an indication if the problem of three-dimensional deviation does not involve *Yaw*. Intra-oral photographs show a malocclusion characterized by mild bimaxillary crowding, anterior open bite, and short tongue frenulum (Figure 12.3.24). The pretreatment lateral cephalometric radiograph and the profile photograph show mild bimaxillary protrusion, mild mandibular plane angle with an anterior open bite tendency, and slightly protruded lips (Figure 12.3.25). The pretreatment panoramic radiograph presents the impaction of the upper third molars in front of the zygomatic fissure area thus, indicating that they should be removed to make the en-masse distalization of the dentition possible (Figure 12.3.26). The treatment plan aimed to produce a better profile and appearance, and included the following.

Lingual fixed appliances were used in the upper dental arch because of patient's preference but labial devices were placed in the lower. The treatment plan included distalization of the entire upper and lower dentition. The palatal placement of TADs in the maxilla can be combined with the lingual fixed appliances. As far as for the mandible concerned, distalization of the entire dentition can be done with the TADs placed in the molar alveolar mandibular crest region. Care should be taken during the distalization to prevent opening of the bite. Therefore, distalization of the molars should be combined with their intrusion to close the bite. Myofunctional therapy sessions are necessary during the treatment for better adaptation of the muscle environment since the existing tongue trust will work against the effort to retract both upper and lower teeth posteriorly.

The treatment started with expansion of the maxilla with a Hybrid-Hyrax appliance followed by placement of the lingual fixed appliances to align the teeth. Next, the labial fixed appliances were placed in the lower teeth to correct the crowding. Placement of TADs on the mandible were needed, but the molar alveolar region is covered with flabby mucosa, and single-standing TADs will be difficult or impossible to survive. Also other things of concern were the amount of intrusion of the lower molars. The intrusion of molars will be difficult in a shallow buccal fold where loose mucosa occupied most of the area (Figure 12.3.27). The use of a plate may solve the problem by implanting submucosally TADs with an extended arm in the region of the buccal fold between the first and second molars. The extended arm has a hook for both molars working toward their intrusion and en-masse distalization. Therefore, the Benefit plates were implanted on both left and right side of the mandible (Figure 12.3.28). The Benefit plate used in this case had a refinement to make it ready to use and versatility to help the three-dimensional movement possible in the correction of the canted occlusal plane. The apparatus is called the Anka-Jorge plate, which is illustrated in the figure. This device was developed due to the need for

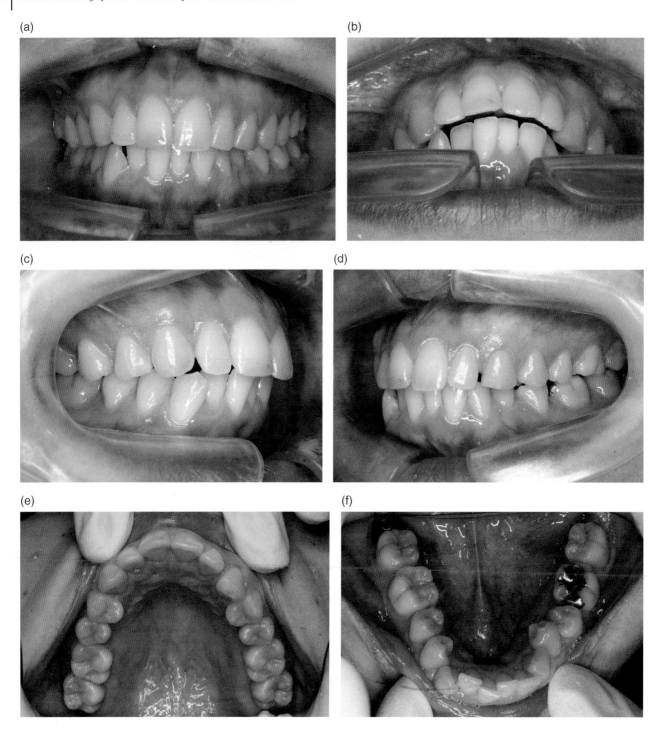

(a) (b)

(c) (d)

(e) (f)

Figure 12.3.24 (a)–(f) Pretreatment intraoral photographs show a malocclusion characterized by crowding, anterior open bite, and short tongue frenulum.

moving teeth from the buccal side, where single-standing TADs may have some limitations in terms of reach and maneuverability. In the maxilla, a lingual appliance was a suitable choice combined with the Benefit plate on the palatal bone to manipulate the upper occlusal plane and with the use of elastics to do the multi-purpose task of controlling the occlusal plane (Figure 12.3.29).

Following the above-mentioned mechanotherapy the following tasks were accomplished:

- Correction of the canted occlusal plane and intrusion of molars to close the anterior open bite. As a result, the force of intrusion of the right and left were in different proportions to correct the occlusal cant.

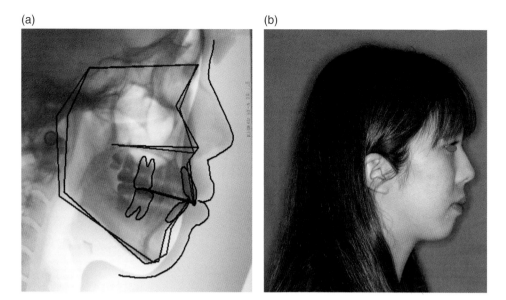

Figure 12.3.25 (a) Pretreatment lateral cephalometric radiograph (the black line tracing is the patient's and the blue line the average value for adult females) and (b) profile photograph revealing mild bimaxillary protrusion, mild high mandibular plane angle with an anterior open bite tendency, and slightly protruded lips.

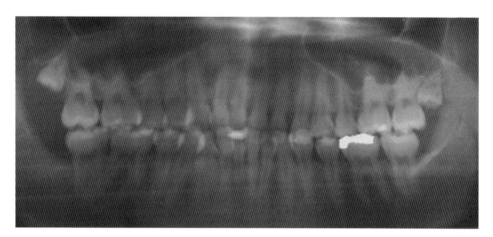

Figure 12.3.26 Pretreatment panoramic radiograph shows the impaction of the upper third molars in front of the zygomatic fissure area thus requiring their removal to make the en-masse distalization of the dentition possible.

(a)   (b)

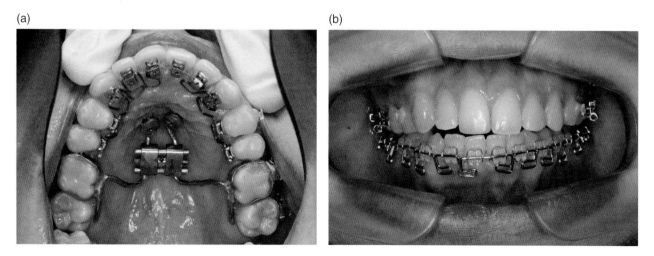

Figure 12.3.27 (a) and (b) Views of the biomechanics with upper lingual appliance including Benefit plates and lower labial appliance.

(a)

(b)

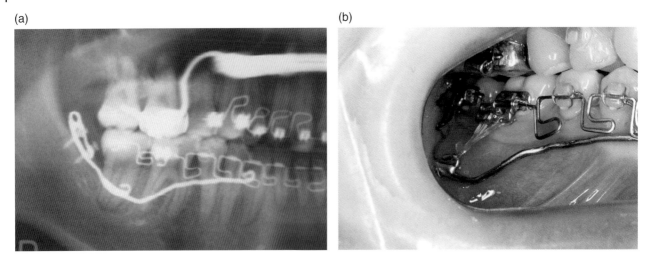

Figure 12.3.28 (a) and (b) Lateral right view from a panoramic radiograph and intraoral right photograph. The Benefit plate with the extended arm has a hook for both working molar intrusions as well as for performing mass distalization.

(a)

(b)

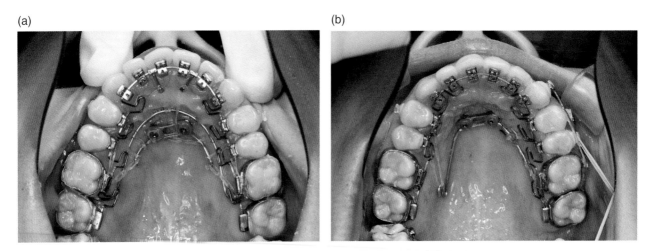

Figure 12.3.29 (a) and (b) Intraoral occlusal photographs of the maxilla with a lingual appliance combined with a Benefit plate to manipulate the upper occlusal plane. Elastics were used to do the multi-purpose task of controlling the occlusal plane. The gummy smile correction was accomplished by using two hooks placed between the lingual wire's central and lateral region. The hooks were linked to the Benefit plate with elastics for intrusion of the four incisors.

- The en-masse retraction was done by engaging the hooks of the Benefit plate directly to the multi-loop archwire (Figure 12.3.29b).
- Gummy smile correction took place by placing two hooks between the lingual wire's position of central and lateral incisors. The hooks were connected to the Bebefit plate with elastics, thus performing intrusion of the four incisors (Figure 12.3.29a). The result is shown in Figure 12.3.30b with comparison with the initial gummy smile showed in Figure 12.3.30a. Within 1 year intrusion and en-masse, retraction of the mandibular dentition took place by engaging the hooks of the Benefit plate directly to the loops of the multi-loop archwire (Figure 12.3.31). The entire

treatment lasted 2 years and 3 months of fixed appliance mechanotherapy, and the final outcome is shown in Figures 12.3.23b, 12.3.30 and 12.3.32. The case remained stable after 2 years of retention (Figure 12.3.33). Comparison of the frontal cephalometric radiographs is illustrated in Figure 12.3.34.

The TPA plus hooks can be used for most cases that do not include the *Yaw* movement. Many cases associated with a more complex three-dimensional deformity and camouflage treatment are challenging to be correct. Therefore, it is necessary to develop several other devices to cope with the camouflage treatment of the canted occlusal plane.

(a) 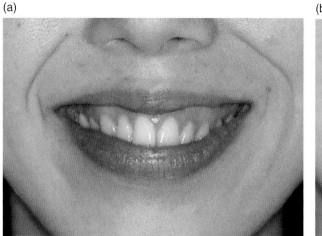 (b)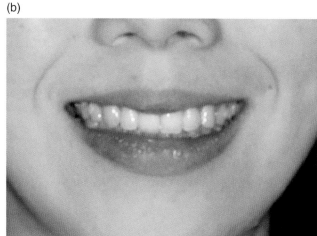

Figure 12.3.30 (a) and (b) Pretreatment and posttreatment photographs showing gummy smile correction.

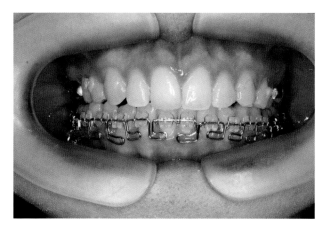

Figure 12.3.31 The en-masse retraction in the mandible was done by engaging the hooks of the Benefit plate directly to the loops of the multi-loop archwire.

The Propeller

The device that the first author uses in asymmetries expressed as discrepancies on the sagittal plane is the Propeller, a stainless steel or titanium coil spring device with a 0.016″×0.016″ rectangular wire as the main structure. The force of the coil springs will generate pressure from 150 g up to 250 g, with an average of around 200 g since movement of three to four teeth at once is expected. The loops of the multi edgewise arch wire (MEAW) will help making the archwire flexible enough to correct the dental arch form, when necessary, while pushing the dental arch into one direction by the Propeller. The whole structure is intended to move the entire dental arch. The Propeller is perhaps the only biomechanical system designed to do the *Yaw* movement of the three-dimensional camouflage

treatment, which is one of the most problematic tasks for performing the orthodontic–orthopedic effect. By this means, the effect is limited to the alveolar bone envelope, the teeth can move with their surrounded alveolar bone, and all the mandibular and maxillary teeth will occlude to one direction or contralateral direction and align with each other. This maneuver should overcome the multifactorial obstacle of muscle force, deviated oral function, and limitation of the bone structure itself, which are all against it.

The Propeller consists of a 0.016″×0.016″ stainless steel wire with a hook on one side to hold the screw, a stainless steel or titanium spring used to generate force, and a stopper with a hook on the other side that attaches to the primary wire bracket (Figure 12.3.35).

The *Yaw* movements induced by the Propeller are illustrated in Figures 12.3.36 and 12.3.37. Between the first and second right premolars, a hook is placed on the rectangular stainless steel wire of 0.016″×0.016″ to retract the right segment distally, which is a relatively easy dental arch form correction. Force used to retract the right buccal segment will depend on the necessity. Usually a force of 250 g is the average to be used for arch form correction, mainly on the premolars' area. The Propeller force drifts the wire with enough power, the main wire will bow and deflect, and the distalization force controls the amount of deflection. If it is desirable to decrease the amount of bow, more retraction of the right buccal side distally is needed, and this case bowing will decrease. This Propeller of bowing and flattening form will adapt to the configuration of the upper dental arch form to the objective of an ideal arch for the case. The left posterior teeth will move mesially using an elastic chain in order to produce interdigitation with the upper teeth. The maneuver will move all the teeth from one side to the other, from left to right, while correcting the midline

(a)

(b)

(c)

(d)

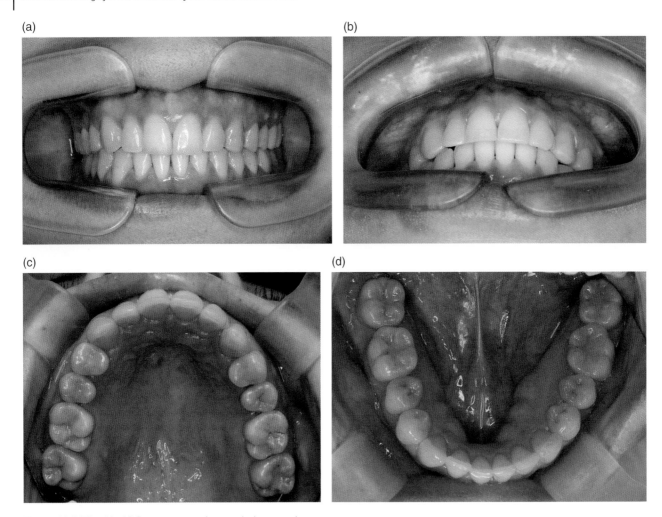

Figure 12.3.32   (a)–(d) Posttreatment intraoral photographs.

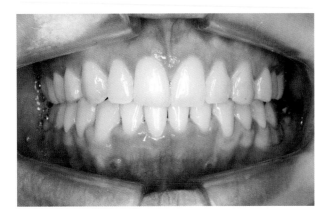

Figure 12.3.33   Intraoral photograph 2 years after retention.

and the arch form. It will also synchronize the upper and lower dental arch forms by making the orthopedic *Yaw* correction motion linked to the canted occlusal plane treatment. Although specific devices are needed to correct the

canted occlusal plane, most of the problems are expressed on the mandible that may shift to either left or right. The Propeller can be also helpful in the maxillary dental arch.

In synchronizing, the form of both dental arches it may need to put the Propeller on both of them. Midline deviation of one jaw will lead to a contralateral direction of the midline of the opposite jaw thus, drifting the midlines against each other. To minimize the complexity, it should be decided whether to move the upper midline to meet the lower or move the lower midline or both approaching each other to make the result less conspicuous. Although often the etiology of the problem is known, sometimes moving one side improves harmony and balance without the final outcome always being perfect. The Propeller can be used horizontally as well as vertically. As explained above, the horizontal use drifts the row of teeth from one side to the other (Figure 12.3.38), and the vertical use is to elongate teeth in the vertical dimension. The vertical use of the Propeller can be utilized on the premolars and

(a) (b) (c)

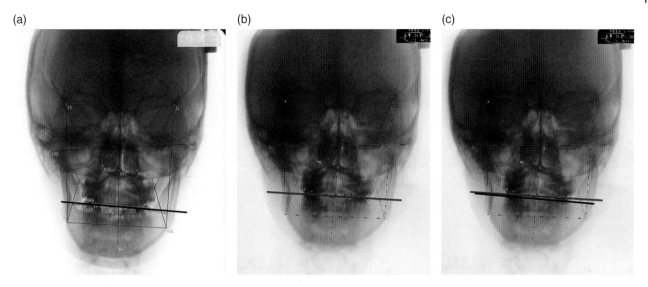

Figure 12.3.34 (a)–(c) The frontal cephalometric radiographs taken before the start (a) and at the end of treatment (b) show successful correction of the canted occlusal plane as much as 2° (c).

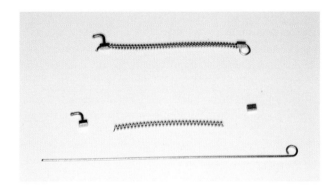

Figure 12.3.35 The entire Propeller (top) and its components.

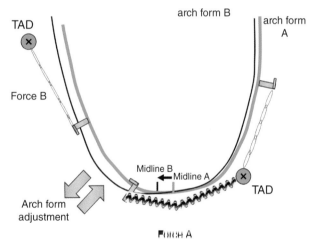

Figure 12.3.37 Dental arch form correction by connecting the premolar area of the main wire when using Propeller. Between the first and second right premolars, a hook was placed on the rectangular stainless steel wire of 0.016″ × 0.016″ to retract the right segment distally.

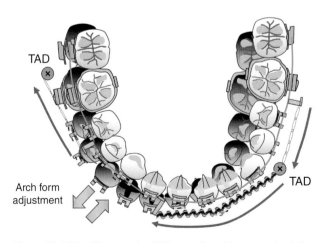

Figure 12.3.36 The anterior TAD was placed between the left canine and the left first premolar. The Propeller was fixed on one end to the TAD, and the other hook was tied on the right lateral incisor; the force being used can up 200 g.

the anterior region only; the excess of the height of the buccal alveolar bone restrict its use in the posterior region (Figure 12.3.39).

The *Yaw* deformity is usually in the opposite direction between mandible and maxilla. Therefore, the direction of forces in many cases will be approaching both jaws to lessen the problem and make it less evident. However, it will be more frustrating when it comes to *Yaw* deformity, in which upper and lower jaws deviate toward the same direction but the midline has shifted. It is a great challenge to move both upper and lower jaws in the same direction but less on one side to correct the midline.

(a)　　　　　　　　　　　　(b)　　　　　　　　　　　　(c)

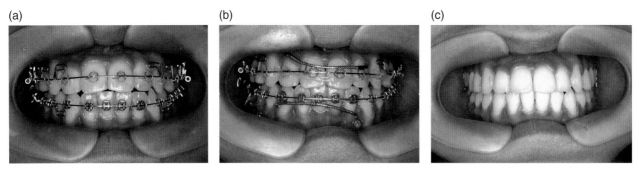

Figure 12.3.38　(a)–(c) The horizontal use of the Propeller is shown in the left and middle figures and the result in the right one.

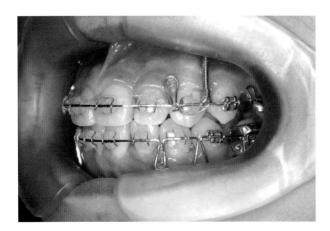

Figure 12.3.39　The vertical use of the Propeller can be utilized on the premolars and the anterior region only; the excess of the height of the buccal alveolar restrict its use on the posterior region.

The Propeller and TPA plus hooks were used in a case of a young male with complaint of upper anterior teeth protrusion with lip incompetency and canted occlusal plane with *Yaw* to the right side in which maxillary and mandibular teeth should be moved to the left (Figure 12.3.40).

The treatment plan included the following:

- Retraction of the entire upper dentition distally.
- Correction of the upper and lower teeth and jaws relationship, anterior–posteriorly, including the midlines.
- Correction of the canted occlusal plane.
- Maneuvering by means of TADs.
- Myofunctional therapy.

In the beginning, third molars were removed to provide space to move the teeth.

The jumping appliance Forsus Fatigue Resistant Device (3M, St. Paul, Minnesota, USA) was used to decrease overjet, reduce the protrusion, and correct the inclination of the upper teeth. The jumping appliance also functions as a pacifier to the TMJs by unloading them. By adjusting left

and right forces of the device correction of the lower midline was accomplished (Figure 12.3.41).

As appears in Figure 12.3.42, TPA plus hooks were constructed to correct left and right molar positions as well as the *Yaw* movement. The right side of the hook helps to extrude the right side or to correct the *Roll* movement. This biomechanical action depends on the ability of the maxillary bone to adapt when the lower jaw moves forward. This maneuver also helps to align the midline to a certain degree, but there is still a need to use the Propeller after Forsus is removed as there will be some tendency for relapse (Figure 12.3.43). Instructions were given to the patient for biting on both left and right sides equally during chewing and eating. The final treatment result at the age 15Y11M is shown in Figure 12.3.44. Growth has helped a lot when treatment biomechanics took advantage of the vertical direction of facial changes as shown in Figure 12.3.45. The changes of the canted occlusal plane are shown in Figure 12.3.46 and they are expressed in the pretreatment and posttreatment extraoral photographs, respectively (Figure 12.3.47).

Correction of the canted occlusal plane can be done efficiently at a younger age. Therefore, attempts should be made to identify and diagnose the problem so that its correction can facilitate better function of the stomatognathic system. It has been claimed that steep canting of the occlusal plane can affect normal occlusion and articulation thus, contributing to the development of signs and symptoms of TMD (Trpkova et al. 2000).

The Ulysses and the Anka-Jorge Plate

When the depth of the buccal mucosa of the vestibule is reduced, it is obvious that the use of the Propeller for extrusion of the posterior tooth is contraindicated. Therefore, a different method is needed, especially when extrusion of the posterior teeth is needed. The easiest way is using the Ulysses system as it includes one TAD screw, usually placed

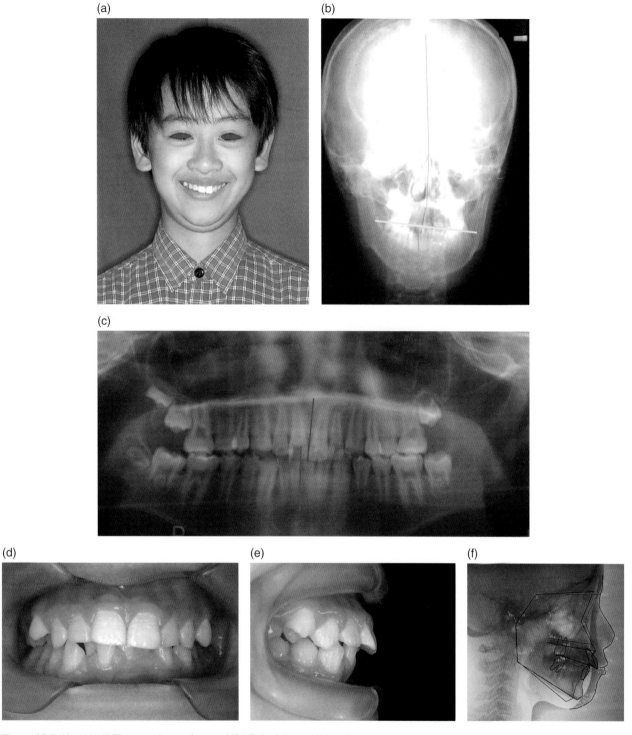

Figure 12.3.40 (a)–(f) The case is a male, age 11Y10M, with complaint of upper anterior teeth protrusion with lip incompetency. In the extraoral frontal with smile photograph, the canted occlusal plane can be observed and a similar finding is seen in the frontal cephalometric radiograph. The deviated to the right lower dental arch midline is noted in the panoramic radiograph where third molars are present in all quadrants except the upper left side. Intraoral photographs show proclination of maxillary anterior teeth, increased overjet and overbite, tooth alignment problems, and a scissor bite of the upper right first premolar. The lateral cephalometric radiograph shows the dental and skeletal protrusion of the maxilla (blue line is the average value for 11-year-old male and black line is patient's tracing).

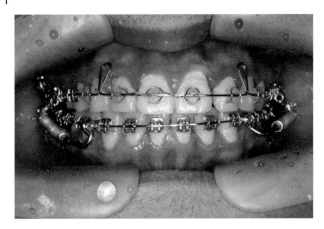

Figure 12.3.41 The bite jumping appliance Forsus has been used to correct the overjet, reduce the protrusion and improve the inclination of the upper anterior teeth.

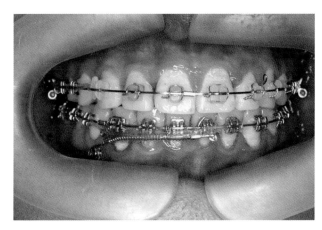

Figure 12.3.43 The use of the Propeller after the removal of Forsus is necessary since some relapse may occur.

(a)

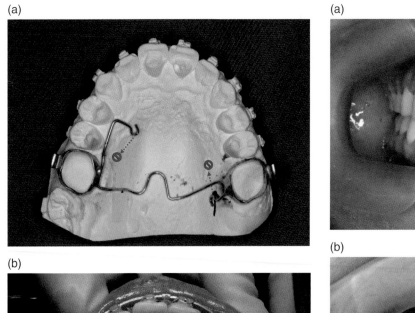

(b)

Figure 12.3.42 (a) and (b) A TPA with hooks was constructed on the palate to correct left and right molar position and perform the *Yaw* movement.

(a)

(b)

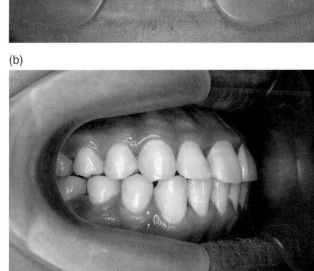

Figure 12.3.44 (a) and (b) Posttreatment intraoral photographs.

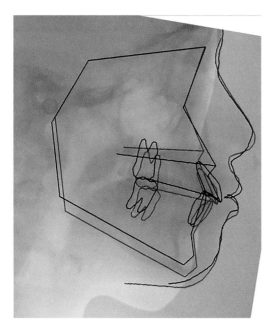

Figure 12.3.45 Superimposition of the lateral cephalometric tracings (black line before treatment and red line after treatment.

on the buccal crest of the mandible between the first molar and the second molar or in the maxilla between the first molar and the second premolar. These anatomic regions are crucial because the buccal ridge gradually gets thicker as it extends posteriorly. Gender consideration should take place per case as females tend to have a less developed alveolar ridge than males. The buccal ridge implantation and

the management of TADs screw can be challenging for anatomical reasons. Inserting the screw in this area may bear a consequence for root damage since the crest is not fully developed; many operators prefer the use of a surgical guide as safety precaution. Certain difficulties are also imposed when this area is occupied by flabby mucosa. For the above reason, a sub-mucosa plate has been introduced, namely the Anka-Jorge plate, to be placed on the buccal site on the ridge behind the second molar and extend its head just in front of the first molars. The insertion place was chosen for easy manipulation of the head of the plate, which has a screw to fix different auxiliaries. The auxiliaries can be made quickly and set to the head of the Anka-Jorge plate, such as the Ulysses wire (Figure 12.3.48). The Anka-Jorge plate before its placement appears in Figure 12.3.49. The head of the plate has a cap, receives any wire auxiliaries that can be screwed, and makes the entire construction stable. The Anka-Jorge plate is a submucosa appliance; placement on the flabby mucosa is possible and at a distant area to avoid sensitive anatomical structures. The corner of the mandible where ascending and descending ramus meet is an ideal site for its placement in terms of preventing damage to the neighboring anatomical structures. In the maxilla, the zygomatic buttress can be perfect for controlling the maxillary teeth in three dimensions of space (Figure 12.3.50). In patients with abnormal swallowing patterns, palatal implantation of the plate is sometimes very uncomfortable. Since this kind of patients cannot tolerate its placement on the palate, the use of the buccal zygomatic buttress as the site of insertion can be a substitute for such a situation.

(a)　　　　　　　　　(b)　　　　　　　　　(c)

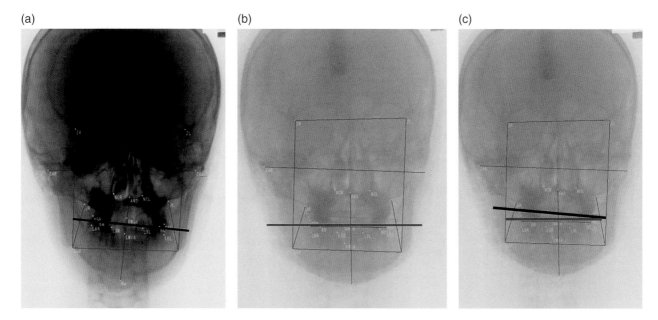

Figure 12.3.46 (a)–(c) The frontal cephalometric radiographs taken before the start and at the end of treatment show successful correction of the canted occlusal plane as much as 3°.

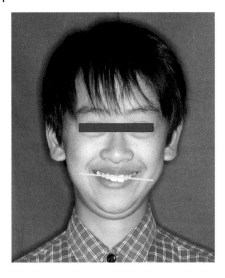
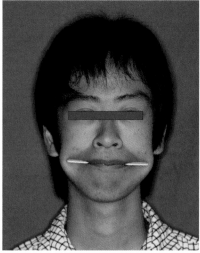

Figure 12.3.47 Extraoral frontal photographs presenting the significantly improved canted occlusal plane.

(a)

(b)

(c)

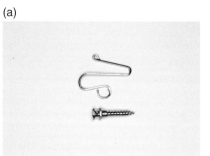
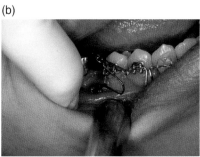
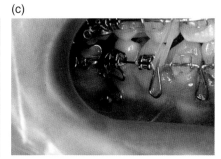

Figure 12.3.48 (a)–(c) The Ulysses wire when is placed on the mandible.

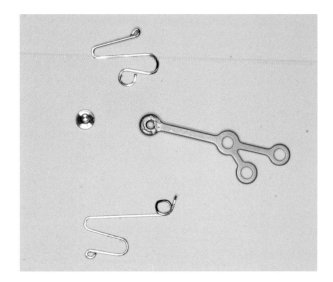

Figure 12.3.49 The Anka-Jorge plate.

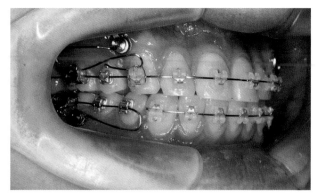

Figure 12.3.50 The Anka-Jorge plate placed in the zygomatic buttress for controlling maxillary teeth in the three dimensions.

The Anka-Jorge plate can be used primarily in a patient with a decreased mandibular plane angle when the correction with the use of a single-standing TAD is not strong enough to overcome the excessive bite forces. In a brachycephalic patient, the bite force can go up to 70 kg and for this reason, two or three screws and a plate are needed to tackle the bite force and make three-dimensional movements of substantial effects.

Figure 12.3.51 present the occlusion of a transfer case in which the Anka-Jorge plate was used to correct the canted

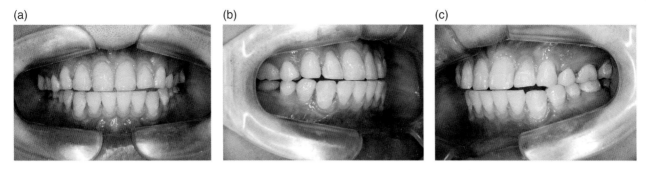

Figure 12.3.51 (a)–(c) Patient has a bruxism habit resulting to a flattening of posterior occlusal surfaces and wear of anterior teeth. Despite the presence of a low mandibular plane angle and strong bite force, a generalized open bite extends from premolars to incisors combining with a tongue thrust habit.

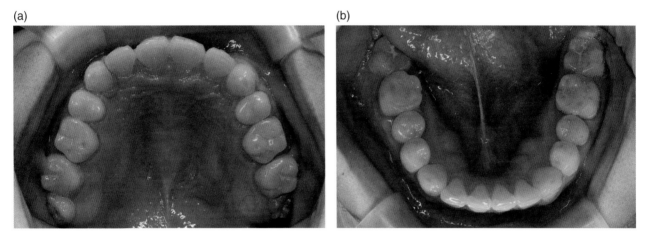

Figure 12.3.52 (a) and (b) Intraoral photographs of occlusal views show the wear of the molars.

occlusal plane. The patient is a male 20Y5M old, having fixed appliances in place on the first visit to the clinic, which were removed to check the condition of the teeth and periodontium. The patient has a bruxism habit and both posterior and anterior occlusal surfaces present severe wear thus indicating significant loading of the TMJs (Figure 12.3.52). Despite the presence of a decreased mandibular plane angle and strong bite force, a generalized open bite exceeds from premolars to incisors combined with a tongue thrust habit. Extraoral profile and un-face photographs as well as lateral and frontal cephalometric radiographs show the brachycephalic pattern and the canted occlusal plane (Figure 12.3.53).

The treatment plan includes oral hygiene instructions, treatment of caries and periodontal problems, start of myofunctional therapy to correct the swallowing pattern, open-close functional exercises, and use of acrylic splint to manage the TMD.

All problems were explained to the patient who requested correction of the canted occlusal plane and the curling of lips as seen on the profile photograph because of the low mandibular plane angle. It was explained that increase in the vertical dimension of the face cannot be easily achieved, as expected by the patient, but the challenge was agreed to be undertaken.

For achieving elongation of the four quadrants of the posterior teeth together with their alveolar bone there is a need for a robust device to complete the task and, therefore, the Anka-Jorge plate is used. The Anka-Jorge plate is placed in the mandible below the ridge on the left and right side. In the maxilla, they are placed on the zygomatic buttress. Adjustment using the wire springs attached to the plates of the four quadrant and tie directly to the brackets will be able to elongate and correct the canted occlusal plane. The patient used to lean on one side when sitting and sleeping, which prevents the effort to extend the vertical dimension of the face. Advice in correcting the body posture when sitting and sleeping was given to eliminate the resistance forces as related to the goals of the treatment without any resistance from the habitual posture.

The auxiliaries used with the Anka-Jorge plate are modified as shown in Figure 12.3.54. The spring wire is

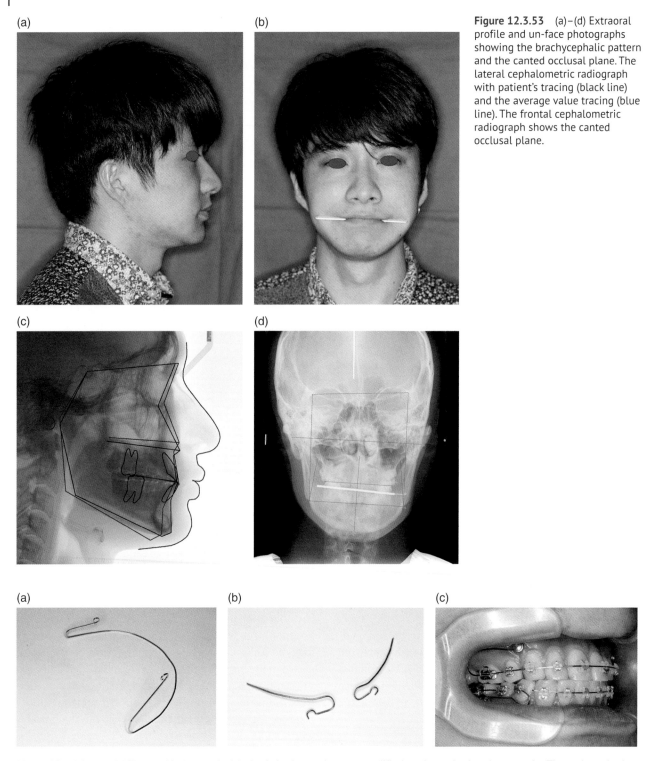

(a)

(b)

Figure 12.3.53 (a)–(d) Extraoral profile and un-face photographs showing the brachycephalic pattern and the canted occlusal plane. The lateral cephalometric radiograph with patient's tracing (black line) and the average value tracing (blue line). The frontal cephalometric radiograph shows the canted occlusal plane.

(c)

(d)

(a)

(b)

(c)

Figure 12.3.54 (a)–(c) The auxiliaries used with the Anka-Jorge plate are modified as shown in the photographs. The spring wire is directly tied to the bracket for efficiency and simplification of the appliance.

directly tied to the bracket for efficiency and simplification of the appliance.

Extraoral photographs taken 6 months after using the devices show improvement in facial appearance

(Figure 12.3.55), the mandibular plane to Frankfort plane angle increased from 19.9° to 24.6° (normal: 26.3°) and the N-Me linear measurement increased from 125.2 to 128.6 mm. The increase in linear measurement is not so

(a)   (b)   (c)

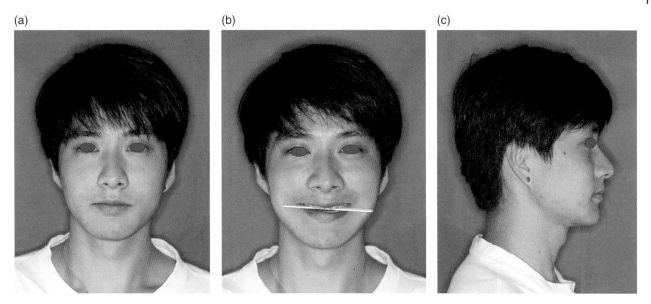

Figure 12.3.55   (a)–(c) Posttreatment extraoral photographs.

substantial, perhaps due to the resistance of the muscle that bounced back every effort to increase the vertical dimension of the face.

The elevator springs increased the vertical dimension and improved the canted occlusal plane. The curl of the lower lip showed significant improvement.

The changes shown in the superimposed cephalometric radiographs are noticeable but not significant (Figure 12.3.56).

Extrusion

Intrusion is inductive to the masticatory muscles, and successful intrusion of the posterior teeth has been reported in many publications from the beginning of the use of TADs in clinical practice. However, extrusion of the posterior teeth to increase the vertical dimension is challenging because of the counteracting effect of the muscles of mastication. Hence, the ability to do extrusion of the posterior teeth is crucial in dealing with the correction of the canted occlusal plane. There have been several biomechanical systems that have been used for the extrusion of posterior teeth. Approaches from the buccal side using single standing TADs with Propeller coil spring, with the Anka-Jorge plate and Ulysses spring, and from the palatal side with TPA plus hooks and the Benefit plate have been demonstrated. However, the demand of a simple design to extrude continuously is necessary for a patient during the relatively long-term period of orthodontic treatment. Otherwise, relapse may occur if the increased vertical height cannot be kept in the position for a long time until the oral muscle environment adapts to the new morphology. For this purpose, a finger spring, called an elevator spring that is soldered on the arm of the Benefit plate has been added (Figure 12.3.57).

Opening of the bite works against the masticatory muscle forces and is a great challenge. A substantial force that can extrude the molars is necessary thus the additional use of an anterior bite plate is essential. In this way, extrusion of the posterior teeth can be less stressful and it will keep the extruded molar in position for a considerable time until oral musculature and function adapt to the new place.

If there are missing teeth or teeth with poor prognosis, restorative works such as crowns, bridges, or onlays can help maintain the vertical dimension rather promising and easily.

If bringing the teeth in an ideal occlusion has been accomplished, then the new occlusal plane and the new mandibular plane have a better chance to stay in place; the perfect form and oral function will help increase the stability. The time and capability of individual adaptation play an important role in future stability.

The elevator spring increases the mandibular plane angle by extruding the upper molars and by bringing the upper occlusal plane downward. The aim is to let the brachycephalic face to be less conspicuous, and as the mandible turns clockwise toward a more extended lower anterior facial height it results in a mesocephalic facial pattern.

The elevator spring can generate 200–300 g and is made out of 0.7 mm diameter stainless steel wire soldered on the left and right of the Benefit plate, which is screwed and positioned median or para-median of the mid-palatal suture; the

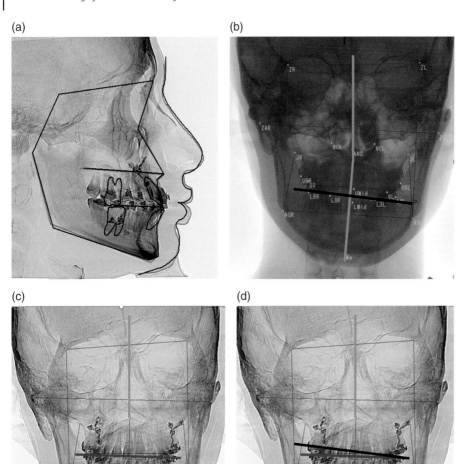

Figure 12.3.56 (a)–(d) Lateral cephalometric tracing superimposition 6 months after of the start of treatment. Comparison of the frontal cephalometric tracings for the same period revealed a noticeable improvement close to 2°.

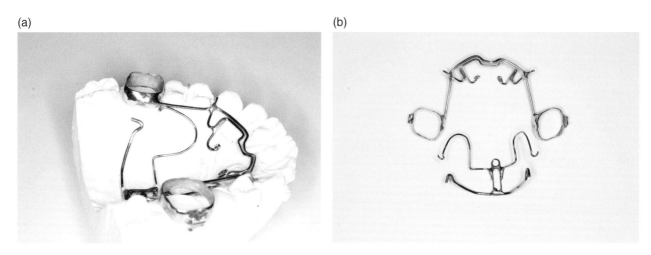

Figure 12.3.57 (a) and (b) For better vertical control a finger spring (elevator spring) is soldered on the arm of the Benefit plate.

spring moves the arms of the TPA upward as in Figure 12.3.57a. The set of the device consists of two parts, as seen in Figure 12.3.57b. The elevator springs will extrude the posterior region (molars and premolars) and move the upper occlusal plane downward. The spring is adjustable and easy to engaged and disengage, replace, and activate. The twin elevator left and right can be adjusted to a different force to meet the requirement for correcting the canted occlusal plane. A single spring can also be used (Figure 12.3.58).

The single spring is to simplify the palatal device to ease the patient. Since orthodontic devices on the palate may disturb swallowing and speech to some degree, simplifying design is called for patient's comfort. The treatment of the case presented in this part of the chapter is in progress, but improvement of the facial appearance as related to the cant of occlusal plane (Figure 12.3.59), of the occlusion (Figure 12.3.60), and the profile (Figure 12.3.61) is evident. The use of the anterior bite plate is essential to slightly

open the posterior bite (less than 1 mm) and by doing so, the device's extrusion of the posterior teeth can be done relatively quickly. The anterior bite plate should be checked each month and its increase should take place as necessary. Excessive height of the bite plate may cause traumatic occlusion of the lower anterior teeth. Obviously, the lower anterior teeth will be intruded for a certain degree as a result, but the overall outcome will be the extrusion of the posterior teeth. The anterior teeth can be enhanced as necessary later on by using the labial fixed appliances.

Pretreatment and progress frontal cephalometric tracings show minor improvement of the tilted occlusal plane as the case is still in progress (Figure 12.3.62).

This method is also effective in cases treated with lingual orthodontic fixed appliances. In these cases, the TPA is not used, as the brackets are on the lingual side, but the spring is utilized directly between the brackets and the wire (Figure 12.3.63).

Figure 12.3.58 A single spring (elevator spring) can be used in selected cases.

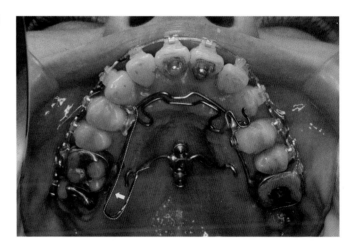

Figure 12.3.59 (a) and (b) Pretreatment and progress frontal photographs showing improvement of the canted occlusal plane.

(a) (b)

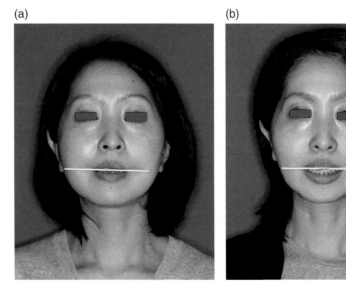

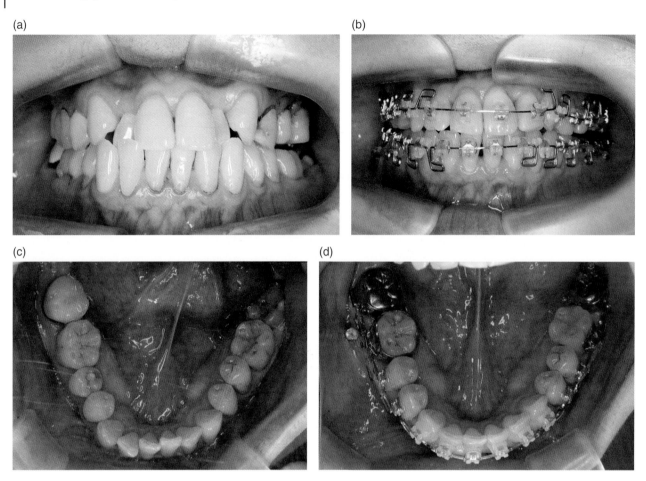

Figure 12.3.60 (a)–(d) Pretreatment and progress intraoral photographs showing significantly improved occlusal relations.

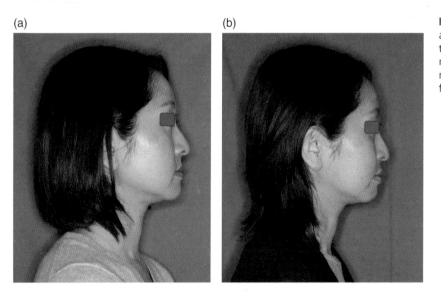

Figure 12.3.61 (a) and (b) Pretreatment and progress profile photographs showing the increased vertical dimension that resulted in a clockwise rotation of the mandible and corrected lips' relationship for a more pleasing profile.

(a)

(b)

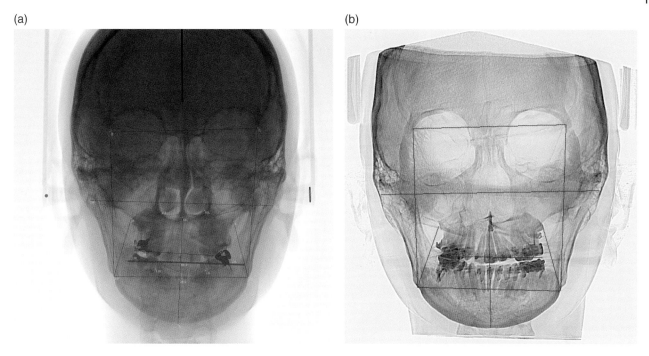

Figure 12.3.62 (a) and (b) Pretreatment and progress frontal cephalometric tracings showing minor improvement of the tilted occlusal plane.

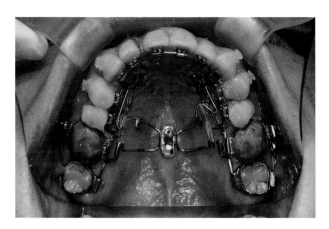

Figure 12.3.63 Lingual fixed orthodontic appliance combined with the spring placed directly between the brackets and the wire.

Cases of the canted occlusal plane in a severe brachycephalic skeletal patterns will impose a great challenge to increase the vertical dimension and correct the canted occlusal plane.

Figure 12.3.64 present pretreatment and progress un-face photographs after the elevator spring moved the occlusal plane downward. In this case, both left and right arms of the TPA are hooked to elevator springs to extrude both left and right posterior teeth (Figure 12.3.65a). The right side of the elevator spring activates more than the left side to give a more protrusion effect to the right side. On the other hand, the bite plane covered the left side occlusal surfaces so that the right side may have a bite opening, which will result with more extrusion of the right region (Figure 12.3.65b). Some intrusion of the left side caused by the bite plane is canceled by the elevator spring. The result is an increase of occlusal plane downward and the correction of the occlusal plane. Although the change in the inclination of the occlusal plane is minimal (Figure 12.3.66), the left and right jaw balance is corrected, and patient presented a balanced facial profile (Figures 12.3.67 and 12.3.68). The bite plate was then removed, and the elevator springs continued to function for another 6 months, waiting for the muscles and condylar structures to adapt to the new environment.

Conclusion

This chapter has no intention to disregard orthognathic surgery for patients with severe malocclusions and skeletal deformities. Selection of a combined orthodontic–surgical approach has specific indications and should be chosen when appropriate to help the patient rather than to challenge both patient and orthodontist by doing orthodontic

(a)　　　　　　　　　(b)

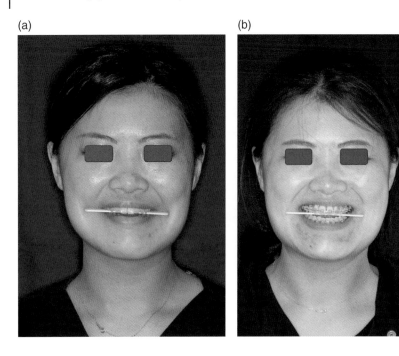

Figure 12.3.64 (a) and (b) Pretreatment and progress un-face photographs after the elevator springs moved the occlusal plane downward and corrected the canted occlusal plane.

(a)　　　　　　　　　(b)

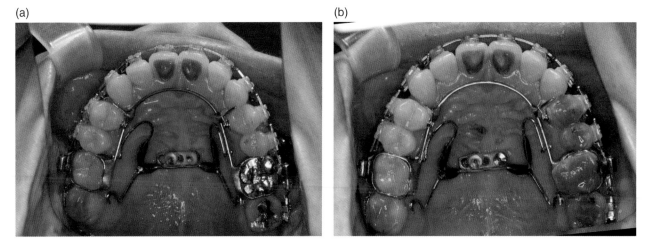

Figure 12.3.65 (a) and (b) Left and right arms of the TPA are hooked the elevator springs to extrude both left and right posterior teeth. The right side of the elevator spring activates more than the left side to give a more protrusion effect to the right side. On the other hand, the bite plane covered the left side occlusal plane so that the right side may have a bite opening, which will give more extrusion of the right region.

therapy alone. This statement is for the benefit of both patients and clinicians. On the other hand, the clinical concepts and cases presented show that camouflage treatment can benefit patients with skeletal problems of moderate severity involving the canted occlusal plane.

This chapter presents various orthodontic treatment options for the correction of the canted occlusal plane. The final position and direction of the occlusal plane can be made and controlled in a predictable manner so as to achieve a satisfactory and stable result of the orthodontic treatment. With the advantage of using the TADs, this section presents devices, techniques, and information advocated to help and recognize the effect of dentofacial orthopedics in the correction of moderate skeletal problems. It is hoped that continuous research will follow in searching better ways to help people who are in need in solving their various orthodontic problems presented in this section of the book.

(a)

(b)

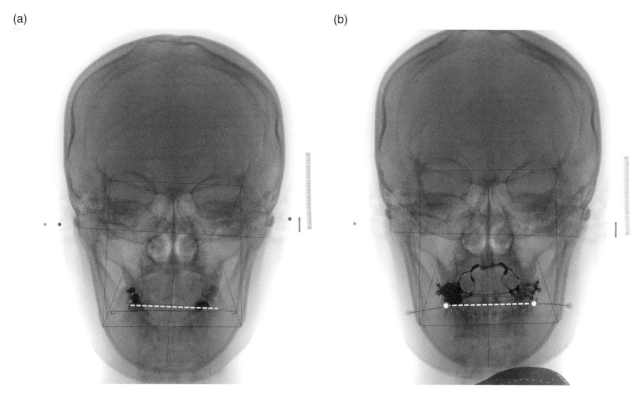

Figure 12.3.66 (a) and (b) Pretreatment (yellow color line of occlusal plane) and progress after the use of the elevator spring (white color line of occlusal plane) frontal cephalometric radiographs. The difference between the yellow and the white lines is 0.5°.

Figure 12.3.67 Superimposition of pretreatment (black line) and progress after the use of elevator spring (red line) lateral cephalometric radiographs. ANS-Me increased from 62.9 to 65.6 mm.

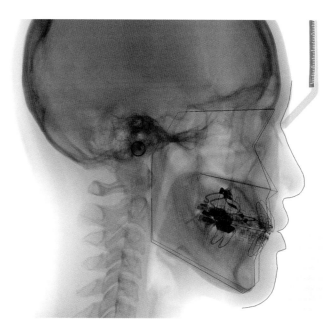

(a)   (b)

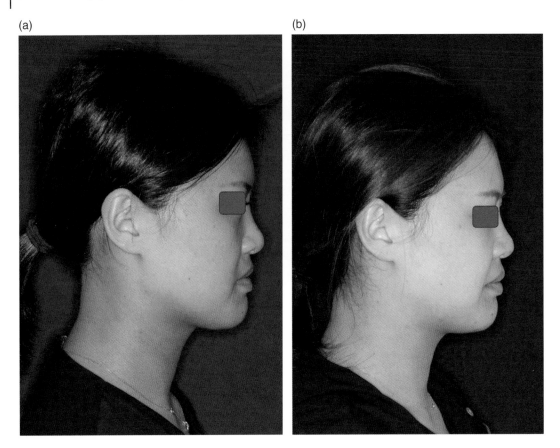

Figure 12.3.68   (a) and (b) Pretreatment and progress after the use of elevator springs profile photographs.

References

Anka G, Grummons D 2009. Treatment of canted occlusal plane. Retrieved from https://www.drgrummons.com/2016/05/23/treatment-of-canted occlusal-plane/.

Barthélemi S, Desoutter A, Souaré F, Cuisinier F. Effectiveness of anchorage with temporary anchorage devices during anterior maxillary tooth retraction: a randomized clinical trial. Korean J Orthod. 2019;49:279–285.

Becker K, Pliska A, Busch C, Wilmes B, Wolf M, Drescher D. Efficacy of orthodontic mini implants for en-masse retraction in the maxilla: a systematic review and meta-analysis. Int J Implant Dent. 2018;4:35.

Bhuvaneswaran M. Principles of smile design. J Conserv Dent. 2010;13:225–232.

Bishara SE, Burkey PS, Kharouf JG. Dental and facial asymmetries: a review. Angle Orthod. 1994;64:89–98.

Chihiro S, Intoy J, Shimojo S. Visual attractiveness is leaky: the asymmetrical relationship between face and hair. Front Psychol. 2015;6:377.

Graber TM. The three M's: muscles, malformation, and malocclusion. Am J Orthod. 1963;49:418–450.

Graber LW, Varnarsdall RL Jr, Vig KWI. Orthodontics Current Principles and Techniques. St. Louis: Elsevier, 2011.

Grayson BH, Santiago PE. Treatment planning and biomechanics of distraction osteogenesis from an orthodontic perspective. Semin Orthod. 1999;5:9–24.

Kanomi R. Mini-implant for orthodontic anchorage. J Clin Orthod. 1997;31:763–767.

Kavitha M. Cant in the interpupillary line. Br Dent J. 2019;227:762.

Kheir NA, Kau CH. The use of three-dimensional imaging to evaluate the effect of conventional orthodontic approach in treating a subject with facial asymmetry. Ann Maxillofac Surg. 2016;6:105–112.

Khlef HN, Hajeer MY, Ajaj MA, Heshmeh O. En-masse retraction of upper anterior teeth in adult patients with maxillary or bimaxillary dentoalveolar protrusion: a systematic review and meta-analysis. J Contemp Dent Pract. 2019;20:113–127.

Kokich VO Jr, Kiyak HA, Shapiro PA. Comparing the perception of dentists and lay people to altered dental esthetics. J Esthet Dent. 1999;11:311–324.

Kondo E. Muscle Wins! Treatment in Clinical Orthodontics. Tokyo: Ishiyaku Publishers, 2007.

Liou EJ-W, Tsai W-C. A new protocol for maxillary protraction in cleft patients: repetitive weekly protocol of alternate rapid maxillary expansions and constrictions. Cleft Palate Craniofac J. 2005;42:121–127.

McGuire MK, Scheyer ET, Gallerano RL. Temporary anchorage devices for tooth movement: a review and case reports. J Periodontol. 2006;77:1613–1624.

Meneghini F, Biondi P. Clinical Facial Analysis: Elements, Principles, and Techniques. Berlin: Springer, 2012.

Moyers RE, Riolo ML, Guire KE, Wainright RL, Bookstein FL. Differential diagnosis of Class II malocclusions. Part 1. Facial types associated with Class II malocclusions. Am J Orthod. 1980;78:477–494.

Olivares A, Vicente A, Jacobo C, Molina S-M, Rodríguez A, Bravo L-A. Canting of the occlusal plane: perceptions of dental professionals and laypersons. Med Oral Patol Oral Cir Bucal. 2013;18:e516–e520.

Proffit WR. On the aetiology of malocclusion. The Northcroft Lecture, 1985 presented to the British Society for the Study of Orthodontics, Oxford, April 18, 1985. Br J Orthod. 1986;13:1–11.

Raghuraj MB, Scindhia R, Amin V, Shetty S, Mascarenhas R, Shetty N. Orthodontic camouflage treatment in skeletal Class II patient. J Orthod Res. 2015;3:57–60.

Revilla-León M, Meyer MJ, Barrington JJ, Sones A, Umorin MP, Taleghani M, Zandinejad A. Perception of occlusal plane that is nonparallel to interpupillary and commissural lines but with the maxillary dental midline ideally positioned. J Prosthet Dent. 2019;122:482–490.

Rifkin R. Facial analysis: a comprehensive approach to treatment planning in aesthetic dentistry. Pract Periodontics Aesthet Dent. 2000;12:865–871.

Saccucci M, Tettamanti L, Mummolo S, Polimeni A, Festa F, Tecco S. Scoliosis and dental occlusion: a review of the literature. Scoliosis. 2011;6:15.

Tan JM, Liu Y-M, Chiu H-C, Chen Y-J. Molar distalization by temporary anchorage devices (TADs) – a review article. Taiwan J Orthod. 2017;29(1): 2.

Trpkova B, Major P, Nebbe B, Prasad N. Craniofacial asymmetry and temporomandibular joint internal derangement in female adolescents: a posteroanterior cephalometric study. Angle Orthod. 2000;70:81–88.

Vibhute PJ. Optimizing anterior en masse retraction with miniscrew anchorage. Case Rep Dent. 2011;2011:475638.

Visscher CM, Lobbezoo F, de Boer W, van der Zaag J, Naeije M. Prevalence of cervical spinal pain in craniomandibular pain patients. Eur J Oral Sci. 2001;109:76–80.

White TC, Gardiner J, Leighton B. Malocclusion. Orthodontics for Dental Students. London: Red Globe Press, 1976.

Yáñez-Vico R-M, Iglesias-Linares A, Torres-Lagares D, Gutiérrez-Pérez J-L, Solano-Reina E. Association between craniofacial asymmetry and unilateral temporomandibular joint sounds in adult patients using 3D-computed tomography. Oral Dis. 2013;19:406–414.

12.4

Managing the Class II Subdivision Malocclusion with Extraction Camouflage: Case Reports

Cesare Luzi and Emese Szabò

Introduction

One of the most common daily challenges for the orthodontist is dealing with the Class II malocclusion. Although standard treatment protocols are well-known to clinicians, they are generally intended for symmetric malocclusions. But how many symmetric Class II patients are encountered in the daily clinical practice? It has been estimated that subdivision cases account to up to 50% of all Class II malocclusions (Rose et al. 1994).

The Class II subdivision malocclusion is known as a primarily dentoalveolar malocclusion (Alavi et al. 1988; Janson et al. 2001). However, analyses carried out with 3D diagnostic methods have highlighted often the presence of skeletal components (Sanders et al. 2010). Once the asymmetry has been located and quantified, the type of treatment should be proposed. Moderate to severe skeletal asymmetries often require surgical correction, nevertheless when these are ruled out and a mild-to-moderate asymmetry is diagnosed, dentoalveolar correction might be the most appropriate treatment.

Malocclusions are often characterized by dental crowding. If a certain amount of crowding exists and/or dental protrusion is present in the Class II subdivision malocclusion, extraction treatment can be the strategy of choice and asymmetric extractions can be beneficial and often successful for a camouflage approach (Janson et al. 2004; Turpin 2005).

The present chapter describes camouflage orthodontic treatment with asymmetric extractions of two patients featuring Class II subdivision malocclusions.

Case 1

A healthy 15-years-old boy, concerned about his crooked teeth, presented a Class II subdivision right malocclusion with bimaxillary crowding in the full permanent dentition (Figure 12.4.1a–h). The extra-oral appearance displayed absence of evident asymmetries (apart from a slightly lower left orbit compared to the right one), good lip competence, and a convex profile with a slight protrusion of the upper lip.

The intra-oral view was characterized by coinciding upper and lower midlines, although the patient presented a full Class II canine and molar relationships on the right side and Class I relationships on the left side. The degree of maxillary crowding was moderate, while mandibular anterior crowding was minimal. The upper and lower dental midlines were coincident, also with the facial midline. The panoramic radiograph displayed a complete permanent dentition with normal condylar anatomy, absence of periodontal pathology and developing buds of the third molars (Figure 12.4.2).

Lateral cephalometric radiographic assessment revealed a Class II normo-divergent skeletal pattern with increased

Dentofacial and Occlusal Asymmetries, First Edition. Edited by Birte Melsen and Athanasios E. Athanasiou.
© 2025 John Wiley & Sons Ltd. Published 2025 by John Wiley & Sons Ltd.

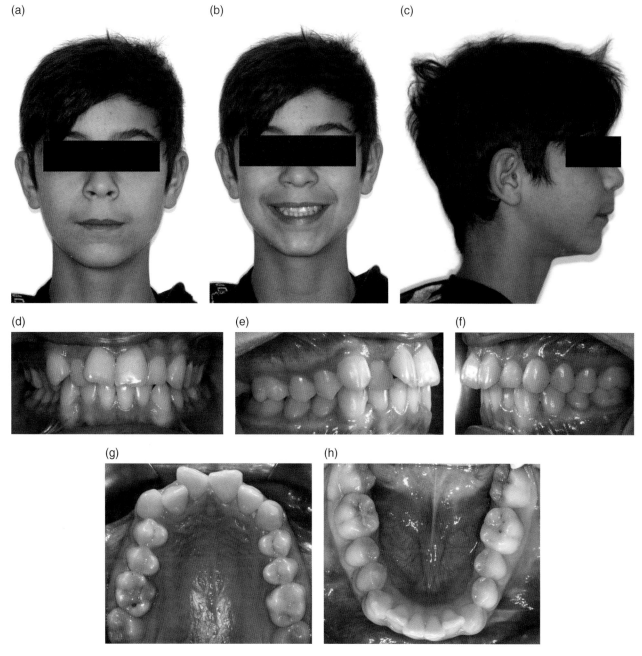

Figure 12.4.1 (a–h) Pre-treatment photographs of case 1. The subdivision right malocclusion displays bimaxillary crowding and centered midlines.

inclinations of both the upper and especially the lower incisors (Figure 12.4.3; Table 12.4.1).

Nonextraction treatment was initially considered.

The first option considered was a direct straight-wire approach. The coinciding upper and lower midlines, with different amount of crowding of the right and left sides of the maxillary dental arch, contraindicated an indiscriminate levelling and alignment phase, which would unmask

the asymmetry. Furthermore, incisor proclination to unravel the crowding was contraindicated due to the initial cephalometric parameters.

The second option considered was again nonextraction with a monolateral upper molar distalization on the Class II side. This option required a fixed intra-oral distalizer and the use of skeletal anchorage. The amount of distalization required and the proclination of the lower incisors during

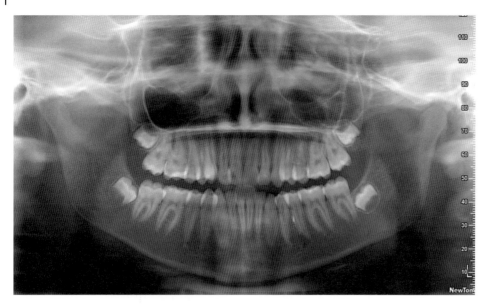

Figure 12.4.2 Pre-treatment panoramic radiograph.

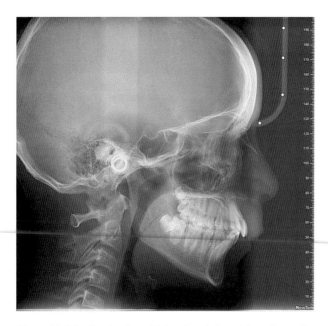

Figure 12.4.3 Pre-treatment lateral cephalometric radiograph displaying mild upper protrusion.

the alignment phase, increasing the initial values, were the main reasons to discard this option.

Camouflage extraction treatment was then considered. A Class II extraction protocol (upper first premolar and lower second premolar) was decided for the right side, while two second bicuspids would be extracted on the left side. This option would allow to alleviate both crowding and dentoalveolar protusion, maintaining midlines symmetry.

This last option became the treatment of choice.

Table 12.4.1 Pre-treatment cephalometric values of case 1.

Cephalometric morphological assessment I			
	Pre-treatment	Mean	SD
Sagittal skeletal relations			
Maxillary position S-N-A	81°	82°	3.5
Mandibular position S-N-Pg	77°	80°	3.5
Sagittal jaw relation A-N-Pg	4°	2°	2.5
Vertical skeletal relations			
Maxillary inclination S-N/ANS-PNS	8°	8°	3.0
Mandibular inclination S-N/Go-Gn	36°	33°	2.5
Vertical jaw relation ANS-PNS/Go-Gn	28°	25°	6.0
Dentobasal relations			
Maxillary incisor inclination ^{1}/ANS-PNS	122°	110°	6.0
Mandibular incisor inclination $_{1}$/Go-Gn	106°	94°	7.0
Mandibular incisor compensation $_{1}$/A-Pg (mm)	5	2	2.0
Dental relations			
Overjet (mm)	7	3.5	2.5
Overbite (mm)	3	2	2.5
Interincisal angle $^{1}/_{1}$	104°	132°	6.0

(a)　　　　　　　　　　(b)　　　　　　　　　　(c)

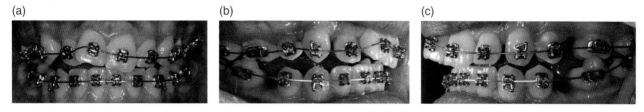

Figure 12.4.4　(a–c) Levelling and alignment phase following extractions of teeth #14, #25, #35, and #45 with super-elastic wires.

(a)　　　　　　　　　　(b)　　　　　　　　　　(c)

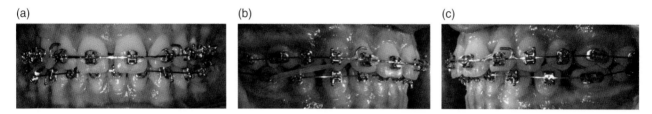

Figure 12.4.5　(a–c) Working phase with stainless steel wires and monolateral right Class II inter-maxillary 4.5 oz. elastics. .

Figures 12.4.4a–c and 12.4.5a–c describe the progress of the treatment, which lasted overall 23 months.

The final result (Figure 12.4.6a–h) displays a symmetric and aligned final occlusion with Class I molar and canine relationships, normal overjet and overbite values and coincident midlines. The extra-oral photos reveal a balanced face with good proportions, a natural smile, and a slightly convex profile.

The final panoramic radiograph demonstrates acceptable root parallelism and absence of detectable root resorption, with developing buds of the third molars (Figure 12.4.7). The final lateral cephalogram displays normalization of the overjet and overbite values (Figure 12.4.8) (Table 12.4.2).

The 24 months post-treatment follow-up displays a stable result (Figure 12.4.9a–f).

Case 2

A highly motivated healthy 32-years-old female came to a first orthodontic consultation concerned about the protrusion of her dentition. Her words, describing her chief complaint were "my teeth are too much forward and I cannot close my lips." She presented a Class II subdivision right malocclusion in the full permanent dentition with increased overjet and overbite without crowding (Figure 12.4.10). The upper dental midline was coinciding with the facial midline while the lower midline was deviated to the Class II side, therefore classifying her as a type 2 subdivision (Janson et al. 2007). Patient had previously lost the lower first molar on the right side, and this had generated spontaneous distal migration of the anterior teeth in the extraction site by means of mesial movement

with tipping of the second and third molars. The extra-oral view showed absence of significant asymmetries, a full smile, and a very convex and bi-protruded profile with lip incompetence at rest. The panoramic radiograph displayed a permanent dentition with absence of tooth 4.6 and mesially inclined teeth 4.7 and 4.8, normal condylar anatomy and absence of periodontal pathology (just a minor pocket could be identified mesial to tooth 4.7, due to the inclined position of the molar) (Figure 12.4.11).

Lateral cephalometric parameters revealed a Class II hyper-divergent skeletal pattern with dentoalveolar bi-protrusion and increased inclinations of both the upper and lower incisors (Figure 12.4.12; Table 12.4.3).

Even though tooth size/arch length discrepancies were not present, the only possible therapeutic strategy for effective reduction of the dentoalveolar bi-protrusion was removing tooth substance and retracting, with maximum posterior anchorage, the anterior limit of the dentition. In cases with a mandibular dental midline deviation with skeletal symmetry, if extractions are an acceptable option for the patient, a three-premolar extraction plan may be the treatment of choice (Rebellato 1998). In order to maintain the centered position of the upper midline and to correct the deviation of the lower midline a decision was taken to extract three first premolars, two maxillary and one lower left bicuspid. This would generate a final occlusion with centered midlines, correct overjet and overbite values, Class I bilateral canine and left molar relationship and a Class II molar relationship on the right side (with the lower right second molar in place of the first molar).

Three orthodontic TADs (Aarhus System™, American Orthodontics) with 6.0 mm thread length and 1.6 mm

(a)　　　　　　　　　(b)　　　　　　　　　(c)

(d)　　　　　　　　　(e)　　　　　　　　　(f)

(g)　　　　　　　　　(h)

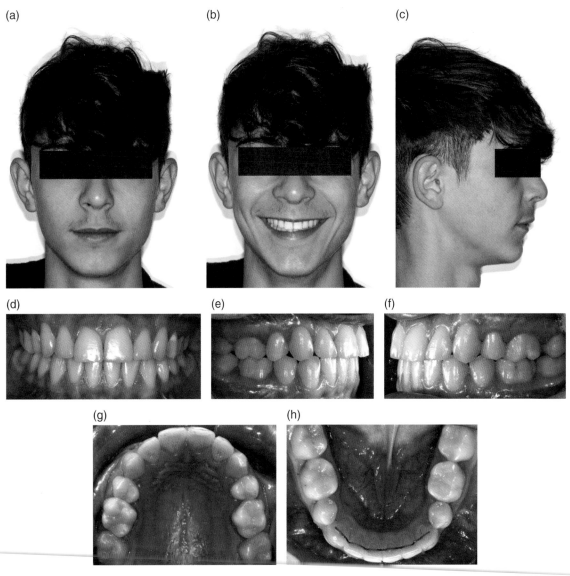

Figure 12.4.6 (a–h) Post-treatment photographs of case 1 displaying bilateral Class I relationships and normal occlusion, symmetric, and well balanced facial aspect.

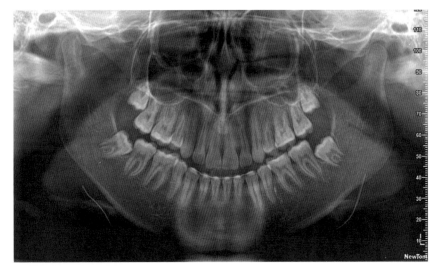

Figure 12.4.7 Post-treatment panoramic radiograph.

Figure 12.4.8 Post-treatment lateral cephalometric radiograph.

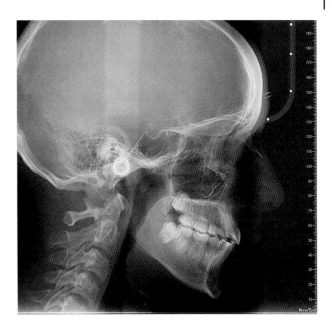

Table 12.4.2 Pre- and post-treatment cephalometric values of case 1.

Cephalometric morphological assessment II				
	Pre-treatment	**Post-treatment**	**Mean**	**SD**
Sagittal skeletal relations				
Maxillary position S-N-A	81°	81°	82°	3.5
Mandibular position S-N-Pg	77°	79°	80°	3.5
Sagittal jaw relation A-N-Pg	4°	2°	2°	2.5
Vertical skeletal relations				
Maxillary inclination S-N/ANS-PNS	8°	7°	8°	3.0
Mandibular inclination S-N/Go-Gn	36°	36°	33°	2.5
Vertical jaw relation ANS-PNS/Go-Gn	28°	29°	25°	6.0
Dentobasal relations				
Maxillary incisor inclination ^{1}/ANS-PNS	122°	114°	110°	6.0
Mandibular incisor inclination $_1$/Go-Gn	106°	94°	94°	7.0
Mandibular incisor Compensation $_1$/A-Pg (mm)	5	1	2	2.0
Dental relations				
Overjet (mm)	7	3	3.5	2.5
Overbite (mm)	3	2	2	2.5
Interincisal angle ^{1}/$_1$	104°	123°	132°	6.0

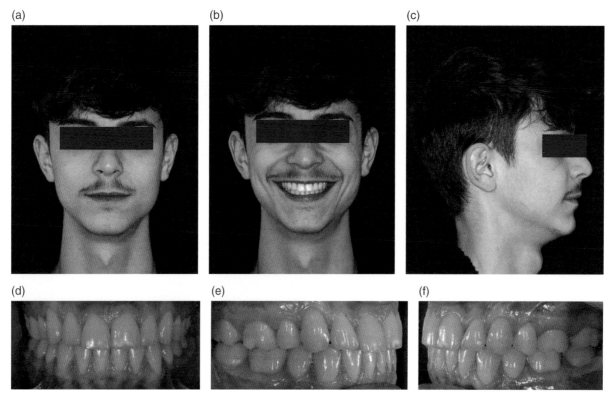

Figure 12.4.9 (a–f) Post-retention records displaying stability 2 years post-treatment.

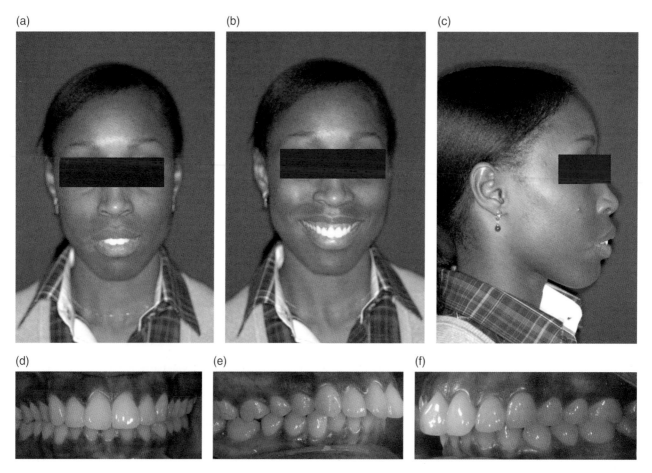

Figure 12.4.10 (a–h) Pre-treatment photographs of case 2. The subdivision right malocclusion displays excessive protrusion of the dentition with lip incompetence, increased overjet and previous loss of tooth #36 with lower midline deviation.

(g) (h)

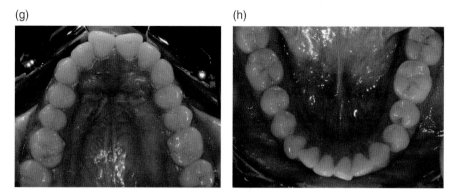

Figure 12.4.10   (Continued)

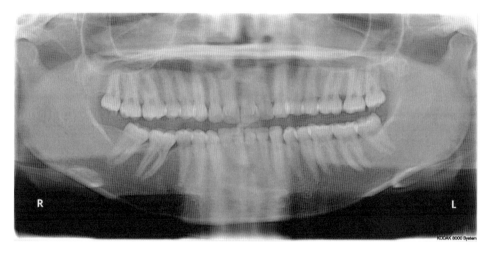

Figure 12.4.11   Pre-treatment panoramic radiograph. The previous loss of tooth #46 was followed by spontaneous space closure with mesial tipping of the lower molars on the right side.

Figure 12.4.12   Pre-treatment lateral cephalometric radiograph displaying severe bi-protrusion and increased inclinations of both the upper and lower incisors.

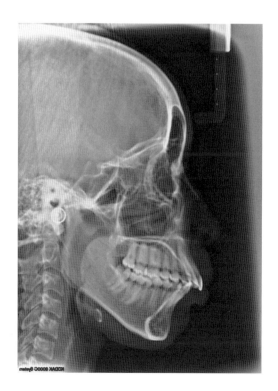

Table 12.4.3 Pre-treatment cephalometric values of case 2.

Cephalometric morphological assessment I			
	Pre-treatment	Mean	SD
Sagittal skeletal relations			
Maxillary position S-N-A	92°	82°	3.5
Mandibular position S-N-Pg	83°	80°	3.5
Sagittal jaw relation A-N-Pg	9°	2°	2.5
Vertical skeletal relations			
Maxillary inclination S-N/ANS-PNS	4°	8°	3.0
Mandibular inclination S-N/Go-Gn	36°	33°	2.5
Vertical jaw relation ANS-PNS/Go-Gn	32°	25°	6.0
Dento-basal relations			
Maxillary incisor inclination ^{1}/ANS-PNS	119°	110°	6.0
Mandibular incisor inclination $_1$/Go-Gn	100°	94°	7.0
Mandibular incisor compensation $_1$/A-Pg (mm)	7	2	2.0
Dental relations			
Overjet (mm)	9	3.5	2.5
Overbite (mm)	6	2	2.5
Interincisal angle $^1/_1$	110°	132°	6.0

diameter were inserted in the first, second, and third quadrant to be used as absolute anchorage devices during the retraction phase.

Figures 12.4.13a–c, 12.4.14a–c, and 12.4.15a–c describe the progress of the case, which lasted overall 26 months.

The final result reveals a normal and aligned final occlusion with Class I bilateral canine and left molar relationships, Class II right molar relationship, normal overjet and overbite values, and coincident midlines (Figure 12.4.16). The extra-oral photos reveal a balanced face with a clear reduction of the pre-treatment bi-protrusion, good proportions, a natural smile with appropriate tooth exposure, and a slightly convex profile (Figure 12.4.16). Lip competence has been successfully achieved together with appropriate tooth exposure during smile (Figure 12.4.17a, b). The post-treatment panoramic radiographs display good root parallelism and absence of detectable apical root resorption (Figure 12.4.18) with a significant distal repositioning of the anterior limit of the dentition (Figure 12.4.19) and reduction of the dentoalveolar bi-protrusion (Table 12.4.4).

Conclusions

The treatment of asymmetries is one of the major challenges in orthodontics. The key to success is a correct diagnostic procedure with precise localization of the asymmetry

(a)　　　　　　　　　(b)　　　　　　　　　(c)

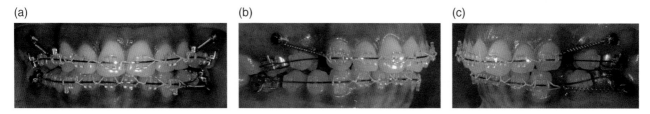

Figure 12.4.13 (a–c) Working phase. The three orthodontic miniscrews are inserted and immediately loaded with 150 g super-elastic coil springs. Retraction of the anterior teeth is performed with sliding mechanics on rectangular stainless-steel wires.

(a)　　　　　　　　　(b)　　　　　　　　　(c)

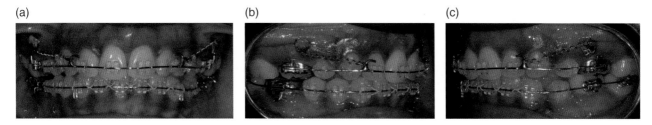

Figure 12.4.14 (a–c) Working phase. The end of the space closure phase (the lower TAD has been removed).

(a)　　　　　　　　　(b)　　　　　　　　　(c)

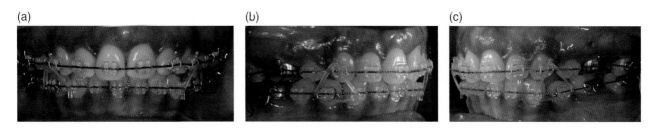

Figure 12.4.15 (a–c) Finishing phase following miniscrews removal in the maxilla. Use of vertical bilateral inter-maxillary 4.5 oz. elastics to enhance final intercuspation.

(a)　　　　　　　　　(b)　　　　　　　　　(c)

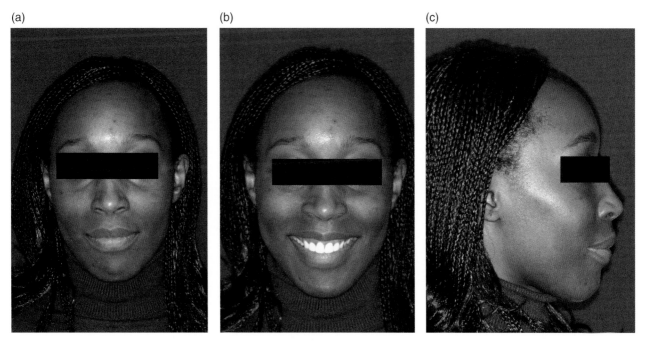

Figure 12.4.16 (a–h) Post-treatment photographs of case 2 displaying a well-balanced facial aspect with lip competence, an asymmetric final occlusion with centered midlines, Class I bilateral canine and left molar relationship and Class II right molar relationship. The overjet and overbite values have been normalized.

(d)   (e)   (f)

(g)   (h)

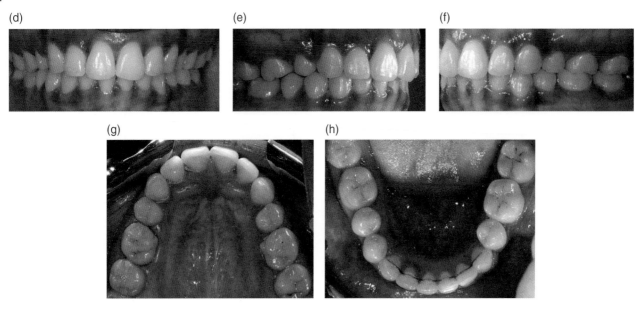

Figure 12.4.16   (Continued)

(a)   (b)

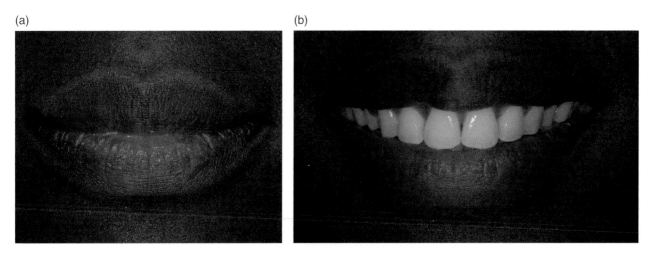

Figure 12.4.17   (a, b). Post-treatment photographs of spontaneous lip competence and tooth display during smile.

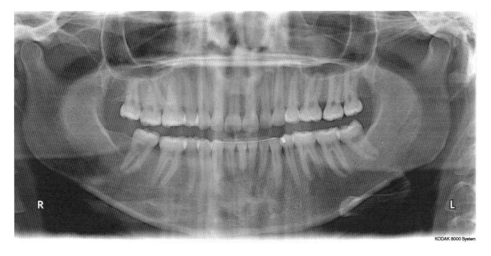

Figure 12.4.18   Post-treatment panoramic radiograph.

Figure 12.4.19 Post-treatment lateral cephalometric radiograph.

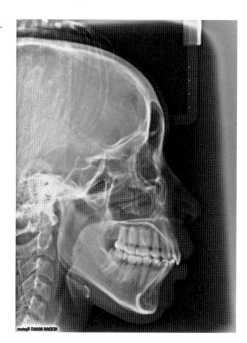

Table 12.4.4 Pre- and post-treatment cephalometric values of case 2.

Cephalometric morphological assessment II				
	Pre-treatment	**Post-treatment**	**Mean**	**SD**
Sagittal skeletal relations				
Maxillary position S-N-A	92°	91°	82°	3.5
Mandibular position S-N-Pg	83°	83°	80°	3.5
Sagittal jaw relation A-N-Pg	9°	8°	2°	2.5
Vertical skeletal relations				
Maxillary inclination S-N/ANS-PNS	4°	5°	8°	3.0
Mandibular inclination S-N/Go-Gn	36°	38°	33°	2.5
Vertical jaw relation ANS-PNS/Go-Gn	32°	33°	25°	6.0
Dento-basal relations				
Maxillary incisor inclination ^{1}/ANS-PNS	119°	104°	110°	6.0
Mandibular incisor inclination $_{1}$/Go-Gn	100°	95°	94°	7.0
Mandibular incisor Compensation $_{1}$/A-Pg (mm)	7	5	2	2.0
Dental relations				
Overjet (mm)	9	3	3.5	2.5
Overbite (mm)	6	4	2	2.5
Interincisal angle $^{1}/_{1}$	110°	130°	132°	6.0

and the subsequent use of the correct biomechanics for treatment. Skeletal asymmetries most often require surgical procedures for correction. Dentoalveolar asymmetries can be camouflaged with ordinary orthodontic treatment, with or without extractions. If some degree of crowding and/or protrusion exist, and extractions are an acceptable offer to the patients, the strategic removal of permanent teeth can be the most successful strategy to overcome the problem and reach a final successful outcome. The Class II subdivision malocclusion, an extremely common problem for every orthodontist, can often be successfully camouflaged with asymmetric extractions. Since several different asymmetric extraction protocols exist (one, three, or four teeth), only a precise and thorough diagnosis and treatment goal definition will allow the most appropriate choice of teeth to be extracted.

References

Alavi DG, BeGole EA, Schneider BJ. Facial and dental asymmetries in Class II subdivision malocclusion. Am J Orthod Dentofac Orthop. 1988;93:38–46.

Janson G, Cruz KS, Woodside DG, Metaxas A, de Freitas MR, Henriquez JF. Dentoskeletal treatment changes in Class II subdivision malocclusions in submentovertex and posteroanterior radiographs. Am J Orthod Dentofac Orthop. 2004;126:451–463.

Janson G, de Lima KJ, Woodside DG, Metaxas A, de Freitas MR, Henriquez JF. Class II subdivision malocclusion types and evaluation of their asymmetries. Am J Orthod Dentofac Orthop. 2007;131:57–60.

Janson GRP, Metaxas A, Woodside DG, de Freitas MR, Pinzan A. Three dimensional evaluation of skeletal and dental asymmetries in Class II subdivision malocclusions. Am J Orthod Dentofac Orthop. 2001;119:406–418.

Rebellato J. Asymmetric extractions used in the treatment of patients with asymmetries. Semin Orthod. 1998;4:180–188.

Rose JM, Sadowsky C, BeGole EA, Moles R. Mandibular skeletal and dental asymmetry in Class II subdivision malocclusion. Am J Orthod Dentofac Orthop. 1994;105:489–495.

Sanders DA, Rigali PH, Neace WP, Uribe F, Nanda R. Skeletal and dental asymmetries in Class II subdivision malocclusions using cone-beam computed tomography. Am J Orthod Dentofac Orthop. 2010;138(542):e1–e20.

Turpin D. Correcting the Class II subdivision malocclusion. Am J Orthod Dentofac Orthop. 2005;128:555–556.

12.5

The Use of Aligners for Correction of Asymmetries

Eugene Chan and M. Ali Darendeliler

Introduction

Skeletal and dental asymmetries have been well described in the orthodontic literature. These innate features could range from severe facial deformities with various etiologies, to indiscernible mild discrepancies. We live with asymmetries and embrace it in nature. However, beauty can be rather subjective and individuals with specific requests to achieve perfect symmetry will seek treatment for the mildest form of irregularity.

Facial symmetry seem to be an important aspect of facial beauty, although mild asymmetry is essentially normal (Grammer and Thornhill 1994). The term describing ordinary, typical facial symmetry known as "averageness" was first introduced in the late 19th century (Galton 1879). Although facial symmetry was an important factor in facial attractiveness, "averageness" appears to be more important (Rhodes et al. 1999).

Treatment with clear aligners has seen a steep uptake in the last decade. Through material advancement, software improvements, and further education, many clinicians are now comfortable treating more complex orthodontic cases with clear aligners.

Severe facial deformity can contribute to the development of an uneven malocclusion (Gorlin et al. 2001). This could be attributed to the expression of genetically linked

Dentofacial and Occlusal Asymmetries, First Edition. Edited by Birte Melsen and Athanasios E. Athanasiou.
© 2025 John Wiley & Sons Ltd. Published 2025 by John Wiley & Sons Ltd.

phenotype (Corruccini et al. 1986), or an early childhood injury (Proffit et al. 1990). The child could also have a normal dentofacial development up until a stage whereby an unusual development or a parafunctional habit contributes to a functional shift (Moss 1980). When early functional shifts in a growing child are not detected and eliminated early, a deviation from normal growth occurs and may contribute to a subsequent irreversible skeletal asymmetry (Pirttiniemi et al. 1990; Thilander 1986) and jaw joint-related disorders (Pullinger et al. 1993; Sonnesen et al. 1998).

Dental Corrections (Non-extraction Therapies)

Asymmetrical dental discrepancies should be detected early. An early loss of deciduous tooth or teeth when left unnoticed, may lead to a reduction in arch length and/or collapse of the dental arch contributing to the development of an asymmetrical malocclusion. Usually, early detection with the placement of appropriate space maintainer will prevent subsequent lengthy orthodontic treatment. It may also be appropriate to regain the space, if necessary prior to the placement of the space maintainer.

Correction of Functional Shift in Mixed Dentition

The early detection of a functional shift and identifying any premature contacts is essential in the mixed dentition. If left uncorrected, the functional shift may develop into a severe skeletal discrepancy. Using a routine method such as the "Dawson bimanual technique" (Dawson 1995), will manipulate the patient into a relaxed centric jaw position, will locate the premature contact, and will identify the functional shift. The most commonly seen functional shift is a unilateral crossbite, either anteriorly, posteriorly, or both (Figure 12.5.1a).

An 11-year-old child in her late mixed dentition presented with concerns of a median diastema, a unilateral posterior crossbite, and an underbite. She had a Class III dental malocclusion on a mild skeletal 3 pattern with a normal direction of growth with no family history of large lower jaws. The child had a normal midface but a prognathic mandible. The upper and lower permanent incisors and the first molars were present and fully erupted. The deciduous canines were slightly mobile while the molars were firm. There was a unilateral crossbite on the right, the upper and lower dental midlines were non-coincidental with the lower midline and chin point both deviated to the right side (Figure 12.5.1b). There was a functional shift detected with premature contact on tooth #21, which subsequently led the mandible to shift anteriorly, as well as laterally to the right.

The panoramic radiograph demonstrated routine findings with a full complement of teeth, with the premolars, permanent second and third molars developing (Figure 12.5.1c).

Stage I interceptive orthodontic treatment was indicated to commence immediately. The primary treatment objectives were to eliminate the functional shift, correct the posterior crossbite, close the upper median diastema, coordinate the arches to realign the dental midlines and mandible, correct the underbite, and to normalize her subsequent facial growth and development. The plan also included the redistribution of spaces along the dental arches to allow the uneventful eruption of the other remaining permanent dentition.

She was treated with clear aligners. The Invisalign First™ product allowed optimized attachment designs and velocity of dental movement for both deciduous and permanent dentition. With shorter clinical crown heights, it is essential to plan sufficient attachments to maintain good retention of the aligners in these mixed dentition cases. We requested for an "elastic simulation" in the ClinCheck plans and executed that clinically with Class II elastics on the right side and Class III elastic on the left side (Figure 12.5.1d). The aligners were worn full-time with the exception of brushing, flossing, and eating and had a weekly change regime.

After 27 out of 29 active aligners and approximately 7 months of treatment, the posterior crossbite on the right side was corrected, the dental midlines were co-ordinated, overjet, overbite was normalized, and the median diastema was closed (Figure 12.5.1e). New intra-oral scans were done and additional aligners were ordered for final detailing to improve the occlusal contacts. The additional aligners were also changed weekly. The stage I treatment was completed in 12 months (Figure 12.5.1f, g). All primary objectives of the interceptive treatment were achieved. The functional shift was eliminated, median diastema closed, unilateral posterior crossbite, overjet, and overbite corrected. Most importantly, her facial balance and asymmetry, and the prognathic mandibular posture were normalized (Figure 12.5.1h). Upper and lower fixed retainers were placed on the incisors and an upper Hawley retainer was prescribed to be worn during her sleep hours.

Subsequent plans were to continue to monitor the child's growth and development periodically 3–6 monthly, until she is in her full permanent dentition. Phase two treatment may then be indicated and planned if necessary.

Congenitally Missing Tooth in Teen Treatment

Congenitally missing tooth/teeth commonly contributes to the formation of an asymmetrical malocclusion (Fekonja 2017). Depending on the severity of the discrepancy, and

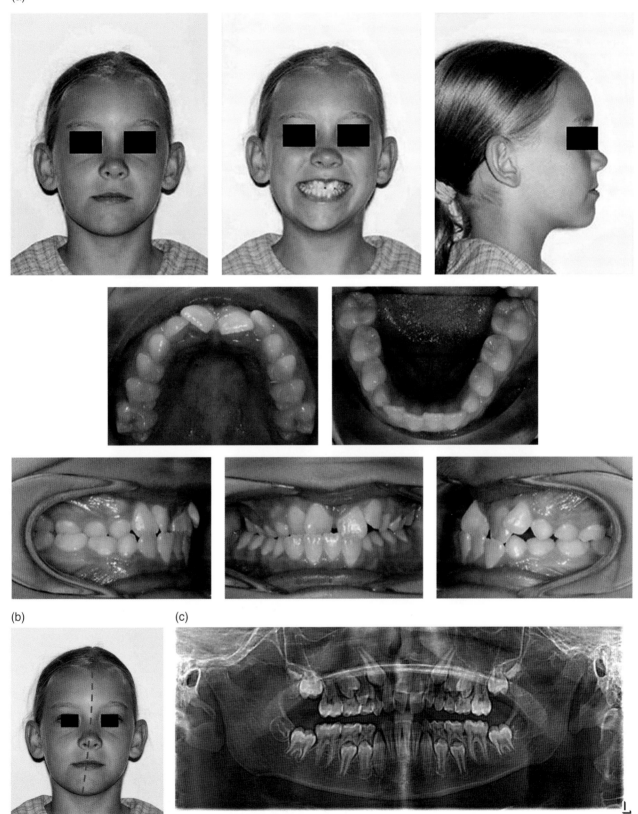

Figure 12.5.1 (a) Pre-treatment images of a child in mixed dentition showing a functional shift with mandibular deviation resulting in a Class III dental malocclusion and a unilateral posterior crossbite. (b) Functional shift contributing to mandibular deviation and facial asymmetry. (c) Pre-treatment OPG radiograph. (d) ClinCheck plans showing (I) pre-treatment and (II) simulated final position of the dentition with attachment designs and precision cuts for elastic wear. (e) Mid-treatment images after wearing 27/29 aligners at 7 months into treatment. (f) Post-treatment images after 12 months of aligner treatment. (g) Post-treatment OPG radiograph. (h) Comparison of frontal and side facial profile of (I) pre-treatment and (II) post-treatment images demonstrating normalization of the facial balance and harmony.

(d)

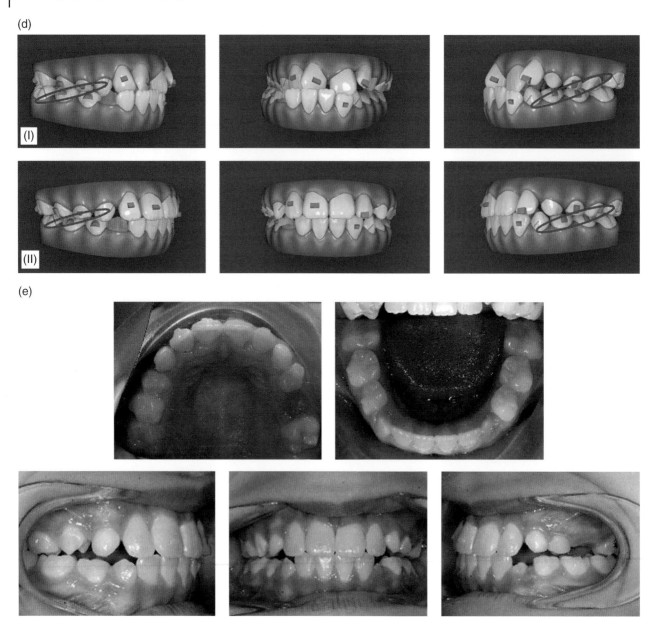

(e)

Figure 12.5.1 (Continued)

which tooth/teeth are missing; it may affect the patient's smile and facial symmetry remarkably. Cases may range from just a single missing tooth to multiple missing teeth associated with certain syndromes.

A 12 years 7 months old female in her permanent dentition presented with a congenitally missing upper right lateral incisor (tooth #12). It contributed to a Class II subdivision left-sided dental malocclusion. There were upper dental spaces, the upper dental midline was deviated to the right side with a half-unit Class II dental relationship on the right side, and a good Class I interdigitation on the left (Figure 12.5.2a, b).

The two obvious treatment options discussed with the child and the parents were to either (i) open and reestablish the #12 space for a future prosthetic tooth. Or alternatively, (ii) to close the space and substitute the #13 for the #12. This option would not require any future prosthetic replacements. The pros and cons of these options should be discussed intimately.

With option (i), the mechanics and treatment duration for the orthodontics could be simpler and shorter, respectively. Dentally, the end result could potentially be more symmetrical and aesthetically pleasing. However, we have to wait for the child to complete her vertical dentoalveolar

(f)

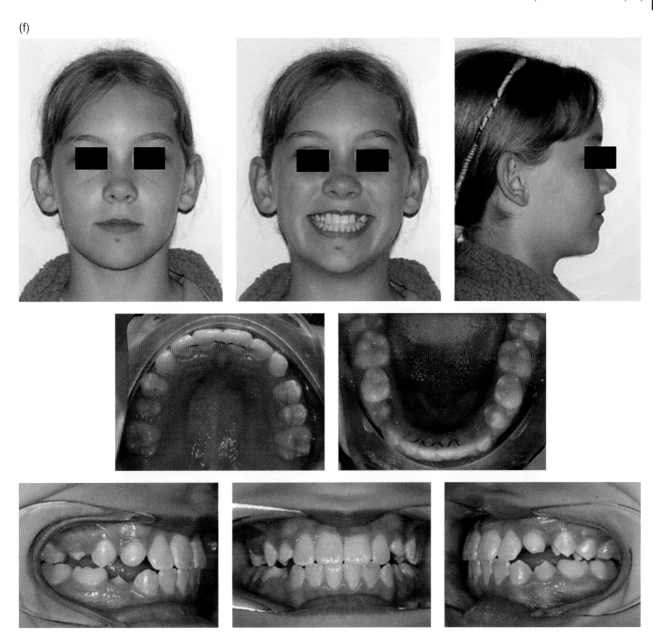

Figure 12.5.1 (Continued)

growth before the placement of a prosthetic tooth such as an implant. That age is usually about 18 years old (Oesterle et al. 1993). The space has to be maintained with an aesthetic temporary solution in the meantime. This could be in the form of resin-bonded bridge or a denture. There would also be the chance of vertical and/or bucco-lingual bone loss during this time (Dietschi and Schartz 1997). Further bone augmentation might then be required before the dental implant is inserted. Such potential complications and surgical procedures need to be made known to the patient as part of informed consent prior to the commencement of the orthodontic treatment.

Option (ii) may offer a less esthetically balanced end result. The shape, color, and size of the #13 substituting as the #12 may require a certain degree of cosmetic enhancement and camouflage. The orthodontic treatment duration and mechanic designs might be longer and more complex. The final occlusion will be a therapeutic Class II relationship on the right while maintaining the Class I relationship on the left. However, this option would negate the need for any future surgery and dental prostheses. In this particular case, after much deliberation and considering all factors, treatment option (ii) was chosen.

(g)

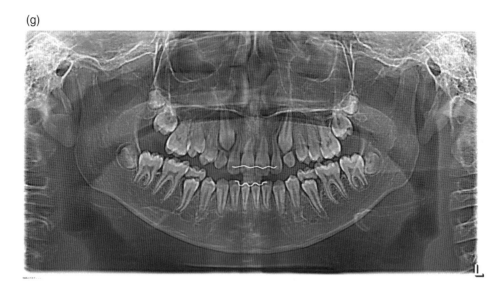

(h)

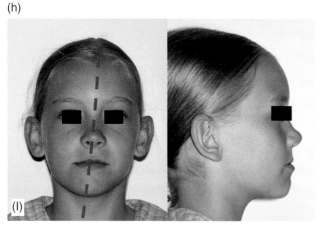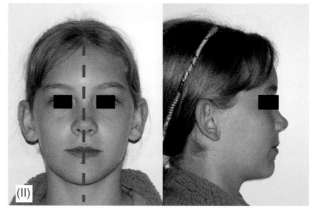

Figure 12.5.1 (Continued)

The ClinCheck plan was set up with a simultaneous staging pattern, optimized, and conventional attachments were designed (Figure 12.5.2c). This plan was supported with concurrent wear of Class II and Class III elastics on the right and left sides, respectively. The patient was instructed to wear her aligners full time with a 2-weekly change regime. She was reviewed at every 8–10 weeks intervals. During these review appointments, ensure to not only check on the compliance of the patient's aligner wear, but also to remove the aligners, get the patient to bite down to check on the dental midlines and the sagittal correction done so far. The clinician needs to adjust the strength and consistency of elastic wear in order to achieve the desired outcome. Progressive records showed the gradual correction of the dental midlines (Figure 12.5.2d). The anchorage design was mainly the judicious adjustment of strength and length of wear of the dental elastics.

With conventional fixed appliance therapy, prolonged use of asymmetrical elastics may contribute to the canting of the occlusal plane and/or opening of the vertical occlusal dimensions. The benefit of the clear aligner system is that the aligners cover the occlusal surfaces of the dentition throughout treatment. This allows a biased distribution of force, diverting the forces from the elastics to a more horizontal vector, and suppressing the vertical component. This phenomenon makes the clear aligner system the appliance of choice when such mechanics need to be applied.

Due to the therapeutic Class II completion on the right side, the molar relationship on the right side was completed to a full unit Class II (Figure 12.5.2e, f) (Nangia and Darendeliler 2001). The active treatment completed in 18 months. Upper and lower fixed retainers, and upper and lower vacuum-formed retainers were prescribed to maintain the orthodontic correction. The upper and lower

(a)

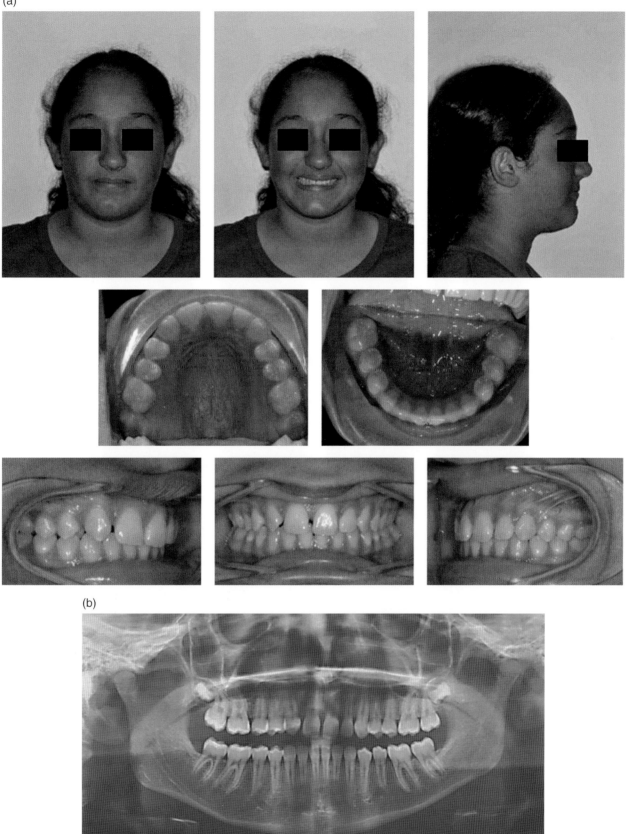

(b)

Figure 12.5.2 (a) Pre-treatment images of a teenager with a congenitally missing #12. (b) Pre-treatment OPG radiograph. (c) ClinCheck plans showing (I) pre-treatment and (II) simulated final position of the dentition, with attachment designs and precision cuts for elastic wear. (d) Mid-treatment images showing progressive correction of dental midlines with judicious control of Class II and Class III elastics. (e) Post-treatment images showing #13 canine substitution and midline correction. (f) Post-treatment OPG radiograph. (g) Comparison of (I) pre-treatment and (II) post-treatment images demonstrating canine substitution and midline correction.

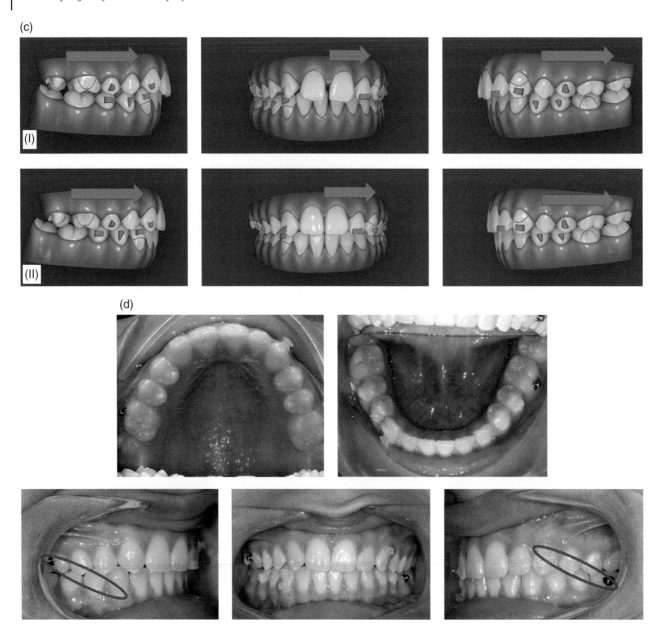

Figure 12.5.2 (Continued)

dental midlines were aligned to restore some degree of dental symmetry. The #13 was judiciously adjusted to mimic the appearance of a lateral incisor (Figure 12.5.2g). There would be an option for the patient to have some dental whitening to further lighten the color of #13 in the future, if she chooses.

Dental Correction in Adult Treatment

Many dental asymmetries in adults are caused by either congenitally missing teeth or teeth that were previously extracted. The reasons for extraction usually include severe dental crowding, irreversible dental decay, or periodontal problems (Cahen et al. 1985; Morita et al. 1994; Richards et al. 2005). The loss of such teeth may lead to the asymmetrical collapse of the dental arch toward the extraction site. Non-coincident dental midlines, asymmetrical archforms, uneven occlusal contacts, and dental crossbites are the usual consequences. These may further contribute to irregular facial muscular changes and other jaw joint-related problems if left untreated (Pirttiniemi et al. 1990; Thilander 1986).

(e)

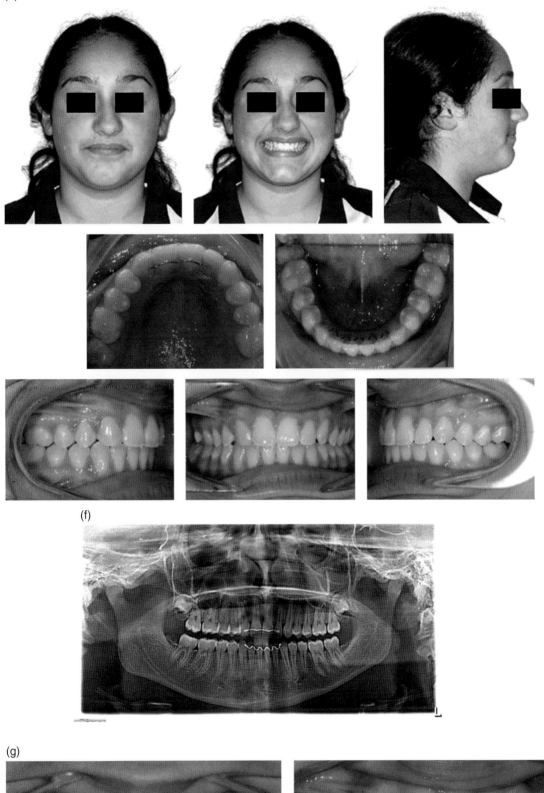

(f)

(g)

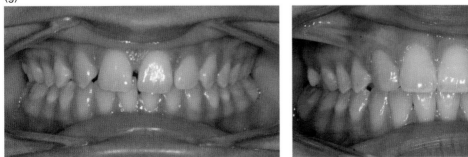

Figure 12.5.2 (Continued)

Class II Correction

An adult female patient presented with concerns of a deep dental overbite and she would like to improve her smile (Figure 12.5.3a). She had teeth #14 and #44 previously extracted due to crowding when she was young and her dentition had slowly drifted over the years. She presented as a Class II division 2 dental malocclusion on a mild skeletal 2 base. The OPG radiograph showed a normal healthy periodontium with all the wisdom teeth previously removed (Figure 12.5.3b). There was a deep dental overbite with evidence of increased wear and attrition on the anterior teeth. The upper dental midline was deviated to right with the Class II dental relationship was more severe on the left.

Upper molar distalization using clear aligners is a common and effective mechanism in correcting Class II dental malocclusions. Corrections of up to a half-unit dental relationship are usually predictable. Sequential staging pattern is the default staging pattern in upper molar distalization in the correction of a Class II dental relationship using Invisalign® clear aligners. The terminal molars are first moved followed by the premolars, canines, and the anterior teeth, sequentially. This staging pattern could be time consuming, while the posterior teeth are being distalized, the anterior crowding is usually not corrected until the later stages of treatment. This may contradict our patients' chief concerns, which usually is the anterior crowding. To overcome this roadblock, clinicians may request for an "aesthetic start" while planning the ClinCheck treatment. This allows the commencement of simple alignment of the anterior teeth while the terminal molars and premolars are distalizing (Chan and Darendeliler 2021).

When a sequential staging pattern is engaged (Figure 12.5.3c), the aligners have a "stopped arch" effect and this cross intra-arch anchorage, supported clinically with inter-arch Class II elastics contributes to the efficiency of this mechanism (Figure 12.5.3d). It is important to ensure minimal resistance to the upper molar distalization by removing any upper wisdom teeth. Start the clinical use of Class II elastics early in the treatment. First, commence with a lighter force and as treatment progresses and as the distance between the points of engagement of the elastics decreases, change to an elastic of a smaller diameter to maintain the strength of the traction. Understanding the variation of the biology of tooth movement is essential. Commence with 2-weekly aligner change and if patient compliance is good and the teeth are tracking well, the clinician may indicate a gradually switch to a 10-day or a 7-day aligner change regime. At each 8–10 weekly appointment, the clinician needs to check the aligner fit, remove the aligners, and check the occlusion in maximum intercuspation. Monitor the progress of the molar distalization and the direction of the midline correction (Figure 12.5.3e). Increase or decrease the strength and intensity of the elastics where necessary.

With an uneven number of premolars on the left and right side of the arches, it is still possible to complete the case with a balanced occlusion and a good dental interdigitation. The key reference is an ideal overjet, overbite, coincident midlines (dentally as well as facially), and a socked-in Class I canine relationship (Figure 12.5.3f). Once these are achieved, the buccal segments will usually fall into a good interdigitated occlusion.

Class III Correction

Molar distalization in correcting Class III dental malocclusion can be less compelling. The mandibular alveolar bone has a higher density and offers a greater resistance to this mechanism of correction. Movements can be less predictable (Chugh et al. 2013; Roberts 2005). However, with the right candidate, good biological response and good compliance from the patient, it can still be well managed.

A male adult patient had the upper right second premolar (tooth #15) previously extracted when he was younger. He presented with an asymmetrical occlusion; the upper dental midline was deviated to right, and the lower dental midline off to the left. There was an anterior crossbite at the lower right canine region with Class III canine relationship on the right side. There were mild and moderate degrees of upper and lower dental crowding, respectively (Figure 12.5.4a). The OPG radiograph showed a full complement of teeth, including lower impacted #38 and #48, and overly erupted #18 and #28 (Figure 12.5.4b). The treatment plan required the removal of all wisdom teeth. Using Invisalign® clear aligners, the ClinCheck plans involved mechanics with lower right and upper left molar distalization, asymmetrical use of Class II and Class III elastics (left and right sides respectively), and asymmetrical reduction (IPR) to achieve the desired results (Figure 12.5.4c).

The monitoring of treatment progress involved regular reviews every 8–10 weeks, with close monitoring of dental midlines, canine, and molar relationships (Figure 12.5.4d). The strength of the elastics was adjusted accordingly to the biological response of the patient, and the amount of dental movement achieved. Aligners were worn full-time with a 2-weekly change regime. Additional aligners worn at the later stage of treatment were changed weekly. The final occlusion achieved showed a therapeutic Class II molar and Class I canine relationship on the right side, Class I molar and canine relationships on the left side, coincident dental and facial midlines, and an ideal overjet

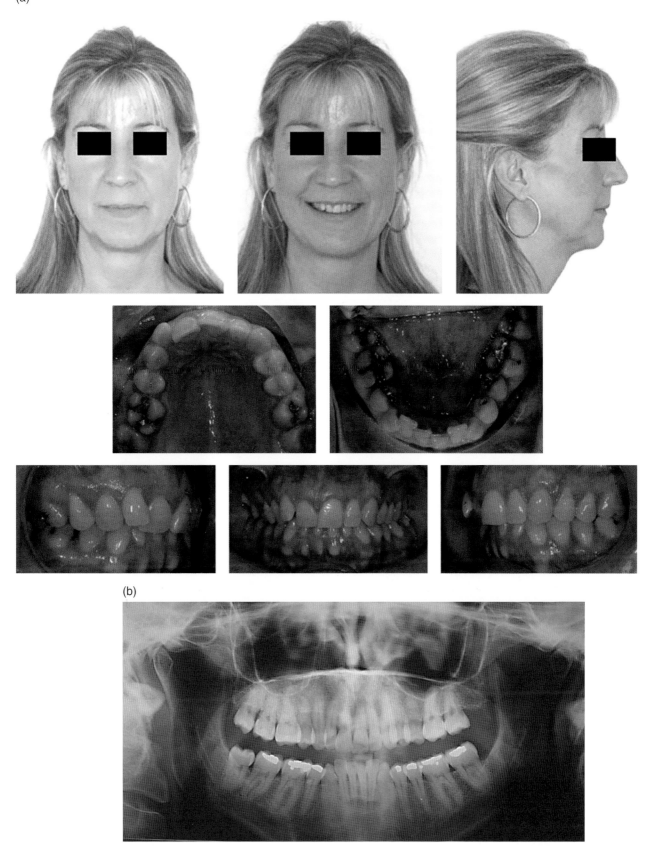

Figure 12.5.3 (a) Pre-treatment images of an adult showing an asymmetrical Class II division 2 dental malocclusion with the upper dental midline deviated to the right side. (b) Pre-treatment OPG radiograph. (c) ClinCheck staging plan showing sequential staging pattern of the upper molar distalization. (d) ClinCheck plans showing (I) pre-treatment and (II) simulated final position of the dentition, with attachment designs and precision cuts for elastic wear. (e) Progressive treatment images showing upper molar distalization and midline correction. (f) Post-treatment images showing a balanced, symmetrical occlusion with coincident dental and facial midlines.

(c)

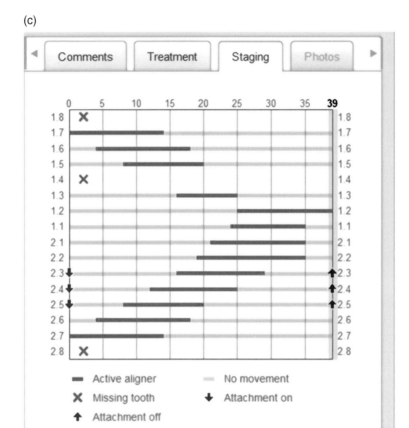

(d)

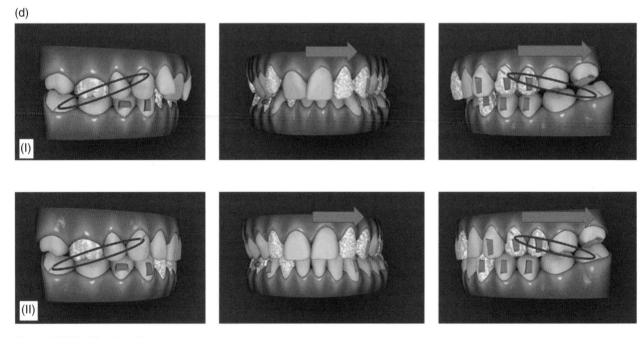

Figure 12.5.3 (Continued)

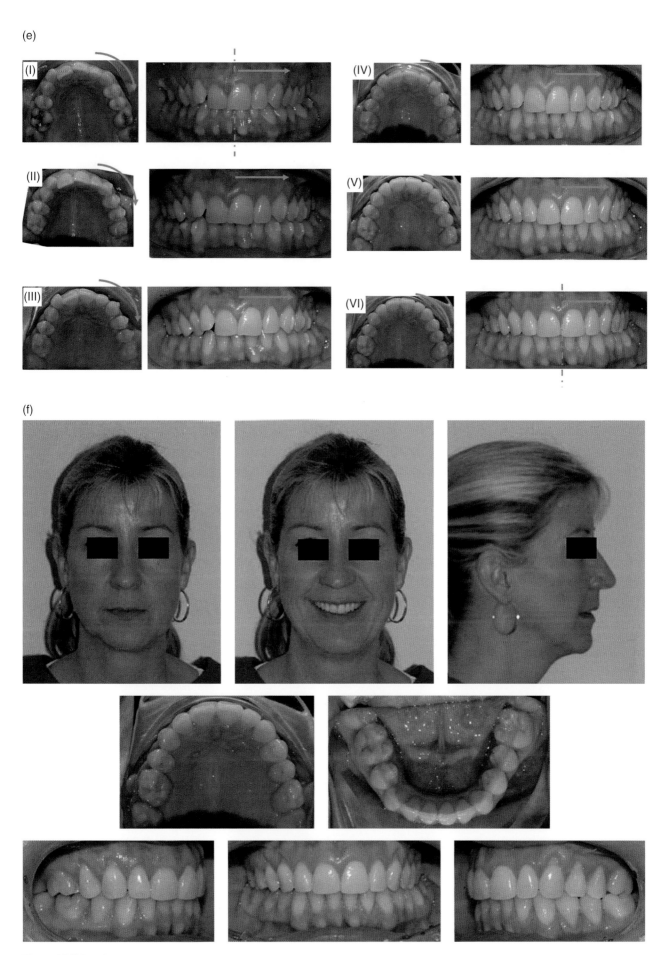

Figure 12.5.3 (Continued)

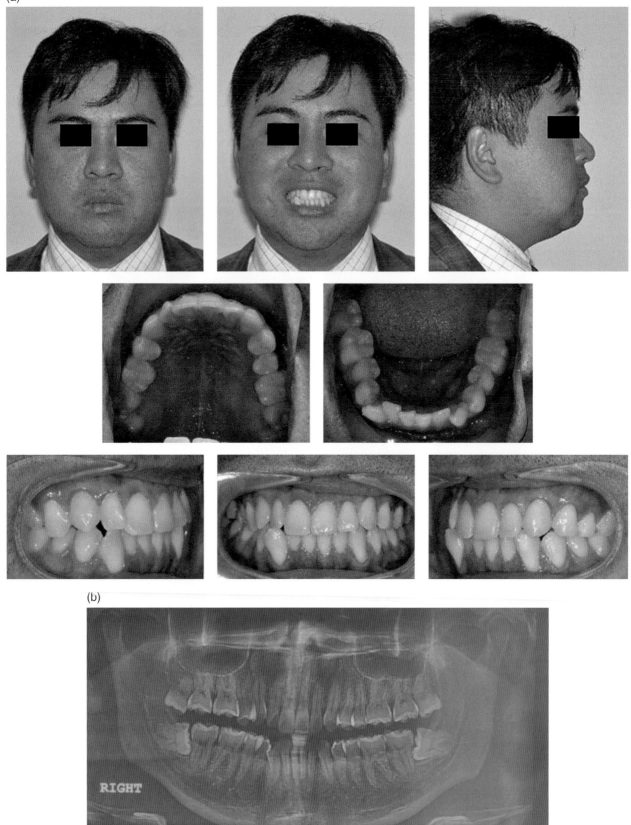

Figure 12.5.4 (a) Pre-treatment images of an adult showing an asymmetrical Class III dental malocclusion after the loss of #15. There was an anterior crossbite with non-coincidental midlines. (b) Pre-treatment OPG radiograph. (c) ClinCheck plans showing (I) pre-treatment and (II) simulated final position of the dentition, with attachment designs and precision cuts for elastic wear. (d) Progressive treatment images showing molar distalization, crossbite correction, and midline correction. (e) Post-treatment images showing a balanced, symmetrical occlusion with coincident dental and facial midlines. (f) Post-treatment OPG radiograph. (g) Superimposition of lateral cephalometric tracings showing molar movements.

(c)

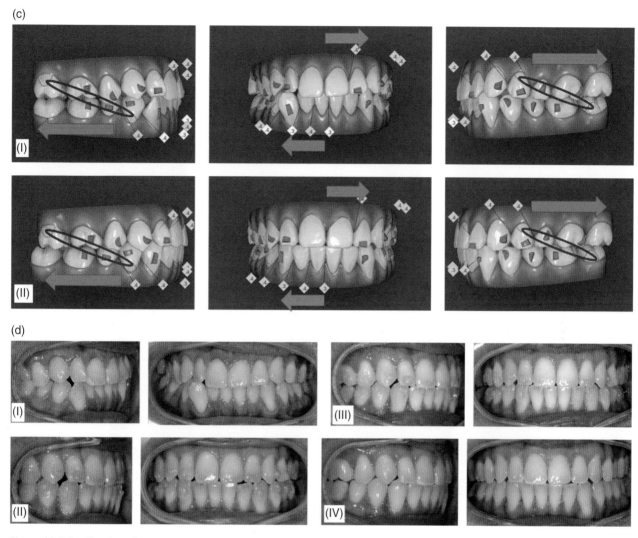

(d)

Figure 12.5.4 (Continued)

and overbite (Figure 12.5.4e, f). The total treatment duration was 16 months. Overall and regional superimpositions of this case showed a successful 2–3 mm of molar distalization achieved for the lower right quadrant (Figure 12.5.4g). It is important to note that the absence of any wisdom teeth in such cases reduces the resistance of dental movement, allowing a more efficient molar distalization.

Dental Implants

Missing tooth/teeth anteriorly or posteriorly contribute to a collapse of the dental archform over time. This creates an asymmetrical dental malocclusion often presenting with deviated dental midlines and/or an overly increased or decreased dental overjet.

Mechanically, reestablishing these dental spaces orthodontically is often easier than to attempt their closure and/or the camouflage of the asymmetry. The distraction of the dentition, creating a dental space creates good bone development interproximally, often allowing successful implant placement without the need for any bone graft or other forms of bone augmentation (Gündüz et al. 2004).

Missing anterior teeth (congenitally or previously extracted), or patients with an anterior Bolton's discrepancy may present an "edge to edge" bite or even a reverse dental overjet. The upper anterior segments are usually more retrusive and retroclined, with the upper dental midline often deviated to the side with the missing dentition (Figure 12.5.5a). The notion of planning Class III elastics, and/or lower anterior IPR, and opening up the dental space to replace the missing tooth with a dental prosthesis

(e)

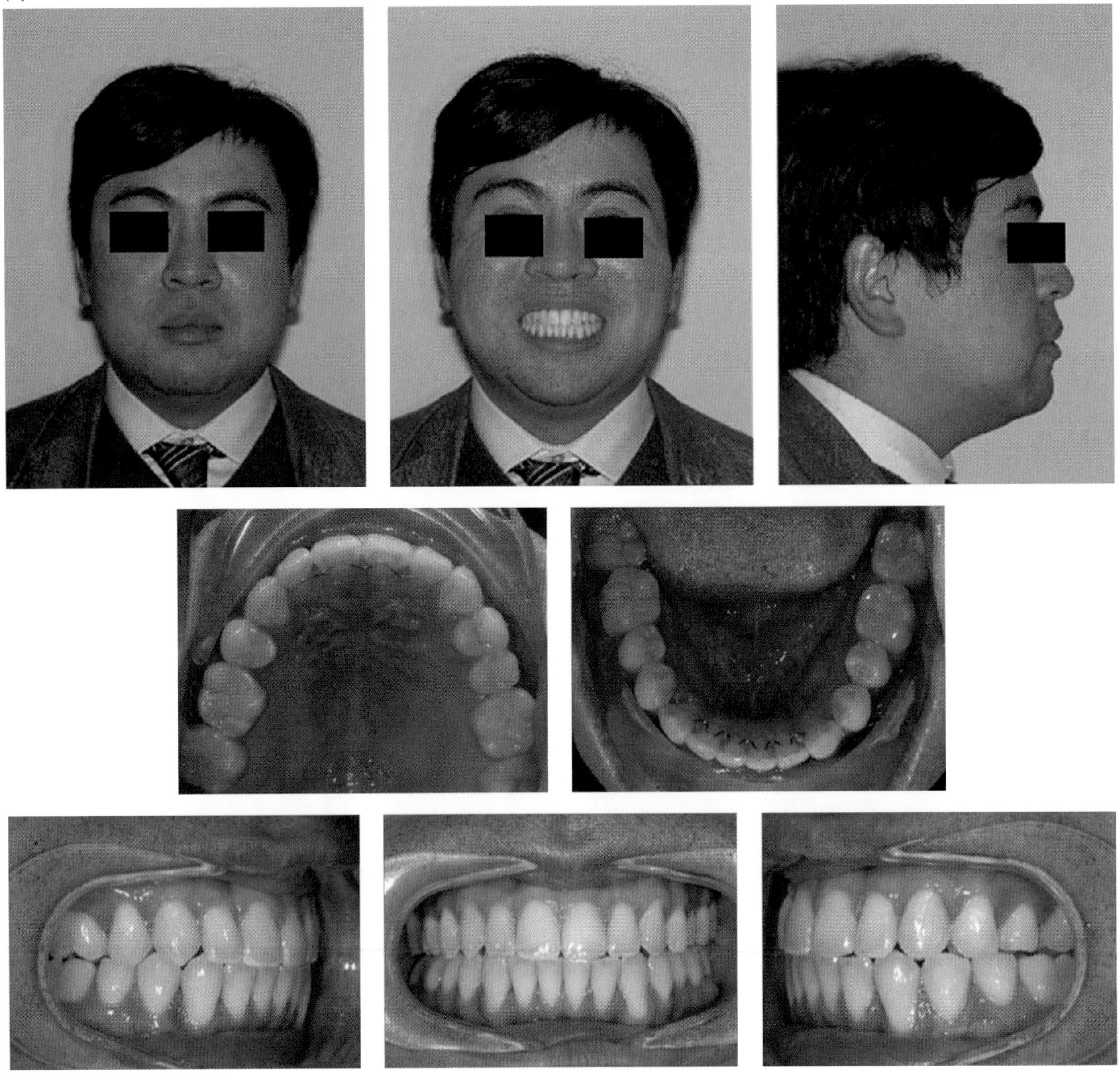

(f)

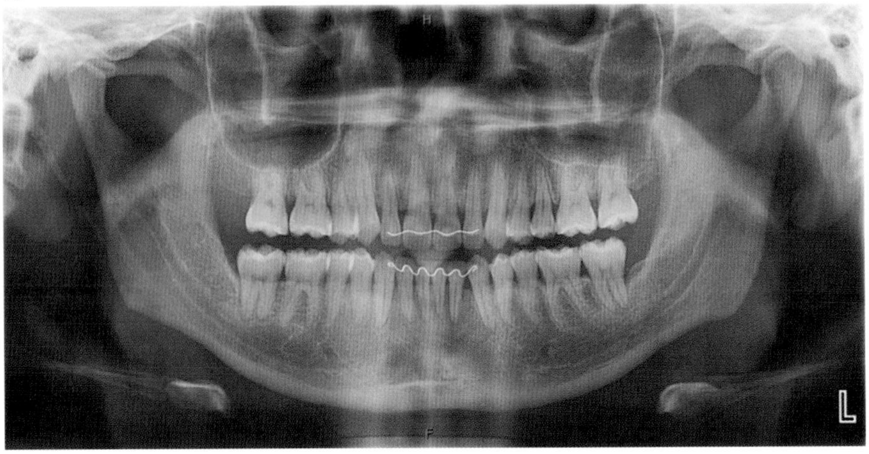

Figure 12.5.4 (Continued)

(g)

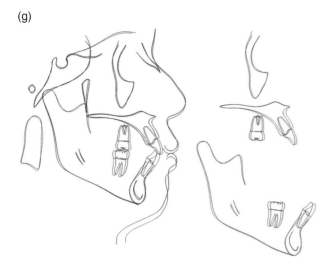

Figure 12.5.4 (Continued)

(dental implant, cantilever bridge, full veneer bridge, resin-bonded bridge, or even a single tooth denture – depending on case suitability) can restore the functionality as well as aesthetics of the case (Figure 12.5.5b). The deviated dental midlines, reverse overbite, and the poor inter-incisor angulation would be corrected simultaneously (Figure 12.5.5c–e).

A previously extracted second premolar (tooth #34) on the lower arch contributed to the collapse of the lower dental archform in an adult female patient (Figure 12.5.6a, b). The lower dental midline deviated toward the side of the missing tooth and resulted in an increased dental overjet. There could be quite a few different treatment options in this particular situation. Options: (i) leave the lower deviated dental midline uncorrected, IPR on the upper dental arch to reduce the overjet, or (ii) extract three other premolar teeth to compensate for the missing #34, or (iii) open the #34 dental space and reestablish the archform for a future prosthetic replacement tooth.

The decision lies firstly on the patient's profile; extracting three other premolars in a delicate profile with mild dental crowding will overly retract the lips and increase the facial concavity. This is not an ideal aesthetic outcome. Although option (iii) allows for the reestablishment of a symmetrical, balanced, and functional occlusion, the clinician has to first evaluate if the periodontium is able to support such dental arch expansion and increase in dental arch length. The mental nerve and canal may be in close proximity to the potential implant site. It is essential to ensure that there would be no obstruction/interference of these structures before adopting this plan. The patient must also be informed of the extra costs and surgical involvement with the implant and prosthesis placement.

The anchorage design in this case was Class II elastics on the left side, supporting the protraction and mesialization of the lower anterior teeth planned in the ClinCheck movements (Figure 12.5.6c). Light lower IPR anteriorly was performed to allow space for alignment, elimination of black triangles, and the prevention of overly proclining the lower incisors. The gradual distraction of the lower premolar space allowed good dentoalveolar bone formation at the edentulous space (Figure 12.5.6d). The completed result presented a harmonious facial and occlusal balance (Figure 12.5.6e, f). The dental arch expansion presented a good smile width and eliminated the buccal corridors. The dental midlines were coincident with a good Class I canine and molar relationship. The profile of the patient was also well protected.

Dental Corrections (Extraction Therapies)

The three-dimensional control of dental movements and space closure in extraction cases using clear aligners remains one of the more challenging treatment modalities in clear aligner therapy. However, armed with a good knowledge of the biology of tooth movement, understanding truly, how the dentition responds to the forces expressed by aligners, together with careful planning, it is not impossible to achieve excellent results.

Canine Substitution

Undetected delayed or ectopic eruption of permanent canines during childhood may contribute to its impaction and subsequent failure of eruption. It is essential to take routine OPG radiographs when the child visits the family dentist for their regular routine dental check-ups. Lengthy delay in detection and treatment may lead to asymmetrical dental changes.

A teenager presented with an increased dental overjet and upper dental spacing (Figure 12.5.7a). The OPG showed an impacted #23, and an otherwise healthy, full complement of teeth (Figure 12.5.7b). The upper dental midline was deviated to the left; there were non-coincidental midlines with a deep dental overbite. Two treatment plans were presented to the parents and child.

Option (i): reestablish the #23 space orthodontically, surgically expose the impacted #23, and tract the tooth back to its rightful position. This allowed a more symmetrical occlusion at completion however there might still be a small risk of the #23 being ankylosed. If ankylosis does occur, there would need to be a second surgery to have the ankylosed #23 removed, and either have that space closed, or be left for a future prosthetic replacement. This could be in the form of a dental implant. However, as the child was still a teenager with existing dentoalveolar growth, it was not advisable to have a dental implant placed until that

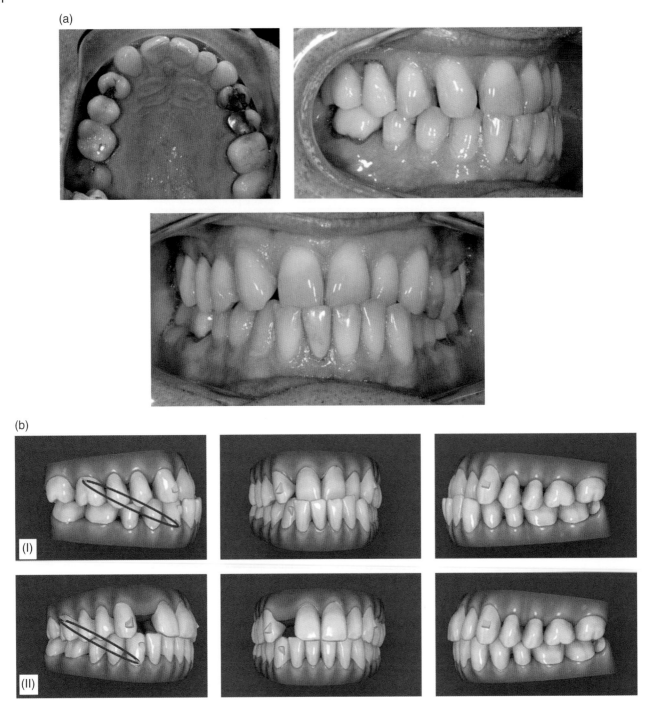

Figure 12.5.5 (a) Pre-treatment Images of an adult showing a missing #12 contributing to a Class III dental malocclusion with reverse overjet and deviated dental midlines. (b) ClinCheck plans showing (I) pre-treatment and (II) simulated final position of the dentition, with attachment designs and precision cuts for Class III elastic wear. (c) Post-treatment images with reestablishment of dental space for a dental implant. (d) Post-prosthetic images with the placement of dental implant and final restoration. (e) Post-prosthetic periapical radiograph showing implant and crown placement.

(c)

(d)

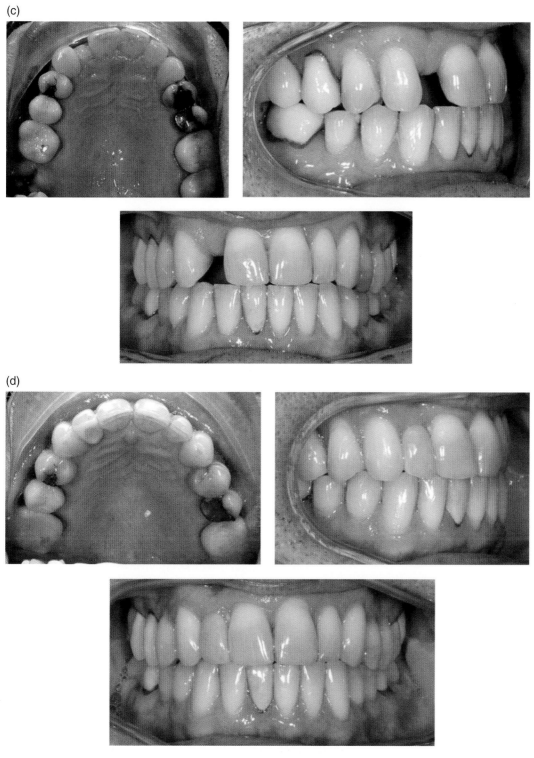

Figure 12.5.5   (Continued)

(e)

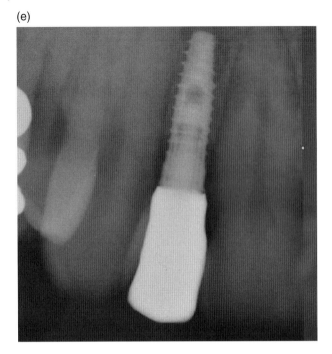

Figure 12.5.5   (Continued)

growth has ceased in her late teen years (Dietschi and Schartz 1997; Oesterle et al. 1993). She would need an interim temporary prosthesis such as a denture or a resin-bonded bridge. These options may not be aesthetically acceptable and may be costly to maintain. Other complications may include alveolar bone loss that requires further surgery with bone augmentation before implant placement.

Option (ii): have the impacted #23 surgically removed and the space closed orthodontically. This would negate the potential need for a second surgery if the tooth was ankylosed, and would avoid any need for future prosthetic replacement and the associated procedures (Figure 12.5.7c). After much weighing of the pros and cons with the child and parents, option (ii) was selected. The tooth #23 was surgically removed and clear aligner therapy with Invisalign commenced. The ClinCheck plans show attachment, anchorage designs, and the mesial root tip of the posterior teeth emphasizing the need for compensatory movements in closure of extraction spaces (Chan and Darendeliler 2017) (Figure 12.5.7d). Class II elastics were used on the right while Class III elastics on the left (Figure 12.5.7e).

In cases with canine substitution, the first premolar needs to mimic the missing/extracted canine. It is pertinent to plan these extra movements on the #24 in the ClinCheck plans: (i) increase the buccal root torque to mimic the canine bulge to accentuate the buccal gingival eminence, and (ii) increase the mesial rotation to hide

the palatal cusp of the premolar (Figure 12.5.7f). The completed result presented a harmonious facial and occlusal balance (Figure 12.5.7g–i). The upper dental spaces were closed, overjet was reduced with the upper and lower dental midlines coincident with the mid-sagittal facial plane. The occlusion on the right is a good Class I canine and molar relationship, while on the left, with the first premolar substituting as the canine, a Class I canine and full Class II molar relationship (Nangia and Darendeliler 2001). It should be noted that although the option to remove the impacted canine and close the extraction was more predictable, it was by no means an easier option. The compliant cooperation of the patient with a favorable dentoalveolar growth has contributed much to the success of this case.

Single Premolar Extraction

In adult patients with upper midline deviations resulting from previously extracted teeth (Figure 12.5.8a, b), correction may include various options. Half-unit correction with molar distalization is often predictable and is a common treatment modality with clear aligners. However, due to the sequential staging pattern involved, treatment duration may be long and protracted. The extraction of a contralateral premolar tooth will allow instantaneous space required for the midline correction and may provide a quicker solution. Due to the lack of overjet in this case, the plan was to extract the #25 instead of #24. The ClinCheck plans show the attachment and anchorage designs with compensatory movements (Figure 12.5.8c) and a simultaneous staging pattern. Class II elastics were used on the left while Class III elastics on the right (Figure 12.5.8d). The completed result presented a harmonious facial and occlusal balance (Figure 12.5.8e–g). The upper dental midline can be successfully moved across the median plane, with the upper and lower dental midlines coincident with each other and the mid-sagittal facial plane.

Single Lower Incisor Extraction

Skeletal asymmetrical Class III malocclusions can often be camouflaged with a single lower incisor extraction without the need for orthognathic surgery. The diagnostic key is the detection of any premature contacts and functional shifts. An adult female patient presented with a Class III dental malocclusion on a skeletal 3 base (Figure 12.5.9a). She had a remarkable reversed overjet with her chin point slightly deviated to the left. The upper second molars were supra-erupted with premature

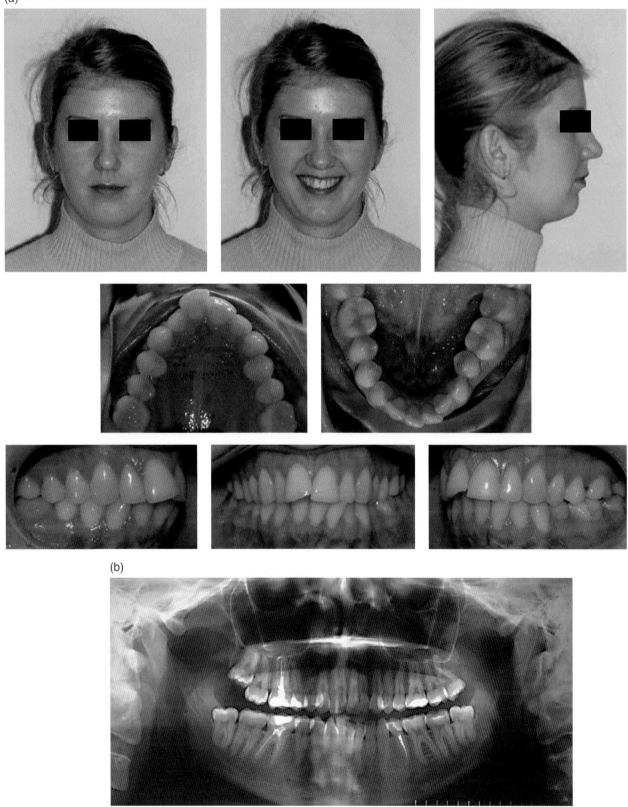

Figure 12.5.6 (a) Pre-treatment images of an adult showing an asymmetrical Class II dental malocclusion after the loss of #34. (b) Pre-treatment OPG radiograph. (c) ClinCheck plans showing (I) pre-treatment and (II) simulated final position of the dentition, with attachment designs and precision cuts for elastic wear. (d) Progressive treatment images showing reestablishment of dental space for a #34 prosthesis and lower midline correction. (e) Post-treatment images showing a balanced, symmetrical occlusion with coincident dental and facial midlines. (f) Post-treatment radiograph showing the placement of dental implant and final restoration. (g) Comparison of (I) pre-treatment and (II) post-treatment profile images demonstrating the maintenance of the profile with treatment.

(c)

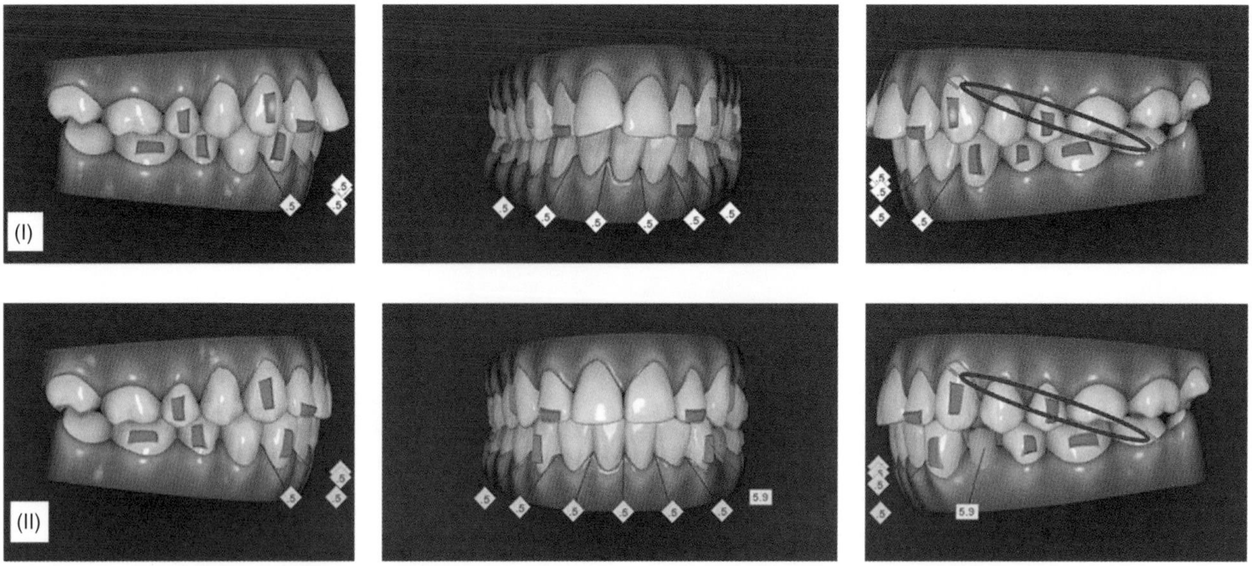

(d)

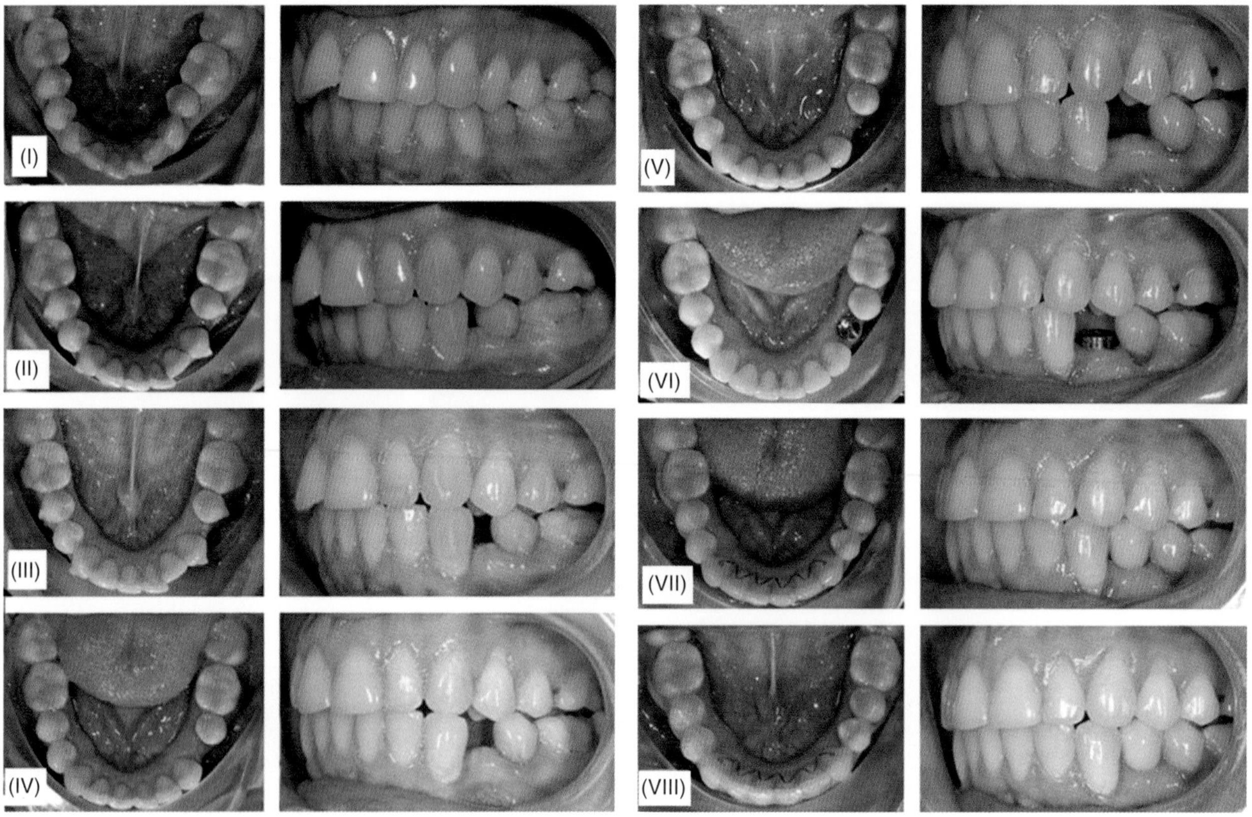

Figure 12.5.6 (Continued)

(e)

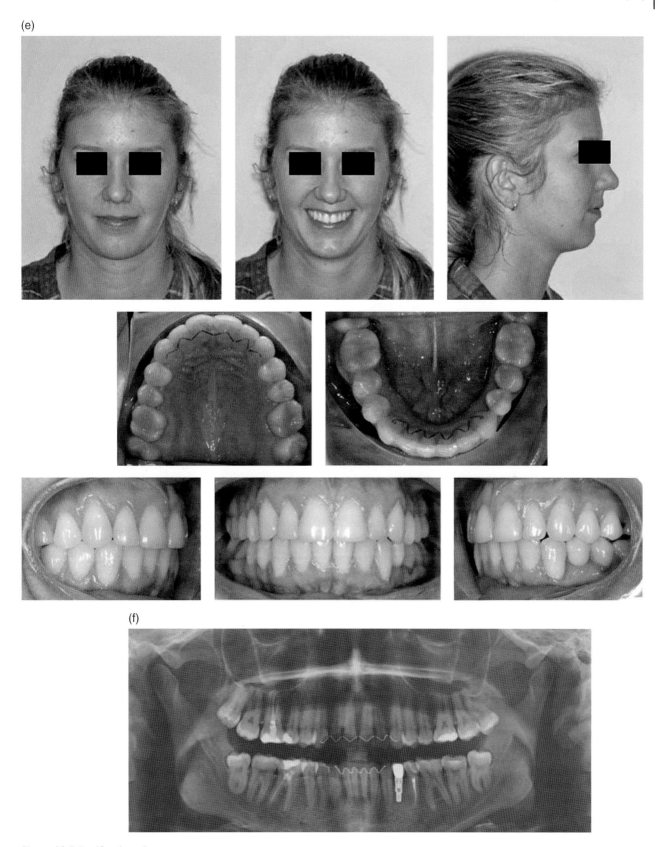

(f)

Figure 12.5.6 (Continued)

(g)

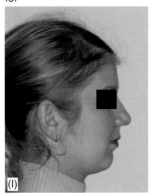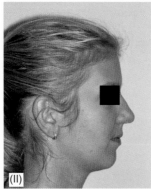

Figure 12.5.6   (Continued)

contact with the lower second molars (Figure 12.5.9b). After manipulating the mandible into a centric relation, the functional shift was detected. The preliminary plan was to eliminate this shift in order to visualize the true anterior–posterior (A–P) relationship before finalizing the treatment plans. Upper left and right sectional fixed appliances were placed on the upper left and right second premolars, first molars, and second molars to intrude the second molars to eliminate the shift. After 3 months of active treatment, the true A–P relationship with a less pronounced reverse overjet was obtained (Figure 12.5.9c). Under such new conditions, a single lower incisor extraction camouflage plan without the need for orthognathic surgery became plausible.

In treatment plans that required a lower incisor extraction, the clinician should consider extracting the incisor that was the most compromised. Select the tooth with either low gingival attachments, marked bone loss or dehiscence, heavily filled or root canal treated, heavily attrited and worn, or ones with the most relapse potential. The ClinCheck plans show the attachment and anchorage designs, with the extraction of #32 (Figure 12.5.9d). The anchorage design was supported with Class III elastics (Figure 12.5.9e). The completed result presented a good overjet and overbite with a normalized facial balance (Figure 12.5.9f–h). The camouflage treatment had successfully corrected the patient's chief concerns without the need for orthognathic surgery.

Asymmetrical Premolar Extractions to Achieve Symmetry

Camouflage treatment in Class III corrections may also involve the extraction of two lower premolar teeth. In asymmetrical Class III corrections, the clinician may consider the asymmetrical extraction of the premolars in order to make the biomechanics symmetrical and easier to design and manage.

An adult female patient presented as a Class III dental malocclusion on a skeletal 3 base with a vertical direction of growth. Her mandible, chin point, and the lower dental midline were all slightly deviated to the right side. There were bilateral posterior crossbites, with instanding upper lateral incisors contributing to anterior crossbites and a minimal overjet and overbite (Figure 12.5.10a, b). The treatment plan was to extract the #34 which was closer to the midline to facilitate the lower midline correction, and #45 as it was blocked out of the dental arch. The ClinCheck plans showed the attachment and elastic designs and compensatory movements (Figure 12.5.10c). The anchorage was supported with increasing strengths of Class III elastics as treatment progressed. As the distance between the elastic hooks and buttons decreased as the extraction spaces closed, the strength of the elastics had to be increased to maintain the optimal level of forces (3M Unitek Chuck elastics increased to Dwight) (Figure 12.5.10d). This adjustment was monitored closely and adjusted accordingly at every 8–10 weeks appointment. The completed results presented a well-interdigitated, therapeutic Class III occlusion (Class I canine and Class III molar relationship) (Nangia and Darendeliler 2001) with a harmonious and balanced smile, and facial appearance. There was an ideal overjet and overbite achieved, the upper and lower dental midlines were coincident with the facial sagittal plane (Figure 12.5.10e). The completed radiographs and superimpositions showed a good control of dental bodily movements, parallel roots, alleviating the dental crowding, camouflaging the underlying skeletal Class 3 pattern while maintaining the vertical dimensions (Figure 12.5.10f–h).

Symmetrical Premolar Extractions in Asymmetrical Case

Not all correction of dental asymmetries require unilateral or asymmetrical extractions. An adult female patient presented as a Class I dental malocclusion on a skeletal 1 base (Figure 12.5.11a, b). She had severe upper and lower dental crowding with both the upper and lower dental midlines deviated to the right. This was mainly due to the greater degree of crowding on the right side. The treatment plan was to have all four first premolar extracted and to control the asymmetrical biomechanics with differential elastics on the left and right side. The ClinCheck plans showed the attachment and elastic designs, with extraction compensatory movements (Figure 12.5.11c). There was a stronger, normal Class II elastic worn on the left side and a triangular, weaker Class II elastic worn on the right

(a)

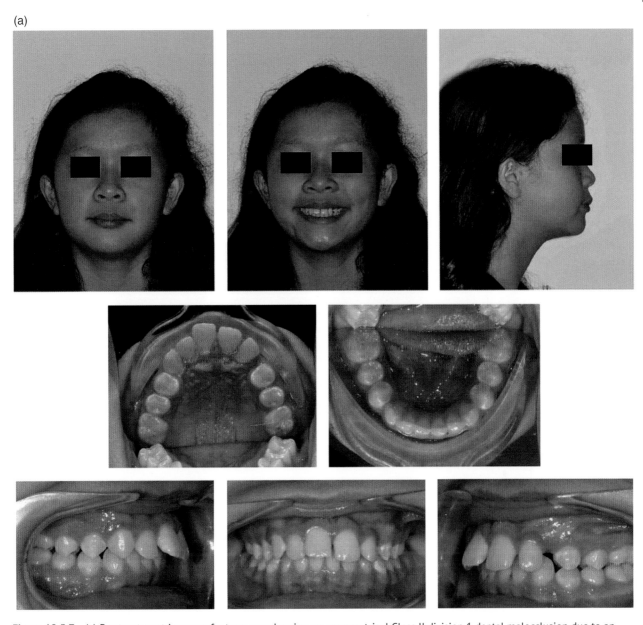

Figure 12.5.7 (a) Pre-treatment images of a teenager showing an asymmetrical Class II division 1 dental malocclusion due to an impacted #23. (b) Pre-treatment OPG radiograph. (c) Different treatment options showing (I) the opening of space, surgical exposure of #23 and tracking it down, and (II) the surgical removal of the impacted #23, and closure of dental space. (d) ClinCheck plans showing (I) pre-treatment and (II) simulated final position of the dentition, with attachment designs, precision cuts for elastic wear and compensatory movements. (e) Progressive treatment images showing space closure and midline correction. (f) Increase the mesial rotation and buccal root torque hides the palatal cusp of the premolar and increases the buccal gingival eminence to mimic the canine bulge. (g) Post-treatment images showing a balanced occlusion with coincident dental and facial midlines. (h) Post-treatment OPG radiograph. (i) Comparison of (I) pre-treatment and (II) post-treatment images demonstrating the premolar substituting a canine, and midline correction.

throughout most of the treatment (Figure 12.5.11d). This adjustment was monitored closely and adjusted accordingly at every 8–10 weeks appointment. The completed results presented a well-interdigitated Class I occlusion. There was an ideal overjet and overbite, with the upper and lower dental midlines coincident with the facial

sagittal plane (Figure 12.5.11e). The completed radiographs and superimpositions showed a good control of dental bodily movements, parallel roots, correcting the dental crowding without overly retracting the lips and profile, while also maintaining the vertical dimensions (Figure 12.5.11f–h).

(b)

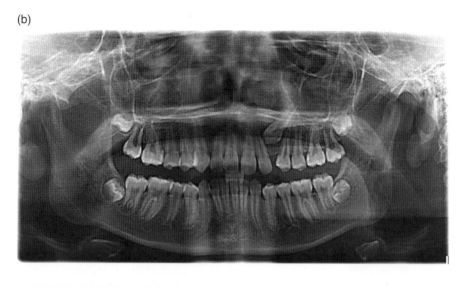

(c)

(d)

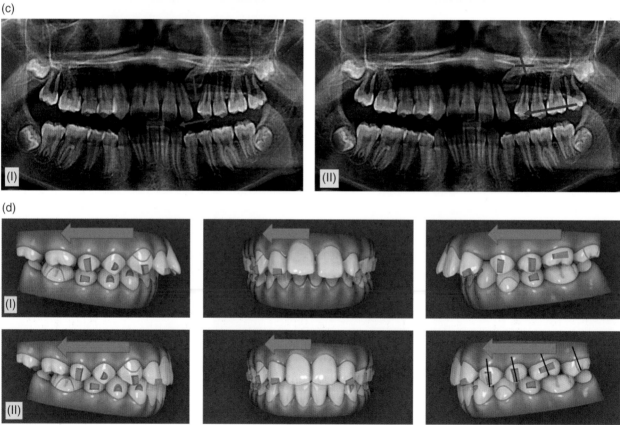

Figure 12.5.7 (Continued)

Skeletal Anchorage Therapies

Anchorage control relying solely on tooth-borne mechanics has its limitations. This has recently been alleviated by the advent of bone-borne devices. Skeletal anchorage devices have gained popularity in obscure cases that require movement otherwise impossible, or very difficult to achieve with conventional treatment modalities. Incorporating these skeletal anchorage devices into clear aligner therapy requires some imagination and creative planning.

(e)

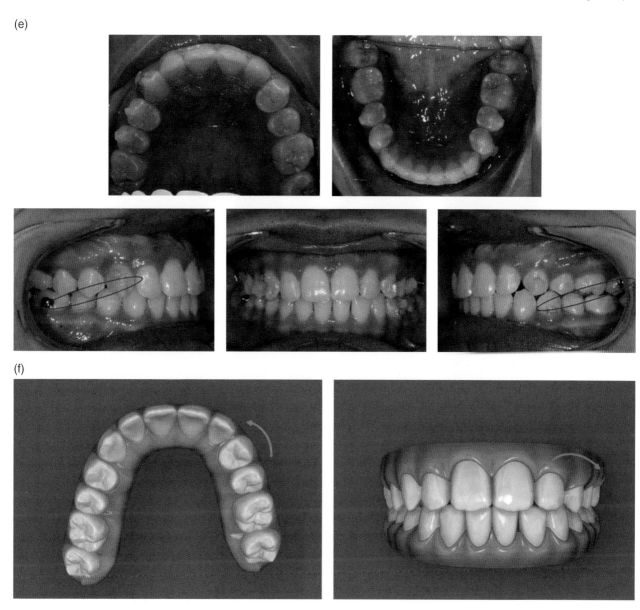

(f)

Figure 12.5.7 (Continued)

Molar Mesialization

An adult patient with a failed restoration and hence extracted #36, would like to have that space closed, mesializing the #37 and #38 (Figure 12.5.12a, b). The case presented with a congenitally missing lower incisor, evident with a Class III dental relationship on the right side. Space closure using clear aligners with a minimal anchorage design is often contraindicated. The mesialization of the posterior teeth is ineffective with aligners alone and bodily movement is difficult to achieve. The treatment plan in this case was to have a temporary anchorage device (TAD, Aarhus 8 mm, American Orthodontics) placed in the interdental space between the #34 and #35, and lower left sectional fixed appliances placed in concurrent with invisalign treatment. The ClinCheck plans showed the attachment designs; position of the placement of the TAD, buccal button cutouts to accommodate the sectional fixed appliances, and Class III elastics on the right side to support the dental movements (Figure 12.5.12c). Clinically, as the case progressed and as the #37 and #38 migrated forward, buttons were placed on the #13 and #15, and a triangular elastic was added to control the vertical anchorage as the TAD supported the space closure with intra-arch elastomeric chains (Figure 12.5.12d). All the dental movements were

(g)

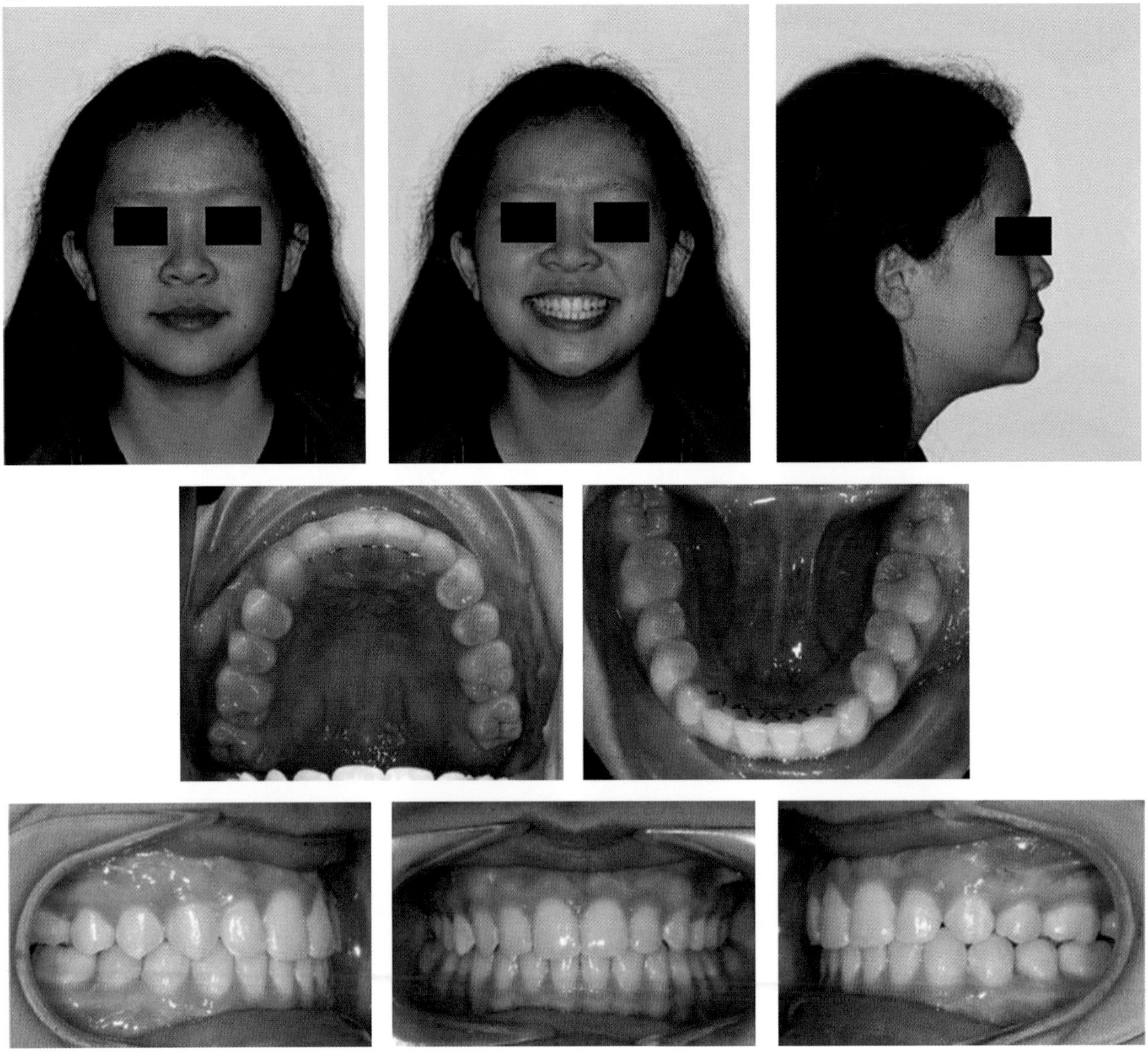

(h)

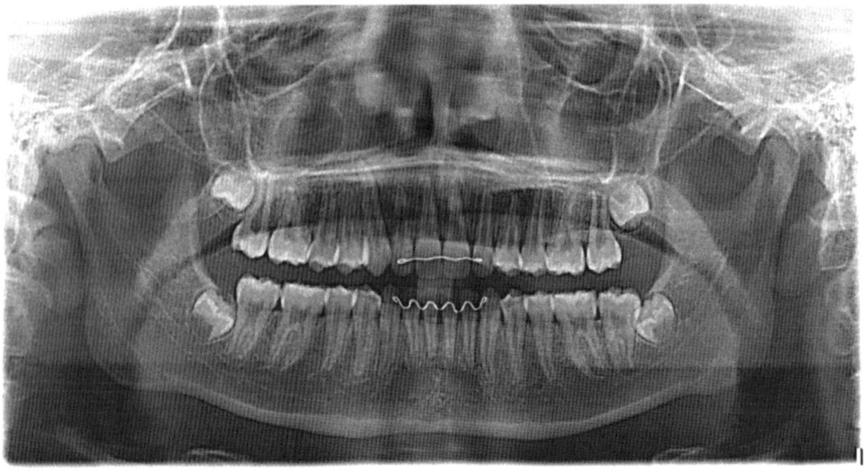

Figure 12.5.7 (Continued)

(i)

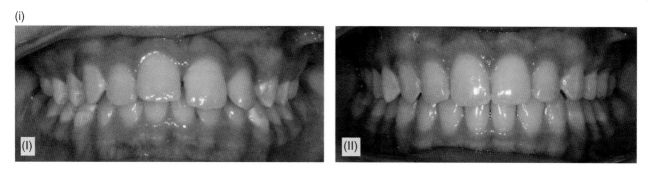

Figure 12.5.7 (Continued)

(a)

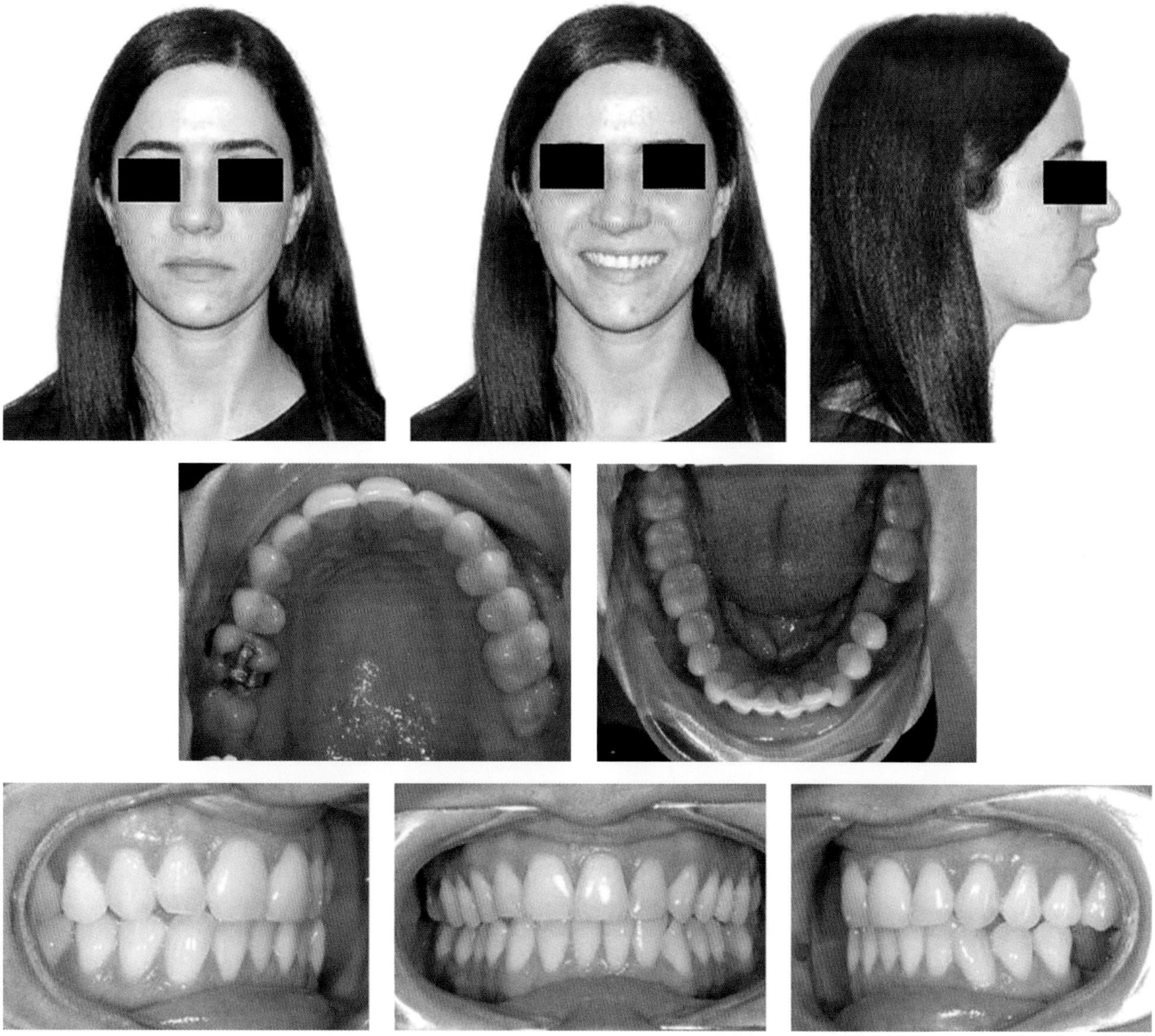

Figure 12.5.8 (a) Pre-treatment images of an adult showing an asymmetrical Class II dental malocclusion after the early loss of the #15. The upper dental midline was deviated to the right, with a minimal dental overjet. (b) Pre-treatment OPG radiograph. (c) ClinCheck plans showing (I) pre-treatment and (II) simulated final position of the dentition, with attachment designs, precision cuts for elastic wear and compensatory movements. (d) Progressive treatment images showing space closure and midline correction e Post-treatment images showing a balanced occlusion with coincident dental and facial midlines. (f) Post-treatment OPG radiograph. (g) Comparison of (I) pre-treatment and (II) post-treatment images demonstrating the re-alignment of the dental midlines.

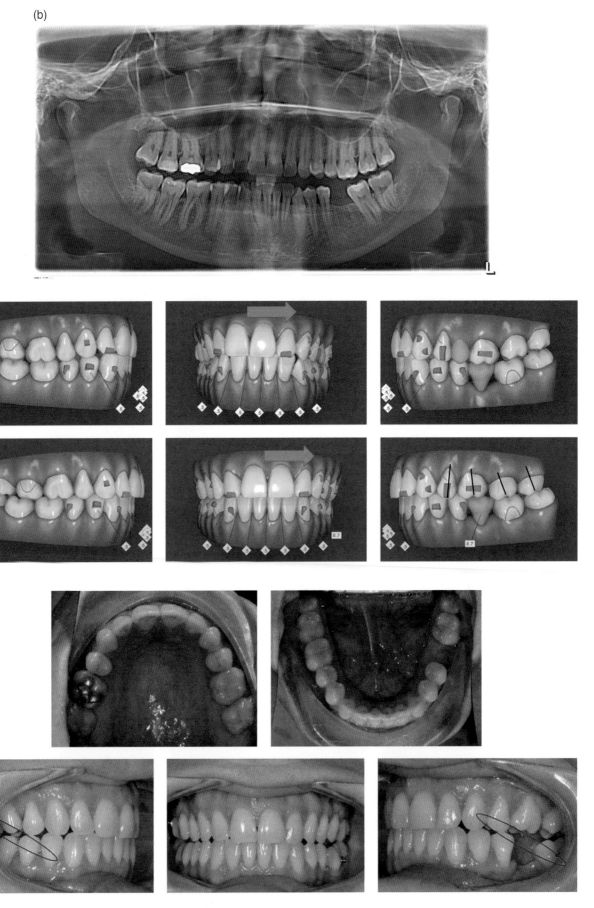

Figure 12.5.8 (Continued)

(e)

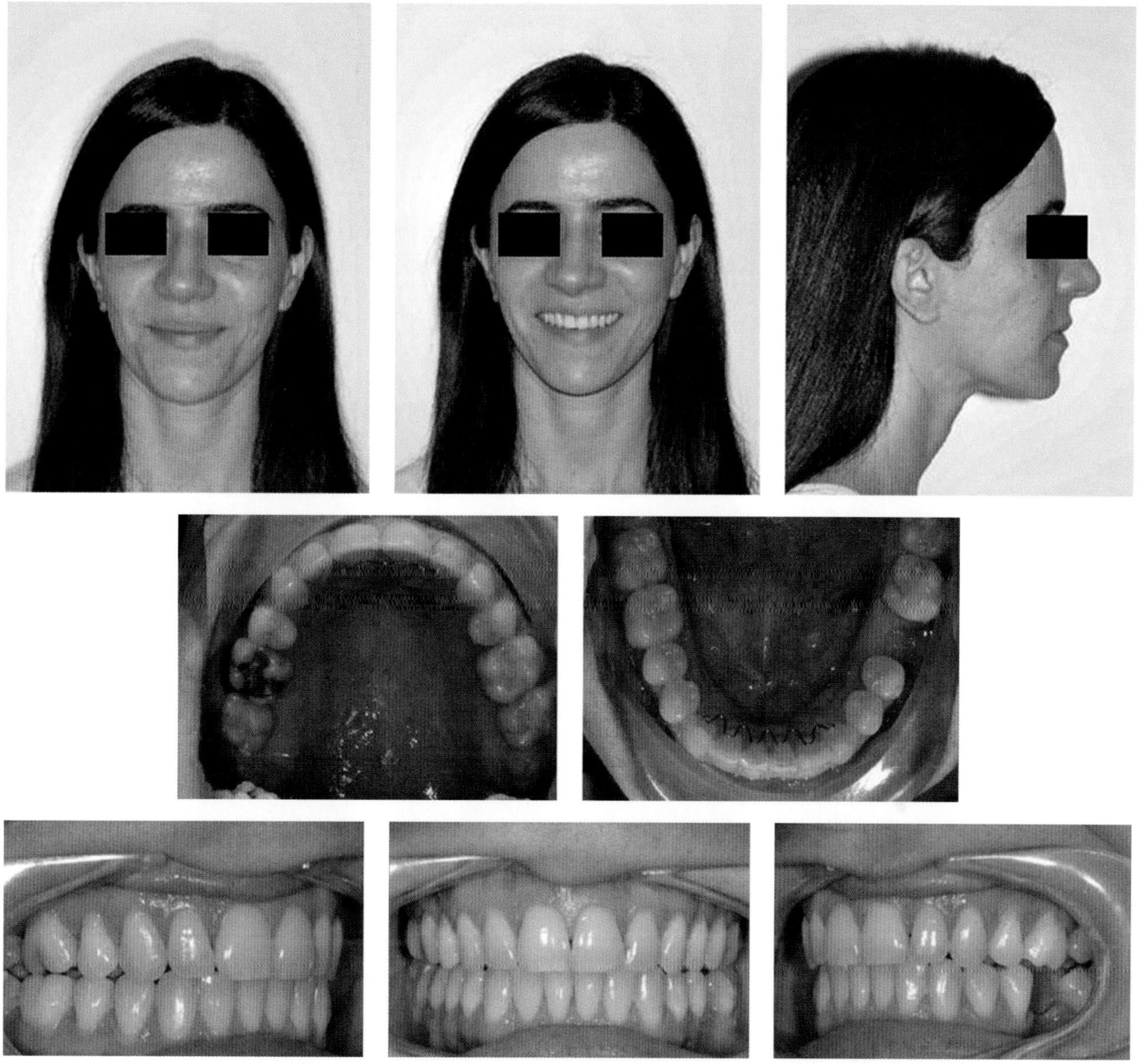

(f)

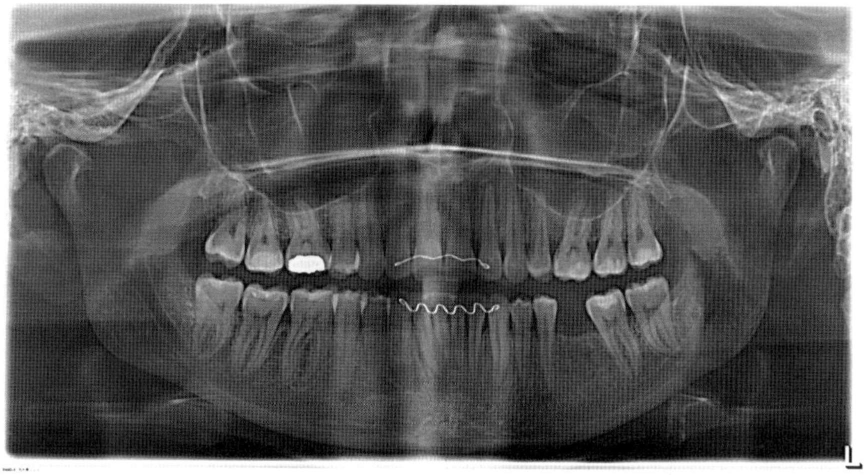

Figure 12.5.8 (Continued)

(g)

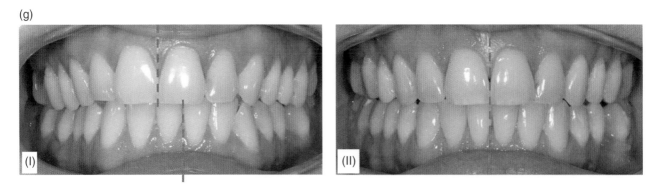

Figure 12.5.8 (Continued)

(a)

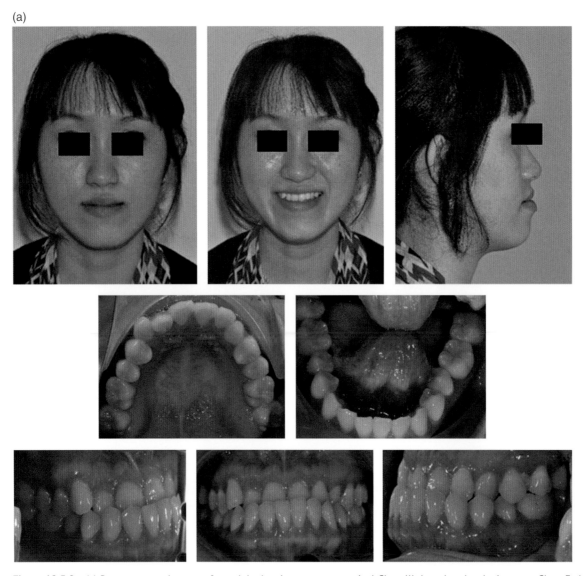

Figure 12.5.9 (a) Pre-treatment images of an adult showing an asymmetrical Class III dental malocclusion on a Class 3 skeletal base. There was a lower dental midline deviation to the left with a severe reverse overjet. (b) Pre-treatment OPG and lateral cephalometric radiograph (indicating the premature contacts at the overly erupted upper second molars). (c) Progressive treatment images showing occlusion after the elimination of the premature contacts and functional shift. (d) ClinCheck plans showing (I) pre-treatment and (II) simulated final position of the dentition, with the extraction of #31, attachment designs and precision cuts for elastic wear. (e) Progressive treatment images showing, direction of elastic wear, space closure, and overjet correction. (f) Post-treatment images showing a balanced occlusion with a normalized dental overbite and overjet. (g) Post-treatment OPG and lateral cephalometric radiograph. (h) Comparison of (I) pre-treatment and (II) post-treatment images demonstrating the non-surgical correction of a severe Class III with the normalization of the overbite and overjet.

(b)

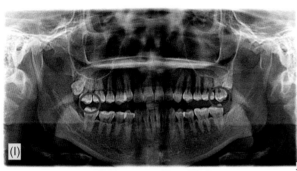 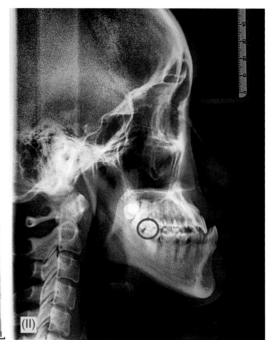

(c)

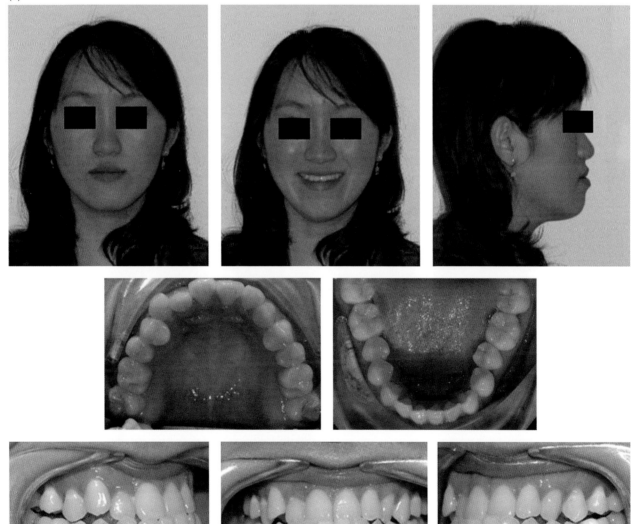

Figure 12.5.9 (Continued)

(d)

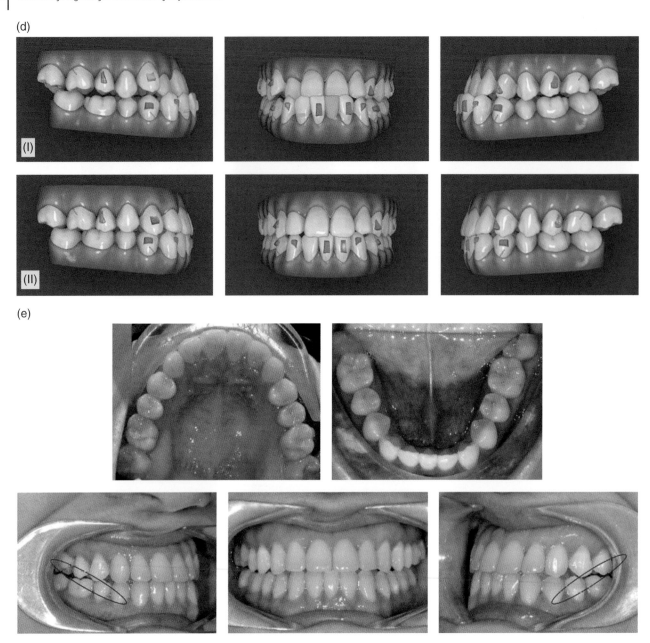

(e)

Figure 12.5.9 (Continued)

designed into the ClinCheck plans and the aligners were directing and supporting the correction with routine 1–2 weekly changes. The completed result showed bodily movement of the #37 and #38, full space closure of the #36 space, while maintaining the dental midlines, and a normal overjet and overbite (Figure 12.5.12e, f).

Unilateral Segmental Distalization

Sequential dental movement is the default staging pattern in most Class II dental corrections requiring molar distalization. However, cases with a thicker dentoalveolar bone mass, and/or larger roots, may contribute to more resistance to such movements. The placement of a single TAD tips the balance and provides the mechanical advantage.

An adult patient presented with the upper dental midline deviated to the left and a Class II dental relationship on the right side. There was an increased overjet and moderate degree of upper dental crowding (Figure 12.5.13a). The ClinCheck plans showed the direction of molar distalization of the upper right quadrant, the placement of the TAD (Vector 8 mm, Ormco) in the high interproximal space between the #16 and 17, attachment designs and positions of the precision cuts (Figure 12.5.13b). The

(f)

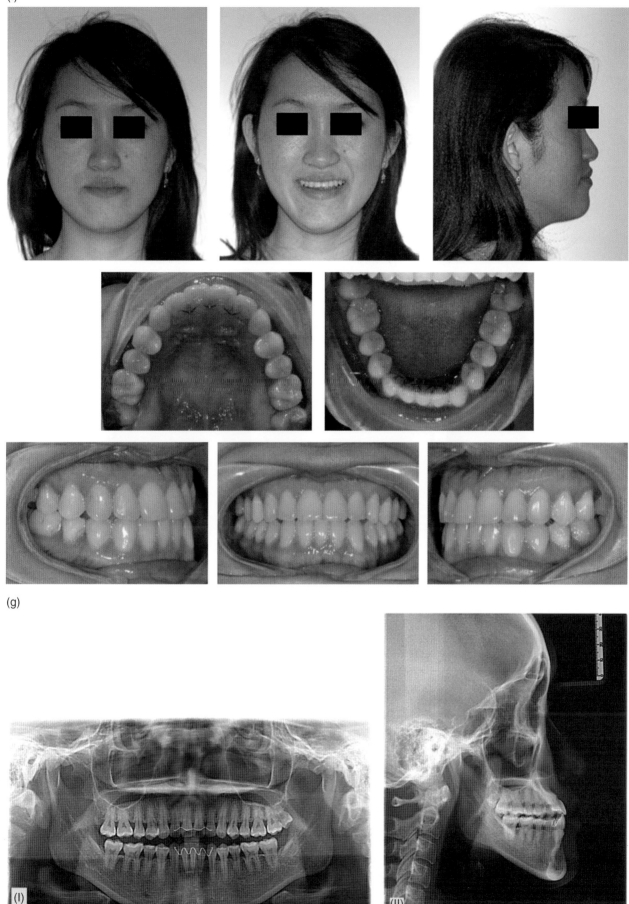

(g)

Figure 12.5.9 (Continued)

(h)

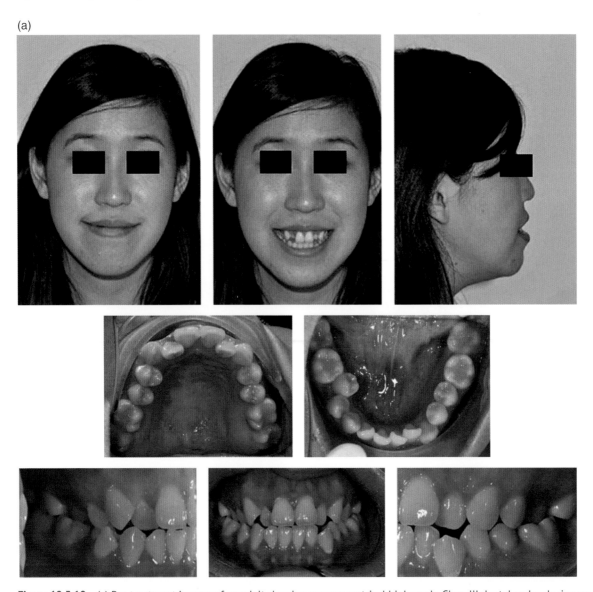

(I) (II)

Figure 12.5.9 (Continued)

(a)

Figure 12.5.10 (a) Pre-treatment images of an adult showing an asymmetrical high angle Class III dental malocclusion on a Class 3 skeletal base. There were anterior and posterior crossbites bilaterally with non-coincident dental midlines. (b) Pre-treatment OPG and lateral cephalometric radiograph. (c) ClinCheck plans showing (I) pre-treatment and (II) simulated final position of the dentition, with the asymmetrical extraction of #34 and #45, attachment designs, and precision cuts for elastic wear. (d) Progressive treatment images showing space closure and dental alignment. (e) Post-treatment images showing a balanced occlusion with the correction of the anterior and posterior crossbites, achieving a Class I canine and Class III molar relationship. (f) Post-treatment OPG and lateral cephalometric radiograph. (g) Superimposition of lateral cephalometric tracings showing vertical control and dental changes with treatment. (h) Comparison of (I) pre-treatment and (II) post-treatment images demonstrating a camouflage treatment plan with asymmetrical extractions of lower premolars.

(b)

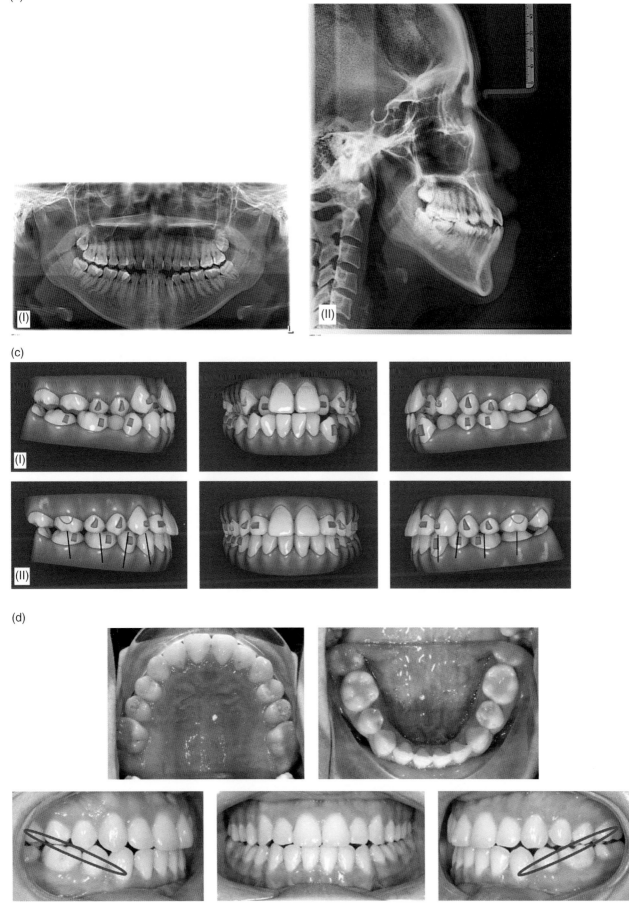

(c)

(d)

Figure 12.5.10 (Continued)

(e)

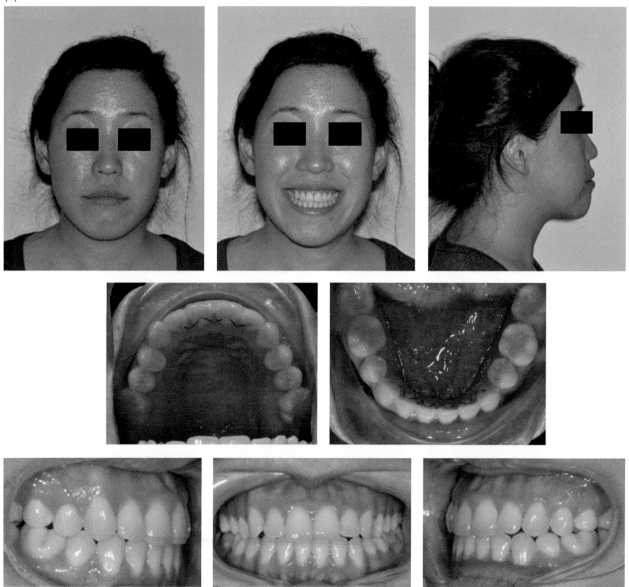

Figure 12.5.10   (Continued)

patient wore intra-arch elastics directly from the TAD to a button bonded on #13. An attachment was also affixed to #13 to prevent the tooth from spinning out of the aligners. No fixed appliances were utilized in this case. As the TAD was placed more apical to the #13, during the distalization process, there was also an unintended intrusion of the #13. Therefore, a night-time triangular elastic was also worn in order to counter such an effect (Figure 12.5.13c). The completed occlusion showed a slightly overcorrected #13 with an otherwise balanced occlusion with coincident dental midlines.

Correction of Occlusal Plane Canting

An adult female patient presented with a Class II division 2 subdivision right-sided dental malocclusion with a skeletal 1 base. There was a unilateral posterior crossbite on the right side, likely contributing to the over-eruption of the upper right quadrant and occlusal plane canting (Figure 12.5.14a). The treatment plan was to align her dentition and correct her Class II dental relationship with clear aligners, and concurrently correct her occlusal plane cant with a TAD (Aarhus, 8 mm, American

(f)

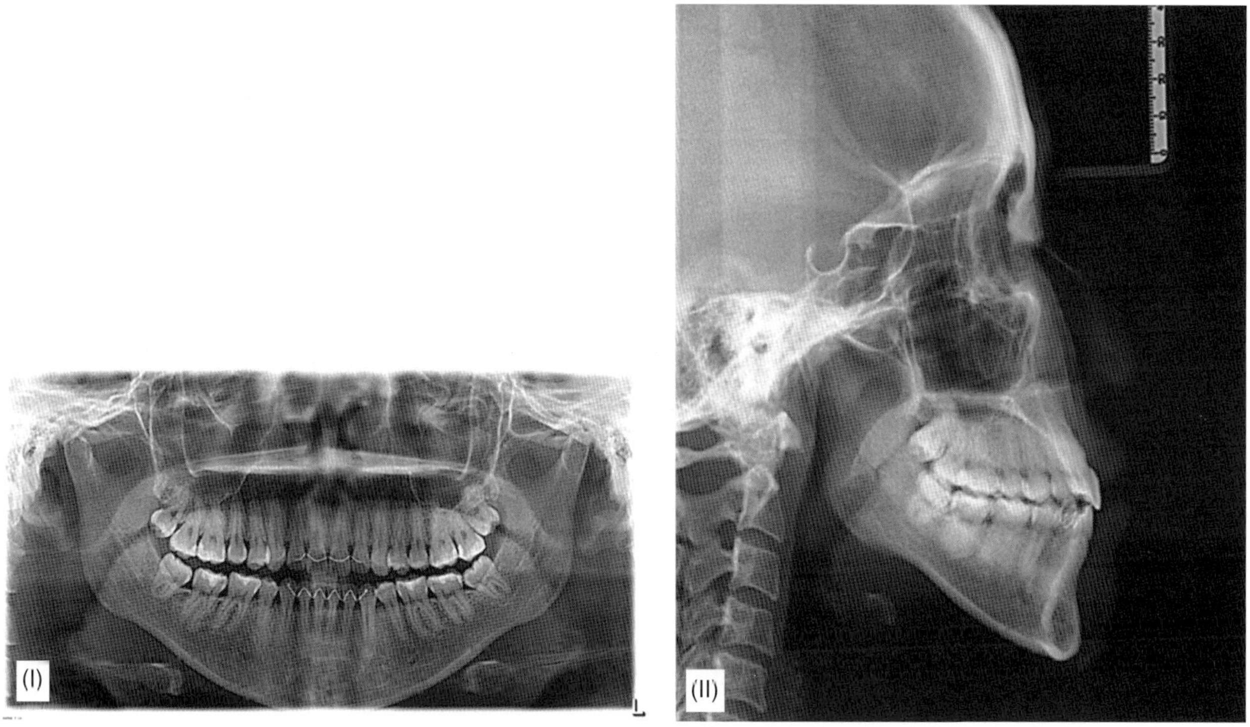

(g)

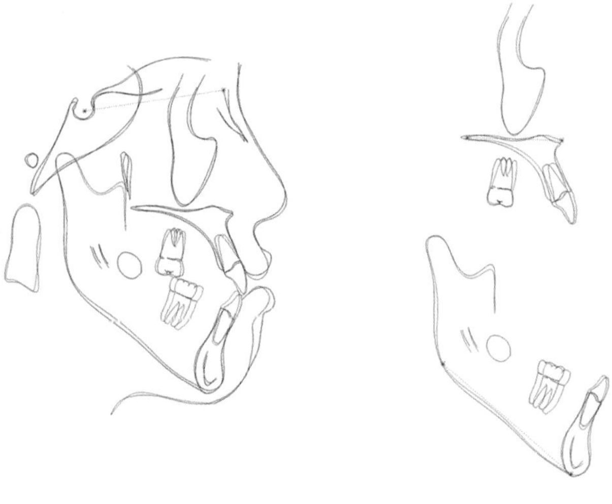

(h)

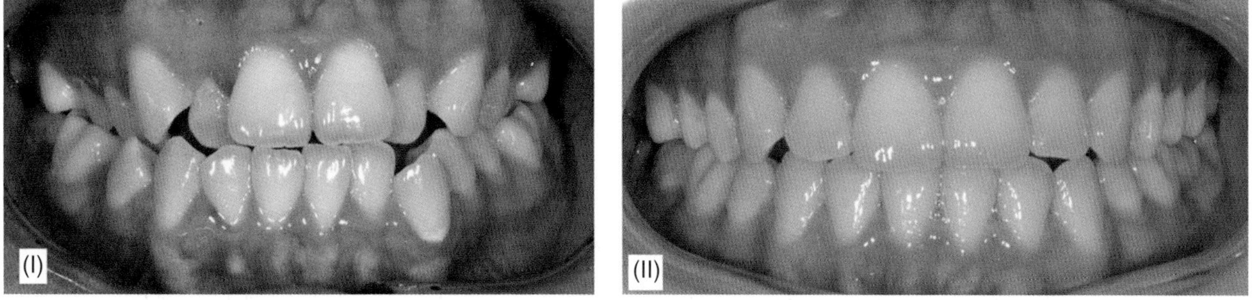

Figure 12.5.10 (Continued)

(a)

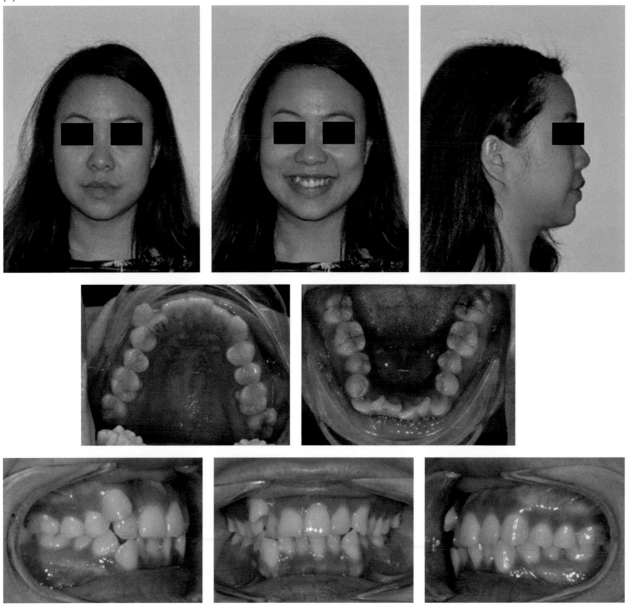

Figure 12.5.11 (a) Pre-treatment images of an adult showing an asymmetrical Class I dental malocclusion on a Class 1 skeletal base. There was a marked deviation of the upper and lower dental midlines to the right side. (b) Pre-treatment OPG and lateral cephalometric radiograph. (c) ClinCheck plans showing (I) pre-treatment and (II) simulated final position of the dentition, with the extraction of four first premolar teeth, attachment designs, precision cuts for elastic wear, and compensatory movements. (d) Progressive treatment images showing space closure and dental alignment. (e) Post-treatment images showing a balanced occlusion with harmonious smile and improved aesthetics. (f) Post-treatment OPG and lateral cephalometric radiograph. (g) Superimposition of lateral cephalometric tracings showing dental changes with treatment. (h) Comparison of (I) pre-treatment and (II) post-treatment images demonstrating the alignment of a severely crowded case with the extraction of four first premolars.

Orthodontics) and sectional fixed appliances. The ClinCheck plans showed the attachment designs, placement of the TAD at the high interproximal space between #14 and #15, and button cutouts to accommodate the sectional fixed appliances (Figure 12.5.14b). Intra-arch elastomeric chain was placed directly from the TAD to the fixed appliance while aligners were concurrently prescribed and changed every 1–2 weekly. After the upper right quadrant was intruded sufficiently, there was a visible inter-arch space. When additional aligners were

(b)

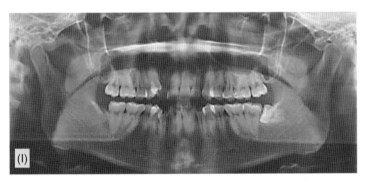
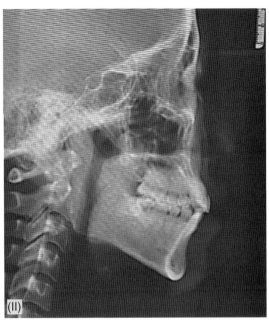

(c)

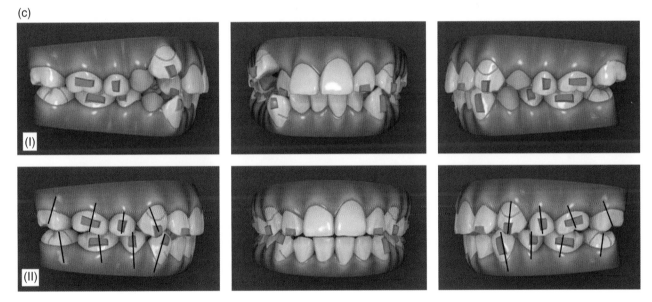

Figure 12.5.11 (Continued)

ordered, new buttons and button cutouts were designed on the #44 and #46 and inter-arch elastics were worn from the TAD to the buttons to extrude the dentition on the lower right quadrant to improve the occlusion (Figure 12.5.14c). The progressive images showed an effective intra-oral correction of the occlusal plane cant. As the cant was isolated more toward the posterior region, there were no obvious changes seen extra-orally with a casual smile (Figure 12.5.14d).

Surgical Intervention

Successful orthodontic correction of dental asymmetries and camouflage treatment of skeletal asymmetries rely on factors such as the age of the patient, potential growth, as well as the extent of dental movements within the boundaries of the envelope of discrepancy. Outside of this scope, surgical intervention may be incorporated with clear aligner therapy and should be considered.

(d)

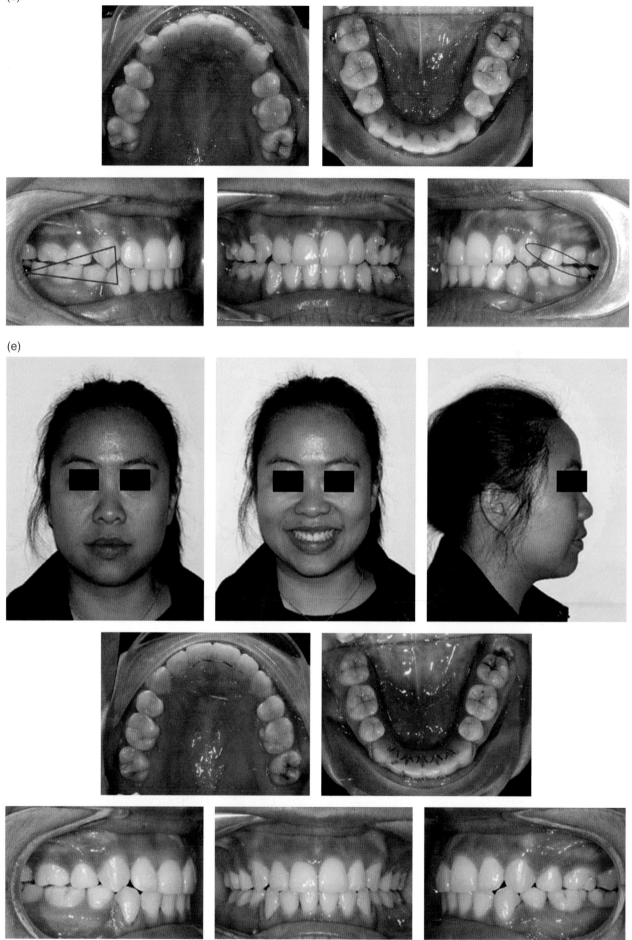

(e)

Figure 12.5.11 (Continued)

(f)

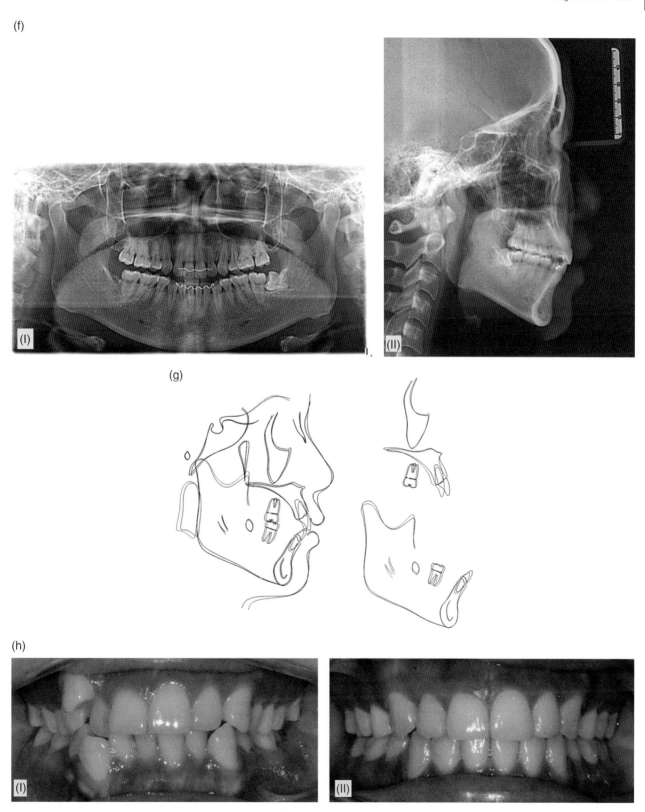

(g)

(h)

Figure 12.5.11 (Continued)

(a)

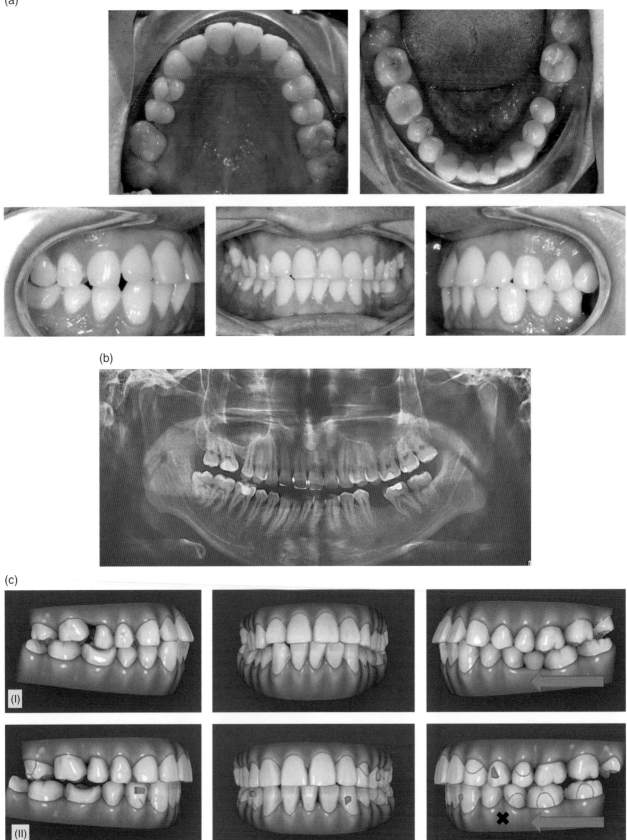

(b)

(c)

Figure 12.5.12 (a) Pre-treatment images of an adult showing an asymmetrical Class I dental malocclusion with a congenitally missing lower incisor and #36 previously extracted. (b) Pre-treatment OPG radiograph. (c) ClinCheck plans showing (I) pre-treatment and (II) simulated final position of the dentition, with cutouts for the placement of sectional fixed appliances, attachment designs, and precision cuts for elastic wear. "X" marks the position of the TAD placement. (d) Progressive treatment images showing (I) initial, (II) space closure with TAD, button and elastics, and sectional fixed appliance, (III) completion. (e) Post-treatment images showing the maintenance of an ideal overbite and overbite, with the complete space closure of #36. (f) Post-treatment OPG radiograph.

(d)

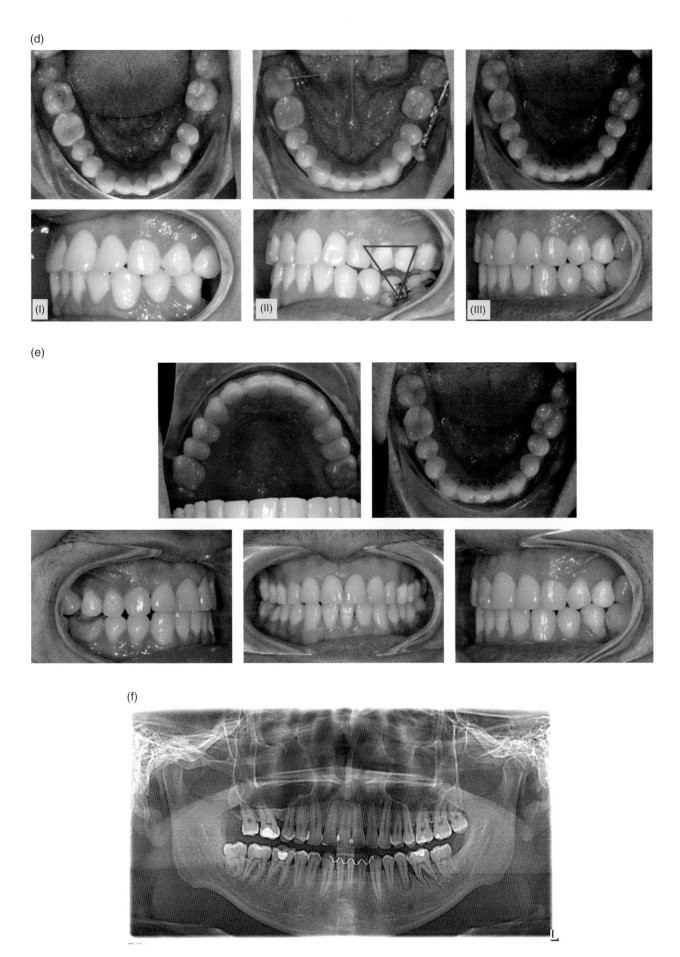

(I)

(II)

(III)

(e)

(f)

Figure 12.5.12 (Continued)

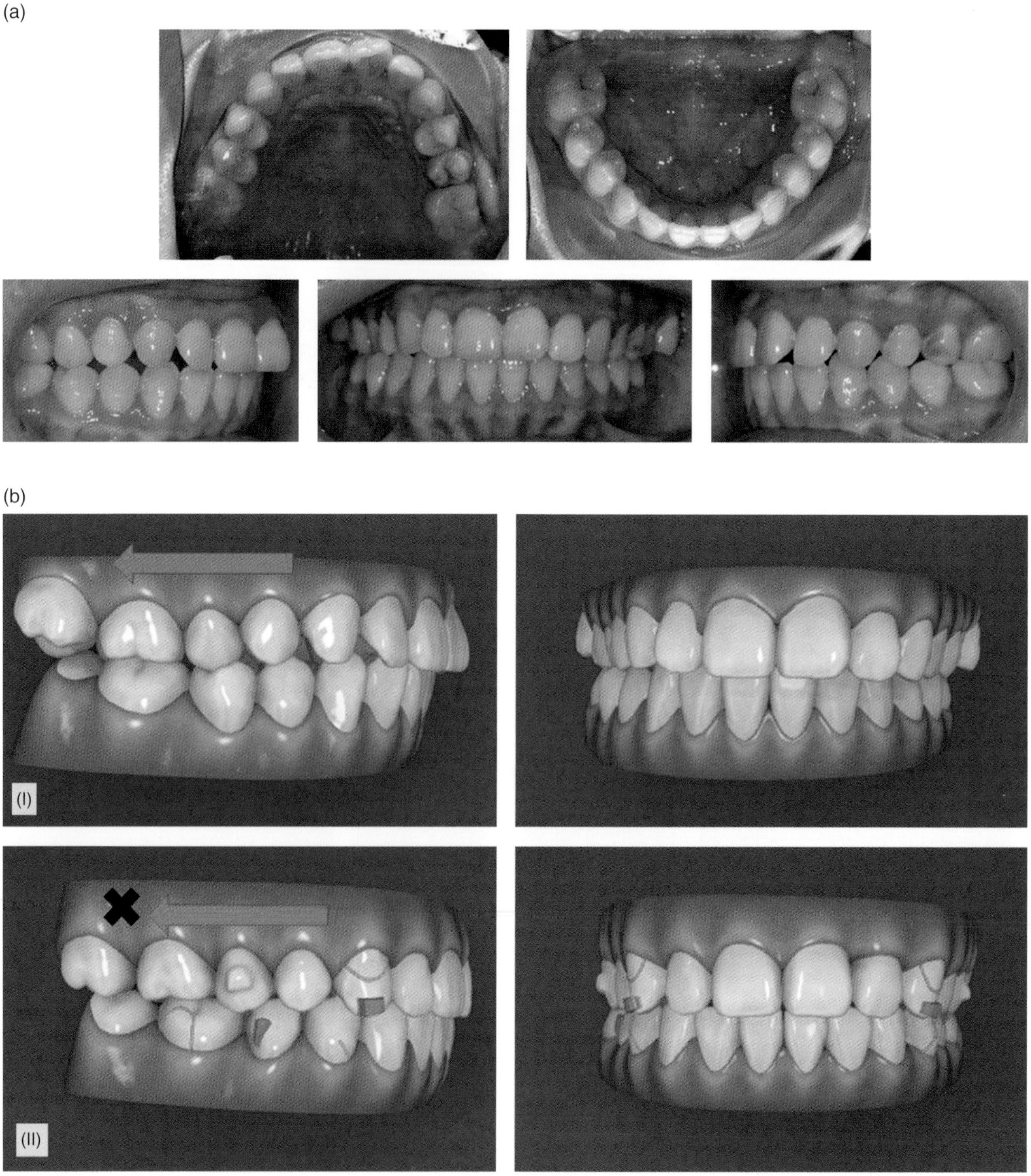

(a)

(b)

Figure 12.5.13 (a) Pre-treatment images of an adult showing an asymmetrical Class II dental malocclusion with an increased overjet and non-coincident dental midlines. (b) ClinCheck plans showing (I) pre-treatment and (II) simulated final position of the dentition with attachment designs and precision cuts for elastic wear to the TAD. "X" marks the position of the TAD placement. (c) Progressive images (I) initial, (II) quadrant distalization and overjet retraction with TAD and elastic, (III) completion with slight canine overcorrection.

(c)

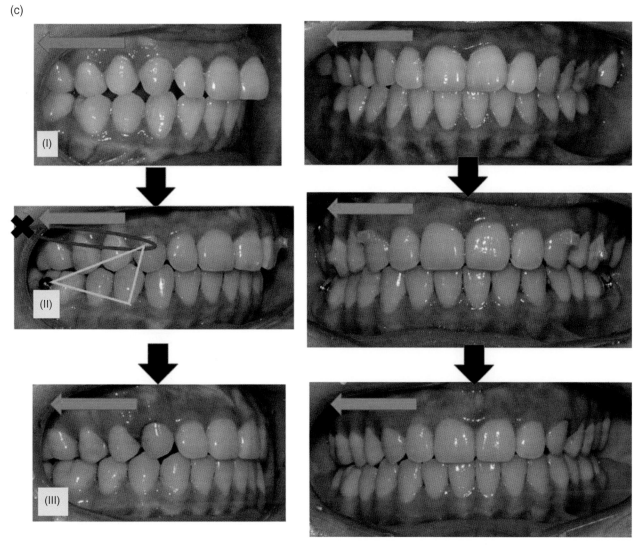

Figure 12.5.13 (Continued)

Asymmetrical Class III Correction

Surgeons involved with orthognathic surgical procedures are used to operating on patients with fixed appliances and may not be familiar performing the surgery with clear aligners alone. Under such circumstances, the pre-surgical decompensation orthodontics can still be done with clear aligners; further additional aligners may be ordered to complete the pre-surgical orthodontics if necessary. Fixed appliances may be placed two to 3 months prior to the surgery to stabilize the arches. After the initial months of recovery from the surgery, the fixed appliances may be removed and additional aligners ordered to complete the case.

An adult female patient presented with a prognathic mandible. She was concerned with her facial imbalance and reverse bite, and would like to seek orthodontic treatment incorporating orthognathic surgery. There was a deficient midface, an asymmetric prognathic mandible with the chin point deviated to the right side. There was mild upper and lower dental crowding with the lower dental midline deviated to the right (Figure 12.5.15a, b). Decompensation pre-surgical orthodontics was performed with clear aligners for approximately 8 months (Figure 12.5.15c). Full fixed appliance was placed approximately 3 months before surgery and once the arches were stabilized with full dimensional stainless steel rectangular archwires, she was ready for surgery. The orthognathic surgical movements performed were maxillary posterior impaction, maxillary advancement, and asymmetrical mandibular bilateral sagittal split osteotomy (BSSO) setback. After the patient regained full jaw movements (approximately 2–3 months after surgery), the fixed appliances were removed,

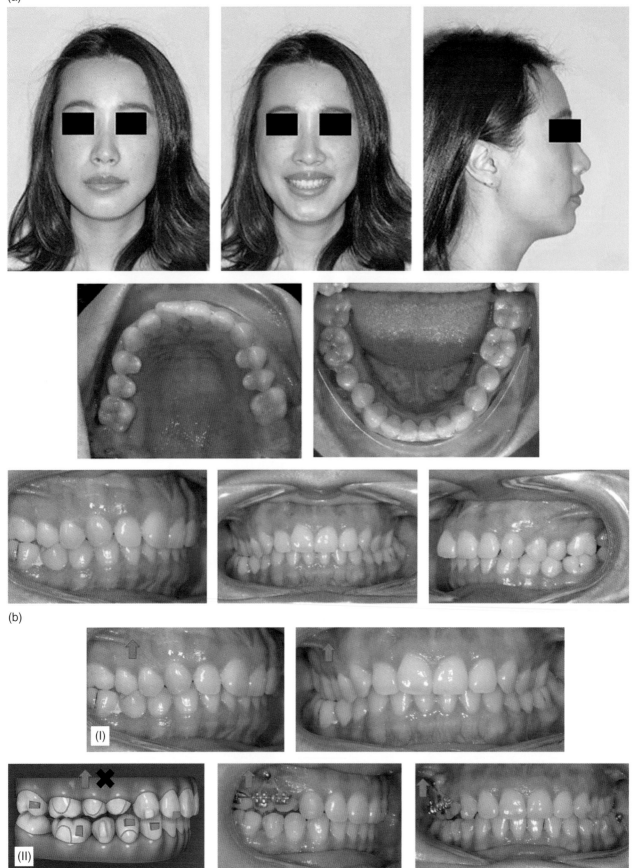

Figure 12.5.14 (a) Pre-treatment images of an adult showing a Class II dental malocclusion with an upper occlusal plane cant. (b) Progressive treatment images showing (I) initial, (II) ClinCheck setup and correction of upper occlusal plane canting with the intrusion of the upper right quadrant with partial fixed appliances and a TAD. "X" marks the position of the TAD placement. (c) Progressive treatment images showing (III) triangular elastics worn to buttons on the lower right dentition to extrude that quadrant to match the upper right intrusion, (IV) ClinCheck setup and clinical comparison to show elastics to settle the occlusion. (d) Comparison of (I) pre-treatment and (II) correction of upper occlusal plane cant.

(c)

(d)

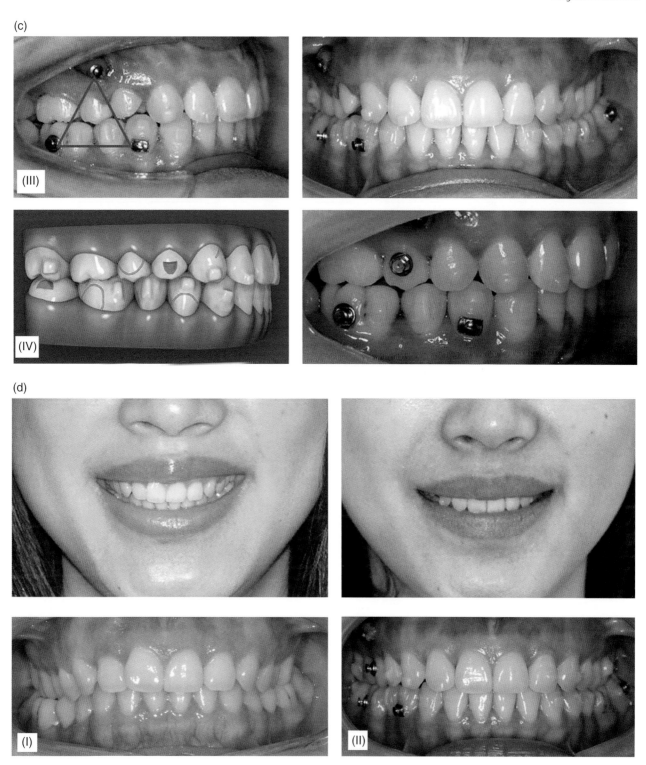

Figure 12.5.14 (Continued)

(a)

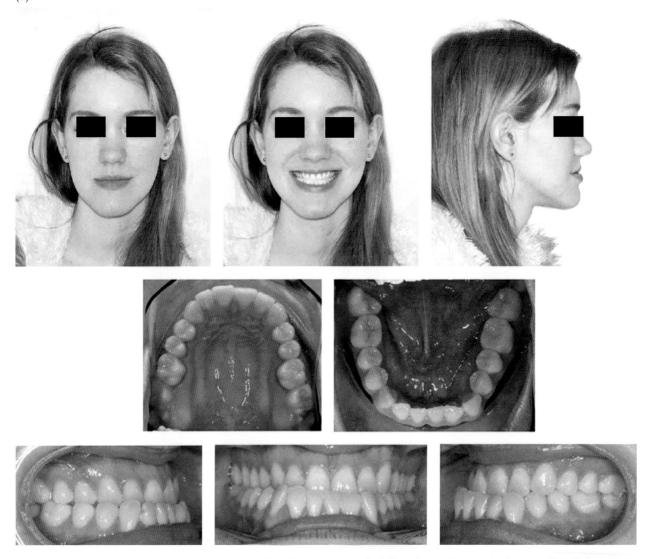

Figure 12.5.15 (a) Pre-treatment images of an adult showing an asymmetrical Class III dental malocclusion on a Class 3 skeletal base. There was a reverse overjet, non-coincident dental midlines with the chin point deviated to the right. (b) Pre-treatment OPG and lateral cephalometric radiograph. (c) ClinCheck plans showing (I) pre-treatment and (II) simulated final position of the dentition with attachment designs. The wisdom teeth were removed during the orthognathic surgery. (d) Progressive treatment images showing post-surgery recovery with fixed appliances just removed and additional aligners ordered. (e) Post-treatment images showing a balanced occlusion and harmonious facial balance with the correction of the anterior crossbites, achieving a Class I canine and molar relationship. (f) Post-treatment OPG and lateral cephalometric radiograph. (g) Superimposition of lateral cephalometric tracings showing skeletal and dental changes with treatment. (h) Comparison of (I) pre-treatment and (II) post-treatment images demonstrating the correction of asymmetry through orthognathic surgery.

and new scans were done for additional aligners to detail and complete the case (Figure 12.5.15d). The completed images showed a balanced and harmonious facial change. The deficient midface, prognathic mandible, and the deviated chin point were normalized (Figure 12.5.15e–h).

Asymmetrical Class II Correction

There are advantages for patients undergoing orthognathic surgery without the need to have fixed appliances placed. The digital planning could be seamless, with no transition and re-adaptation to a different appliance. Without the

(b)

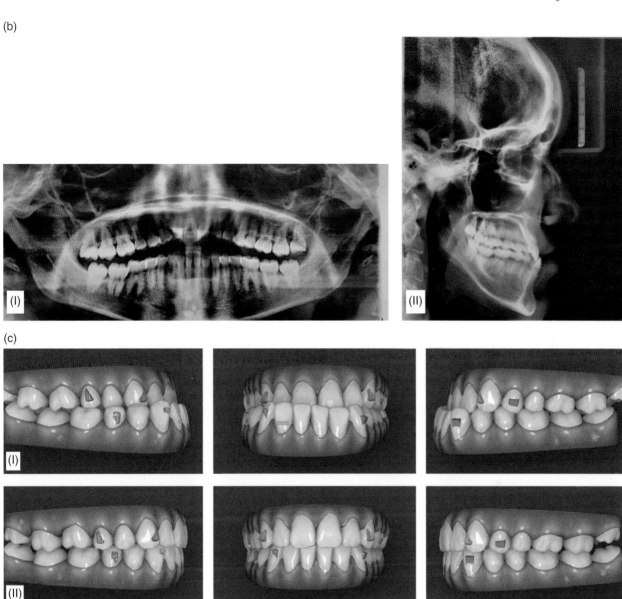

(c)

Figure 12.5.15 (Continued)

presence of fixed appliances and surgical wire fixations, oral hygiene could be much better managed. This promotes patient comfort and optimises wound healing.

An adult male patient presented with a deep dental overbite and a recessive chin (Figure 12.5.16a, b). He was concerned with his retrognathic mandible and would like to seek orthodontic treatment incorporating orthognathic surgery. There was a deep dental overbite, retroclined upper incisors, and rather constricted archforms with mild to moderate upper and lower dental crowding. The lower dental midline was deviated to the right. Decompensation pre-surgical orthodontics was performed with clear aligners for approximately 14 months (Figure 12.5.16c). Once the arches were ready for surgery, buttons were bonded on the upper and lower, left and right canines and first molars with corresponding "button cutouts" placed in the aligners (Figure 12.5.16d). The orthognathic surgical movements

(d)

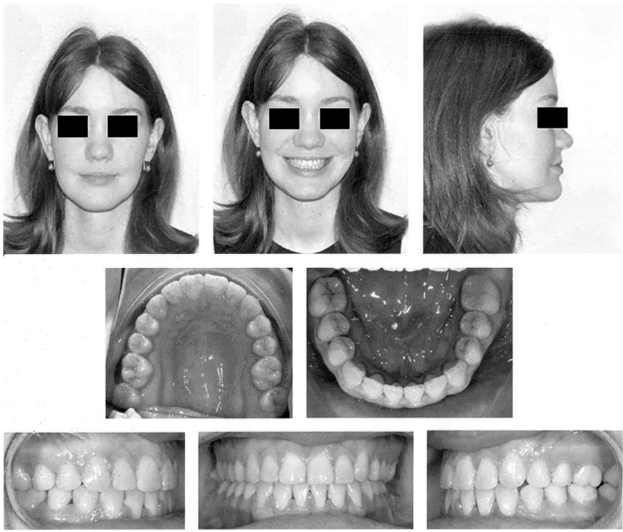

Figure 12.5.15 (Continued)

performed were maxillary posterior impaction, asymmetrical mandibular BSSO advancement, and an advancement genioplasty. Without the need to have fixed appliances placed during the orthognathic surgical procedure, oral hygiene was immaculately maintained (Figure 12.5.16e). Once the patient had regained full jaw movements, new additional aligners were ordered to detail and complete the treatment. The completed images showed a balanced and harmonious facial change. The deep dental overbite, dental crowding, deviated midlines, recessive mandible, and chin were normalized (Figure 12.5.16f–j).

(e)

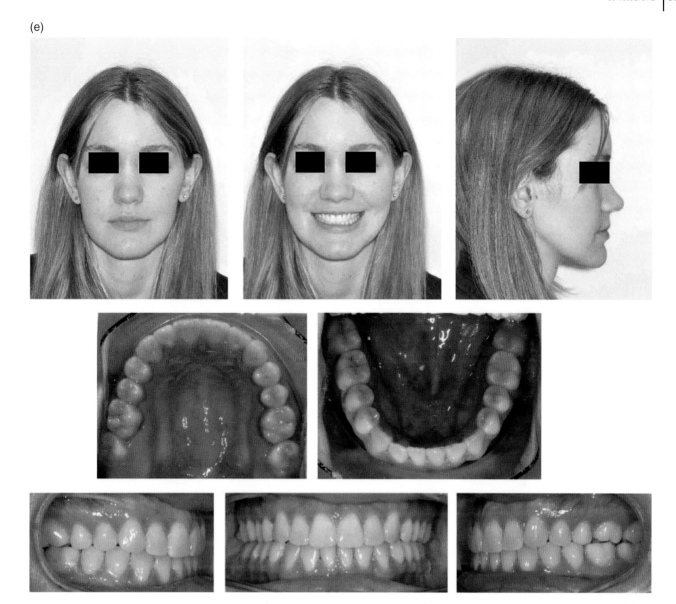

Figure 12.5.15 (Continued)

Conclusions

Using clear aligners to treat complex comprehensive orthodontic cases is still relatively new. Shifting the mindset and applying knowledge and biomechanics learned from fixed appliances to clear aligners requires time. This brief chapter introduces what clear aligners can do with dental and skeletal asymmetrical cases under different contexts and conditions. Incorporating the clinician's knowledge, embracing digital technology in orthodontics and with co-operative subjects, treatment with clear aligners in complex comprehensive cases can eventuate with excellent results.

(f)

(g)

(h)

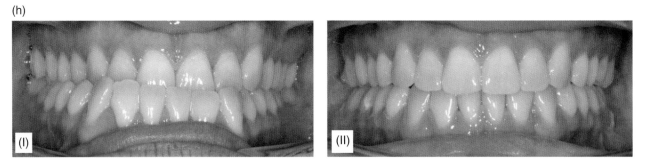

Figure 12.5.15 (Continued)

(a)

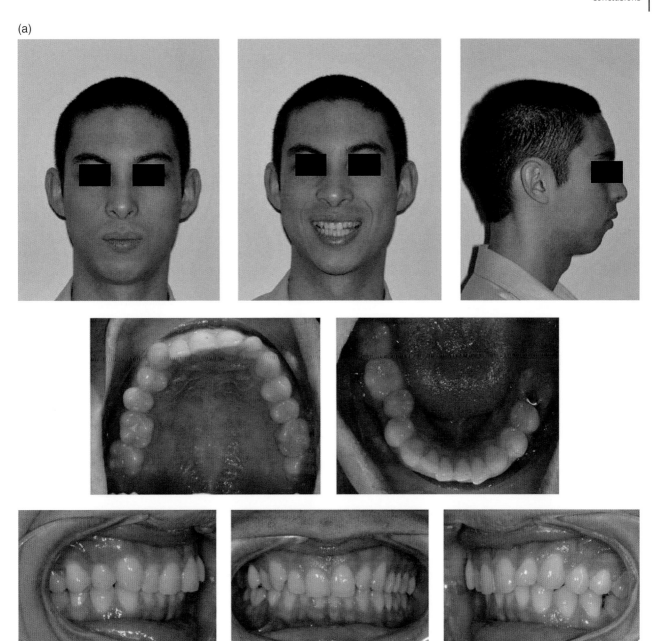

Figure 12.5.16 (a) Pre-treatment images of an adult showing an asymmetrical Class II division 2 dental malocclusion on a Class 2 skeletal base. There was an increased dental overbite and non-coincident dental midlines. (b) Pre-treatment OPG and lateral cephalometric radiograph. (c) ClinCheck plans showing (I) pre-treatment and (II) simulated final position of the dentition with attachment designs. Eight buttons were placed with "button cutouts" on the aligners just prior to orthognathic surgery. (d) Progressive treatment images showing occlusion prior surgery comparing (I) ClinCheck designs and (II) clinically with aligners and buttons in place. (e) Progressive treatment images showing 3 weeks post-surgical recovery with excellent oral hygiene. (f) Post-treatment images showing a balanced occlusion and harmonious facial balance with the correction of the deep dental overbite and dental midlines. (g) Post-treatment OPG and lateral cephalometric radiograph. (h) Superimposition of lateral cephalometric tracings showing skeletal and dental changes with treatment. (i) Comparison of (I) pre-treatment and (II) post-treatment images demonstrating facial profile changes with orthognathic surgery. (j) Comparison of (I) pre-treatment and (II) post-treatment images demonstrating the correction of asymmetry and dental overbite achieved with clear aligners and orthognathic surgery.

(b)

(c)

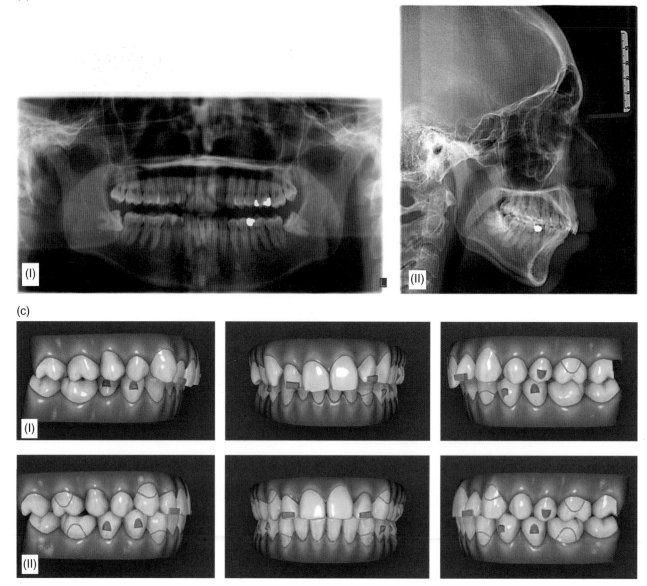

Figure 12.5.16 (Continued)

(d)

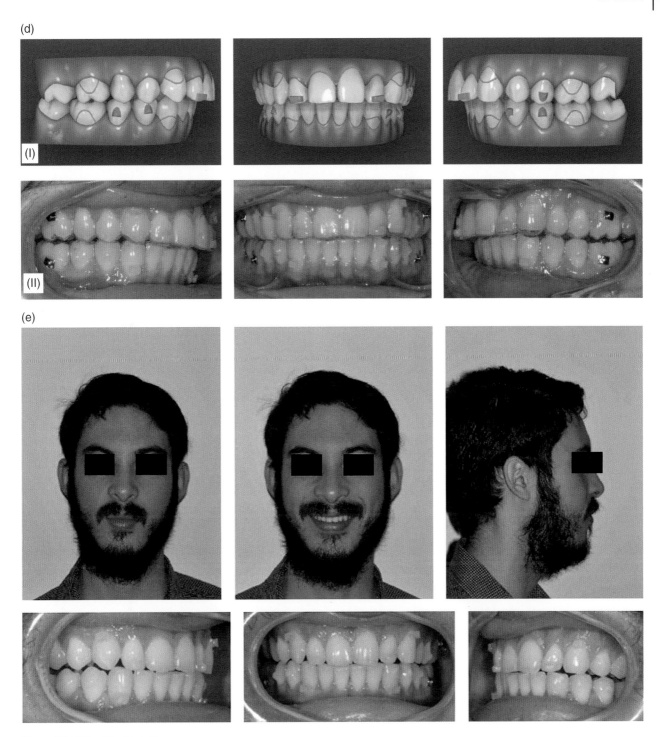

(e)

Figure 12.5.16 (Continued)

(f)

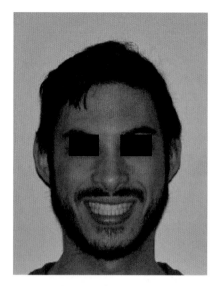
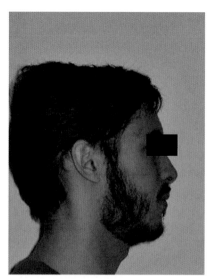

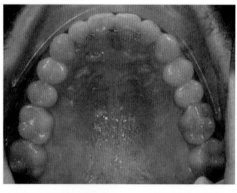
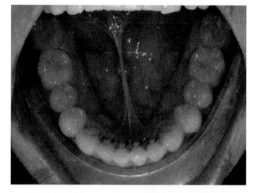

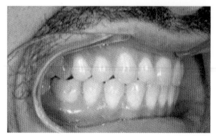
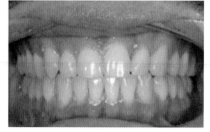
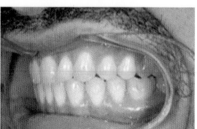

Figure 12.5.16 (Continued)

(g)

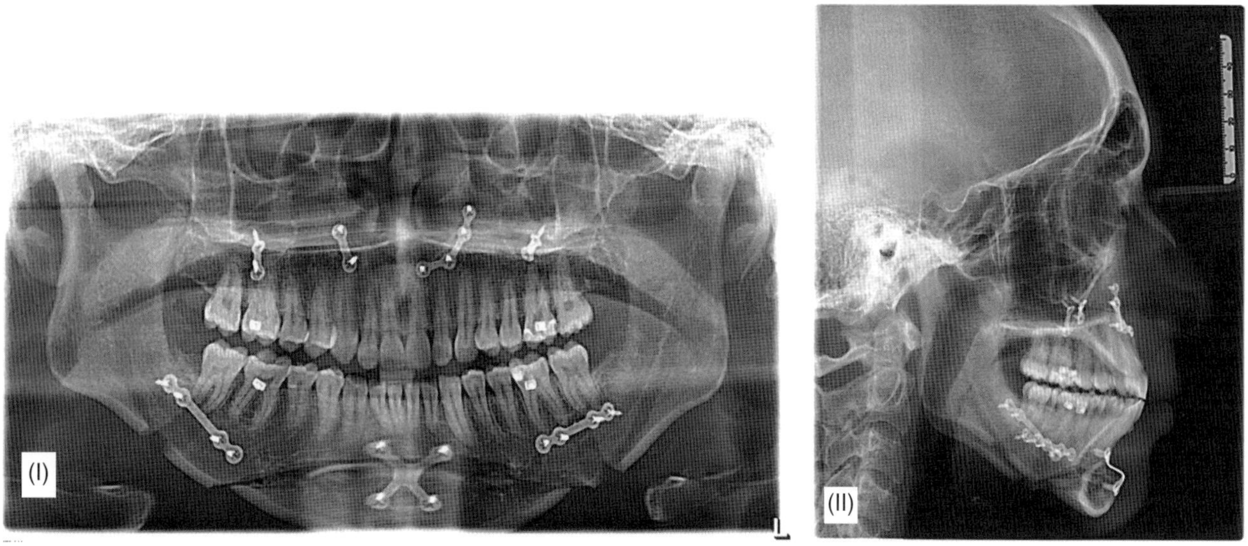

(h)

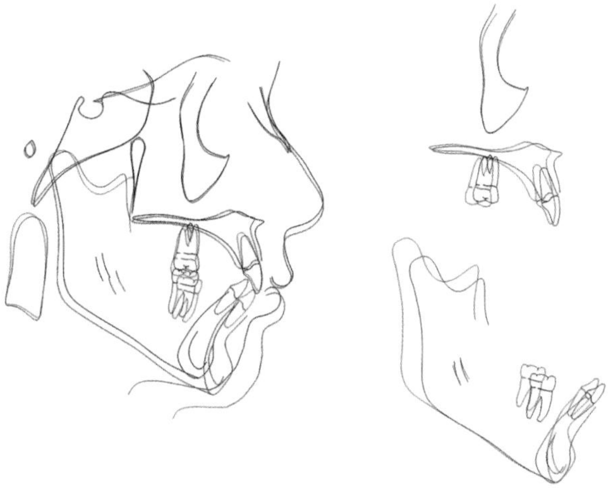

(i)

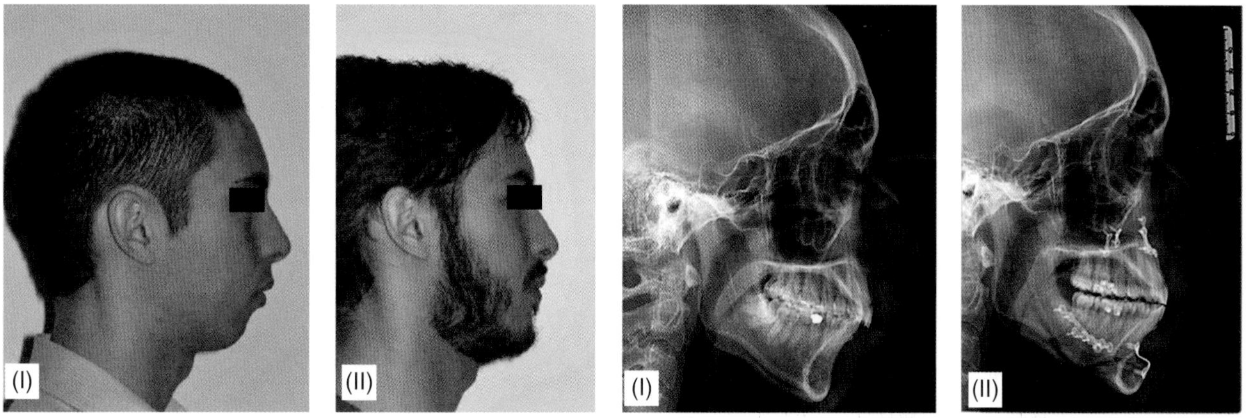

Figure 12.5.16 (Continued)

(j)

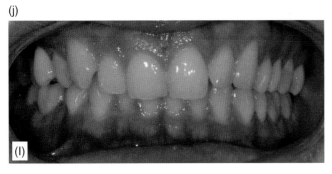

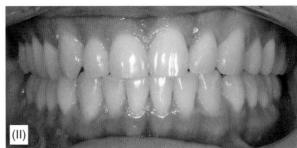

Figure 12.5.16 (Continued)

References

Cahen PM, Frank RM, Turlot JC. A survey of the reasons for dental extractions in France. J Dent Res. 1985;64:1087–1093.

Chan E, Darendeliler MA. The Invisalign appliance today: a thinking person's orthodontic appliance. Semin Orthod. 2017;23:12–64.

Chan E, Darendeliler MA. Routine mechanics and aligners (extraction/non-extraction). In: Eliades T, Athanasiou AE, eds. Orthodontic Aligner Treatment, A Review of Materials, Clinical Management, and Evidence. New York: Thieme, 2021:69–94.

Chugh T, Jain AK, Jaiswal RK, Mehrotra P, Mehrotra R. Bone density and its importance in orthodontics. J Oral Biol Craniofac Res. 2013;3:92–97.

Corruccini RS, Sharma K, Potter RHY. Comparative genetic variance and heritability of dental occlusal variables in U.S. and north-west Indian twins. Am J Phys Anthropol. 1986;70:293–299.

Dawson PE. New definition for relating occlusion to varying conditions of the temporomandibular joint. J Prosthet Dent. 1995;74:619–627.

Dietschi D, Schartz JP. Current restorative modalities for young patients with missing anterior teeth. Pediatr Dent. 1997;28:231–240.

Fekonja A. Prevalence of dental developmental anomalies of permanent teeth in children and their influence on aesthetics. J Esthet Restor Dent. 2017;29:276–283.

Galton F. Composite portraits, made by combining those of many different persons in a single resultant figure. J Anthropol Inst Great Br Ireland. 1879;8:132–144.

Gorlin RJ, Cohen MM, Hennekam RCM, Cohen MM Jr. Syndromes of the Head and Neck. London: Oxford University Press, 2001.

Grammer K, Thornhill R. Human facial attractiveness and sexual selection: the role of symmetry and averageness. J Comp Psychol. 1994;108:233–242.

Gündüz E, Rodríguez-Torres C, Gahleitner A, Heissenberger G, Bantleon HP. Bone regeneration by bodily tooth movement: dental computed tomography examination of a patient. Am J Orthod Dentofac Orthop. 2004;125:100–106.

Morita M, Kimura T, Kanegae M, Ishikawa A, Watanabe T. Reasons for extraction of permanent teeth in Japan. Comm Dent Oral Epidem. 1994;22:303–306.

Moss JP. The soft tissue environment of teeth and jaws: an experimental and clinical study. Br J Orthod. 1980;7:107–137.

Nangia A, Darendeliler MA. Finishing occlusion in Class II or Class III molar relation: therapeutic Class II and III. Aust Orthod J. 2001;17:89–94.

Oesterle LJ, Cronin RJ Jr, Ranly D. Maxillary implants and the growing patient. Int J Oral Maxillofac Implants. 1993;8:377–387.

Pirttiniemi P, Kantomaa T, Lahtela P. Relationship between craniofacial and condyle path asymmetry in unilateral cross-bite patients. Eur J Orthod. 1990;12:408–413.

Proffit WR, Vig KWL, Dann C IV. Who seeks surgical-orthodontic treatment? The characteristics of patients evaluated in the UNC Dentofacial Clinic. Int J Adult Orthodon Orthognath Surg. 1990;5:153–160.

Pullinger AG, Seligman DA, Gornbein JA. A multiple regression analysis of the risk and relative odds of temporomandibular disorders as a function of common occlusal features. J Dent Res. 1993;72:968–979.

Rhodes G, Roberts J, Simmons L. Reflections on symmetry and attractiveness. Psychol Evol Gender. 1999;1:279–295.

Richards W, Ameen J, Coll A. Reasons for tooth extraction in four general dental practices in South Wales. Br Dent J. 2005;198:275–278.

Roberts WE. Bone physiology, metabolism, and biomechanics in orthodontic practice. In: Graber TM, Vanarsdall RL, Vig KWL, eds. Orthodontics: Current Principles and Techniques. St. Louis: Mosby, 2005:221–292.

Sonnesen L, Bakke M, Solow B. Malocclusion traits and symptoms and signs of temporomandibular disorders in children with severe malocclusion. Eur J Orthod. 1998;20:543–559.

Thilander B. Temporomandibular joint dysfunction in children. In: Graber LW, ed. Orthodontics, State of the Art, Essence of the Science. St. Louis: The C V Mosby Co., 1986:342–351.

12.6

TMJ Conditions Causing Facial Asymmetry: Diagnosis and Treatment

Larry M. Wolford

CHAPTER MENU

Introduction

All individuals express facial asymmetry (FA) of varying degrees; some are unperceivable while others have severe deformities. Etiology can include: genetics, birth molding, congenital and developmental deformities, abnormal growth, tumors or other pathology of facial structures, trauma, neurological or neuromuscular disorders, vascular anomalies, iatrogenic injury, temporomandibular joint (TMJ) pathology, etc. TMJ conditions causing FA can affect the dentoalveolar, skeletal, and soft tissues structures (Gorlin et al. 2001; Wolford 2008, 2012; Wolford and Goncalves 2017). Patient surgical workup includes history, clinical evaluation, dental model analysis, imaging, etc. The author has previously published the comprehensive patient analysis and treatment planning with specifics for FA (Wolford 2008, 2012; Wolford and Goncalves 2017), so this information will not be reiterated here.

In the presence of TMJ pathology, FA correction with only orthognathic surgery may result in the asymmetry and malocclusion redeveloping post-surgery, with worsening TMJ-associated symptoms including pain and jaw dysfunction (Fuselier et al. 1998; Wolford et al. 2003b; Goncalves et al. 2008; Al-Moraissi and Wolford, 2016, 2017; Al-Moraissi et al. 2017; Bianchi et al. 2018; Gomes et al. 2018). In FA, the TMJs should always be evaluated to determine if the joints are: The etiological factor; developed because of FA; coexisting condition; or normal and healthy. This chapter will focus on the common TMJ conditions that cause FA, divided into two basic categories: (i) Unilateral overdevelopment and (ii) Unilateral underdevelopment.

Overdevelopment

Enlargement or overgrowth of the mandibular condyle is defined as condylar hyperplasia (CH) of which there are several etiologies. Wolford et al. (2014c) developed a simple classification based on the specific pathology. CH Type 1 is an accelerated and often prolonged over-growth of the "normal" growth center of the condyle. CH Type 1A occurs bilaterally and CH Type 1B unilaterally. CH Type 2 is the most common benign unilateral condylar tumor (osteochondroma). CH Type 3 are other benign pathologies and CH Type 4 are malignant tumors.

Condylar Hyperplasia Type 1

CH Type 1 creates mandibular prognathism (Figures 12.6.1a–c, 12.6.2a–c, 12.6.3a) usually beginning during pubertal growth causing the mandible to grow at an accelerated rate, occurring more frequently in females (2:1 ratio). Growth is self-limiting but can continue into the early to mid-20s before cessation (Obwegeser and Makek 1986; Wolford and LeBanc 1986; Wolford 2002; Wolford et al. 2002c, 2009, 2014c). Patients begin with a Class I skeletal and occlusal relationship and develop into a Class III relation, or start as Class III, but develop a worse Class III relationship as the mandible grows predominantly in a horizontal direction, although sometimes there can be a vertical growth vector (Obwegeser and

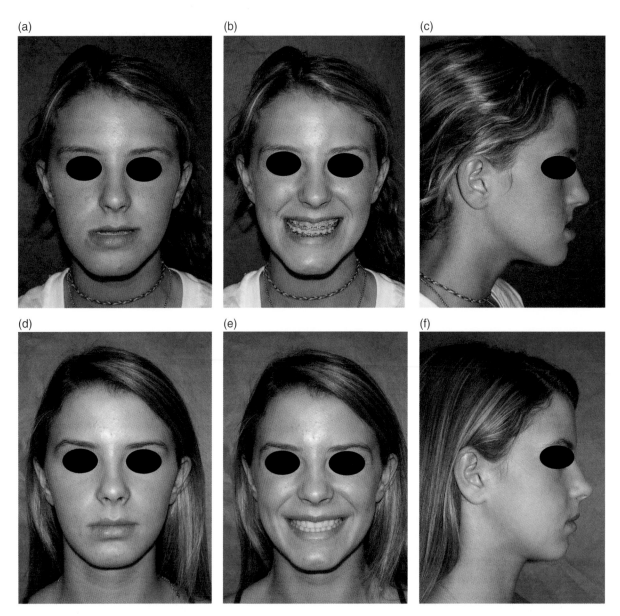

Figure 12.6.1 Case 1. (a–c) A 14-year-old female presents with condylar hyperplasia type 1A with the left side growing faster than the right side creating a progressive deviated mandibular prognathism shifted to the right side; (d–f) two-years post-surgery the patient demonstrates good facial balance and stability with elimination of the condylar hyperplasia growth pathology by the bilateral high condylectomies and double jaw orthognathic surgery performed in one operation.

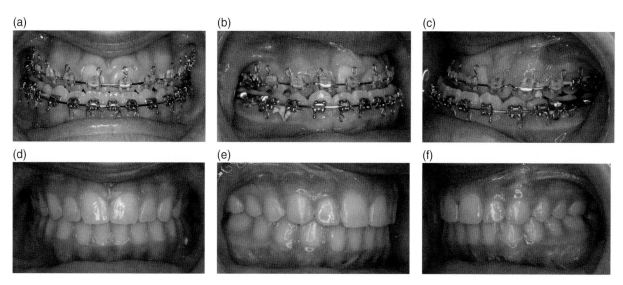

Figure 12.6.2 Case 1. (a–c) Presurgery occlusion views showing mandibular dental midline shifted to the right, right-sided posterior crossbite as well as Class III occlusion greater on the left than the right side; (d–f) two-years post-surgery shows the significant improvement and stability of the occlusal outcome.

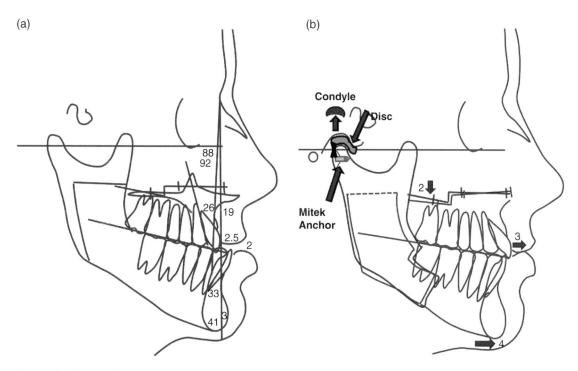

Figure 12.6.3 Case 1. (a) Cephalometric analysis shows a Class III skeletal and occlusal relationship, mandibular prognathism, and elongated mandibular condylar heads and necks consistent with condylar hyperplasia type 1A; (b) the prediction tracing plan included bilateral mandibular high condylectomies with disc repositioning using Mitek anchors, bilateral mandibular ramus sagittal split osteotomies, and multiple maxillary osteotomies performed in a single stage.

Makek 1986; Wolford et al. 2009, 2014c). Asymmetry of the mandible can occur by CH Type 1B (Obewegeser's hemi-mandibular elongation) (Obwegeser and Makek 1986) or CH Type 1A where one condyle grows at a faster rate than the opposite side. The mandible, dental midline, and chin

become deviated toward the contralateral side; there is a Class III occlusion on the ipsilateral side and a crossbite on the contralateral side. Pubertal onset of CH Type 1 strongly suggests a hormonal etiology. However, trauma, infection, heredity, intrauterine factors, and hypervascularity have also been implicated as causative factors (Wolford et al. 2009, 2014c). Approximately 1/3 of CH Type 1 cases have a familial history (Gottlieb 1951).

Cone-beam computed tomography (CBCT) and computed tomography (CT) scans usually show a relatively normal condylar architecture, although an increased length of the condylar head, neck, and mandibular body (Figure 12.6.3a). In the coronal view, the top of the ipsilateral condyle may have a more global morphology (Wolford et al. 2009, 2014c). The normal pubertal growth rate measuring from condylion to point B in females is a mean of 1.6 mm per year with 98% of growth complete by the age of 15 years. Males grow at a mean rate of 2.2 mm per year with 98% of growth complete by the age of 17–18 years (Riolo et al. 1974). An increased rate and prolonged growth may indicate active CH Type 1. Bone scans may not be of value in diagnosing CH Type 1 because the growth center (proliferative layer) is very narrow where the cellular activity is located (Chan and Leung 2018; Xiao et al. 2022) with minimal differentiation in the amount of isotope uptake compared to a normal joint. Serial radiographs (lateral cephalograms, cephalometric TMJ tomograms, etc.), dental models, and clinical evaluations are usually the best methods to determine if the growth process is active. Magnetic resonance imaging (MRIs) may show thin discs that may be difficult to identify. On the ipsilateral side, the disc can become posteriorly displaced. About 62% of these patients will show a displaced disc on the contralateral side from increased joint loading created by the ipsilateral CH (Wolford et al. 2009, 2014c).

Histologically, CH Type 1 condyles appear similar to normal condylar architecture, but in some cases, the proliferative layer may demonstrate greater thickness with cartilage-producing cells prevalent at the lower level. In normal condyles, the cartilage formation from the proliferative layer and the replacement of cartilage by bone ceases by approximately age 20, where the marrow cavity is occluded from the remaining cartilage by the closure of the bone plate. The inability of this plate to close in the presence of an active proliferative cartilage layer may be a major etiological factor for prolonged growth in CH Type 1 (Wolford 2002; Wolford et al. 2002c, 2009, 2014c).

Treatment of this deformity depends on whether the condylar growth is active or quiescent. If jaw growth has stopped, orthognathic surgery can correct the asymmetry. TMJ surgery would only be indicated if disc displacement is present. If active growth is confirmed, then there are two predictable treatment options. The most predictable option is to perform a high condylectomy removing 4–5 mm of the top of the condylar head on the involved side(s), reposition the articular discover the remaining condyle

using the Mitek anchor (Mitek Products, Westwood, MA, USA) technique (Wolford et al. 1995, 2002c; Mehra and Wolford 2001) and perform orthognathic surgery to correct the associated dentofacial deformity (Figure 12.6.3b) (Wolford and LeBanc 1986; Wolford 2002; Wolford et al. 2002c, 2009, 2014c). This will stop mandibular growth with stable long-term functional and esthetic outcomes (Figures 12.6.1d–f and 12.6.2d–f) (Wolford and LeBanc 1986; Wolford 2002; Wolford et al. 2002c, 2009, 2014c). The recommended age for unilateral CH surgery is 15 years for females and 17 years for males. Performing a unilateral high condylectomy earlier during normal growth will result in arresting the growth on the CH side, but the normal side can continue to grow until normal cessation, with the potential of causing asymmetry by the mandible shifting toward the original CH side (Wolford et al., 2001a, 2001b; Wolford and Rodrigues, 2012a, 2012b; Mehra and Wolford 2016).

The second option is to delay surgery until growth is complete. However, since these cases often continue to grow into the early to mid-20s, the surgery would be delayed until it is confirmed that the growth has stopped. The longer the asymmetric growth proceeds, the worse the facial deformity, asymmetry, and dental compensations affecting both the hard and soft tissues. This may increase the difficulties in obtaining an optimal functional and esthetic result, as well as adversely affect the patient's psychosocial development.

Wolford et al. (2009) presented a study of 54 CH Type 1 patients with confirmed active growth divided into two groups. Group 1 (12 patients) only had orthognathic surgery without high condylectomy, and all grew into Class III skeletal and occlusal relationships. Group 2 (42 patients) treated with high condylectomies and orthognathic surgery maintained stable Class I skeletal and occlusal relationships, confirming the efficacy of this treatment protocol.

Condylar Hyperplasia Type 2

CH Type 2 is a unilateral mandibular benign condylar tumor (osteochondroma, also referred to as hemimandibular hyperplasia) (Obwegeser and Makek 1986; Wolford et al. 2002a, 2014b, 2014c) initiated at any age, although 67% of cases start between ages 10 and 20 years (Wolford et al. 2014b), creating unilateral vertical enlargement of the condyle and mandible, creating facial asymmetry (Wolford et al. 2002a, 2014b, 2014c). Common characteristics of CH type 2 include: (i) enlarged, elongated, deformed ipsilateral condyle (CH type 2A; Figures 12.6.4a–c, 12.6.5a–c, 12.6.6a), often with exophytic extensions of the tumor of the condyle (CH type 2B; (ii) increased

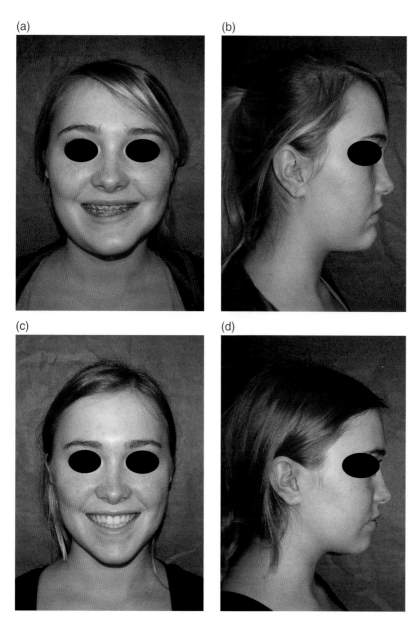

Figure 12.6.4 Case 2. (a, b) An 18-year-old female with significant vertical elongation of the right side of her face and jaws related to right condylar hyperplasia type 2A. Facial asymmetry is noted with the chin shifted to the left and a transverse cant in the occlusal plane with the right side lower than the left. In profile, the patient does have fairly good A–P facial balance but the right side is significantly elongated vertically; (c, d) the patient is seen 2-years post-surgery showing improvement in facial symmetry and maintenance of a good profile.

thickness of the ipsilateral condylar neck; (iii) progressive increasing vertical height of the ipsilateral mandibular condyle, neck, ramus, body, symphysis, and dentoalveolus; (iv) an increased vertical height of the ipsilateral maxillary dentoalveolus; (v) transverse cant in the occlusal plane; (vi) coronoid process will be a normal size and displaced below the zygomatic arch; (vii) loss of ipsilateral antigonial notching with downward bowing of the inferior border of the mandible; (viii) the inferior alveolar nerve canal commonly positioned toward the inferior border of the mandible; and (ix) the chin vertically longer on the ipsilateral side and prominent in profile. Bone scintigraphy may show increased uptake, particularly, in the more active tumors. MRI will show the enlarged ipsilateral condyle (Figure 12.6.7a). Usually, the articular disc will be in position. The contralateral TMJ will commonly have an anteriorly displaced disc (76% of cases) and associated arthritic condylar changes created by the

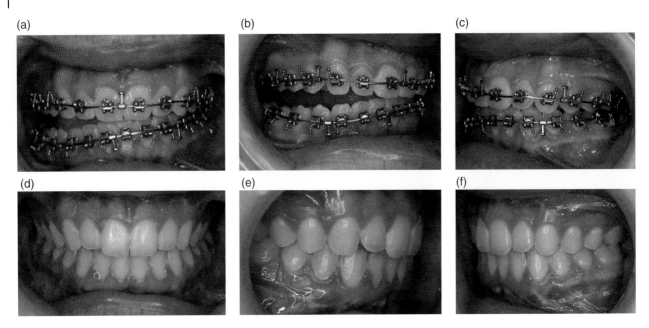

Figure 12.6.5 Case 2. (a–c) Presurgery occlusion shows mandibular dental midline shifted to the right 3 mm with a large posterior open bite on the right side related to the excessive vertical down growth of the right mandibular condylar tumor (osteochondroma); (d–f) the patient is seen 2-years post-surgery follow-up with a very stable occlusal outcome.

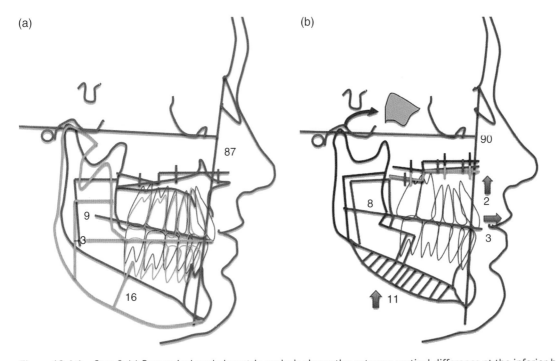

Figure 12.6.6 Case 2. (a) Presurgical cephalometric analysis shows the extreme vertical difference at the inferior border of the mandible with the right side 16 mm longer vertically than the left side. There is a significant transverse cant in the occlusal plane. The anteroposterior facial balance is reasonably good; (b) prediction tracing shows the treatment including a right TMJ low condylectomy and repositioning of the articular discs in both joints with Mitek anchors, bilateral mandibular ramus sagittal split osteotomies, maxillary osteotomies, and an additional 11 mm of bone removed from the inferior border of the right mandible with preservation of the inferior alveolar nerve.

(a)

(b)

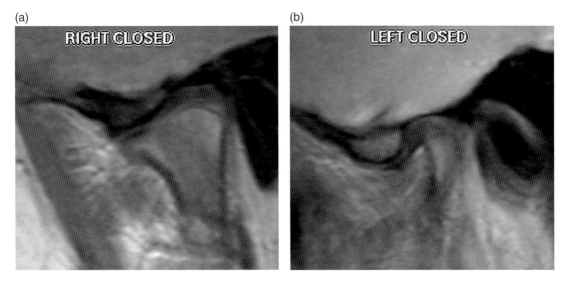

Figure 12.6.7   Case 2. (a) MRI shows the vertical and anteroposterior enlargement of the right mandibular condyle. The articular disc is in position. During surgery, the right condyle was treated with a low condylectomy and the disc repositioned with Mitek anchors; (b) left TMJ MRI shows that the disc is anteriorly displaced as commonly seen in about 62% of these cases. During surgery, the left TMJ was treated with the disc repositioned with Mitek anchor.

functional overload (Figure 12.6.7b). In CH type 2A, the articular disc can become posteriorly displaced on the ipsilateral side (Wolford et al. 2002a, 2014b, 2014c).

Histologically, CH type 2 will include a cartilaginous cap similar to that seen in normal growth cartilage, endochondral ossification, and cartilaginous islands in the subcortical bone. The cartilage islands are mini-growth centers producing bone, causing enlargement of the condyle. As more bone is produced from these islands, additional separation occurs between them, making it more difficult to identify these islands histologically in larger and older tumors (Wolford et al. 2002a, 2014b, 2014c).

The highly predictable treatment protocol for CH Type 2 includes: Ipsilateral low condylectomy recontour the condylar neck (neo-condyle), reposition the disc over the neo-condyle, and reposition the articular disc on the contra-lateral side, if displaced, with the Mitek anchor technique; orthognathic surgery to correct the maxillary and mandibular asymmetries; and an inferior border ostectomy on the ipsilateral side if indicated, with preservation of the inferior alveolar nerve, to reestablish vertical balance of the mandible (Figure 12.6.6b) (Wolford et al. 2002a, 2014b, 2014c). This treatment approach will allow removal of the tumor yet still use the enlarged condylar neck as the new condyle thus providing predictable and stable outcomes (Figures 12.6.4c, d and 12.6.5d–f). Other treatment considerations include condylar replacement with autogenous tissue grafts (not recommended by the author because of complications), or preferably, total joint

prostheses, particularly if the articular disc(s) are non-salvageable (Wolford et al. 2002a, 2014a).

Wolford et al. (2014b) evaluated 37 CH Type 2 patients. The study showed that 74% of the patients were females, 68% had onset between ages 10 and 20 years, left and right sides equally involved, and 76% had displaced discs on the contralateral side. The treatment protocol of single-stage surgery for low condylectomy, disc repositioning with Mitek anchor, double jaw orthognathic surgery, and ipsilateral inferior border ostectomy when indicated, resulted in stable skeletal and occlusal outcomes, as well as significant improvement in TMJ pain, headaches, myofascial pain, jaw function, diet, and disability.

Unilateral Facial Under-development

The most common causes of unilateral facial under-development include:

1) Adolescent internal condylar resorption (AICR).
2) TMJ reactive (inflammatory) arthritis.
3) Acquired: i.e. trauma; infection; ankylosis; Iatrogenic (e.g. tumor resection, radiation, unstable orthognathic procedure, adverse surgical event, etc.); failed TMJ alloplastic implants; failed autogenous tissue grafts, etc.
4) Congenital deformities, i.e. hemifacial microsomia (HFM).
5) Connective tissue/autoimmune diseases.

The commonly used term, idiopathic condylar resorption (ICR), is a catch-all phrase to describe several conditions that cause condylar resorption, but does not identify the specific pathology. The three most common causes of "idiopathic condylar resorption" include: AICR, reactive arthritis, and connective tissue/autoimmune diseases.

Surgical considerations for TMJ pathologies involving condylar resorption are dependent on the specific TMJ pathology. For example, patients with TMJ articular disc dislocation, with no previous TMJ surgeries and without significant other joint or systemic disease involvement, and treated within 4 years of onset of the disc displacement, may benefit from articular disc repositioning and ligament repair with Mitek anchors to achieve a stable treatment outcome (Wolford et al. 1995, 2002b; Mehra and Wolford 2001). Patients who do not meet this criteria, or with 2 or more previous TMJ surgeries, or end-stage TMJ conditions such as severe arthritis, ankyloses, TMJ damage from trauma, connective tissue/autoimmune diseases, failed TMJ alloplastic implants, etc., will have a high failure rate using autogenous tissues for TMJ reconstruction (Badrick and Indresano 1992; Henry and Wolford 1993; Wolford 2019). A patient-fitted TMJ total joint prosthesis, such as the TMJ Concepts system (TMJ Concepts Inc., Ventura, CA, USA) will have a much higher rate of success (Henry and Wolford 1993; Wolford 2019).

Growing FA patients with unilateral TMJ pathology can be treated in a single operation by limiting treatment of the jaws and TMJ-related deformities to one major operation with high predictability by waiting until growth is relatively complete; females age of 15 years and males age of 17–18 years, although there are individual variations (Riolo et al. 1974).

Performing surgery at earlier ages may result in the need for additional surgery at a later time to correct asymmetry and malocclusion that may develop during the completion of growth. Indications for surgery during growth include ankylosis, masticatory dysfunction, tumor removal, airway obstruction, etc. The author and his coauthors have previously published on the effects of orthognathic surgery on maxillary and mandibular growth (Wolford et al., 2001a, 2001b; Wolford and Rodrigues 2012a; Mehra and Wolford 2016) as well as effects of TMJ pathology and surgery on jaw growth, with guidelines for age when considering surgical intervention (Wolford and Rodrigues 2012b).

Adolescent Internal Condylar Resorption (AICR)

AICR is a specific TMJ pathology causing condylar resorption and is one of the most common TMJ conditions affecting teenage females (Wolford and Cardenas 1999; Wolford 2001; Galiano et al. 2019; Wolford and

Galiano 2019). This TMJ pathology occurs with a 8:1 female-to-male ratio, no apparent genetic etiology, and usually develops between the ages of 11 and 15 years during pubertal growth (hormonal mediated), and rarely initiated outside of that time frame. Average rate of condylar resorption is 1.5 mm per year. Although this condition usually occurs bilaterally, it can occur unilaterally, or occur at a more rapid rate on one side causing asymmetry (Wolford and Cardenas 1999; Wolford 2001; Galiano et al. 2019; Wolford and Galiano 2019).

Specific clinical characteristics of AICR include: high occlusal plane angle and mandibular plane angle facial morphology; predominance of Class II skeletal and occlusal relationship with or without anterior open bite (Figures 12.6.8a–c, 12.6.9a–c, 12.6.10a); TMJ symptoms could include clicking, popping, TMJ pain, headaches, myofascial pain, earaches, tinnitus, vertigo; but no other joints in the body involved. However, 25% of AICR patients have no symptoms except changes in their occlusion and retrusion of the mandible (Wolford and Cardenas 1999; Wolford 2001; Galiano et al. 2019; Wolford and Galiano 2019). AICR rarely occurs in low occlusal and mandibular plane angle facial types or in Class III skeletal relationships. When it occurs unilaterally or one side has greater condylar resorption than the other, then additional FA characteristics include: Mandible deviated toward the affected side; progressive worsening facial deformity and occlusion; premature contact on the ipsilateral side; and may develop an anterior and contralateral open bite (Figures 12.6.8a–c and 12.6.9a–c) (Wolford and Cardenas 1999; Wolford 2001; Galiano et al. 2019; Wolford and Galiano 2019). Since this condition occurs only in teenagers, condylar resorption that is initiated in late teens or at a later age is not AICR and may require a different treatment protocol. AICR can progress for a while and then may go into remission or proceed on until a significant amount of the condylar head has resorbed. In cases where it goes into remission, excessive joint loading (i.e. parafunctional habits, trauma, orthodontics, orthognathic surgery etc.) can reinitiate the resorption process later in life.

CBCT, CT, and MRI features include: small condyle on the affected side compared to a normal condyle; decreased vertical height of the ramus and condyle on the involved side; disc anteriorly displaced and commonly nonreducing with amorphous appearing tissue surrounding the condyle, with or without an increased joint space (Wolford and Cardenas 1999; Wolford 2001; Galiano et al. 2019; Wolford and Galiano 2019).

The highly predictable and stable protocol for treating AICR, if performed within 4 years of onset, includes; removal of the bilaminar tissue surrounding the condyle, repositioning the disc with a Mitek anchor, and perform the indicated

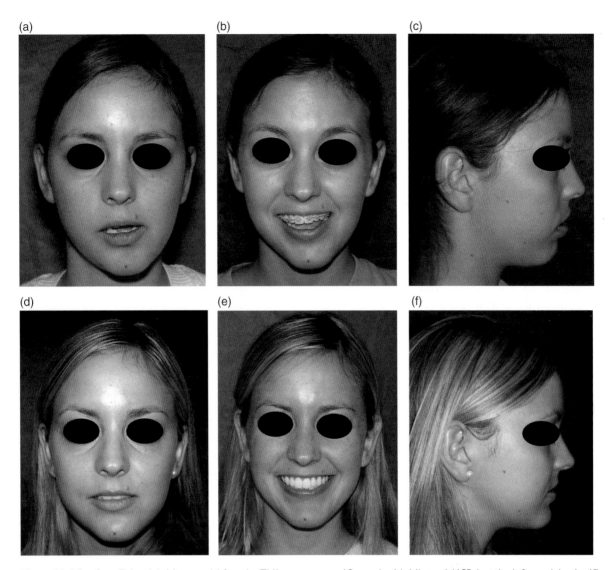

Figure 12.6.8 Case 3. (a–c) A 16-year-old female (TMJ onset at age 12 years) with bilateral AICR, but the left condyle significantly more resorbed and progressive than the right side resulting in a retruded mandible, Class II occlusion, anterior open bite, transverse cant in the occlusal plane and significant facial asymmetry; (d–f) the patient is seen 2-years post-surgery with a stable outcome following bilateral TMJ disc repositioning with Mitek anchors, bilateral mandibular ramus sagittal split osteotomies, and maxillary osteotomies for counterclockwise rotation of the maxillomandibular complex.

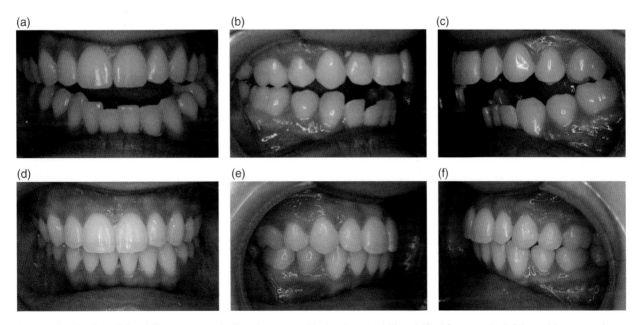

Figure 12.6.9 Case 3. (a–c) Presurgery occlusion shows mandibular dental midline shifted 2 mm to the left but with an anterior open bite and transverse cant in the occlusal plane; (d–f) two-years post-surgery demonstrates a stable occlusion.

(a)

(b)

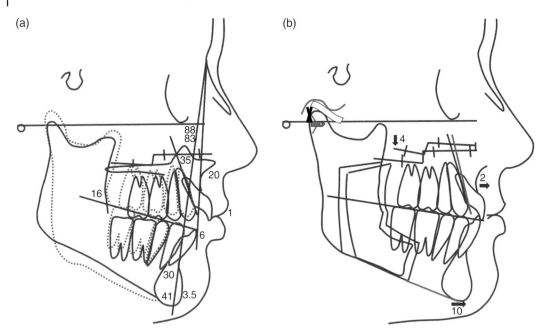

Figure 12.6.10 Case 3. (a) Cephalometric tracing shows a retruded mandible, Class II skeletal and occlusal relationship, high occlusal plane facial morphology, and a large anterior open bite; (b) Prediction tracing shows the intended treatment of bilateral TMJ articular disc repositioning with Mitek anchors, bilateral mandibular ramus osteotomies, and multiple maxillary osteotomies to advance the maxillomandibular complex in a counterclockwise direction.

orthognathic surgery (Figure 12.6.10b) (Wolford and Cardenas 1999; Wolford 2001; Goncalves et al. 2015; Wolford and Goncalves 2015; Bodine et al. 2016; Galiano et al. 2019; Wolford and Galiano 2019). This protocol stops the disease process and allows the orthognathic surgery to be done at the same operation, usually requiring double jaw surgery with counterclockwise rotation of the maxillo-mandibular complex to achieve optimal results (Figures 12.6.8d–f, 12.6.9d–f, and 12.6.10b). In growing patients, condylar growth will begin again (Wolford and Cardenas 1999; Wolford 2001; Bodine et al. 2016; Galiano et al. 2019; Wolford and Galiano 2019). In cases where the disc is non-salvageable because of severe deformation/degeneration or there is severe condylar resorption, then total joint prostheses may be the best treatment method where the TMJ can be reconstructed and the mandible advanced in a counterclockwise direction with the prostheses, along with maxillary osteotomies (Mercuri et al. 1995, 2002; Wolford 1997, 2016b, 2018; Mercuri 2000; Wolford and Mehra 2000; Wolford et al. 2003a; Coleta et al. 2009; Dela Coleta et al. 2009; Pinto et al. 2009; Perez et al. 2016).

Reactive Arthritis

Reactive arthritis usually involves bacterial or viral microorganisms within the tissues of the TMJ that stimulate the production of substrates that cause breakdown of the joint structures and pain. Although this condition can occur at any age, it is more commonly seen in the late teens up through the fourth decade, predominately in females and often when the discs are displaced (Wolford 2014). These bacteria include Chlamydia and Mycoplasma species may be in the bilaminar tissues in 70% of patients with TMJ symptoms. This could be the etiology or simply a contributing factor to the pathological process. It is known that these bacteria produce cytokines substance P, tissue necrosis factor, etc. that are pain mediators (Henry et al. 1999, 2000, 2001, 2002; Hudson et al. 2000; Henry and Wolford 2001; Wolford et al., 2001c, 2004; Wolford 2014). There may be a genetic predisposition to susceptibility to TMJ disorders and pathology as well as to these bacteria (Henry et al. 2002).

Although this condition commonly occurs bilaterally, it can occur unilaterally where the following features may be observed: Mandible will deviate toward the ipsilateral side; progressive worsening skeletal and occlusal deformity; Class II occlusion and crossbite as well as premature contact of the posterior occlusion on the ipsilateral side; commonly develops an anterior and contralateral open bite relationship; common associated TMJ symptoms include clicking, popping, crepitus, TMJ pain, headaches, myofascial pain, jaw dysfunction, earaches, tinnitus, vertigo, etc., and other joints or systems may be involved.

CBCT and CT will usually show arthritic condyle on the affected side with loss of vertical dimension; articular surface of the condyle and fossa may be eroded with loss of the fibrocartilage covering; decreased vertical height of the ramus and condyle on the ipsilateral side; and the mandible may be retruded and asymmetric. MRI may show the articular disc anteriorly displaced or in position, with joint effusion and inflammation present.

If the TMJ condition is identified within the first 4 years of the onset of the disc dislocation, the destruction is not significant, and there are no other joints or systemic conditions present; then repositioning the articular disc with the Mitek anchor technique (Wolford et al. 1995, 2002b; Mehra and Wolford 2001) may work, preserving the normal anatomical structures, but there is a significant risk of continued joint degeneration. The orthognathic surgery can be done at the same time as the joint repair is performed or done as a separate procedure. If there is significant destruction of the condyle and the disc is not salvageable or multiple other joints are involved, then the most predictable procedure is the total joint prosthesis (TMJ Concepts system) to reconstruct the condyle as well as reposition the mandible to its proper position (Coleta et al. 2009; Dela Coleta et al. 2009; Pinto et al. 2009; Wolford et al. 2014a; Perez et al. 2016; Wolford 2016b, 2018). Fat grafts packed around the total joint prosthesis are an important component to help prevent fibrous tissue and heterotopic bone from forming (Wolford and Karras 1997; Mercuri et al. 2008; Wolford et al. 2008; Wolford and Cassano 2010).

Trauma

Patients with a unilateral displaced subcondylar fracture will develop FA exhibiting the following: mandible deviated toward the affected side; pain and jaw dysfunction; may exhibit deficient growth on the affected side when occurring in growing patients; Class II skeletal and occlusal relationships; premature posterior occlusal contact and crossbite on the ipsilateral side; open bite tendency anteriorly and on the contralateral side; chin shifted toward the ipsilateral side (Figures 12.6.11a–c and 12.6.12a–c).

Imaging may show evidence of a displaced subcondylar fracture with decreased vertical ramus/condyle length (Figure 12.6.13a). When identified early, condylar fractures may be best treated by open reduction for moderate to significantly displaced segments or closed reduction for minimally displaced segments to achieve a symmetric face, stable occlusion, and good growth potential in growing patients. If the condylar segment is not significantly displaced, it may grow relatively normally with conservative, nonsurgical management. If the condyle is minimally to moderately displaced, still salvageable along with its articular disc but already healed, then it is possible that orthognathic surgery could realign the jaw structures properly. If the condyle is significantly displaced and non-salvageable, then reconstruction of the TMJ and mandible may be indicated using a total joint prosthesis (Figures 12.6.11d–f, 12.6.12d–f, 12.6.13b) (Mercuri et al. 1995, 2002; Wolford 1997; Mercuri 2000; Wolford and Mehra 2000; Wolford et al. 2003a; Coleta et al. 2009; Dela Coleta et al. 2009; Pinto et al. 2009; Perez et al. 2016; Wolford 2016a, 2018). If TJP is not available, then sternoclavicular or rib graft could be considered, but outcomes are less predictable (Wolford et al. 1994a; Tompach et al. 2000; Wolford 2019).

TMJ Ankylosis

TMJ ankylosis usually develops as a result of trauma, inflammation, sepsis, and/or systemic diseases (Wolford et al. 2016; Wolford 2017). Fibrous ankylosis usually allows some rotational jaw opening, but minimal translation. Bony ankylosis is caused by bony fusion or by reactive or heterotopic bone formation between or around the condyle and fossa causing severely limited jaw function as well as oral hygiene and nutritional problems. When this condition occurs during the growing years, it can severely affect jaw growth and development. In unilateral ankylosis, the other joint will continue to grow but may be retarded in its true growth potential. The common clinical and radiographic characteristics of unilateral TMJ ankylosis, particularly when occurring in children, include: Decreased jaw mobility and function; decreased growth on the involved side; facial asymmetry with the mandible shifted toward the ipsilateral side; retruded mandible; decreased vertical height of the maxilla and mandible on the ipsilateral side; usually a Class II occlusion and crossbite tendency on the ipsilateral side; transverse cant in the occlusal plane; evidence of bony ankylosis between the condyle and the fossa; and decreased oropharyngeal airway (Figures 12.6.11a–c, 12.6.12a–c, 12.6.13a) (Wolford et al. 2016; Wolford 2017).

CBCT, CT, or other imaging in fibrous ankylosis may appear as decreased joint space with adhesions creating limited jaw mobility. Bony ankylosis will usually appear as bony confluence between the condyle and fossa or heterotopic bone that has grown around the articular elements of the TMJ (Wolford et al. 2016; Wolford 2017).

The most predictable treatment protocol for TMJ ankylosis includes: Release of the ankylosed joint; removal of the heterotopic and reactive bone, condylectomy, thorough debridement of the TMJ and adjacent areas; reconstruct the TMJ (and if indicated, advance the mandible) with a

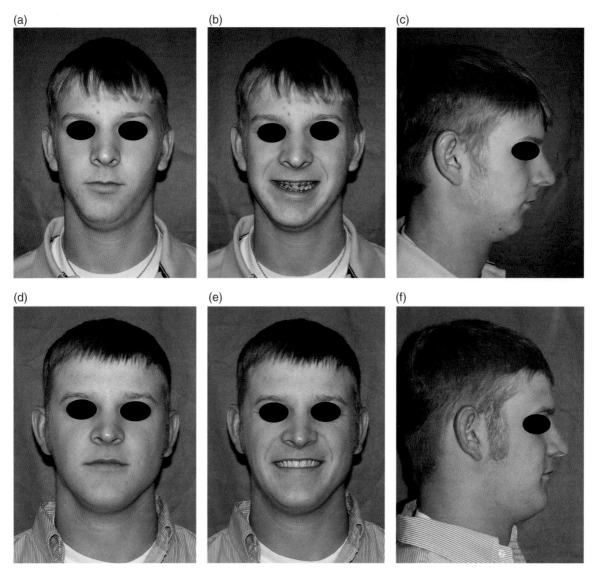

Figure 12.6.11 Case 4. (a–c) An 18-year-old male sustained a unilateral displaced right subcondylar fracture, non-reduced at the age of 10 years, with subsequent ankylosis. The mandible is deviated off to the right side and in profile both the maxilla and mandible are retruded; (d–f) the patient is seen 2-years post-surgery following right TMJ reconstruction and mandibular advancement with TMJ concepts total joint prostheses, left mandibular ramus sagittal osteotomy, and multiple maxillary osteotomies to advance the maxillomandibular complex forward in a counterclockwise direction.

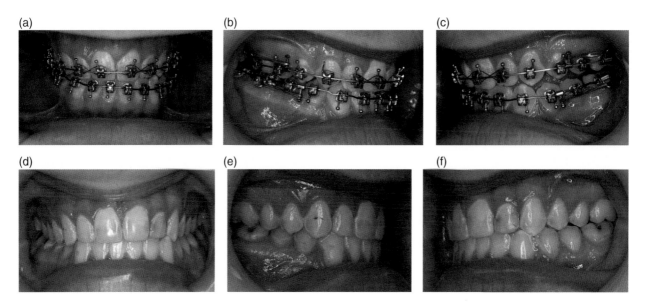

Figure 12.6.12 Case 4. (a–c) Presurgery occlusion demonstrates a transverse cant in the occlusal plane with the right side higher than the left side, Class I cuspid-molar relationship, and open bite tendency left posterior; (d–f) shows a good stable occlusal outcome.

(a) (b)

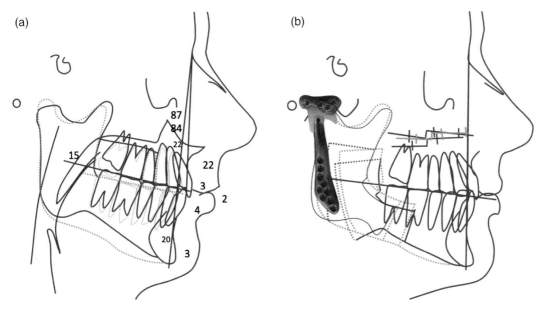

Figure 12.6.13 Case 4. (a) Presurgical cephalometric analysis demonstrates a significant difference in the vertical height of the inferior border of the mandible and occlusal plane, with the right side higher than the left side. Related to the right subcondylar fracture. There is a steep occlusal plane angle with retrusion of the maxilla and mandible; (b) prediction tracing shows right TMJ reconstructed and advanced with a TMJ Concepts total joint prostheses, left side mandibular ramus sagittal split osteotomy for advancement, and multiple maxillary osteotomies to advance the maxillomandibular complex in a counterclockwise direction. The mandible was advanced at pogonion 12 mm.

patient-fitted total joint prosthesis (TMJ concepts system) (Figure 12.6.13b); ipsilateral coronoidectomy if the ramus is significantly advanced or vertically lengthened with the prosthesis; and importantly, autogenous fat graft (usually harvested from the abdomen or buttock) packed around the prosthesis in the TMJ articulation area to prevent reankylosis (Wolford and Karras 1997; Mercuri et al. 2008; Wolford et al. 2008, 2016; Wolford and Cassano 2010; Wolford 2017); additional orthognathic surgery if indicated including a ramus osteotomy on the contralateral side and maxillary osteotomies; and any additional adjunctive procedures indicated (i.e. genioplasty, rhinoplasty, turbinectomies, septoplasty, etc.) (Figures 12.6.11d–f, 12.6.12d–f, 12.6.13b) (Coleta et al. 2009; Dela Coleta et al. 2009; Pinto et al. 2009; Perez et al. 2016; Wolford 2016a; 2016b; Wolford 2017, 2018). Orthodontics can be performed presurgery in some cases by using bonded brackets on the teeth. In some cases, it may be necessary to reconstruct the TMJ first followed by secondary orthognathic surgery.

When treating growing patients, the patient-fitted total joint prosthesis and fat grafts are still the best option to eliminate ankylosis. However, since there is no growth potential on the ipsilateral side of the mandible, orthognathic surgery will likely be necessary but can be delayed until the patient has most of the facial growth complete

(females age 15 years, males age 17–18 years) (Riolo et al. 1974). Then double jaw orthognathic surgery can be performed, including a ramus sagittal split on the side of the prosthesis to reposition the jaws into the best alignment, or the ipsilateral side can be advanced by repositioning the mandibular component of the prosthesis or fabrication of a new, longer mandibular component (Wolford et al. 2016a; Wolford 2017).

Hemifacial Microsomia (HFM)

HFM is also known as Goldenhar's syndrome, oculo-auriculo-vertebral spectrum, and branchial arch syndrome. HFM is present at birth and occurs sporadically with extreme variability of expression is characteristic of this disorder (Gorlin et al. 2001). Clinical and radiographic features of HFM may include: Unilateral hypoplasia or aplasia of the mandible and condyle as well as hypoplasia of the maxilla, zygomatico-orbital complex, and temporal bone; decreased ipsilateral facial height; retruded chin deviated toward the ipsilateral side; eye, ear, and vertebral anomalies; Class II malocclusion; premature occlusal contact on the ipsilateral side; transverse cant in the occlusal plane and skeletal structures; hypo-eruption of the teeth on the ipsilateral side; significant soft tissue deficiency on the involved side affecting muscles, subcutaneous tissues, and skin volume, and decreased oropharyngeal airway (Figures 12.6.14a–c, 12.6.15a–c, 12.6.16a). With growth, the facial deformity, asymmetry, and malocclusion worsen (Gorlin et al. 2001; Wolford 2002; Wolford et al. 2012).

The patient's age can affect the treatment protocol including the surgical options. For patients 12 years old with absence of the TMJ may benefit from a growth center transplant, sternoclavicular or rib grafts have been advocated (Tompach et al. 2000). However, these grafts are unpredictable relative to growth and stability, with risk of ankylosis. Teenage or older patients with significant deformity of the condyle and ramus will have a much better outcome using a patient-fitted TMJ total joint prosthesis

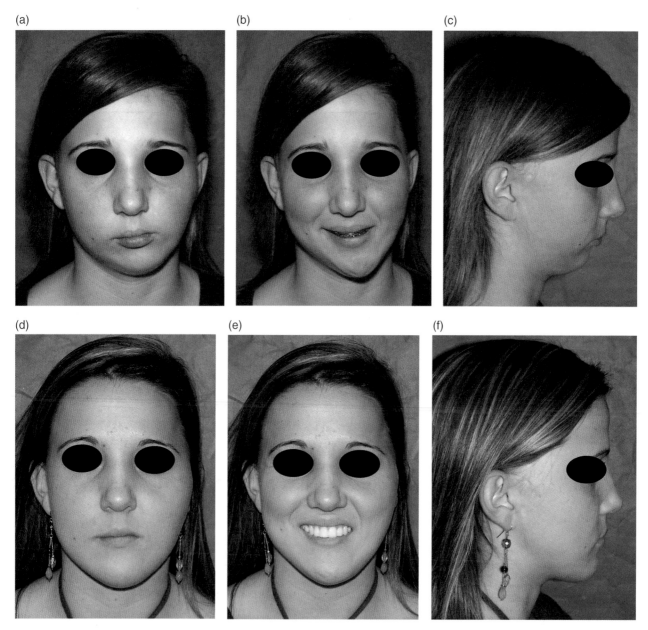

Figure 12.6.14 Case 5. (a–c) This 14-year-old female was born with left-sided hemifacial microsomia. She was absent the left mandibular condyle and the ramus was hypoplastic. She has significant transverse asymmetry, retruded mandible, and Class II occlusion; (d–f) the patient is 2-years post-surgery for left TMJ reconstruction and mandibular advancement in a counterclockwise direction with TMJ Concepts total joint prostheses, advancement of the right mandible with ramus sagittal split osteotomy, and maxillary osteotomies for counterclockwise rotation of the maxillomandibular complex. She had significant improvement in her facial symmetry, pain free with an incisal opening of 42 mm.

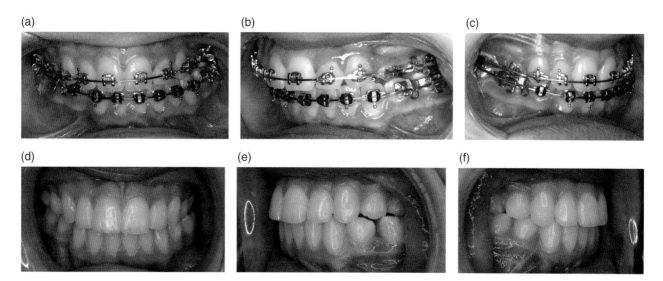

Figure 12.6.15 Case 5. (a–c) Presurgery occlusion has a transverse cant, left-sided posterior crossbite, mandibular dental midline shifted to the left 6 mm, and a Class III end-on cuspid relationship on the right side and Class II cuspid relationship on the left side. She has a displaced disc in the right TMJ that can occur in about 33% of these patients; ☹ d–f) at 2-years post-surgery there is significant improvement in her occlusion with the dental midlines aligned, transverse leveling of the occlusion, and a Class I cuspid relationship bilaterally.

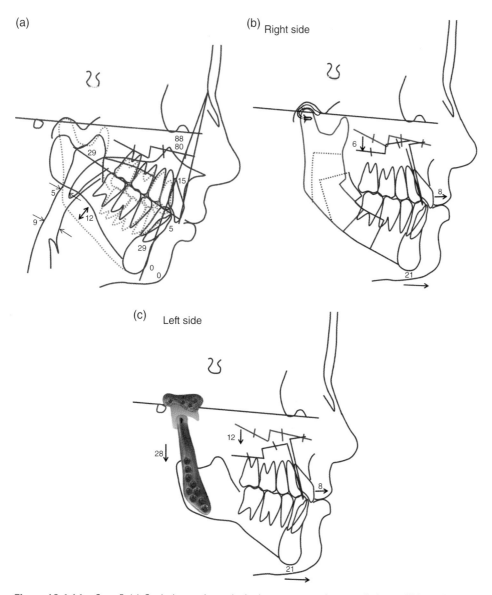

Figure 12.6.16 Case 5. (a) Cephalometric analysis demonstrates the retruded mandible and maxilla, vertical facial asymmetry, high occlusal plane angle, skeletal and occlusal Class II relationship, and decreased oropharyngeal airway; (b) the prediction tracing shows the right TMJ disc repositioned with a Mitek anchor and mandible advance with a sagittal split osteotomy; (c) the left TMJ was reconstruction and mandible advanced in a counterclockwise rotation with a patient-fitted TMJ Concepts total joint prosthesis, and multiple maxillary osteotomies with the posterior maxilla down grafted 12 mm on the left side. Pogonion advanced 21 mm.

(TMJ concepts system) to advance and lengthen the ramus on the ipsilateral side (Figure 12.6.16b) (Wolford et al. 2012; Wolford and Perez 2015; Polley et al. 2019). Deferring treatment until the patient is closer to completion of facial growth (females 15 years old, males 17–18 years old) will help minimize subsequent contralateral normal growth effect on the treatment outcome. A mandibular ramus sagittal split osteotomy can be performed on the contra-lateral side and the indicated maxillary osteotomies completed as well as any other adjunctive procedures (i.e. genioplasty, rhinoplasty, turbinectomies, nasoseptoplasty, etc.) (Figures 12.6.14d–f, 12.6.15d–f, 12.6.16b). A unilateral TMJ prosthesis is highly successful and should not have an adverse effect on the contralateral TMJ if that joint is healthy (Perez et al. 2016). Additional reconstruction may be necessary using bone grafts, synthetic bone, alloplastic implants, etc. to build up the residual deformed skeletal structures. Soft tissue reconstructed using fat grafts, tissue flaps, free vascularized grafts, etc., may be necessary to fill out the soft tissue defects (Wolford et al. 2012; Wolford and Perez 2015; Polley et al. 2019; Wolford 2022; Wolford et al. 1994b).

Connective Tissue/Autoimmune Diseases (CT/AI)

Connective tissue/autoimmune diseases (CT/AI) diseases that can affect the TMJs include: Juvenile idiopathic arthritis, rheumatoid arthritis, psoriatic arthritis, ankylosing spondylitis, Sjogren's syndrome, systemic lupus erythematosus, scleroderma, mixed connective tissue disease, etc. The triggers and precise pathophysiology are unknown for most of these disorders. Multiple systems are usually involved. Joint damage may be mediated by cytokines, chemokines, and metalloproteases. Peripheral joints are usually symmetrically inflamed resulting in progressive destruction of articular structures (Petty et al. 2004; Ravelli and Martini 2007). FA can occur with unilateral involvement or if one TMJ is more severely affected than the other causing greater unilateral condylar resorption.

Clinical features when occurring unilaterally or one TMJ is affected greater than the other side includes: Deviation of the mandible toward the ipsilateral side; progressive worsening facial and occlusal deformity; Class II occlusion, crossbite tendency, and premature contact on the ipsilateral side; commonly develops an anterior and contralateral open bite relationship; TMJ symptoms could include clicking, popping, crepitus, TMJ pain, headaches, myofascial pain, earaches, tinnitus, vertigo, etc.; jaw and jaw joint dysfunction, and other joints and systems involved (Figures 12.6.17a–c, 12.6.18a–c, 12.6.19a) (Wolford 2021; Trivedi et al. 2022; Wolford and Kesterke 2022).

Radiographic and MRI features when occurring unilaterally or one side resorbs at a faster rate than the other side include: condylar loss of vertical dimension, significant medio-laterally narrowing, but may become broad in the anterior–posterior (A–P) direction; articular disc may be in position but surrounded by a reactive pannus that eventually destroys the disc but also causes the condylar and articular eminence resorption; in more severe cases, the condylar stump may function beneath the remaining articular eminence; and decreased vertical height of the ramus and condyle. The mandible becomes progressively retruded with development of a Class II occlusion and an anterior open bite (Figure 12.6.19a) (Wolford 2021; Wolford and Kesterke 2022).

The most predictable treatment for the TMJ affected by CT/AI diseases includes: reconstruction of the TMJ (and if indicated, advance the mandible) with a patient-fitted total joint prosthesis (TMJ concepts system), usually required bilaterally (Mehra et al. 2009, 2018; Wolford 2021; Trivedi et al. 2022; Wolford and Kesterke 2022); ipsilateral or bilateral coronoidectomy if the ramus is significantly advanced or vertically lengthened with the prosthesis; autogenous fat graft packed around the prostheses in the articulation area (Wolford and Karras 1997; Mercuri et al. 2008; Wolford et al. 2008; Wolford and Cassano 2010); additional orthognathic surgery if indicated including sagittal split osteotomy on opposite ramus if no TMJ pathology in the contralateral joint; maxillary osteotomies (Figures 12.6.16b, 12.6.17d–f, 12.6.18a–c); and any additional adjunctive procedures indicated (Mehra et al. 2009, 2018; Wolford 2021; Trivedi et al. 2022; Wolford and Kesterke 2022). With the development of computer-assisted surgical simulation, virtual surgical planning (VSP), the surgical accuracy for these complex cases has been significantly improved (Movahed et al. 2013; Movahed and Wolford 2015; Wolford 2016a, 2021; Gupta et al. 2019; Wolford and Kesterke 2022). Orthognathic surgery can be performed at the same time as the TMJ is reconstructed or performed at a later surgery. Autogenous tissues such as temporal fascia and muscle flaps, rib grafts, sternoclavicular grafts, vertical sliding osteotomy, etc. are contraindicated because the disease process that created the original TMJ pathology can attack the autogenous tissues used in the TMJ reconstruction causing failure of the grafts (Mehra et al. 2018; Wolford 2019).

The TMJ total joint prosthesis with a fat graft packed around it is a superior technique relative to elimination of the disease process in the TMJ, improves function, and esthetics, and eliminates or decreases pain in end-stage TMJ pathology (Mehra et al. 2009, 2018; Wolford 2021; Trivedi et al. 2022; Wolford and Kesterke 2022). Wolford and Goncalves (2015) have demonstrated that at 21-year follow-up, the TMJ Concepts devices provide good quality-of-life outcomes and do not require replacement for

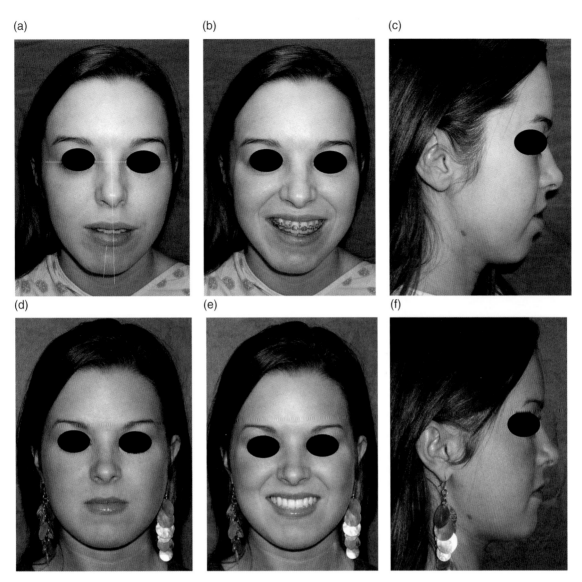

Figure 12.6.17 Case 6. (a–c) A 16-year-old female with bilateral TMJ juvenile idiopathic arthritis (JIA) with greater condylar resorption on the right side. Other joints and systemic systems were involved. She had facial asymmetry, a retruded mandible, Class II skeletal and occlusal relationship, and anterior open bite; (d–f) the patient is seen 2 years after treatment following orthodontics and surgery that included: Bilateral TMJ reconstruction and mandibular advancement with TMJ Concepts total joint prostheses, bilateral coronoidectomy, and maxillary osteotomies to level the occlusal plane, and counterclockwise rotation of the maxillomandibular complex.

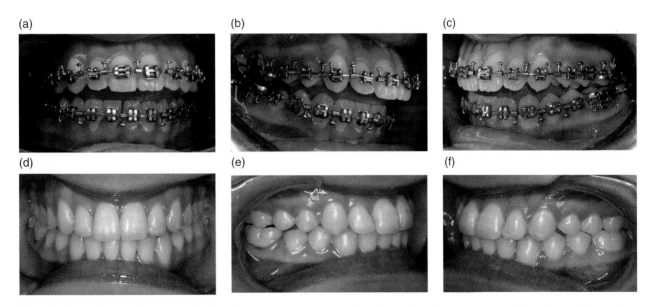

Figure 12.6.18 Case 6. (a–c) The occlusion demonstrates asymmetry with the mandibular midline shifted 4 mm to the right of the maxillary midline, anterior open bite, right posterior crossbite, with occlusion predominantly on the molars; (d–f) two-years post-surgery the occlusion is aligned with a stable Class I cuspid-molar relationship and closure of the anterior open bite.

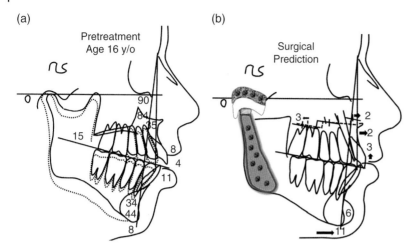

Figure 12.6.19 Case 6. (a) Cephalometric analysis shows the vertical difference of the inferior borders of the mandible and the occlusal plane, as well as the retruded mandible, posterior maxillary vertical hypoplasia, and anterior open bite; (b) the prediction tracing shows the surgical changes including bilateral TMJ reconstruction and mandibular advancement in a counterclockwise direction with TMJ concepts total joint prostheses and multiple maxillary osteotomies with counterclockwise rotation of the maxillomandibular complex.

material failure or wearing out. When treating young growing patients (10 years or older), the total joint prosthesis may still be the best option to eliminate the disease process. However, since there would be no growth potential on the involved side of the mandible, orthognathic surgery may be necessary but can be delayed until the patient has most of the facial growth completed. Then double jaw surgery can be performed, including the sagittal split on the side of the prosthesis to reposition the jaws into the best alignment, or repositioning of the mandibular component of the prosthesis, or manufacturing a new mandibular component to allow advancement of the mandible on the involved sides (Wolford 2021).

There are numerous etiologies for FA including TMJ pathologies as discussed in this chapter. Accurate diagnosis of the TMJ pathology and associated hard and soft tissue involvement are paramount to develop a comprehensive treatment plan to achieve optimal results for FA patients.

References

Al-Moraissi EA, Wolford LM, Perez D, Laskin DM, Ellis E 3rd. Does orthognathic surgery cause or cure temporomandibular disorders? A systematic review and meta-analysis. J Oral Maxillofac Surg. 2017;75:1835–1847.

Al-Moraissi EA, Wolford LM. Does temporomandibular joint pathology with or without surgical management affect the stability of counterclockwise rotation of the maxillomandibular complex in orthognathic surgery? A systematic review and meta-analysis. J Oral Maxillofac Surg. 2017;75:805–821.

Al-Moraissi EA, Wolford LM. Is counterclockwise rotation of the maxillomandibular complex stable compared with clockwise rotation in the correction of dentofacial deformities? A systematic review and meta-analysis. J Oral Maxillofac Surg. 2016;74:2066.e12.

Badrick JP, Indresano AT. Failure rates of repetitive temporomandibular joint surgical procedures. 74th Annual Meeting of the American Association of Oral and Maxillofacial Surgeons. Scientific Poster Session III, Honolulu, Hawaii, USA, 1992 (abstract).

Bianchi J, Porciuncula GM, Koerich L, Ignacio J, Wolford LM, Goncalves JR. Three-dimensional stability analysis of maxillomandibular advancement surgery with and without articular disc repositioning. J Craniomaxillofac Surg. 2018;46:1348–1354.

Bodine TP, Wolford LM, Araujo E, Oliver DR, Buschang PH. Surgical treatment of adolescent internal condylar resorption (AICR) with articular disc repositioning and orthognathic surgery in the growing patient. Prog Orthod. 2016;17:2.

Chan BH, Leung YY. SPECT bone scintigraphy for assessment of condylar growth activity in mandibular asymmetry: is it accurate? Int J Oral Maxillofac Surg. 2018;47:470–479.

Coleta KE, Wolford LM, Goncalves JR, Pinto Ados S, Cassano DS, Goncalves DA. Maxillo-mandibular counter-clockwise rotation and mandibular advancement with TMJ Concepts total joint prostheses: part II - airway changes and stability. Int J Oral Maxillofac Surg. 2009;38:228–235.

Dela Coleta KE, Wolford LM, Goncalves JR, dos Santos Pinto A, Pinto LP, Cassano DS. Maxillo-mandibular counter-clockwise rotation and mandibular advancement with TMJ concepts total joint prostheses: part I - skeletal and dental stability. Int J Oral Maxillofac Surg. 2009;38:126–138.

Fuselier C, Wolford LM, Pitta M, Talwar R. Condylar changes after orthognathic surgery with untreated TMJ internal derangement. J Oral Maxillofac Surg. 1998;56(Suppl 4):61.

Galiano A, Wolford L, Goncalves J, Goncalves D. Adolescent internal condylar resorption (AICR) of the temporomandibular joint can be successfully treated by disc repositioning and orthognathic surgery, part 2: treatment outcomes. Cranio. 2019;37:111–120.

Gomes LR, Soares Cevidanes LH, Gomes MR, Carlos de Oliveira Ruellas A, Obelenis Ryan DP, Paniagua B, Wolford LM, Goncalves JR. Three-dimensional quantitative assessment of surgical stability and condylar displacement changes after counterclockwise maxillomandibular advancement surgery: effect of simultaneous articular disc repositioning. Am J Orthod Dentofac Orthop. 2018;154:221–233.

Goncalves JR, Cassano DS, Rezende L, Wolford LM. Disc repositioning: does it really work? Oral Maxillofac Surg Clin North Am. 2015;27:85–107.

Goncalves JR, Cassano DS, Wolford LM, Santos-Pinto A, Marquez IM. Postsurgical stability of counterclockwise maxillomandibular advancement surgery: effect of articular disc repositioning. J Oral Maxillofac Surg. 2008;66:724–738.

Gorlin RJ, Cohen MM Jr, Hemekam RCM. Syndromes of the Head and Neck. Oxford: Oxford University Press, 2001:405–408,790–797.

Gottlieb OP. Hyperplasia of the mandibular condyle. J Oral Surg. 1951;9:118–135.

Gupta RJ, Schendel SA, Wolford LW. Concomitant custom-fitted temporomandibular joint reconstruction and orthognathic surgery. In: Connelly S, Tartaglia G, Silva R, eds. Contemporary Management of Temporomandibular Disorders. New York: Springer, 2019:233–285.

Henry CH, Hudson AP, Gerard HC, Franco PF, Wolford LM. Identification of chlamydia trachomatis in the human temporomandibular joint. J Oral Maxillofac Surg. 1999;57:683–688.

Henry CH, Hughes CV, Gerard HC, Hudson AP, Wolford LM. Reactive arthritis: preliminary microbiologic analysis of the human temporomandibular joint. J Oral Maxillofac Surg. 2000;58:1137–1142.

Henry CH, Nikaein A, Wolford LM. Analysis of human leukocyte antigens in patients with internal derangement

of the temporomandibular joint. J Oral Maxillofac Surg. 2002;60:778–783.

Henry CH, Pitta MC, Wolford LM. Frequency of chlamydial antibodies in patients with internal derangement of the temporomandibular joint. Oral Surg Oral Med Oral Pathol Oral Radiol Endod. 2001;91:287–292.

Henry CH, Wolford LM. Substance P and mast cells: preliminary histologic analysis of the human temporomandibular joint. Oral Surg Oral Med Oral Pathol Oral Radiol Endod. 2001;92:384–389.

Henry CH, Wolford LM. Treatment outcomes for TMJ reconstruction after Proplast-Teflon implant failure. J Oral Maxillofac Surg. 1993;51:352–358.

Hudson AP, Henry C, Wolford LM, Gerard HC. Chlamydia psittaci infection may influence development of temporomandibular joint dysfunction. J Arthritis Rheumatism. 2000;43:S174.

Mehra P, Henry CH, Giglou KR. Temporomandibular joint reconstruction in patients with autoimmune/connective tissue disease. J Oral Maxillofac Surg. 2018;76:1660–1664.

Mehra P, Wolford LM, Baran S, Cassano DS. Single-stage comprehensive surgical treatment of the rheumatoid arthritis temporomandibular joint patient. J Oral Maxillofac Surg. 2009;67:1859–1872.

Mehra P, Wolford LM. Early orthognathic surgery: considerations for surgical management. In: Naini FB, Gill DS, eds. Orthognathic Surgery Principles, Planning and Practice. London: John Wiley & Sons, Ltd, 2016:347–360.

Mehra P, Wolford LM. The Mitek mini anchor for TMJ disc repositioning: surgical technique and results. Int J Oral Maxillofac Surg. 2001;30:497–503.

Mercuri LG, Ali FA, Woolson R. Outcomes of total alloplastic replacement with periarticular autogenous fat grafting for management of reankylosis of the temporomandibular joint. J Oral Maxillofac Surg. 2008;66:1794–1803.

Mercuri LG, Wolford LM, Sanders B, White RD, Giobbie-Hurder A. Long-term follow-up of the CAD/CAM patient fitted total temporomandibular joint reconstruction system. J Oral Maxillofac Surg. 2002;60:1440–1448.

Mercuri LG, Wolford LM, Sanders B, White RD, Hurder A, Henderson W. Custom CAD/CAM total temporomandibular joint reconstruction system: preliminary multicenter report. J Oral Maxillofac Surg. 1995;53:106–115.

Mercuri LG. The use of alloplastic prostheses for temporomandibular joint reconstruction. J Oral Maxillofac Surg. 2000;58:70–75.

Movahed R, Teschke M, Wolford LM. Protocol for concomitant temporomandibular joint custom-fitted total joint reconstruction and orthognathic surgery utilizing computer-assisted surgical simulation. J Oral Maxillofac Surg. 2013;71:2123–2129.

Movahed R, Wolford LM. Protocol for concomitant temporomandibular joint custom-fitted total joint reconstruction and orthognathic surgery using computer-assisted surgical simulation. Oral Maxillofac Surg Clin North Am. 2015;27:37–45.

Obwegeser HL, Makek MS. Hemimandibular hyperplasia - hemimandibular elongation. J Maxillofac Surg. 1986;14:183–208.

Perez D, Wolford LM, Schneiderman E, Movahed R, Bourland C, Perez E. Does unilateral temporomandibular total joint reconstruction result in contralateral joint pain and dysfunction? J Oral Maxillofac Surg. 2016;74:1539–1547.

Petty RE, Southwood TR, Manners P, Baum J, Glass DN, Goldenberg J, He X, Maldonado-Cocco J, Orozco-Alcala J, Prieur AM, Suarez-Almazor ME, Woo P. International League of Associations for Rheumatology classification of juvenile idiopathic arthritis: second revision, Edmonton, 2001. J Rheumatol. 2004;31:390–392.

Pinto LP, Wolford LM, Buschang PH, Bernardi FH, Goncalves JR, Cassano DS. Maxillo-mandibular counter-clockwise rotation and mandibular advancement with TMJ Concepts total joint prostheses: part III – pain and dysfunction outcomes. Int J Oral Maxillofac Surg. 2009;38:326–331.

Polley JW, Girotto JA, Fahrenkopf MP, Dietze-Fiedler ML, Kelley JP, Taylor JC, Lazarou SA, Demetriades NC. Salvage or solution: alloplastic reconstruction in hemifacial microsomia. Cleft Palate Craniofac J. 2019;56:896–901.

Ravelli A, Martini A. Juvenile idiopathic arthritis. Lancet. 2007;369:767–778.

Riolo ML, Moyers RE, McNamara JA Jr, Hunter WS. An Atlas of Craniofacial Growth. Ann Arbor: Center for Human Growth and Development, University of Michigan, 1974.

Tompach P, Dodson TB, Kaban LB. Autogenous temporomandibular joint replacement. In: Fonseca R, ed. Oral and Maxillofacial Surgery: Temporomandibular Disorders. Philadelphia: WB Saunders Co., 2000:301–315.

Trivedi B, Wolford LM, Kesterke MJ, Pinto LP. Does combined temporomandibular joint reconstruction with patient fitted total Joint prosthesis and orthognathic surgery reduce symptoms in juvenile idiopathic arthritis patients? J Oral Maxillofac Surg. 2022;80:267–275.

Wolford L, Movahed R, Teschke M, Fimmers R, Havard D, Schneiderman E. Temporomandibular joint ankylosis can be successfully treated with TMJ Concepts patient-fitted total joint prosthesis and autogenous fat grafts. J Oral Maxillofac Surg. 2016;74:1215–1227.

Wolford L. Autogenous tissues versus alloplastic TMJ condylar replacement. In: Connelly S, Tartaglia G, Silva R, eds. Contemporary Management of Temporomandibular Disorders. Cham: Springer, 2019:173–202.

Wolford L. Concomitant TMJ total joint prosthetic reconstruction and orthognathic surgery. In: Turvey TA, Costello BJ, Ruiz RL, eds. Fonseca Oral and Maxillofacial Surgery. St. Louis: Elsevier, 2018:222–245.

Wolford L. Diagnosis and management of TMJ heterotopic bone and ankylosis. In: Bouloux GF, ed. Complications of Temporomandibular Joint Surgery. Cham: Springer, 2017:111–133.

Wolford L. Surgical management of hemifacial microsomia with temporomandibular joint malformation. In: Yates DM, Markiewicz MR, eds. Craniofacial Microsomia and Treacher Collins Syndrome: Comprehensive Treatment of Associated Facial Deformities. Cham: Springer, 2022:93–131.

Wolford LM, Bourland TC, Rodrigues D, Perez DE, Limoeiro E. Successful reconstruction of nongrowing hemifacial microsomia patients with unilateral temporomandibular joint total joint prosthesis and orthognathic surgery. J Oral Maxillofac Surg. 2012;70:2835–2853.

Wolford LM, Cardenas L. Idiopathic condylar resorption: diagnosis, treatment protocol, and outcomes. Am J Orthod Dentofac Orthop. 1999;116:667–676.

Wolford LM, Cassano DS. Autologous fat grafts around temporomandibular joint total joint prostheses to prevent heterotopic bone. In: Shiffman MA, ed. Autologous Fat Transfer. Berlin: Springer, 2010:361–382.

Wolford LM, Cottrell DA, Henry CH. Sternoclavicular grafts for temporomandibular joint reconstruction. J Oral Maxillofac Surg. 1994a;52:119–128.

Wolford LM, Cottrell DA, Henry CH. Temporomandibular joint reconstruction of the complex patient with the techmedica custom-made total joint prosthesis. J Oral Maxillofac Surg. 1994b;52:2–10.

Wolford LM, Cottrell DA, Karras SC. Mitek mini anchor in maxillofacial surgery. Proceedings of SMST-94, the First International Conference on Shape Memory and Superelastic Technologies, Monterey, California, USA, 1995:477–482.

Wolford LM, Galiano A. Adolescent internal condylar resorption (AICR) of the temporomandibular joint part 1: a review for diagnosis and treatment considerations. Cranio. 2019;37:35–44.

Wolford LM, Gerard HC, Henry CH, Hudson AP. Chlamydia psittaci infection may be involved in development of temporomandibular joint dysfunction. J Oral Maxillofac Surg. 2001c;30(Suppl 1):59–60.

Wolford LM, Goncalves JR. Condylar resorption of the temporomandibular joint: how do we treat it? Oral Maxillofac Surg Clin North Am. 2015;27:47–67.

Wolford LM, Goncalves JR. Surgical planning in orthognathic surgery and outcome stability. In: Brennan PA, Schliephake H, Ghali GE, Cascarini L, eds. Maxillofacial Surgery. St. Louis: Elsevier, 2017:1048–1126.

Wolford LM, Henry CH, Goncalves JR. TMJ and systemic affects associated with chlamydia psittaci. J Oral Maxillofac Surg. 2004;62(Suppl 1):50–51.

Wolford LM, Karras SC, Mehra P. Concomitant temporomandibular joint and orthognathic surgery: a preliminary report. J Oral Maxillofac Surg. 2002b;60:356–362.

Wolford LM, Karras SC, Mehra P. Considerations for orthognathic surgery during growth, part 1: mandibular deformities. Am J Orthod Dentofac Orthop. 2001a;119:95–101.

Wolford LM, Karras SC, Mehra P. Considerations for orthognathic surgery during growth, part 2: maxillary deformities. Am J Orthod Dentofac Orthop. 2001b;119:102–105.

Wolford LM, Karras SC. Autologous fat transplantation around temporomandibular joint total joint prostheses: preliminary treatment outcomes. J Oral Maxillofac Surg. 1997;55:245–251.

Wolford LM, Kesterke MJ. Does combined temporomandibular joint reconstruction with patient fitted total Joint prosthesis and orthognathic surgery provide stable skeletal and occlusal outcomes in juvenile idiopathic arthritis patients? J Oral Maxillofac Surg. 2022;80:138–150.

Wolford LM, LeBanc J. Condylectomy to arrest disproportionate mandibular growth. American Cleft Palate Association Meeting, New York, USA, 1986:Abstract.

Wolford LM, Mehra P, Franco P. Use of conservative condylectomy for treatment of osteochondroma of the mandibular condyle. J Oral Maxillofac Surg. 2002a;60:262–268.

Wolford LM, Mehra P, Reiche-Fischel O, Morales-Ryan CA, Garcia-Morales P. Efficacy of high condylectomy for management of condylar hyperplasia. Am J Orthod Dentofac Orthop. 2002c;121:136–151.

Wolford LM, Mehra P. Custom-made total joint prostheses for temporomandibular joint reconstruction. Baylor Univ Med Cent Proc. 2000;13:135–138.

Wolford LM, Mercuri LG, Schneiderman ED, Movahed R, Allen W. Twenty-year follow-up study on a patient-fitted temporomandibular joint prostheses: the techmedica/TMJ concepts device. J Oral Maxillofac Surg. 2014a;73:952–960.

Wolford LM, Morales-Ryan CA, Garcia-Morales P, Cassano DS. Autologous fat grafts placed around temporomandibular joint total joint prostheses to prevent heterotopic bone formation. Baylor Univ Med Cent Proc. 2008;21:248–254.

Wolford LM, Morales-Ryan CA, Garcia-Morales P, Perez D. Surgical management of mandibular condylar hyperplasia type 1. Baylor Univ Med Cent Proc. 2009;22.321–329.

Wolford LM, Movahed R, Dhameja A, Allen WR. Low condylectomy and orthognathic surgery to treat mandibular condylar osteochondroma: retrospective review of 37 cases. J Oral Maxillofac Surg. 2014b;72:1704–1728.

Wolford LM, Movahed R, Percz D. A classification system for conditions causing condylar hyperplasia. J Oral Maxillofac Surg. 2014c;72:567–595.

Wolford LM, Perez DE. Surgical management of congenital deformities with temporomandibular joint malformation. Oral Maxillofac Surg Clin North Am. 2015;27:137–154.

Wolford LM, Pitta MC, Reiche-Fischel O, Franco PF. TMJ concepts/techmedica custom-made TMJ total joint prosthesis: 5-year follow-up. Int J Oral Maxillofac Surg. 2003a;32:268–274.

Wolford LM, Reiche-Fischel O, Mehra P. Changes in TMJ dysfunction after orthognathic surgery. J Oral Maxillofac Surg. 2003b;61:665–660.

Wolford LM, Rodrigues DB. Orthognathic considerations in the young patient and effects on facial growth. In: Preedy VR, ed. Handbook of Growth and Growth Monitoring in Health and Disease. New York: Springer, 2012a: 1789–1808.

Wolford LM, Rodrigues DB. Temporomandibular joint (TMJ) pathologies in growing patients: effects on facial growth and development. In: Preedy VR, ed. Handbook of Growth and Growth Monitoring in Health and Disease. New York: Springer, 2012b:1809–1828.

Wolford LM. Author's response: efficacy of high condylectomy for management of condylar hyperplasia. Am J Orthod Dentofac Orthop. 2002;121:151.

Wolford LM. Computer – assisted surgical simulation for concomitant temporomandibular joint custom-fitted total joint reconstruction and orthognathic surgery. In: Sullivan SM, ed. Techniques in Orthognathic Surgery, An Issue of Atlas of the Oral and Maxillofacial Surgery Clinics of North America. Vol. 24. Philadelphia: Elsevier, 2016a:55–66.

Wolford LM. Concomitant TMJ total joint replacement and orthognathic surgery. In: Mercuri LG, ed. Temporomandibular Joint Total Joint Replacement. Cham: Springer, 2016b: 133–164.

Wolford LM. Facial asymmetry: diagnosis and treatment considerations. In: Fonseca RJ, Marciani RD, Turvey TA, eds. Oral and Maxillofacial Surgery. St. Louis: Elsevier, 2008:272–315.

Wolford LM. Idiopathic condylar resorption of the temporomandibular joint in teenage girls (Cheerleaders syndrome). Baylor Univ Med Cent Proc. 2001;14:246–252.

Wolford LM. Mandibular asymmetry: temporomandibular joint degeneration. In: Bagheri SC, Bell RB, Khan HA, eds. Current Therapy in Oral and Maxillofacial Surgery. St. Louis: Elsevier Saunders, 2012:696–725.

Wolford LM. Surgical correction of the severe jaw deformity in teenagers with juvenile idiopathic arthritis. Plast Aesthet Res. 2021;8:31–43.

Wolford LM. Temporomandibular joint devices: treatment factors and outcomes. Oral Surg Oral Med Oral Pathol Oral Radiol Endod. 1997;83:143–149.

Wolford LM. Understanding TMJ reactive arthritis. Cranio. 2014;35(5):274–275.

Xiao J, Wu Z, Ye W. Using 3D medical modeling to evaluate the accuracy of single-photon emission computed tomography (SPECT) bone scintigraphy in diagnosing condylar hyperplasia. J Oral Maxillofac Surg. 2022;80:285.e1–285.e9.

12.7

Distraction Osteogenesis in Maxillofacial Surgery

Ioannis Iatrou and Nadia Theologie-Lygidakis

Introduction

A primary report about lengthening a fractured or shortened leg with traction, comes from the time of the ancient Greek physician Hippocrates (Peltier 1990). However, only relatively recently, the Russian orthopedic surgeon Gavriil Abramovich Ilizarov developed a successful method to lengthen the lower extremities (fibulas and tibias) by performing an osteotomy, which is followed by gradual dissociation of the bone sides by external fixation (Ilizarov et al. 1969). The efficacy of the method of distraction osteogenesis (DO) which since then has been scientifically proved (Ilizarov et al. 1980), gained popularity and gave the idea to plastic and maxillofacial surgeons to apply the same principles in cases of mandibular deficiencies (McCarthy et al. 1992). McCarthy was the first surgeon who, following extensive experimental studies to the jaws of dogs, applied an extraoral device to lengthen a malformed mandible. Since then DO has been established as an early treatment

of asymmetry in the maxillofacial region, mainly in cases of syndromes (Diner et al. 1996; Moore et al. 1994; Wangerin and Gropp 1994, 1999). DO presents important advantages compared to conventional grafting surgery; especially in mandibular asymmetries, it can safely be applied early in life, in neonates, infants and young children, achieving a significant elongation of the bone usually up to 2.5 cm or even up to 5.0 cm (Rossini et al. 2016), without jeopardizing nerve vitality; new bone develops without the need of a donor site for bone autograft, operation that has a relative morbidity.

Biological Basis

The biological procedure in distraction osteogenesis, that leads to bone production and lengthening, is similar to what follows in case of bone fracture, incidental, or surgical as in corrective osteotomies. Bone formation starts right

Dentofacial and Occlusal Asymmetries, First Edition. Edited by Birte Melsen and Athanasios E. Athanasiou.
© 2025 John Wiley & Sons Ltd. Published 2025 by John Wiley & Sons Ltd.

after osteotomy and stabilization of the distraction device (distractor). A hematoma is formed at the osteotomy region and inflammatory cells and infiltrates arrive there due to the presence of cytokines IL-1 and IL-6. In the beginning, an osteoclastic activity is observed at the osteotomy edges and then pluripotent cells create new tissue and new vessels (angiogenesis). Several chemical agents and particularly transforming growth factors, as TGF-β1, are found in increased quantities, which seem to play a major role in creating collagen and non-collagenous matrix. Mineralization and remodeling follows, ending up to new bone formation (Singh et al. 2016).

Gradual distancing of the bony edges at the osteotomy site does not seem to influence the final ossification result of the produced gap, provided that the distractor offers stability to the osteotomized bony edges.

Staging of Distraction Osteogenesis

DO is a lengthy process, performed in four stages. The first stage refers to the operation, under general anesthesia. Following surgical procedures, the osteotomy of deficient bone is performed and the distractor is fixed in place. A latency phase usually lasting 1–3 days follows for soft tissue wound healing and callus formation procedure.

The second stage is the activation of the device, which is initiated by the gradual widening, 1 mm per day, of the gap created between the bone fragments. There is no need for any type of anesthesia during this phase.

The third stage is a consolidation phase which is initiated once the distracted bone has reached the preselected length and usually lasts twice as long as the activation phase. In maxillary cases, this phase can last up to 1 year.

There is also a short-lasting fourth stage, where the distraction device is removed; it is performed under general anesthesia in children under 14 years of age.

Indications for Distraction Osteogenesis

DO has a wide range of applications in maxillofacial region, such as in cases of asymmetries associated with syndromes, trauma, rheumatoid arthritis, or tumor resection, as well as in pre-implant surgery. DO is most often applied in children, taking additional advantage of the fast-growing process at this period of life, offering both esthetic and functional improvement to young patients.

Mandibular DO most often associated with airway obstruction, is applied in cases of severe retrognathia, micrognathia, mandibular asymmetry, craniofacial syndromes such as Goldenhar, Treacher Collins and Nager syndrome, hemifacial microsomia and P. Robin sequence. As reported in the literature, DO was initially used in children for mandibular elongation and since then has been most often applied in this region, compared to maxillary or mid-facial procedures (Swennen et al. 2001); long-term follow-up results of early mandibular DO cases have been reported and discussed (Ow and Cheung 2008). Findings showed a degree of relapse and the return of asymmetry with growth. In these cases, repetition of DO has been suggested (Ascenceo et al. 2014; Meazzini et al. 2012; Nagy et al. 2009).

Main indications for *maxillary DO* include moderate and major dentofacial deformities, severe maxillary deficiencies of various etiologies, such as syndromic children, with sleep apnea, or with cleft palate as well as cases with failure of previous attempts to solve those problems. Maxillary DO was first reported in 1999; external distractor was applied in the beginning and later an internal device was also introduced (Figueroa et al. 1999; Figueroa and Polley 2007). In cases of maxillary/mid-facial distraction, the main aim is a gradual advancement of the maxilla or the frontomaxillary complex in the posterior–anterior direction. Frontofacial monobloc advancement, in cases of craniosynostoses, has also been reported (Marchac and Arnaud 2012).

Early DO contributes significantly to the relief of upper airway obstruction, due to the posterior position of the mandible or the maxilla, especially in cases of syndromic neonates or infants with severe retrognathia or micrognathia (Shand 2015). In these cases, the tongue not having enough space, takes a posterior position resulting in partial obstruction and early tracheostomy can become necessary. Further treatment with DO will elongate the mandible and will create space for the tongue thus providing a real functional rehabilitation. Mandibular DO is considered as the most indicated therapy to eliminate upper airway obstruction in babies to achieve their decannulation, if present (i.e. removal of their tracheostomy), and relieve them from problems associated with feeding, sleep apnea, and snoring (Iatrou et al. 2010). According to a relatively recent systematic review, obstructive sleep apnea in cases of retrognathia, treated with DO, was successful in 90–100% of the cases (Tsui et al. 2016). Especially in cleft patients, where maxillary advancement with DO has been achieved, a relatively high possibility of skeletal relapse has been reported, indicating the need for overcorrection; the latter is required mostly in cases of incorrect primary procedures and scar formation (Liu and Zhou 2018). Fronto-maxillary distraction can be selected in synostosis patients; in these cases, brain damage is prevented, the upper airway space is enlarged, exophthalmia is corrected, and the face improves esthetically.

DO can be selected to correct mandibular defects caused by severe trauma or tumor resection in children. In addition, cases of temporomandibular joint ankylosis or those of stable juvenile rheumatoid arthritis, leading to asymmetrical development of the mandible, can be improved with DO.

The Distractors and Their Function

Nowadays the distractors are titanium made. They are fabricated in different types, sizes, and shapes to fulfill the previously described needs. Distractors are mainly categorized to those for mandibular lengthening, and those specialized for the maxillary and/or midface and upper-face advancement. The devices are screw or pin retained. Their mechanism, depending on the type of distractor, is either internal with plates and monocortical screws or external with pins; screws or pins, most often three on each osteotomy site, are fixed on each side of the osteotomized bone, allowing the distraction osteogenesis.

The internal devices consist of an expanding mechanism, two malleable plates, one at each side of the mechanism, and a rod within a cylinder which remains approachable postoperatively. The plates, regular, L or T in shape, are scheduled for at least three monocortical screws each, for infants up to 1 year old and for 4–6 screws for older children. The screw length should not exceed 3–5 mm, to protect teeth buds or apices and the inferior mandibular neurovascular bundle. The screws, in difficult to be approached sites as the mandibular angle, can be inserted with special, long, and angulated handpiece. By manually rotating the rod with the screwdriver provided, the device is activated and space is created between the plates and consequently between the edges of the osteotomized bone.

Mandible: Both types of distractors are used for mandibular DO, with internal devices being the first choice; they are inserted and fixed on the buccal mandibular surface intraorally or via a submandibular approach. Depending on the approach, the bar is located intraorally or extraorally. For external distraction, pins are inserted percutaneously and secured in the mandible on one end and the other end is connected to the extraoral distractor. In any case, distractors for mandibular DO are placed either unilaterally in cases of facial hemi-microsomia or bilaterally in cases of mandibular micrognathia.

Maxilla and midface: Maxillary DO is performed most often with external distractors and more recently with internal ones. For external distraction, the concept being to advance the maxilla, one part of the distractor is fixed to the maxilla (to the teeth or to the bone), and the other part to the cranium. During operation, an external metallic wreath is stabilized horizontally with 2–6 screws, on each lateral side of the cranium, 3–4 cm over the ear helix, where the bone is thick enough. The tooth-borne component, in cases of permanent dentition, has been preoperatively adapted by the orthodontist; in cases of mixed dentition, a bone-borne component is intraoperatively adapted to the maxilla. After performing the osteotomy (in LeFort I, II, or even III level), the cranial part of the distractor relates to the maxillary part with external components and shafts which are scheduled for gradual distraction. Upon activation, the osteotomized maxilla moves forward up to the pre-selected point. The same procedure can be applied in cases of frontofacial monobloc advancement. Internal devices for anterior maxillary advancement are based on the same concept and similar devices, as those for mandibular distraction. Recent developments in maxillary distractors include an antirelapse ratchet, hooks on the plates for additional use of guiding elastics, and a swivel joint, to facilitate the cranial adaptation of the distractor and allow compensation of exercised undesirable forces.

More recent publications point out the advantages of internal distractors; they are better tolerated by the patients in comparison to the external ones, which may become intimidating and cumbersome to both patients and clinicians (Combs and Harshbarger 2014).

Resorbable distractors have been introduced for mandibular DO (Burstein 2008); nevertheless, by the experience acquired from resorbable osteosynthesis plates, they probably are not stable and strong enough for DO, compared to metallic ones.

Preoperative Patient Evaluation

A well-organized pediatric maxillofacial surgery unit in a pediatric hospital, with the special armamentarium required for DO, as well as access to the hospital Intensive Care Unit, are the prerequisites to proceed to an osteogenesis distraction operation. For better results, a team collaboration approach between experts is advocated including pediatrician, pediatric maxillofacial surgeon, orthodontist, and pediatric dentist. The operation is performed under general anesthesia.

Patients' selection needs to be careful, as there are several general, anesthesiologic, and surgical limitations. As in every scheduled operation, a thorough preparation is required, including medical and dental history followed by clinical and laboratory findings.

Diagnostic imaging with panoramic X-rays (in children over 4 years of age), cone beam computer tomograms (CBCTs), and CTs with three-dimensional (3D) reconstructions are needed; existing bone volume is evaluated to ensure that it is adequate, before proceeding to bone osteotomy and insertion of the DO device. Photographs of the patient's face are also helpful for evaluation of postoperative changes and possible relapse. Additional contribution to the treatment planning is made nowadays with the 3D virtual models of the jaws of the child; they provide information about the type, vector, and insertion approach of the distraction device.

Preoperative anesthesiologic evaluation in children with severe deficiency or asymmetry of the jaws needs to be thorough. Findings like difficult mouth opening, laryngomalacia, and mechanical airway obstruction due to glossoptosis, need to be preevaluated. Another finding resulting to partial airway obstruction may be laryngeal insufficiency due to grown, very soft laryngeal tissues above the vocal cords, which fall in towards the airway. In this case, a tracheostomy may be needed independently and regardless of the existence of jaw deformities to be corrected with DO. Polysomnography is useful to record any sleep disorders. Intra-operatively, a nasotracheal intubation is preferred; the tube, depending on the patient's needs, can be inserted either using a video laryngoscope or a fiberoptic bronchoscopic device.

Further attention should be given if concomitant neurologic conditions exist, as in the case of hypotonic or hyperkinetic patients. The first patient's type may show delay in recovering from anesthesia. Further hospitalization, in Intensive Care Unit, is required until airway passage is completely free and the whole breathing and swallowing function becomes normal. Patients with sleep apnea due to central deficiencies, will not take advantage by lengthening their jaws. Hyperkinetic, noncompliant, or anxious patients may move or remove the distractor; treatment with sedatives and/or hand bandage will help.

Surgical Procedure

Mandibular Distraction Osteogenesis

The most frequent osteotomy site is the mandibular angle, although others prefer the ramus or the body. When planning the osteotomy, the vector of distraction is taken into consideration to place the device accordingly.

Intraoral distraction: A buccal mucoperiosteal flap is raised at the preselected site. Intraoperatively, the device is adapted at the buccal surface of the mandible before the osteotomy, considering that the osteotomy line will be performed between the two plates; its final position is secured by drilling the screw holes. Then the device is removed, and the osteotomy is performed; a corticotomy is preferred, buccally and lingually, with special attention to preserve the inferior alveolar neurovascular bundle. A reciprocal handpiece with a fine bur or a protected disk is used. The cutting line should remain between the prepared holes of each plate. Then the distraction device is placed and fixed finally with the screws in the prepared holes. Full mobilization of the fragmented bone and good function of the distractor are tested prior to wound closure with 3-0 resorbable suture (Figure 12.7.1). Depending on the type of asymmetry, osteotomies are unilateral or bilateral (Figure 12.7.2).

The main advantages of the intraoral distraction are the avoidance of any type of skin scar on the face of the patient and its possible consequences. Furthermore, the risk of any kind of damage to the marginal branch of the facial nerve is minimal in comparison to the extraoral approach. When intraorally, the device is better protected in cases of noncompliant or anxious patients. However, there are *l*imitations concerning the intraoral insertion, which is not advocated for neonates, babies, and little children up to 4 years of age because of the limited access conditions due to the very small dimensions of the childrens' mouth.

Extraoral distraction: Indications for this approach are related to the selection of devices immobilized with external pins, or to intentional selection of extraoral approach with the use of conventional distractors. For the insertion of a pin-related distractor, an intraoral approach as previously described, is performed without fully completing the corticotomy; then an extraoral percutaneous application of pins, 2 or 3 on each side of the corticotomy, in a safety distance of 5 mm away of it, is performed. The pins are then connected to the extraoral device. At this stage, corticotomy can be completed and the whole system should be tested before wound closure (Walker 2011) (Figure 12.7.3).

In cases of extraoral insertion of a distraction device, a Risdon-type submandibular approach is recommended. The steps of the procedure are carefully followed, by incising through skin, subcutaneous, and platysma muscle, identifying and protecting the marginal branch of the facial nerve, dissecting, clamping, transecting, and ligating the facial artery and vein. After raising the buccal flap, a periosteal incision at the lower rim of the mandible is undertaken. Periosteal elevation follows both at the buccal and lingual side of the mandible so that adequate bony surface is exposed for the insertion of the distraction apparatus. The operation after that is like the previously described osteotomy approach (Figure 12.7.4).

The main advantage of this operation is that the surgeon has a wider operative field compared to a small mouth and a difficult intraoral approach, and at the same time, adaptation and immobilization of the

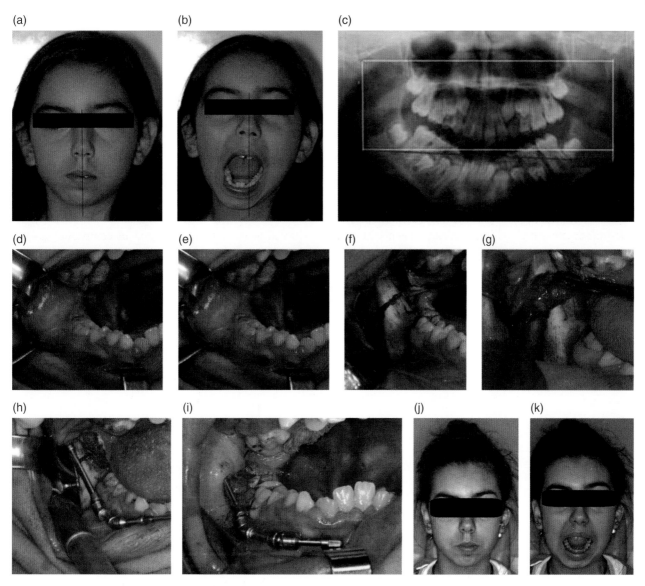

Figure 12.7.1 Girl 11 years old with rheumatoid arthritis affecting the right TMJ and causing asymmetry of the lower part of the face, treated with intraoral distraction. (a) Preoperative image; (b) with mouth opening the asymmetry becomes more obvious; (c) panoramic radiograph view; (d) intraoral view; (e) mucoperiosteal incision; (f) flap elevation and corticotomy at the mandibular angle region; (g) preservation of the inferior mandibular alveolar neurovascular angle; (h) adaptation and insertion of the screw related distraction device; (i) wound closure; (j) improved postoperative view 1 year later; (k) improvement of the asymmetry may be seen with complete mouth opening as well.

apparatus is more convenient. Disadvantages of this method are scar tissue formation at the face of the patient, unintentional removal of the device, paresis, or even paralysis of the marginal mandibular branch of the facial nerve.

Maxillary Distraction Osteogenesis

Treatment planning includes collaboration between surgeon and orthodontist and depends on the patients' age and dentition as well as on the severity of the problem.

Internal distraction: The main steps of this procedure are the placement of fixed orthodontic appliances with wires and surgical hooks, preparation of an acrylic interdental splint and selection and model adaptation of the appropriate maxillary distractor. The acrylic splint is used to maintain intraoperatively the preoperative dental occlusion after the LeFort osteotomy, so that the application of the distractor may be achieved without any tension at the best possible place. The orthodontic appliances will be used after completion of the scheduled maxillary advancement, to achieve the best possible dental occlusion.

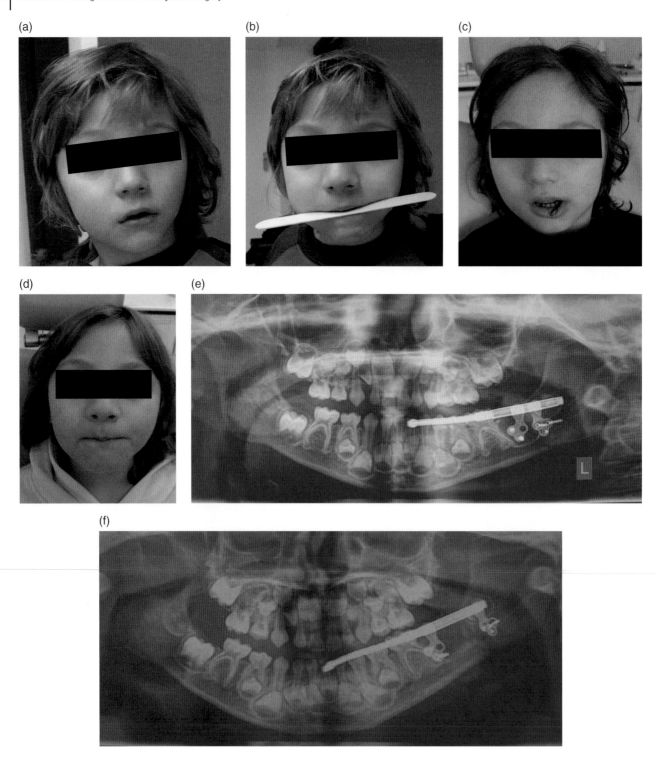

Figure 12.7.2　Boy 5 years old with facial asymmetry due to Goldenhar syndrome. (a) Preoperative image; (b) preoperative image using an occlusal spatula; (c) the intraoral distractor in place. The distraction bar is visible in the mouth of the child; (d) final result after 1 year; (e) panoramic radiograph view immediately after insertion of the device; (f) panoramic radiograph view before removing the distractor. Ossification of the created gap may be seen.

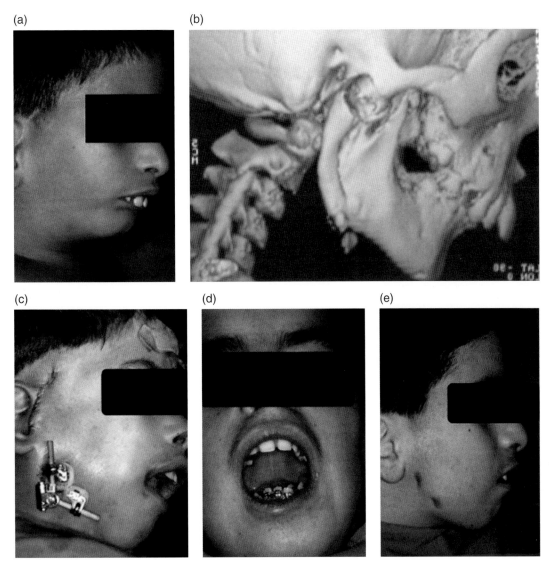

Figure 12.7.3 Boy 5 years old with mandibular hypoplasia due to severe trauma of both temporomandibular joints. (a) Preoperative image; (b) three-dimensional CT showing replacement of the joint with pleural autotransplant; (c) application of an extraoral pin distractor; (d) improvement of mandibular size; (e) however, two scars are visible at the buccal skin of the face, which can easily be corrected with plastic surgery later on.

Intraoperatively, a vestibular incision of the mucosa 5 mm above the mucogingival line between the two zygomatic buttresses is performed. The incision should be limited in the mucosa leaving the underlying muscular tissue undestroyed. An incision of the periosteum is further undertaken and its meticulous detachment cranially follows in order to achieve a clear maxillary and zygomatic osseous surface. Precise adaptation and fixation of the distractors at the zygoma and the maxilla bilaterally follows; then the devices are removed and the osteotomy at the previously selected level, is carried out. The distractors are finally stabilized and an undisturbed mobilization of the bony segment in the predetermined vector is checked. Following hemostasis, the wound is sutured, with the distractor's bar lying gently in the vestibule.

Extraoral distraction: It is selected when the need for an anterior movement of the maxilla is over 1.5 cm. As previously described in the relevant chapter, the distractor is stabilized or anchored with pins or with the use of special plates fixed with screws or a wreath in the lateral cranial vault and in the maxillary bone or in the upper dentition via an arch bar. The operation is performed intraorally for the Le Fort osteotomy and the fixation of the intraoral part of the device and with percutaneous approach at the cranium for the external part (Figure 12.7.5).

Postoperative Procedure – Activation of the Device

The patient should not be extubated in cases of excessive swelling, or in case of any doubt concerning his ability to breathe normally. Transfer to the Intensive Care Unit overnight or for as long as it is required should be considered. Once extubation is carried out the child remains hospitalized for few days for observation and to check its ability for liquid or soft diet intake. Soon the device is activated by the surgeon initially in the presence of the parents; they need to be given instructions and get used to the procedure, which they will perform at home.

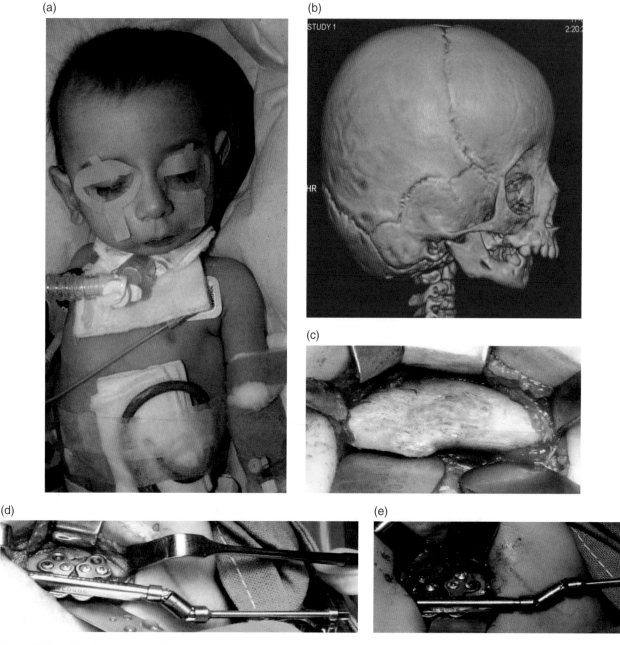

Figure 12.7.4 Boy 6 months old with excessive micrognathia due to P. Robin sequence. Despite the esthetic problem, the situation has caused severe breathing and feeding problems jeopardizing his life and leading to tracheostomy and gastrostomy. (a) preoperative image; (b) three dimensional CT scan, showing a 2.5 cm gap between upper and lower dentition; (c) intraoperative image showing the preparation of the mandibular angle and body; (d) insertion and adaptation of the distractor; (e) corticotomy of the mandible; the prepared holes and the interior alveolar bundle are visible; (f) distraction device back in its place; (g) suture of the wound. The movable bar remains extra orally; (h) radiograph of the patient; (i) operation has achieved 2 cm bilateral lengthening of the mandibular body; (j) the patient at the age of 2 years old, enjoying his milk; (k) the patient at the age of four years old.

(f) (g) (h)

(i) (j) (k)

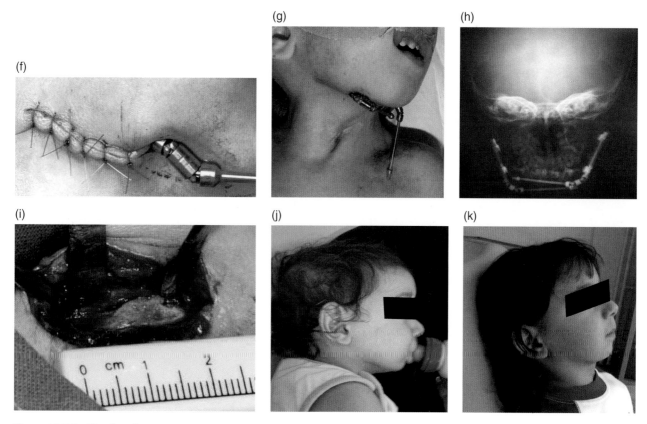

Figure 12.7.4 (Continued)

In case of feeding difficulties, a nasogastric feeding tube should be used for as long as needed (Walker 2011). The procedure is gradual and long-lasting, so a close observation of the patient is recommended to prevent and avoid any kind of complications.

Once the activation phase is finished, a following latency period should last twice as much. In this time interval that usually lasts 2–3 months, time is given to the ossification of the newly formed bone within the osteotomy-produced gap. Good function of the mandible and creation of bone are tested with radiographs. Attention should be given during the consolidation period in cases of maxillary advancement, which usually lasts 3–9 months but may need to last up to 1 year.

The device is removed at this stage, under general anesthesia. Follow-up of the patients should last for at least the end of puberty, since in several cases, especially concerning asymmetries and hemifacial microsomia patients, an additional orthognathic operation may be needed.

For optimal results, orthodontic treatment should take place, especially in cases of mixed or permanent dentition during the distraction and consolidation periods on a monthly basis, to prevent and occasionally correct dental and occlusal discrepancies.

Complications

Surgical complications likely to occur in any operation may include hemorrhage, accidental tooth or bud injury, swelling, formation of hematoma, wound infection, or wound dehiscence; in extraoral approaches, the main possible complications are trauma of the mandibular branch of the facial nerve, hemorrhage and scar tissue formation. All can be minimized with proper surgical techniques, meticulous hemostasis, and careful follow-up. Especially in cases of external pins or the functional device bar, thorough local cleaning with Betadine solution and H_2O_2 will help avoiding local infection.

Midfacial distraction can also be associated, fortunately rarely, with major complications as cerebrospinal fluid leaks or meningitis (Knackstedt et al. 2018).

Device-related complications include infection of the screw area, loss of a screw in the soft tissues, loosening of the device, device malfunction, osseous malunion, failure of the distraction process due to anticlockwise turning of the activation arm. Fortunately, most of those complications can be treated with a second interventional approach.

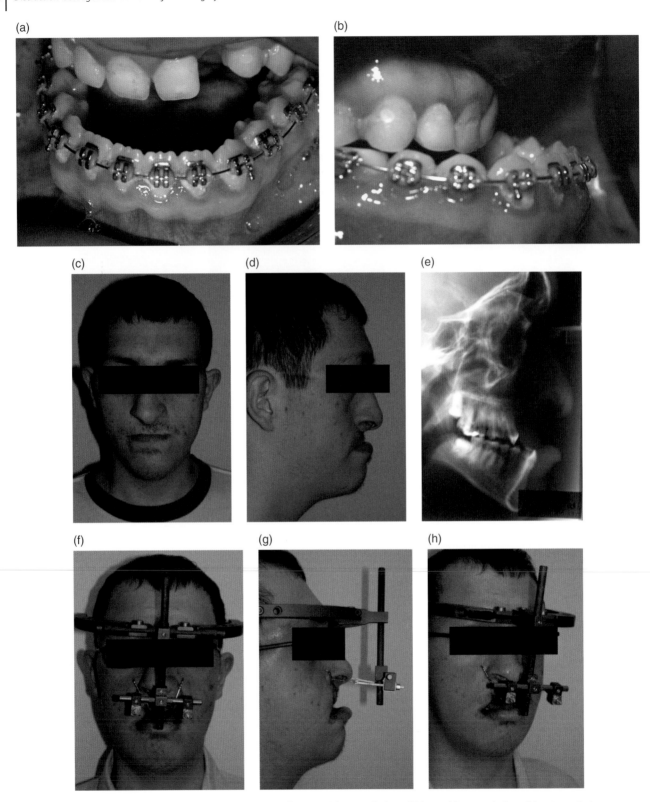

Figure 12.7.5 Boy 13 years old with severe upper micrognathia. (a) Intraoral view; (b) lateral intraoral view; (c) extraoral view; (d) lateral extraoral view; (e) lateral cephalometric radiograph; (f, g, and h) extra-orally pin fixated tooth-borne distractor; (i, j and k) postoperative view 11 months after the operation; (l and m) postoperative intraoral views. (Courtesy of Dr. John Fakitsas).

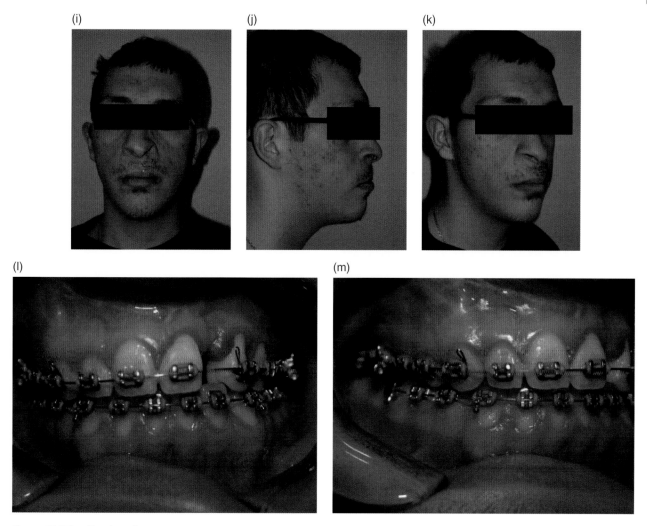

Figure 12.7.5 (Continued)

Possibility of relapse of asymmetry up to 64.8%, during growth, especially in cases of hemifacial macrosomia, as mentioned, can be considered among late complications (Master et al. 2010).

Orthodontic Collaboration

In neonates and infants, the role of the orthodontist is not so important as it is in young children and adolescents. In those ages, orthodontist is the main collaborator of the maxillofacial surgeon.

As in conventional orthognathic surgery cases, for the correction of facial asymmetries, oral and maxillofacial surgeon and orthodontist should work together in planning and supporting the patients. Especially in cases of DO, this collaboration should be maximized. The two specialists proceed to pre-distraction assessment of the

occlusal and skeletal status of the patient. Furthermore, the orthodontist plans both the pre-distraction and post-distraction orthodontic care.

Based on careful clinical examination and all imaging findings, the orthodontist, in collaboration with the oral and maxillofacial surgeon, plan DO, the device placement, and the suitable vectors of distraction. They both follow closely the patient during the distractor activation period. In this phase, additional teeth-borne (teeth-based) measures as use of intermaxillary elastics, sometimes combined with guidance splints, and stabilization arches are used to mold the newly formed bone which will optimize the status of the dental occlusion; the latter, gradually alters during distraction process and needs to be corrected accordingly (Grayson and Santiago 1999). By means of the entire orthodontic procedure, both dental occlusion and newly formed bone are stabilized. However, genetic factors may still influence the final growth process; close long-term follow-up by both specialists is of great value to timely prevent and treat any developing irregularities.

Distraction Osteogenesis and/or Conventional Orthognathic Surgery

Mandible: There is no doubt that mandibular DO is an option for treating Class II malocclusion (Bialobrzeska and Dowgierd 2016). However, if great advancement of the mandible in early ages is required unilateral or bilateral, mandibular DO appears to be the only procedure to achieve it. Conventional orthognathic methods, as sagittal split osteotomy, are not selected during development; additionally, no great extension in one stage, can be exercised to the mandibular neurovascular bundle.

Maxilla: Advancement of the maxillary complex in cases of hypoplasia or retrusion has been used for over 60 years with great success and sufficiency from maxillofacial surgeons who more often applied Le Fort I and rather rarely Le Fort II or Le Fort III osteotomies. However, these osteotomies have limitations concerning the age of the patient and the degree of advancement that can be performed in one step. The age of the patient according to most applied protocols, should be over 16 or 17 years and the amount of the anterior movement of the maxilla should not exceed 1 cm. Furthermore, in several cases a supplementary bone transplant is needed, adding to the morbidity rates of this procedure. Maxillary DO seems to overcome the above-mentioned restrictions; however, there are several differences between the two methods.

In rather extended studies where the treatment of maxillary retrognathia in cleft palate patients, via DO, was compared to orthognathic surgery, better skeletal stability in the distraction group and significant relapse in the conventional surgery group were reported (Cheung et al. 2006). In terms of stability and relapse, as well as about growth after distraction, the results showed greater maxillary advancement with DO with improved stability over time and further maxillary growth in growing patients (Baek et al. 2007; Rachmiel et al. 2012).

It is understood that DO should not be applied in patients who underwent radiotherapy, in cases with insufficient bone quantity and quality, as well as in not collaborating patient and family environment (Guerrero et al. 1999).

Conclusion

There is no doubt that DO, as applied in the facial skeleton, is a very useful and scientifically efficient method of lengthening facial bones. Its help in cases of syndromes needing tracheostomy to breath or gastrostomy to be fed is undisputable. However, the first enthusiastic reports of the 1990s, that this method could be the solution for every problem related to facial asymmetry, either in the coronal or the sagittal plane, have been lately revised with more moderate opinions.

While most of the bilateral asymmetries in the sagittal plane (Pierre Robin sequence, cleft, or micrognathia cases), are adequately treated with DO, in cases of asymmetries in the coronal plane (Goldenhar syndrome and hemifacial macrosomia cases), DO does not provide the definite solution. Although there is a significant improvement, in these latter cases, a final conventional orthognathic surgery procedure, including enlargement of the soft tissues, is usually needed.

References

Ascenceo ASK, Balbinot P, Maluf I Jr, D'Oro U, Busato L, da Silva FR. Mandibular distraction in hemifacial microsomia is not a permanent treatment: a long-term evaluation. J Craniofac Surg. 2014;25:352–354.

Baek SH, Lee JK, Lee JH, Kim MJ, Kim JR. Comparison of treatment outcome and stability between distraction osteogenesis and Le Fort I osteotomy in cleft patients with maxillary hypoplasia. J Craniomaxillofac Surg. 2007;18:1209–1215.

Bialobrzeska A, Dowgierd K. Mandibular sagittal split osteotomy versus mandibular distraction osteogenesis in treatment of non-syndromic skeletal Class II patients. Polish Annals Med. 2016;23:21–25.

Burstein FD. Resorbable distraction of the mandible: technical evolution and clinical experience. J Craniofacial Surg. 2008;19:637–643.

Cheung LK, Chua HDP, Hägg UB. Cleft maxillary distraction versus orthognathic surgery: clinical morbidities and surgical relapse. Plast Reconstr Surg. 2006;118:996–1008.

Combs PD, Harshbarger RJ. Le Fort I maxillary advancement using distraction osteogenesis. Semin Plast Surg. 2014;28:193–198.

Diner PA, Kollar EM, Martinez H, Vazquez MP. Intraoral distraction for mandibular lengthening: a technical innovation. J Craniomaxillofac Surg. 1996;24:92–95.

Figueroa AA, Polley JW. Management of the severe cleft and syndromic midface hypoplasia. Orthod Craniofacial Res. 2007;10:167–179.

Figueroa AA, Polley JW, Ko EW. Maxillary distraction for the management of cleft maxillary hypoplasia with a rigid external distraction system. Semin Orthod. 1999;5:46–51.

Grayson BH, Santiago PE. Treatment planning and biomechanics of distraction osteogenesis from an orthodontic perspective. Semin Orthod. 1999;5:9–24.

Guerrero CA, Bell WH, Meza LS. Intraoral distraction osteogenesis: maxillary and mandibular lengthening. Atlas Oral Maxillofac Surg Clin North Am. 1999;7:111–151.

Iatrou I, Theologie-Lygidakis N, Schoinohoriti O. Mandibular distraction osteogenesis for severe airway obstruction in Robin Sequence. Case report. J Craniomaxillofac Surg. 2010;38:741–747.

Ilizarov GA, Devyatov AA, Kamerin VK. Plastic reconstruction of longitudinal bone defects by means of compression and subsequent distraction. Acta Chir Plast. 1980;22:32–41.

Ilizarov GA, Lediaev VI, Shitin VP. The course of compact bone reparative regeneration in distraction osteosynthesis under different conditions of bone fragment fixation (experimental study). Eksp Khir Anestesiol. 1969;14:3–12.

Knackstedt R, Gharb BB, Papay F, Rampazzo A. Comparison of complication rate between Le Fort III and monobloc advancement with or without distraction osteogenesis. J Craniofac Surg. 2018;29:144–148.

Liu K, Zhou N. Long-term skeletal changes after maxillary distraction osteogenesis in growing children with cleft lip and palate. J Craniofac Surg. 2018;29:349–352.

Marchac A, Arnaud E. Cranium and midface distraction osteogenesis: current practices, controversies, and future applications. J Craniofac Surg. 2012;23:235–238.

Master DL, Hanson PR, Gosaln AK. Complications of mandibular distraction osteogenesis. J Craniofac Surg. 2010;21:1565–1570.

McCarthy J, Schreiber J, Karp N, Thorne C, Grayson B. Lengthening the human mandible by gradual distraction. Plast Recostr Surg. 1992;89:92–95.

Meazzini MC, Mazzoleni F, Bozzeti A, Brusati R. Comparison of mandibular vertical growth in hemifacial microsomia patients treated with early distraction or not treated: follow-up till the completion of growth. J Craniomaxillofac Surg. 2012;40:105–111.

Moore MH, Guzman-Stein G, Proudman TW, Abbott AH, Netherway DJ, David DJ. Mandibular lengthening by distraction for airway obstruction in Treacher-Collins syndrome. J Craniofac Surg. 1994;5:22–25.

Nagy K, Kuijpers-Jagtman AM, Mommaerts MY. No evidence for long-term effectiveness of early osteodistraction in hemifacial microsomia. Plast Reconstr Surg. 2009;124:2061–2071.

Ow ATC, Cheung LK. Meta-analysis of mandibular distraction osteogenesis: clinical applications and functional outcomes. Plast Reconstr Surg. 2008;121:54e–69e.

Peltier LF. Fractures: A History and Iconography of Their Treatment. Norman Orthopedic Series 1. San Francisco: Norman Publishing, 1990.

Rachmiel A, Even-Almos M, Aizenbud D. Treatment of maxillary cleft palate: distraction osteogenesis vs. orthognathic surgery. Ann Maxillofac Surg. 2012;2:127–130.

Rossini G, Vinci B, Rizzo R, Pinho TMD, Deregibus A. Mandibular distraction osteogenesis: a systematic review of stability on hard and soft tissues. Int J Oral Maxillofac Surg. 2016;45:1438–1444.

Shand JM. Mandibular distraction in infancy. In: Kademani D, Tiwana PS, eds. Atlas of Oral and Maxillofacial Surgery. St. Louis: Elsevier, 2015:332–340.

Singh M, Vashistha A, Chaudhary M, Kaur G. Biological basis of distraction osteogenesis – a review. J Oral Maxillofac Surg Med Path. 2016;28:1–7.

Swennen G, Schliephake H, Dempf R, Schierle H, Malevez C. Craniofacial distraction osteogenesis: a review of the literature. Part I: clinical studies. Int J Oral Maxillofac Surg. 2001;30:89–103.

Tsui WK, Yang Y, Cheung LK, Leung YY. Distraction osteogenesis as a treatment of obstructive sleep apnea syndrome. A systematic review. Medicine (Baltimore). 2016;95:e4674.

Walker DA. Mandibular distraction osteogenesis by intraoral and extraoral techniques. In: Langdon J, Patel M, Ord R, Brennan P, eds. Operative Oral and Maxillofacial Surgery. London: Hodder and Stoughton, 2011:659–674.

Wangerin K, Gropp H. Die enorale Distraktionsosteotomie des mikrogenen Unterkiefers zur Beseitigung der Atemwegsobstruktion. Dtsch Z Mund Kiefer Gesichtschir. 1994;18:236–242.

Wangerin K, Gropp H. Mandibular distraction osteogenesis using intraorally applied devices. In: Härle F, Champy M, Terry B, eds. Atlas of Craniomaxillofacial Osteosynthesis: Miniplates, Microplates, and Screws. Stuttgart: Thieme, 1999:200–209.

12.8

Maxillo-mandibular Growth in Hemifacial (or Craniofacial) Microsomia

Maria Costanza Meazzini di Seyssel

Introduction – Clinical Appearance

Hemifacial microsomia (HFM) (or craniofacial microsomia) is characterized by facial asymmetry, even when bilateral (10–30%) (Burglen et al. 2001). There is a great variability in clinical manifestations. Derivatives of the first branchial arch (ramus, mandibular condyle, ramus and body, temporomandibular joint (TMJ), maxilla, masticatory muscles, oral commissure, and some components of the ear), or of both the first and second arch (the facial nerve may be affected, totally or partially and other segments of the ears). The mandibular ramus together with the coronoid process on the affected side, are short, or absent. The mandibular angle is more cranial and medial relative to the contralateral; the chin is deviated to the affected side and the occlusal plane is often oblique (Bettega et al. 2001). The TMJ may be affected with different levels of severity. Its severity has guided the classification of Pruzansky (1969) for the mandibular deformity in HFM, which was later modified by Kaban et al. (1988) (Figure 12.8.1a–d). The cheek is generally flattened because

of the hypoplastic musculature. Often the temporal muscles and the masseter muscles are fused together in the temporo-masseter sling (Marsh et al. 1989).

Gorlin et al. (2001) proposed to group under the denomination "Ocular auricular vertebral spectrum" the isolated asymmetrical forms of oto-mandibular dysostosis and Goldenhar syndrome (10% of the cases) or ocular auricular dysplasia.

Throughout this chapter, we shall keep the classical denomination HFM.

Craniofacial Growth in Hemifacial Microsomia

Long-term Growth in Nontreated Hemifacial Microsomia Patients

One of the most controversial topics in the literature regards the progressive nature of the clinical asymmetry during growth of a patient affected by HFM. It has been

(a)

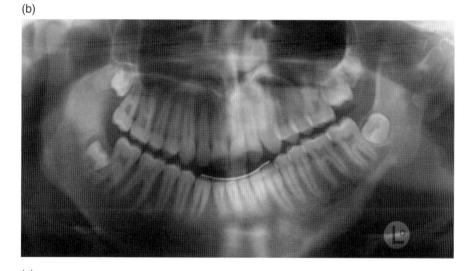

(b)

(c)

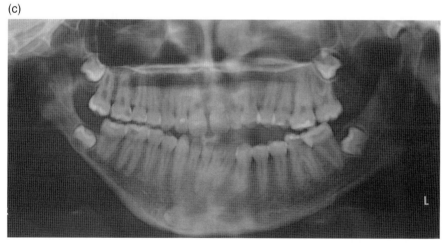

Figure 12.8.1 Patient affected by an HFM with mandibular deformity Type I: the condyle and ramus are normal but smaller (a). Mandibular deformity Type IIa: the condyle is deformed in terms of shape and size, but the relationship with the glenoid fossa is maintained (b). Type IIb: the condyle is severely deformed in terms of shape and size. The TMJ is rudimentary and anteriorly and medially dislocated (c). Type III: the condyle, the coronoid process, the TMJ, and the proximal portion of the ramus are absent (d).

(d)

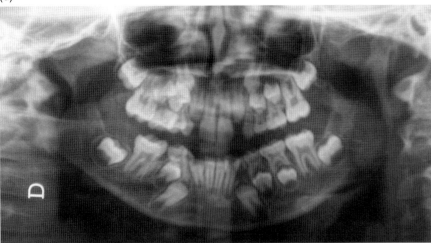

Figure 12.8.1 (Continued)

suggested that the anomaly worsens during growth and the facial asymmetry of the child becomes more severe with time (Converse et al. 1973; Murray et al. 1984; Kearns et al. 2000). This is what occurs, for example, in a child with a unilateral ankylosis of the TMJ. The progressiveness of the asymmetry would dictate the need for surgery as early as possible. Other authors, on the contrary, suggested that the asymmetry in HFM is not progressive. Polley et al. (1997), following the growth from 6 months of age till the end of craniofacial growth of 26 HFM nonoperated patients on serial posteroanterior cephalometric X-rays, collected by Pruzansky, have demonstrated that the affected side of the mandible continues to grow with a rate that maintains the vertical ratio between both sides. The same was concluded in a later longitudinal study on panoramic X-rays, calculating the ratio between affected and nonaffected side, of untreated type I and II patients, from 5 years till the completion of growth (Meazzini et al. 2012). These findings mean that the facial proportion of the patient affected by HFM is maintained throughout the whole process of craniofacial growth (Figure 12.8.2). As noted by Mommaerts and Nagy (2002), much confusion exists between the rate of growth, meaning the yearly amount of growth, and the ratio between the affected and the nonaffected side. Authors who studied patients longitudinally and not cross-sectionally, as Kearns et al. (2000), noted that the growth of the affected side maintains the same proportion, in the same patient, relative to the nonaffected side so that the degree of asymmetry and neuro-muscular architecture remain constant during development (Rune et al. 1981; Polley et al. (1997); Meazzini et al. 2012; Ongkosuwito et al. 2013).

Is Maxillary Growth in Hemifacial Microsomia Inhibited by Mandibular Growth?

Another long-believed "dogma" in HFM literature is that early surgery is also indicated to prevent maxillary and zygomatic deformities, which are believed to be secondary to a primary mandibular deformity (Kaban et al. 1998). Padwa et al. (1998) suggested to perform costochondral grafting (CCG) in early adolescence, to "unlock" maxillary growth. A way to evaluate the hypothesized influence of mandibular hypoplasia on maxillary growth is to look at studies conducted on patients affected by HFM subjected to unilateral mandibular surgical lengthening. In these patients, the "deforming" effect of the hypoplastic mandible on the maxillary complex has been "removed" by mandibular lengthening, consequently, "uninhibited" maxillary growth may be investigated. In a 5-year follow-up study on mandibular distraction osteogenesis (DO) in HFM, conducted on a very homogeneous sample in terms of age at the time of surgery (average age 5.6 ± 0.6 years) and in terms of the initial severity of the mandibular hypoplasia (type I and type II according to Pruzansky) patients were monitored with posteroanterior cephalometric X-rays immediately before surgery, and every year till the longest follow-up, 5.8 ± 0.4 years. After distraction, the asymmetry of the maxillary skeletal base (infra-orbital plane and in the nasal floor) was unchanged. On the contrary, the dentoalveolar component of the maxilla (occlusal plane inclination) was reduced significantly, as the distraction had created a gradually increasing open bite on the affected side, which was closed by eruption guidance. These data suggested that, thanks to DO, a significant dentoalveolar remodeling of the maxilla is possible, as every orthodontist

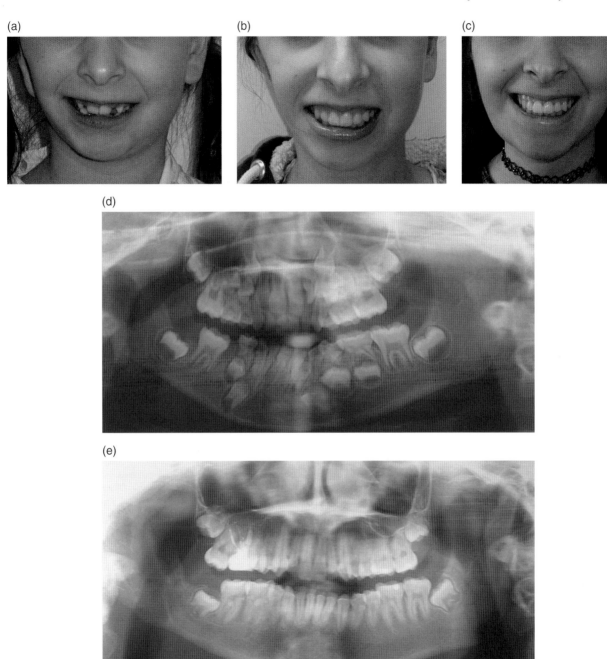

Figure 12.8.2 Nontreated female patient affected by HFM type III. Frontal facial photograph smiling at 6 years of age (a). Frontal smiling photograph of the patient at 16 years of age, never subjected to any surgery, only expansion and orthodontic alignment. Note that the degree of asymmetry did not change with growth and occlusal plane is only mildly canted (b). Frontal smiling photograph of the patient at 17 years of age, only subjected to lipofilling. Very low total burden of care (c). Panoramic radiograph at 6 years of age (d). Panoramic radiograph at 17 years of age. Note that there is no worsening of the asymmetry in 11 years (e).

knows, but no true skeletal modification of the maxilla can be obtained. Additionally, there was a gradual return toward the original occlusal plane inclination in the subsequent 5 years (Meazzini et al. 2005). Another very suitable example of effect of the "removal" of the distorting influence of the mandible on the maxillary bone, was a study after CCG, which showed comparable results to the study after DO, reporting occlusal plane improvement but no nasal floor improvement, thus no skeletal base "catch-up" growth (Padwa et al. 1997).

Therefore, it is reasonable to believe that the maxillary deformity in HFM is primary and associated to the embryological first branchial arch defect (maxilla and zygomatic arch are first branchial arch derivatives), and this is the reason why there is no spontaneous correction of the maxillary skeletal base when the mandibular interference is eliminated. Only the dentoalveolar component of the maxilla may be temporarily remodeled, both after DO and CCG. These data contradict the previous "conviction" that early surgery might actually prevent the "supposed" secondary adaptation of the maxilla, zygoma, and soft tissues to mandibular deformity (David 2018).

Long-term Growth After Distraction Osteogenesis of the Mandible

In the study mentioned (Meazzini et al. 2005), it was also shown that in terms of ratio between the affected ramus and the nonaffected ramus; at the end of distraction, there was excellent facial and mandibular symmetry, with some overcorrection. Nevertheless, 5 years post-distraction already much of the correction in terms of ratio obtained with DO was lost. In a subsequent very long-term study, with a follow-up between 10 and 13 years post-DO, it was demonstrated that 100% of the correction, was lost, and the patients presented the same proportions they had pre-DO (Meazzini et al. 2012). In Figure 12.8.3, a follow-up 15 years post-DO in a patient affected by hemifacial microsomia Type II operated at 5.4 years of age is shown. In parallel, in Figure 12.8.4 a 13-year follow-up of a patient affected by HFM Type II who was never treated, showed maintenance of the same degree of asymmetry.

Can Functional Appliances Increase Postsurgical Stability After Distraction Osteogenesis?

In a very early study, on a small sample of patients subjected to DO, a recurrence of the mandibular morphology during the first year after distraction had already been reported (Meazzini et al. 1997). At the time, it was hoped that the association of functional jaw orthopedics might help reduce this recurrence of the phenotype. It was hypothesized that a pre-DO and post-DO orthopedic treatment, as suggested by Vargervik et al. (1986), might help maintain a better stability of the skeletal correction. The biological hypothesis was that muscles need a slower rate of elongation than bone, thus, early muscle stretching might improve stability (Simpson et al. 1995). In order to demonstrate whether the combined orthopedic-distraction treatment had any real advantage, we compared two groups of patients, treated consecutively with two different protocols. One group (treated in a different hospital) had no orthopedic preparation before or after DO (only occlusal guidance post-DO), while the second group had at least 1 year of orthopedic

treatment, with an asymmetric functional appliance, prior to DO and 1 year post-DO. The results of this study unfortunately eventually demonstrated that orthopedic treatment may initially slow down (Meazzini et al. 1999), but does not stop, the process of "return" to the original pattern of asymmetry and, again, the beneficial influence of orthopedic treatment expresses itself more at the dento-alveolar level then at a skeletal level (Meazzini et al. 2008a).

Final Considerations on Distraction Osteogenesis in Hemifacial Microsomia

Although the term "return" is usually not as clinically clear as the term "relapse," it was preferred, because what is truly happening in these patients, is not an actual relapse. Relapse refers to loss of the regenerate, whereas, in HFM, the return to the original pattern is related to a differential growth which is directly linked to the congenital pathological neuromuscular pattern of growth. Stability of the regenerate is usually measured during the first 6 months to 1 year after DO. The literature agrees that there is little loss of regenerate (relapse) after DO (Hollier et al. 1999). The controversy is more on long-term effects. DO guarantees the achievement of good symmetry in the short-term (Figure 12.8.3c). In the long-term, mandibular morphology is remodeled through a process of re-expression of the syndrome-specific pattern of growth (Figure 12.8.3d). The contradiction in HFM was originated by the belief that the growth of the patients was of a progressive nature. The literature, thanks to long-term longitudinal studies, seems now oriented toward the clinical indication that HFM patients, whether operated or not, present, at the end of growth, an asymmetry which has a very similar proportion to the initial disproportion (Hollier et al. 1999; Kusnoto et al. 1999; Huisinga-Fischer et al. 2003; Meazzini et al. 2005, 2012; Nagy et al. 2009; Suh et al. 2013; Ascenço et al. 2014). It is important to realize that DO is just a tool, extremely efficient in its ability to modify the skeletal structure of young patients, but not their genetic code. This knowledge forces us to select patients with great care and to be honest and transparent with families regarding long-term prognosis, making it very clear, that the hope that an early correction through DO will be a definitive procedure, is extremely unrealistic.

Long-term Results After Costochondral Graft in Growing Patients with Hemifacial Microsomia

CCG has been traditionally used in the growing population with severe mandibular hypoplasia (Type III). The rationale for the use of a CCG is that the cartilaginous portion of the rib graft is considered to have growth potential and adaptive capabilities. Nevertheless, many authors have

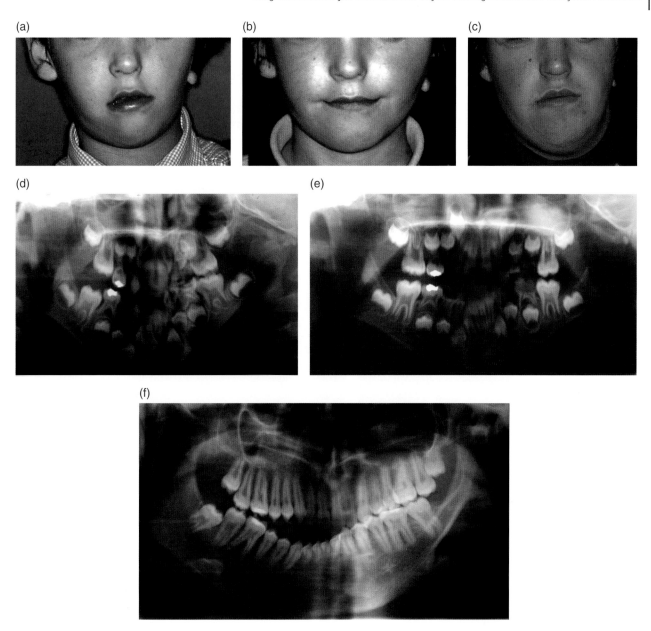

Figure 12.8.3 Male patient affected by HFM IIb treated with early DO: frontal facial photograph before DO at 5 years of age (a). Frontal facial photograph of the patient post-DO: note the symmetry achieved (b). Frontal facial photograph of the patient 15 years post-DO: note the recurrence of the asymmetry (c). Panoramic radiograph before DO (d). Panoramic radiograph 1 year post-DO, note the early tendency toward an asymmetrical growth (e). Panoramic radiograph of the patient 15 years post-DO: the ratio affected/nonaffected side has returned to the pre-DO ratio (f).

shown that the growth of a CCG is unpredictable (Guyuron and Lasa 1992) and not linear (Lindqvist et al. 1988; Mulliken et al. 1989).

In a recent longitudinal retrospective long-term case-control study, the growth after CCG of patients affected by HFM type III was compared with the growth of a non-treated matched type III HFM sample (Meazzini et al. 2020). Out of 70 procedures of ramus condyle reconstruction with CCG, performed between 1995 and 2006, to obtain a truly homogeneous sample in terms of type of pathology, severity, age at surgery, and length of follow-up (8 years post-CCG),

only growing patients (5–8 years) affected by HFM type III where included. A control sample of patients who were never offered or did not accept treatment during growth and were all HFM type III, with records in the early growing period (5–8 years) and records at 15–17 years prior to any other surgical procedure, was retrospectively collected. This was the first study in the literature to report long-term skeletal and soft tissue results in a sample of HFM type III Pruzansky patients treated with CCG at an early age, compared to a nontreated sample. The main limit of this study was the relatively small number of cases, although, this is

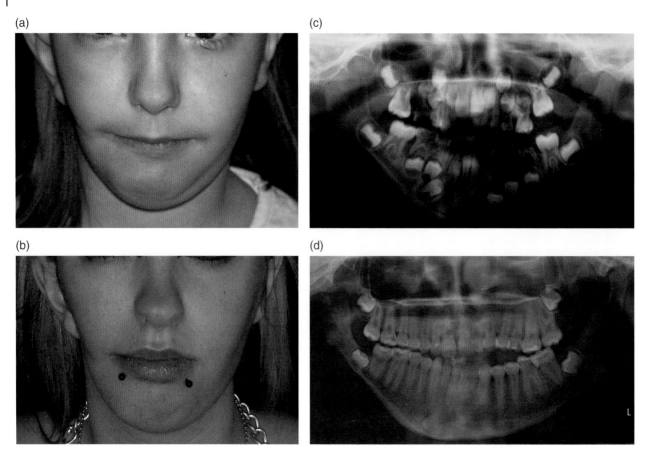

Figure 12.8.4 Nontreated female patient affected by hemifacial microsomia type IIb: frontal facial photograph at 4 years of age (a). Frontal facial photograph at 17 years of age, never subjected to any surgery. Note that the degree of asymmetry did not change with growth (b). Panoramic radiograph at 4 years of age (c). Panoramic radiograph at 17 years of age. Note that the ratio between the rami is identical after 13 years (d).

true in all studies on CCG. Mandibular ratios, calculated on panoramic X-rays, were used as they were available for all patients at all time points and are considered reliable for vertical measurements (Ongkosuwito et al. 2009). Of course, cone-beam computed tomography (CBCT) would have allowed a more accurate evaluation of growth in the vertical and the lateral planes. Unfortunately, given the length of follow-up, in this sample only panoramic X-rays were available in the initial records of most patients, to be compared with the long-term records. In this study, only patients reconstructed between 5 and 8 years of age were selected. Including older children in the study would have introduced a severe bias. Interestingly, 8 years post-CCG the proportion between grafted side and nonaffected side was only mildly reduced, but even though the graft grows, how much does the CCG influence the dental and the facial symmetry in the long-term and is the graft functional in the long-term, could not be answered? The occlusal plane in type III Pruzansky (Ross 1999) is very variable and often not as oblique as in Type II. In most patients, it was essentially flat, while only in 30% of the patients it was canted of 4°–5°, which is considered a moderate canting

(Padwa et al. 1997). In the long-term, the occlusal plane in CCG patients was not corrected. Additionally, facial contour (lateral projection) and chin deviation on the affected side in CCG relapsed almost completely in the long-term follow-up, confirming the tendency in HFM patients to reexpress the congenital facial proportion, as seen after DO in Type I and Type II. Clinically, 8 years post CCG, there was very little difference in terms of facial contour of the affected side, compared to the nonaffected side, whether a CCG has been placed or not (Figure 12.8.5). Most importantly, none of the CCG had kept a functional articulation in time.

Final Considerations on Costochondral Graft in Hemifacial Microsomia

In patients with type III HFM, restoring the height of the ramus with CCG leads to an immediate improvement of facial asymmetry. In the long-term, though the graft grows, a complete return of the asymmetry of the soft tissues and a lack of functionality is seen in most of the patients (Meazzini et al. 2020).

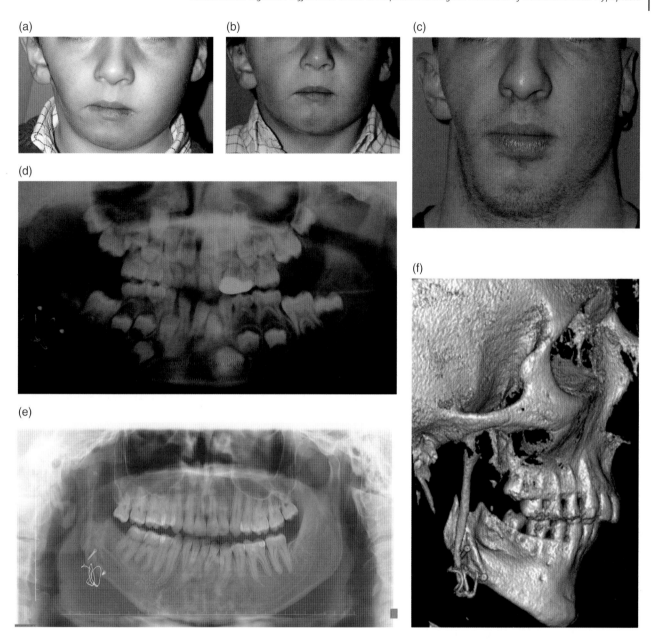

Figure 12.8.5 Male patient affected by HFM type III treated with early CCG: fontal facial photograph before surgery (a). Frontal facial photograph after surgery (b). Frontal facial photograph 12 years after CCG: note the asymmetrical growth (c). Panoramic radiograph before costochondral graft (d). Panoramic radiograph of the patient after CCG (e). Panoramic radiograph 12 years post-CCG (f). Lateral view of CBCT of the patient 12 years after costochondral graft. Note that the graft has grown but is nonfunctional.

Clinical and Prognostic Differences in the Orthopedic and Surgical Treatment of Hemimandibular Hypoplasia in Hemifacial Microsomia versus Pseudo-hemifacial Microsomia (or Condylar Coronoid Collapse Deformity)

Etiologic diagnosis is possibly the most difficult, but certainly also the most important step in orthodontic treatment. Facial asymmetries are a very challenging chapter for both the orthodontist and the maxillo-facial surgeon. HFM, as mentioned, is the best known of the branchial arch syndromes. To understand the difficulty of a correct diagnosis in these patients, it is mandatory to review what is known regarding the biological defect underlying the dysmorphology. In terms of etiology of HFM, the only evidence at this time is that it is one of four conditions defined as Neurocristopathies, which share a major involvement of neural crest cells, together with DiGeorge Syndrome, Retinoic Acid Syndrome, and Treacher Collins Syndrome (Charrier et al. 2001;

Mooney and Siegel 2002). Neural crest cells are a migratory cell population that gives rise to most of the cartilage, bone, connective tissue, and sensory ganglia in the head and play an integral part in facial morphogenesis. Just before the neural folds fuse to form the neural tube, neuroectodermal cells adjacent to the neural plate migrate into the facial region, where they form the skeletal and connective tissue of the face namely bone, cartilage, fibrous, connective tissue, and all dental tissues except enamel. The disruption in the migration or proliferation of neural crest cells can lead to a craniofacial malformation (Engleka et al. 2008). Extremely important for differential diagnosis is the knowledge that the neural crest cells which migrate into the first branchial arch, carry the pattern of information needed for proper morphogenesis of mesodermal derivates such as cranial muscles (Ericsson et al. 2004; Olsson et al. 2005). Extirpation of the mandibular neural crest stream leads to severe alterations of mandibular muscles patterning (Olsson et al. 2001). Therefore, although HFM may be very variable in terms of phenotype, mandibular deformity is always proportionate to the associated muscular deformity (Caix 2008) and this is a fundamental aspect for differential diagnosis.

As stated before, under the diagnosis of HFM, there is a great deal of variability (Figueroa and Pruzansky 1982), thus, treatment may vary. HFM cases with minor mandibular and soft tissue involvement may be treated using a conservative approach obtaining a good dentoalveolar correction/compensation and possibly some mild improvement in the general asymmetry. Treatment with functional appliances was recommended in the 70s to improve muscle function and to stimulate growth of the soft and hard tissues on the affected side (Harvold 1975). For years orthodontic functional appliance therapy during growth has been used even in moderate to severe cases, but there is no consensus about the true effect of such treatment (American Association of Orthodontists Council on Scientific Affairs 2005) and no evidence supporting its efficacy even in "classical" mandibular hypoplasia (Cacciatore et al. 2019). Vargervik et al. (1986) demonstrated that functional appliances improved only the short-term results after costochondral grafting, but there was a return of the asymmetry during subsequent growth. Likewise, it was shown that functional therapy associated to DO, only temporarily slows down the return to the original asymmetry of HFM (Meazzini et al. 2008a).

Moreover, after more than 40 years of functional treatment in HFM, not one single study showing a series of successfully treated patients has ever been published. In contrast, in the literature, we find many case reports describing very successful orthopedic treatment in patients diagnosed as moderate to severe forms of HFM (Melsen et al. 1986; Kaplan 1989; Silvestri et al. 1996; Sidiropoulou et al. 2003).

Mandibular asymmetrical growth is also seen in patients who have suffered postnatal trauma or infection in the condylar region. This deformity differs from HFM in that it is limited to the jaw, without affecting the ear, the soft tissues, or other organs (Lund 1974). Asymmetry can be part of many conditions with different causes. In abnormalities of early embryonic development (lack of neural crest cells migration) such as HFM or micrognathia, an alteration of growth patterns is observed because of the developmental abnormality. Orthopedic treatment has, thus, little probability of changing the pattern. In contrast, abnormalities of late fetal or postnatal growth, where it is presumed that the abnormal process becomes causative after the embryonic period, including trauma, infection, or surgical iatrogenic deformities, often only show involvement of the bony structures of the mandible, but generally the soft tissues or the neuromuscular pattern are not affected. Therefore, these conditions are more likely to show good response to functional stimulation.

In a series of papers, a peculiar type of mandibular asymmetry, frequently misdiagnosed as HFM, has been described (Meazzini et al. 2008b, 2011a, 2011b). The cases shared indeed two main characteristics which distinguish them from the more traditional HFM patients: (i) There is no soft tissue involvement, the external ear is well formed, the musculature well developed and, although the chin point deviates to the affected side, not only the typical flatness of the gonial area seen in HFM patients is not present, but there is usually more fullness on the affected side than on the nonaffected side (Figure 12.8.6). (ii) The shape of the hypoplastic ramus is very peculiar and extremely similar in all cases. The condyle is very short and collapses against the coronoid process (Figure 12.8.6). In this chapter, one case treated surgically with an excellent long-term follow-up is shown (Figure 12.8.7). Two other cases treated orthopedically, with remarkable ramal and condylar deformity correction are also included (Figures 12.8.8 and 12.8.9).

Several long-term studies on mandibular condylar fractures have shown the ability of self-correction (Lund 1974; Larsen and Nielsen 1976; Proffit et al. 1980) or a successful correction with dentofacial orthopedics (Girthofer and Göz 2002). We suggested that all the cases described might be undiagnosed very early trauma cases. These patients present a bony defect, but a normal neuromuscular pattern, which can remodel the damaged bony structure into a new condyle-coronoid complex, with the

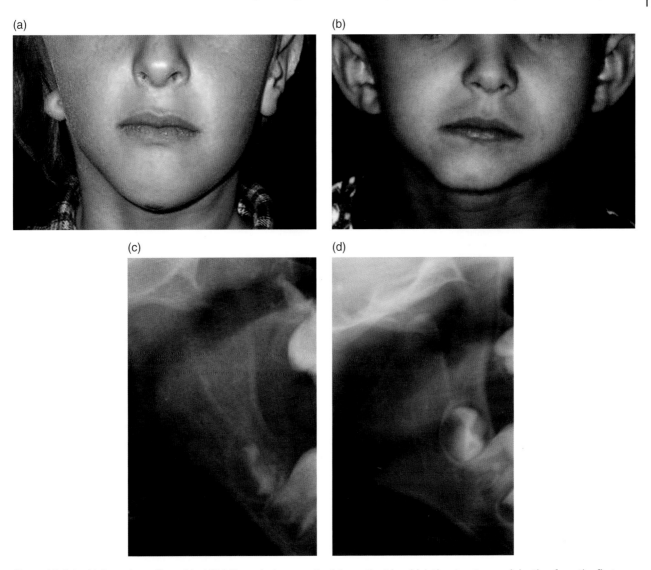

Figure 12.8.6 Male patient affected by HFM. Frontal photograph of the patient in which the structures originating from the first branchial arch as well as those from the second branchial arch are involved. The mandibular angle is more medial and cranial (a). Male patient misdiagnosed as HFM. Frontal facial photograph pretreatment. Note the presence of a normal ear and the fullness of the soft tissues on the affected side, even fuller than the contralateral side. The mandibular angle is more lateral (b). Panoramic radiograph of a patient affected by HFM IIa (c). Panoramic radiograph of a patient affected by misdiagnosed HFM (defined Condylar Coronoid collapse or CCC), where the condyle is shorter and collapsed against the coronoid and the gonial angle is acute (whereas in true HFM it is obtuse) (d).

help of functional stimulation. Even long-term results of surgical treatment are very satisfactory in contrast with what we see in DO in true HFM. More cases with an identical phenotype were recently described (Bertin et al. 2020; Perrotta et al. 2020).

Given the great heterogeneity of HFM phenotype and the little genetic knowledge on the syndrome, the differences between these two types of hemimandibular hypoplasia are not always obvious. Consequently, it is crucial to

correctly recognize those cases which have been mislabelled as HFM and might have great benefit from functional stimulation. True HFM patients, given the very early timing of the offset of the pathology, are more likely to have a bony as well as a neuromuscular deficit, which orthopedics might help improve, but certainly not correct. It is important to correctly identify patients in order not to impose ineffective long orthopedic therapy on those who have a clear embryological deficit.

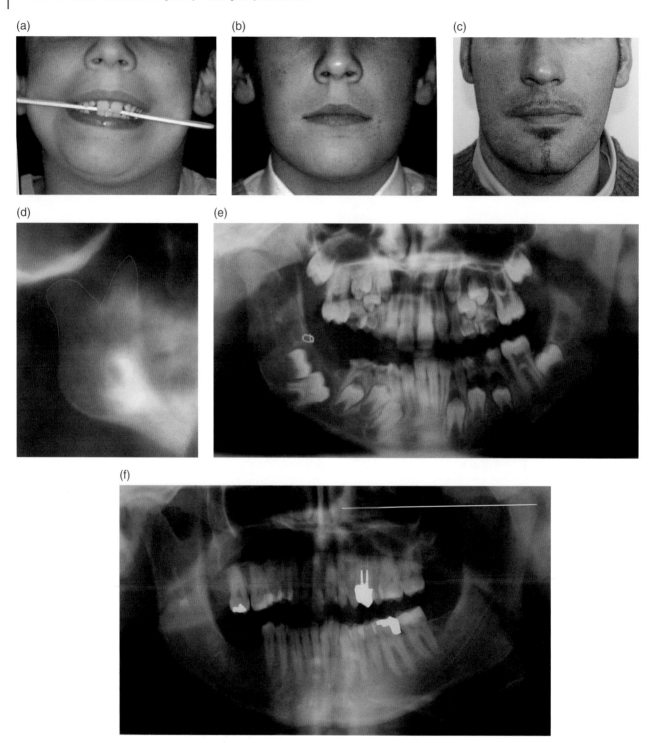

Figure 12.8.7 Male patient mislabeled as HFM, treated with unilateral mandibular osteotomy. Frontal facial photograph presurgery (a). Frontal facial photograph immediately postsurgery (b). Frontal facial photograph 29 years postsurgery (c). Panoramic radiograph presurgery (d). Panoramic radiograph immediately postsurgery (e). Panoramic radiograph 29 years postsurgery depicting the extraordinary stability (f).

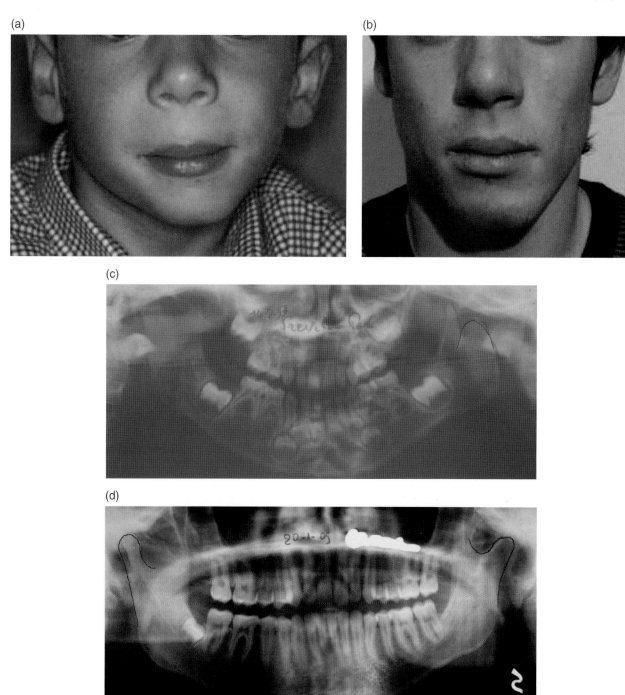

Figure 12.8.8 Male patient mislabeled as HFM, treated with an asymmetrical functional appliance. Frontal facial photograph pretreatment. Note the integrity of the ears and the fullness of the soft tissues on the side of the mandibular deviation (in true HFM there is usually a flatness of the gonial area) (a). Frontal facial photograph posttreatment (b). Panoramic radiograph pretreatment. Note the typical pretreatment shape of the condyle-coronoid relationship, similar in all these cases (c). Panoramic radiograph post-treatment (Courtesy of Professor Ennio Gianni) (d).

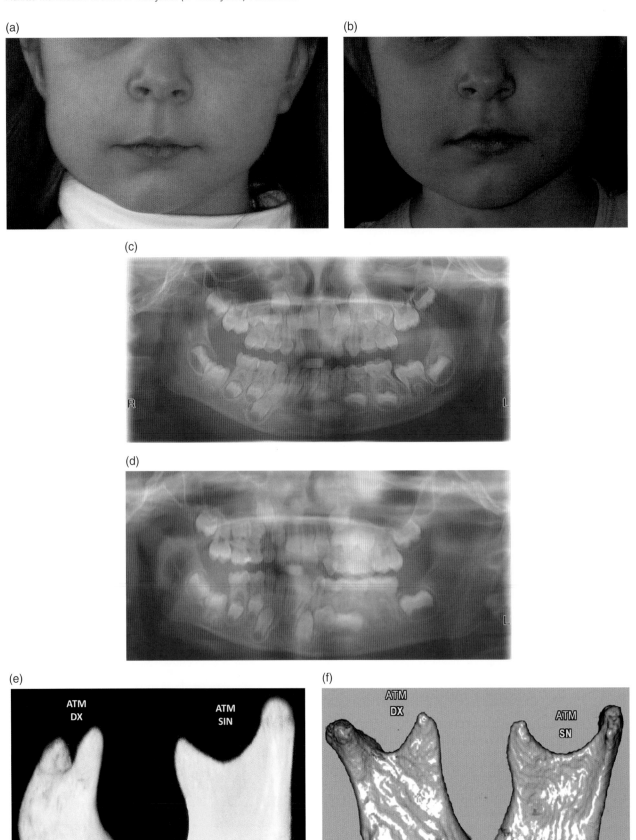

Figure 12.8.9 Female patient correctly diagnosed as CCC deformity treated with a unilateral mandibular functional appliance. Frontal facial photograph at 4 years (a). Frontal facial photograph 26 months post-treatment (b). Panoramic radiograph pretreatment. Note the typical pretreatment shape of the condyle-coronoid relationship, similar in all these cases (c). Panoramic radiograph posttreatment. Note the frequent ankylosis of the first molar in CCC (d). CBCT of the right and left mandibular rami pretreatment (e). CBCT scan of the rami post-treatment (f).

References

American Association of Orthodontists Council on Scientific Affairs. Functional appliances and long-term effects on mandibular growth. Am J Orthod Dentofac Orthop. 2005;128:271–272.

Ascenço AS, Balbinot P, Junior IM, D'Oro U, Busato L, da Silva Freitas R. Mandibular distraction in hemifacial microsomia is not a permanent treatment: a long-term evaluation. J Craniofac Surg. 2014;25:352–354.

Bertin H, Merlet FL, Khonsari RH, Delaire J, Corre P, Mercier J. Dental and maxillofacial features of condylo-mandibular dysplasia: a case series of 21 patients. J Craniomaxillofac Surg. 2020;48:956–961.

Bettega G, Morand B, Lebeau J, Raphaël B. Les altérations morphologiques au cours des syn- dromes oto-mandibulaires (Morphological alterations of oto-mandibular syndromes). Ann Chir Plast Esthet. 2001;46:495–506.

Burglen L, Soupre V, Diner PA, Gonzalès M, Vazquez MP. Dysplasis oto-mandibulaires: Génétique et nomenclature des formes syndromiques (Oto-mandibular dysplasias: genetics and nomenclature of syndromes). Ann Chir Plast Esthet. 2001;46:400–409.

Cacciatore G, Ugolini A, Sforza C, Gbinigie O, Plüddemann A. Long-term effects of functional appliances in treated versus untreated patients with Class II malocclusion: a systematic review and meta-analysis. PLoS One. 2019;14:e0221624.

Caix P. Embryopathology of the Face. Milano: Proceedings of the Italian Society for Cleft Lip and Palate, 2008.

Charrier JB, Bennaceur S, Couly G. Hemifacial microsomia. Embryological and clinical approach. Ann Chir Plast Esthet. 2001;46:385–399.

Converse JM, Coccaro PJ, Becker M, Wood-Smith D. On hemifacial microsomia. The first and second branchial arch syndrome. Plast Reconstr Surg. 1973;51:268–279.

David DJ. A critical analysis of the management of craniofacial microsomia. Australas J Plast Surg. 2018;1:65–78.

Engleka KA, Lang D, Brown CB, Antonucci NB, Epstein CJ. Neural crest formation and craniofacial development. In: Epstein CJ, Erickson RP, Wynshaw-Boris AJ, eds. Inborn Errors of Development: The Molecular Basis of Clinical Disorders of Morphogenesis. Oxford: Oxford University Press, 2008:69–79.

Ericsson R, Cerny R, Falck P, Olsson L. Role of cranial neural crest cells in visceral arch muscle positioning and morphogenesis in the Mexican axolotl, *Ambystoma mexicanum*. Dev Dyn. 2004;231:237–247.

Figueroa AA, Pruzansky S. The external ear, mandible, and other components of hemifacial microsomia. J Maxillofac Surg. 1982;10:200–211.

Girthofer K, Göz G. TMJ remodeling after condylar fracture and functional jaw orthopaedics: a case report. J Orofac Orthop. 2002;63:429–434.

Gorlin RJ, Cohen MM Jr, Hennekam RCM. Syndromes of the Head and Neck. Oxford: Oxford University Press, 2001.

Guyuron B, Lasa CI Jr. Unpredictable growth pattern of costochondral graft. Plast Reconstr Surg. 1992;90:880–886; discussion 887–889.

Harvold EP. New treatment principles for mandibular malformations. In: Cook JT, ed. Transactions of the Third International Orthodontic Congress. St. Louis: Mosby, 1975:148–154.

Hollier LH Jr, Gosain A, Stelnecki E, Longaker M, McCarthy JG. Symposium – craniofacial distraction osteogenesis. J Craniofac Surg. 1999;10:268.

Huisinga-Fischer CE, Vaandrager JM, Prahl-Andersen B. Longitudinal results of mandibular distraction osteogenesis in hemifacial microsomia. J Craniofac Surg. 2003;14:924–933.

Kaban LD, Moses MH, Mulliken JB. Surgical correction of hemifacial microsomia. Plast Reconstr Surg. 1988;82:9–19.

Kaban LB, Padwa BL, Mulliken JB. Surgical correction of mandibular hypoplasia in hemifacial microsomia: the case for treatment in early childhood. J Oral Maxillofac Surg. 1998;56:628–638.

Kaplan RG. Induced condylar growth in a patient with hemifacial microsomia. Angle Orthod. 1989;59:85–90.

Kearns GJ, Padwa BL, Mulliken JB, Kaban LB. Progression of facial asymmetry in hemifacial microsomia. Plast Reconstr Surg. 2000;105:492–498.

Kusnoto B, Figueroa AA, Polley JW. A longitudinal three-dimensional evaluation of the growth pattern in hemifacial microsomia treated by mandibular distraction osteogenesis: a preliminary report. J Craniofac Surg. 1999;10:480–486.

Larsen OD, Nielsen A. Mandibular fractures. II. A follow-up study of 229 patients. Scand J Plast Reconstr Surg. 1976;10:219–226.

Lindqvist C, Jokinen J, Paukku P, Tasanen A. Adaptation of autogenous costochondral grafts used for temporomandibular joint reconstruction: a long-term clinical and radiologic follow-up. J Oral Maxillofac Surg. 1988;46:465–470.

Lund K. Mandibular growth and remodelling processes after condylar fracture. A longitudinal roentgen cephalometric study. Acta Odontol Scand. 1974;32:3–117. (suppl.).

Marsh JL, Baca D, Vannier MW. Facial musculoskeletal asymmetry in hemifacial microsomia. Cleft Palate J. 1989;26:292–302.

Meazzini MC, Battista VMA, Brusati R, Mazzoleni F, Biglioli F, Autelitano L. Costochondral graft in growing patients with hemifacial microsomia case series: long-term results compared with non-treated patients. Orthod Craniofac Res. 2020;23:479–485.

Meazzini MC, Brusati R, Caprioglio A, Diner P, Garattini G, Giannì E, Lalatta F, Poggio C, Sesenna E, Silvestri A, Tomat C. True hemifacial microsomia and hemimandibular hypoplasia with condylar-coronoid collapse: diagnostic and prognostic differences. Am J Orthod Dentofac Orthop. 2011a;139:e435–e447.

Meazzini MC, Brusati R, Diner P, Giannì E, Lalatta F, Magri AS, Picard A, Sesenna E. The importance of a differential diagnosis between true hemifacial microsomia and pseudo-hemifacial microsomia in the post-surgical long-term prognosis. J Craniomaxillofac Surg. 2011b;39:10–16.

Meazzini MC, Caprioglio A, Garattini G, Lenatti L, Poggio CE. Hemandibular hypoplasia successfully treated with functional appliances: is it truly hemifacial microsomia? Cleft Palate Craniofac J. 2008b;45:50–56.

Meazzini MC, Figueroa AA, Polley JW. Maxillary changes in patients with hemifacial microsomia after mandibular distraction osteogenesis. In: Diner PA, Vasquez MP, eds. Proceedings of the 1st International Congress on Cranial and Facial Bone Distraction Processes. Bologna: Monduzzi, 1997:115–119.

Meazzini MC, Mazzoleni F, Bozzetti A, Brusati R. Does functional appliance treatment truly improve stability of mandibular vertical distraction osteogenesis in hemifacial microsomia? J Craniomaxillofac Surg. 2008a;36:384–389.

Meazzini MC, Mazzoleni F, Bozzetti A, Brusati R. Comparison of mandibular vertical growth in hemifacial microsomia patients treated with early distraction or not treated: follow-up till the completion of growth. J Craniomaxillofac Surg. 2012;40:105–111.

Meazzini MC, Mazzoleni F, Bozzetti A, Caronni E. Orthopedic treatment prior to mandibular distraction osteogenesis in growing patients with hemifacial microsomia. In: Diner PA, Vasquez MP, eds. Proceedings of the 2nd International Congress on Cranial and Facial Bone Distraction Processes. Bologna: Monduzzi, 1999:81–86.

Meazzini MC, Mazzoleni F, Gabriele C, Bozzetti A. Mandibular distraction osteogenesis in hemifacial microsomia: long-term follow-up. J Craniomaxillofac Surg. 2005;33:370–376.

Melsen B, Bjerregaard J, Bundgaard M. The effect of treatment with functional appliance on a pathologic growth pattern of the condyle. Am J Orthod Dentofac Orthop. 1986;90:503–512.

Mommaerts MY, Nagy K. Is early osteodistraction a solution for the ascending ramus compartment in hemifacial microsomia? A literature study. J Craniomaxillofac Surg. 2002;30:201–207.

Mooney MP, Siegel MI. Understanding Craniofacial Anomalies: The Etiopathogenesis of Craniosynostoses and Facial Clefting. New York: Wiley, 2002.

Mulliken JB, Ferraro NF, Vento AR. A retrospective analysis of growth of the constructed condyle-ramus in children with hemifacial microsomia. Cleft Palate J. 1989;26:312–317.

Murray JE, Kaban LB, Mulliken JB. Analysis and treatment of hemifacial microsomia. Plast Reconstr Surg. 1984;74:186–199.

Nagy K, Kuijpers-Jagtman AM, Mommaerts MY. No evidence for long-term effectiveness of early osteodistraction in hemifacial microsomia. Plast Reconstr Surg. 2009;124:2061–2071.

Olsson L, Ericsson R, Cerny R. Vertebrate head development: segmentation, novelties, and homology. Theory Biosci. 2005;124:145–163.

Olsson L, Falck P, Lopez K, Cobb J, Hanken J. Cranial neural crest cells contribute to connective tissue in cranial muscles in the anuran amphibian, *Bombina orientalis*. Dev Biol. 2001;237:354–367.

Ongkosuwito EM, Dieleman MMJ, Kuijpers-Jagtman AM, Mulder PGH, van Neck JW. Linear mandibular measurements: comparison between orthopantomograms and lateral cephalograms. Cleft Palate Craniofac J. 2009;46:147–153.

Ongkosuwito EM, van Vooren J, van Neck JW, Wattel E, Wolvius EB, van Adrichem LN, Kuijpers-Jagtman AM. Changes of mandibular ramal height, during growth in unilateral hemifacial microsomia patients and unaffected controls. J Craniomaxillofac Surg. 2013;41:92–97.

Padwa BL, Kaiser MO, Kaban LB. Occlusal cant in the frontal plane as a reflection of facial asymmetry. J Oral Maxillofac Surg. 1997;55:811–816.

Padwa BL, Mulliken JB, Maghen A, Kaban LB. Midfacial growth after costochondral graft construction of the mandibular ramus in hemifacial microsomia. J Oral Maxillofac Surg. 1998;56:122–127; discussion 127–128.

Perrotta S, Bocchino T, D'Antò V, Michelotti A, Valletta R. Pseudo hemifacial microsomia with condylar-coronoid collapse: new therapeutic approach in growing patients. J Craniofac Surg. 2020;31:2128–2131.

Polley JW, Figueroa AA, Liou EJ, Cohen M. Longitudinal analysis of mandibular asymmetry in hemifacial microsomia. Plast Reconstr Surg. 1997;99:328–339.

Proffit WR, Vig KWL, Turvey TA. Early fracture of the mandibular condyles: frequently an unsuspected cause of growth disturbance. Am J Orthod. 1980;78:1–24.

Pruzansky S. Not all dwarfed mandibles are alike. Birth Defects. 1969;5:120–129.

Ross RB. Costochondral grafts replacing the mandibular condyle. Cleft Palate Craniofac J. 1999;36:334–339.

Rune B, Selvik G, Sarnas KV, Jacobsson S. Growth in hemifacial microsomia studied with the aid of roentgen sterophotogrammetry and metallic implants. Cleft Palate J. 1981;18:128–146.

Sidiropoulou S, Antoniades K, Kolokithas G. Orthopedically induced condylar growth in a patient with hemifacial microsomia. Cleft Palate Craniofac J. 2003;40:645–650.

Silvestri A, Natali G, Iannetti G. Functional therapy in hemifacial microsomia: therapeutic protocol for growing children. J Oral Maxillofac Surg. 1996;54:271–278; discussion 278–280.

Simpson AH, Williams PE, Kyberd P, Goldspink G, Kenwright J. The response of muscle to leg lengthening. J Bone Joint Surg Br. 1995;77:630–636.

Suh J, Choi TH, Baek SH, Kim JC, Kim S. Mandibular distraction in unilateral craniofacial microsomia: longitudinal results until the completion of growth. Plast Reconstr Surg. 2013;132:1244–1252.

Vargervik K, Ousterhout DK, Farias M. Factors affecting long-term results in hemifacial microsomia. Cleft Palate J. 1986;23(Suppl 1):53–68.

12.9

Special Treatment Considerations of Face Asymmetries

Giampietro Farronato

CHAPTER MENU

Introduction

Dysgnathic facial patterns characterized by asymmetrical function or morphology have always been a subject of serious debate regarding their orthodontic–surgical management. The reason for this is that asymmetrical dysgnathic patterns lead to different interpretations by clinicians and researchers, and there is no definitive consensus on many aspects of their classification and characteristics. Asymmetries present specific diagnostic, prognostic, and therapeutic challenges that clearly differentiate them from other patterns of facial malformations. Certainly, the etiopathogenetic evaluation of causal etiology also offers cues for various interpretations.

In this section, the most salient diagnostic, etiologic, and therapeutic aspects will be considered thus suggesting the interpretive key in genesis-causal and logical interpretation of treatment. In addition, the various nosological pictures of dentoalveolar and skeletal components in growing and late-growing patients in need of functional,

orthopedic, orthodontic, and orthodontic–surgical treatment will be presented.

Diagnosis

Diagnosis in orthodontics and dentofacial deformities has been based on clinical and cephalometric examination for more than one century. The lateral cephalometric examination of the skull is totally unsuitable for evaluating asymmetrical patterns allowing at most to evaluate the bisection of the lower and posterior border of the mandible. With the advent of posteroanterior cephalometric radiography thanks to the contributions of Ennio Giannì and later of Robert M. Ricketts, the examination was amplified by examining the coincidence of the midpoints with the axis of facial symmetry and the skewness and dysmetria (different distance) of the analogous lateral points.

After the introduction of cone-beam computed tomography (CBCT) in orthodontics and thanks to the studies

---

Dentofacial and Occlusal Asymmetries, First Edition. Edited by Birte Melsen and Athanasios E. Athanasiou.
© 2025 John Wiley & Sons Ltd. Published 2025 by John Wiley & Sons Ltd.

performed at the University of Milan, it became evident that the evaluation of points and segments that lie on the median sagittal plane or are parallel to it are accurately evaluated on two-dimensional radiographs (lateral and posteroanterior cephalometric radiographs) while segments oblique to the median sagittal plane for lateral cephalograms and to the frontal plane for posteroanterior cephalograms undergo underestimation, the greater the obliquity (Farronato et al. 2010a, 2010b, 2015b; Bombeccari et al. 2015; Firetto et al. 2019).

For example, the size of the mandibular body in normal subjects is underestimated by 13 mm when comparing its assessment by lateral cephalograms and CBCT. This underestimation is not a systematic error that can be corrected with appropriate adjustment but it varies as obliquity is different from subject to subject (narrow and long faces, wide and short faces) as well as in the same subject in two successive evaluations as obliquity with growth increases.

Among other things, this limitation may explain why the changes that occur as a result of treatment and growth are not well understood in the literature yet.

Three-dimensional evaluation by using CBCT allows today a good understanding of the changes that characterize symmetric or asymmetric morphology and their precise qualitatively and quantitatively assessment.

Since 2007, faculty of the University of Milan have proposed an 18-point cephalometric analysis from which 36 measurements are calculated and lead to a comprehensive evaluation of the subjects under examination (Figures 12.9.1 and 12.9.2). In addition, clinical evidence of asymmetry well justifies the use of CBCT based on the conservative concepts of ALADAIP, beyond ALARA, and toward a personalized optimization for pediatric patients (Oenning et al. 2021).

To facilitate diagnostic judgment and for educational purposes at our institution, evaluation of dental and skeletal changes takes place in the three planes of space namely sagittal, vertical, and transverse. Furthermore, the path that dysgnathia has taken in its genesis is assessed thus highlighting whether it is linear or rotational in nature.

Following this protocol of evaluation, the following findings, by increasing severity, can be verified:

One-plane, two-planes, three-planes with linear, rotational or linear, and rotational alteration (Figures 12.9.3–12.9.5).

At the one end of the great range of variation, alterations affecting only one plane of space with only linear displacement will represent the most easily diagnosed and treated clinical situation (Maspero et al. 2011; Farronato et al. 2013, 2014a, 2014b, 2015a). At the other end of variation, clinical situations of maximum complexity with involvement of the three planes of space with linear and rotational displacements may present serious diagnostic and management challenges. Clinical appearances of asymmetry often involve two or three planes of space with both linear and rotational displacements.

By describing dysgnathic appearances in this way, the clinician can well understand the path that the deformity has followed in its development and the way to achieve correction. Such a described method allows one to understand how some alterations are able to be corrected using dentofacial orthopedic procedures while others can be managed by performing only orthodontic–surgical treatments.

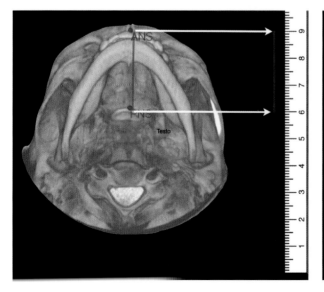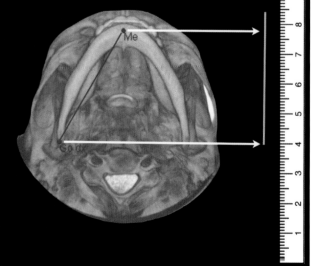

Figure 12.9.1 Everything that is oblique is underestimated in the lateral view.

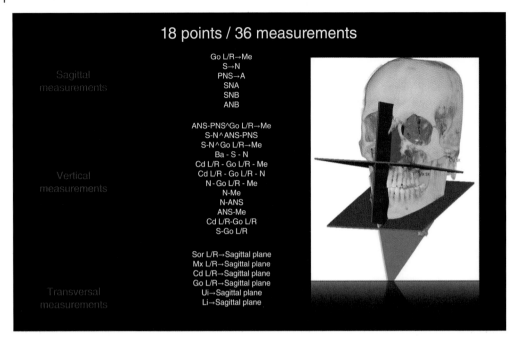

Figure 12.9.2 The University of Milan cephalometric analysis on CBTC including 18 points and 36 measurements.

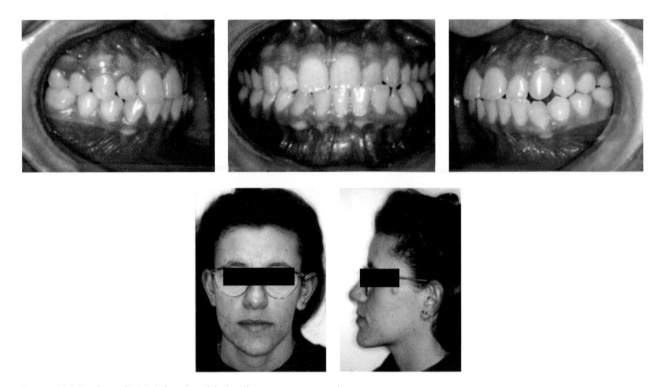

Figure 12.9.3 Dentofacial deformity with the discrepancy on one plane.

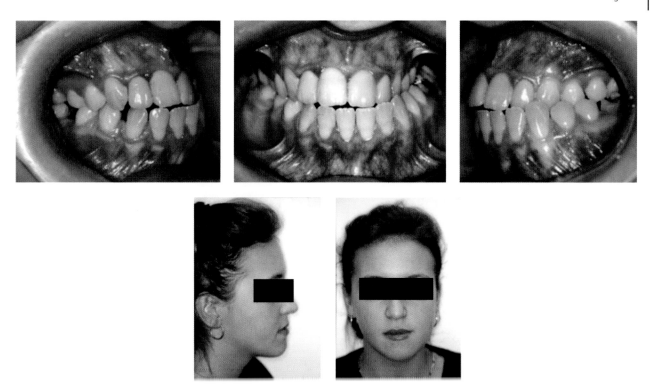

Figure 12.9.4 Dentofacial deformity with the discrepancy on two planes.

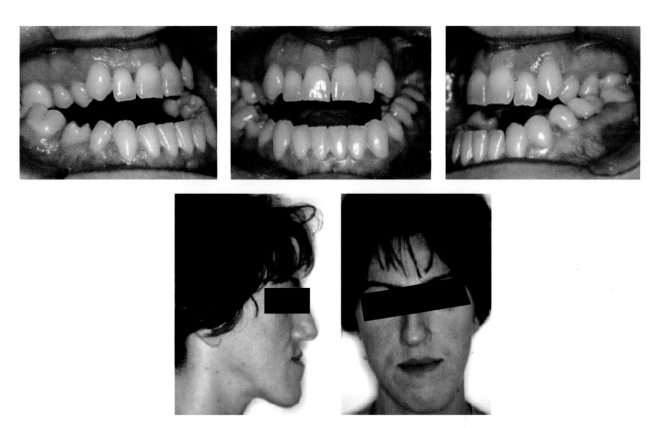

Figure 12.9.5 Dentofacial deformity with the discrepancy on three planes.

Dealing exclusively on complex asymmetry problems by following such a diagnostic-descriptive pathway allows an understanding of whether favorable or unfavorable treatment consequences may occur.

An asymmetrical Class II dentoskeletal deformity can be treated orthopedically in the dynamic phase of growth by modulating through the construction bite the different major activation on one side versus the other.

An asymmetrical Class I dentoskeletal deformity offers cues for more considerations as it is to be considered a false Class I which is actually Class III on one side and Class II on the other. The correction mostly is surgical, reductive on one side, and additive on the other.

In an asymmetrical Class III dentoskeletal deformity, if it coexists with an increase in vertical height, the worst of the unfavorable correlations develops. If the mandible is set back to the center then the Class III relationship is aggravated.

In most of the cases of increased vertical height, if the mandible is rotated up it also goes forward thus further aggravating the Class III relationship.

Therefore, asymmetrical Class III dentoskeletal deformities with increased vertical height find solution only with orthodontic–surgical treatments since only through osteotomies can the complex corrective movements in the three planes of space can be achieved.

Categories of Asymmetry

It is of great importance to address the most frequent conditions that might be encountered by the clinician in identifying the predisposing triggering factors and the developmental course of asymmetry.

Trauma

In children, the situations that can cause face asymmetry and whose origin can be clearly identified are those related to trauma of the maxillomandibular structures. These structures most exposed to trauma can be identified within the areas of the nose and the mandible.

The nasal septum constitutes a growth center in early life that contributes to the forward and downward displacement of the maxilla. Even a traumatic event of no particular intensity can cause its fracture and the deviation of its median axis. Following this trauma, the surrounding structures undergo a series of consequent progressive adaptations that can be characterized as following:

- Elevation of the maxilla on the side of the concavity of the septum, lowering on the side of the convexity, unevenness, and obliquity of the occlusal plane.

- If the pathogenic cause occurs early and persists for a long time, it affects mandibular growth, which exhibits canting of the occlusal plane, obliquity of the chin, rami of different lengths, and unevenness of the gonial angle and mandibular plane.
- The severity of the condition is determined by the earliness of the event, the intensity of the damage, and the greater or lesser susceptibility of the subject determined by the intrinsic factor of growth (more severe in skeletal Class III, less severe in skeletal Class II) as well as additional concomitant unfavorable dysfunctional factors (abnormal breathing and swallowing).
- Impaired respiratory function, if it is established early and persists for a long time, can trigger impaired transverse and vertical development of the maxilla that will influence the downward development of the nasal septum. When associated, as is often noted, with unilateral crossbite, it will lead not only to the deviation of dental arches' midlines but also to an increasingly aggravating and complex asymmetry of the maxillomandibular complex (Figure 12.9.6).

The author's team has amply demonstrated how therapeutic expansion of the maxilla leads to a reduction in nasal septum deviation, correction of unilateral crossbite, and reposition of the mandible to its normal median position. It also allows the resumption of normal respiratory function and normal mandibular kinesiology (Figure 12.9.7).

Occlusal Interference

The mechanism by which an occlusal interference in the transverse plane expresses itself in maxillomandibular growth process deserves further investigation. It has been shown that occlusal interference that intervenes by deviating the path in jaw closure to the side alters the functions of the temporomandibular joint (TMJ) structures in particular. The condyle represents a site of growth, which well demonstrated, responds to functional stimuli that in the norm are symmetrical on the two sides (Andresen 1932; Cozza et al. 2004, 2006).

Deviant interference in the frontal plane leads to a different condylar kinesiology: on the side of the deviation, the movement will be more vertical and reduced in excursion, on the other side, it will be wider vertically and with greater horizontal excursion. This gap will first be expressed by functional positional deviation, and then progressively by structural adaptation and remodeling leading to less predominantly vertical growth of one condyle and more predominantly horizontal growth of the other. The initial positional alteration will become increasingly structural involving not only the mandible but also the maxilla. If the occlusal interference is transient as a result of tooth

(a)

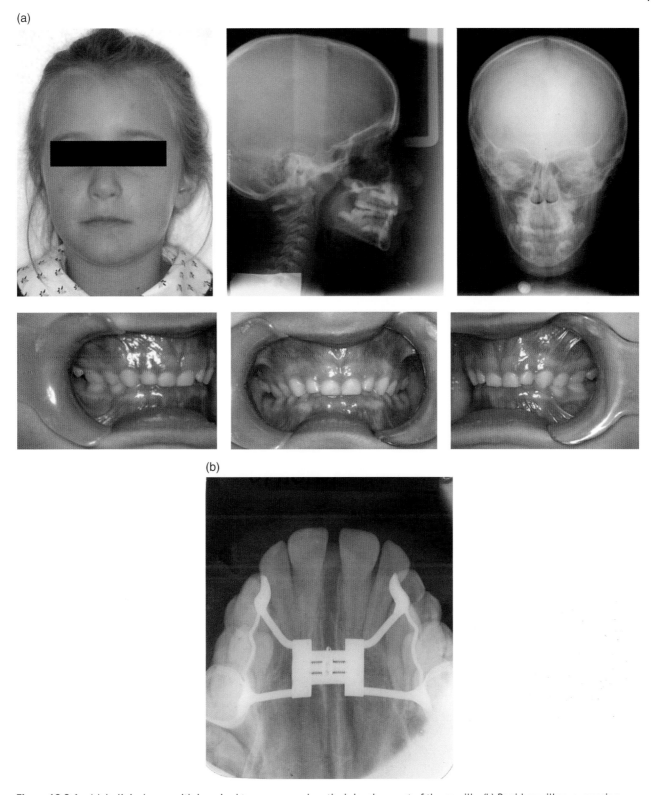

(b)

Figure 12.9.6 (a) A clinical case with impaired transverse and vertical development of the maxilla. (b) Rapid maxillary expansion. (c) As a result of the rapid maxillary expansion, the septum deviation was corrected.

(c)

Figure 12.9.6 (Continued)

(a)

(b)

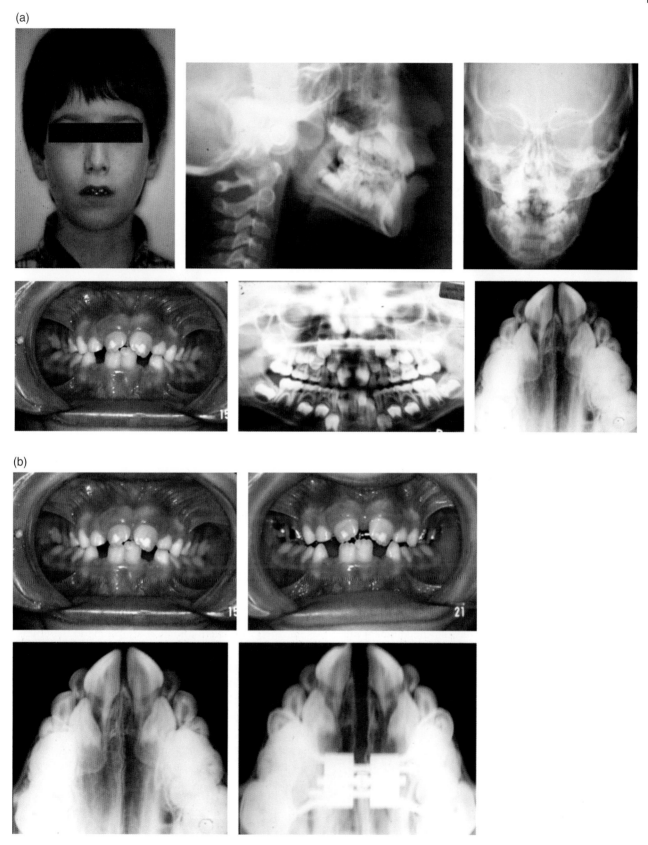

Figure 12.9.7 (a) A patient presenting oral respiration with transversal hypo-development of the maxilla; (b) rapid maxillary expansion; (c) follow-up of the functional restoration; (d) correction of the nasal septum following rapid maxillary expansion.

(c)

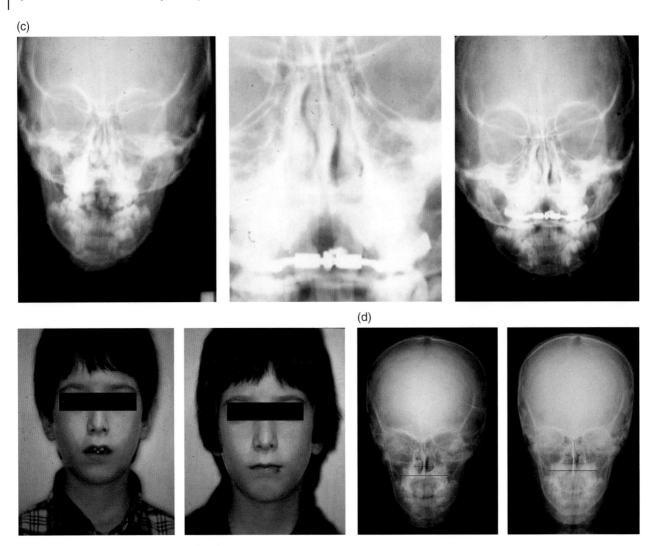

Figure 12.9.7 (Continued)

displacement, exfoliation, occlusal adjustment, or follow-ing appropriate orthodontic correction, the anomaly rap-idly regresses with restitution ad integrum.

The need to monitor and promptly correct alterations in the permutation of the occlusal environment that may cause the establishment of such pathogenic etiology is of great importance.

Condylar Fractures

Regarding the mandible, an event that can have serious reper-cussions and sometimes pass untimely diagnosed is condylar fractures (Farronato et al. 2009a). At a young age, the condylar structure of cartilaginous nature may be damaged by fall trauma involving the chin. Nowadays diagnosis is facilitated by three-dimensional assessment utilizing CBCT.

Following unilateral condylar fracture, mandibular motion is impaired with latero-deviation at opening to the injured side. The injured condyle does not support the mandible at opening. The noninjured condyle always exhibits compensa-tory hyperfunction. In such situations, in the absence of ade-quate treatment, the healthy condyle will exhibit increased growth reflecting the dynamics of movement, predominantly upward and backward. Absent or reduced growth usually characterizes the injured condyle.

In these cases, a situation of progressively increasing asymmetry develops, which will also involve the vertical growth of the occlusal plane and the maxilla, which will be vertically lower on the healthy side than on the frac-tured side.

What causes trauma can also cause therapy in the oppo-site direction. Therapy involves functional treatment that influences the mandibular kinesiology in closure to cause a deviation of the mandible exactly opposite to the deviation it undergoes in opening. An occlusal elevation will be arranged on the side of the fracture that forces the mandible to deviate from the fractured side to the healthy side resulting in a mandibular movement in closure exactly opposite to that in opening.

Such treatment is easier in skeletal Class II because it will partly help compensate for the skeletal situation. In cases of skeletal Class III, the correction of mandibular asymmetries always results in an aggravation of the mandibular protrusion and of the skeletal Class III relationship (Figure 12.9.8).

In our institution, the functional treatment of unilateral and bilateral condylar fractures in childhood has been

(a)

(b)   (c)

(d)   (e)

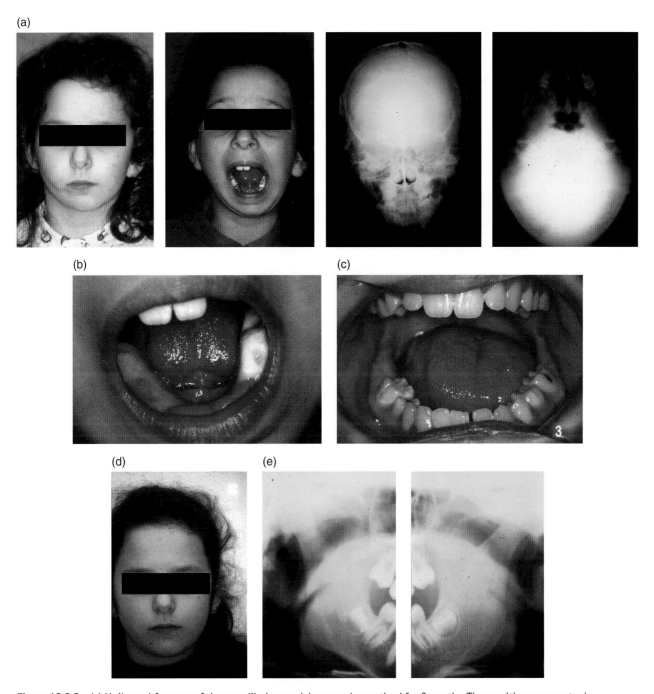

Figure 12.9.8 (a) Unilateral fracture of the mandibular condyle passed unnoticed for 8 months. The resulting asymmetry is noticeable; (b) start of the functional therapy; (c) after 8 months of functional therapy, restoration of normal mandibular kinesiology is evident; (d) restoration of facial symmetry; (e) restoration of condylar morphology resulting from functional therapy.

always favored and affirmed the contraindications to the surgical therapeutic alternative. Surgical treatment becomes mandatory if the small fractured condylar fragment impedes mandibular movement and raises the fear of evolution into ankylosis. Functional treatment is not possible if joint function is impeded. In such cases, surgical removal of the small fragment is performed (intraorally). Once the opening of the mouth has been reestablished, the functional therapy as illustrated in Figure 12.9.9 will be implemented.

(a)

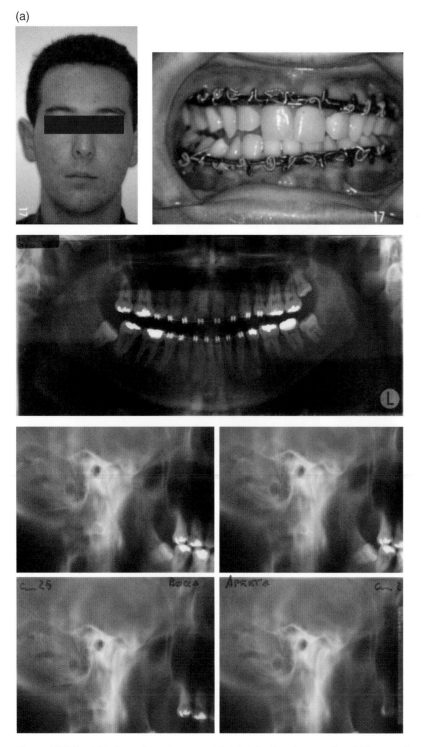

Figure 12.9.9　(a) Left condylar fracture with left joint function restricted. The opening of the mouth is prevented; (b) results of condylectomy and functional treatment; (c) restoration of mandibular kinesiology is evident; (d) 30 years follow-up.

(b)

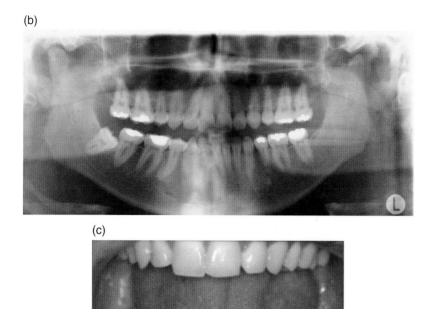

(c)

(d)

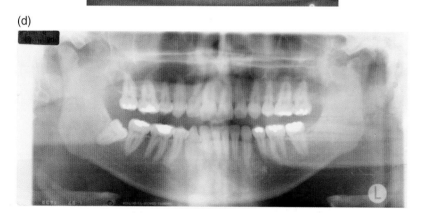

Figure 12.9.9   (Continued)

Juvenile Idiopathic Rheumatoid Arthritis

Juvenile idiopathic rheumatoid arthritis in high percentage of cases (85%) affects the temporomandibular joints (Kreiborg et al. 1990; Bertram et al. 2001; Arvidsson et al. 2010; Farronato et al. 2010c, 2011a; Garagiola et al. 2013, 2019). The damage is due to systemic underlying pathology (sinusitis) but aggravated by altered mandibular kinesiology due to painful symptoms and drug therapies taken.

The University of Milan has been supporting rheumatologists in these situations with dedicated orthodontic therapies for more than 30 years (Bellintani et al. 2002, 2005a).

In subjects with juvenile rheumatoid arthritis, mandibular movement is reduced in amplitude and excursion. The muscles involved are hypotonic and hyporegulated due to reduced predominantly antalgic function and as a result of extensive use of steroidal anti-inflammatory drugs.

Untreated subjects present special characteristics including mandibular hypodevelopment, increased anterior vertical dimension, posterior mandibular rotation, and asymmetry more or less depending on the different joint involvement namely unilateral or bilateral (Brusati and Chiapasco 1999; Ciancaglini 2007; Farronato et al. 2011b).

Functional treatment involves the use of appliances that in closure guide the mandible in a movement forward, upward, and sideways (Bellintani et al. 2005b; Farronato et al. 2009, 2009b, 2011c).

In response to the treatment that is to be continued beyond systemic remission until the end of growth

excellent results have been obtained (Pancherz et al. 1998; Farronato et al. 2010d). In some cases, it has been possible to use the Herbst fixed functional appliance, activated asymmetrically according to clinical indications, with excellent functional and skeletal results (Figure 12.9.10) (Farronato et al. 2011).

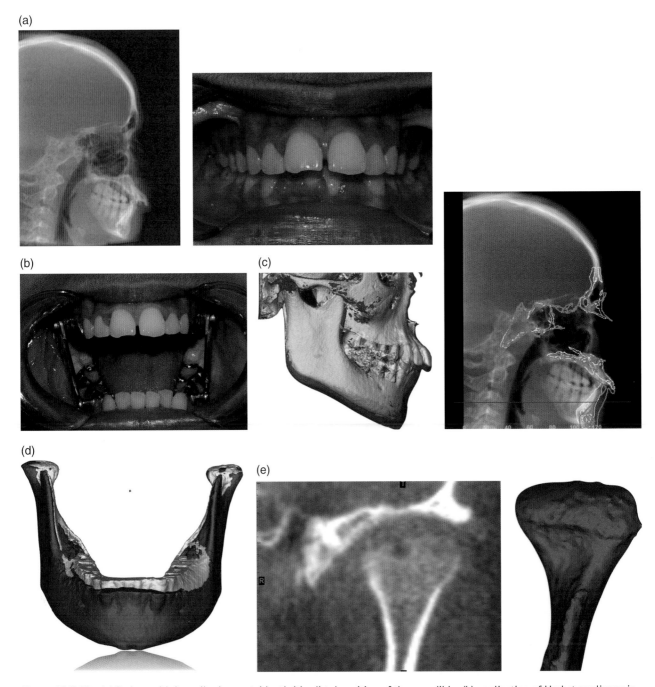

Figure 12.9.10 (a) Patient with juvenile rheumatoid arthritis: distal position of the mandible; (b) application of Herbst appliance in the patient with juvenile rheumatoid arthritis; (c) CBCT presents skeletal changes after 12 months of treatment; (d) before and after treatment; (e) before and after treatment with evident the restoration of condylar morphology post-therapy.

Special Treatment Considerations

In adult subjects, excluding congenital syndromic forms (Franceschetti, hemifacial microsomia, Goldenhar, etc.), is not always possible to reconstruct the "primum movens" and the etiopathogenetic process of face asymmetry (Figure 12.9.11) (Holmström 1986; Greenberg 1991; Draf et al. 2003; Meazzini et al. 2008; Chummun et al. 2012; Defraia et al. 2012; Farronato et al. 2014c; Cossellu et al. 2015).

Severe situations mostly involve a multifactorial etiology in which exogenous and functional epigenetic factors have found fertile ground in an unfavorable genetic predisposition. To be counted as exogenous factors trauma, dysfunctional factors that altered respiratory function and severe deviant occlusal changes should be considered.

In particular, the genetic substrate of severe skeletal Class III predisposes even to the most severe asymmetrical forms. On the other hand, the more reduced mandibular

(a)

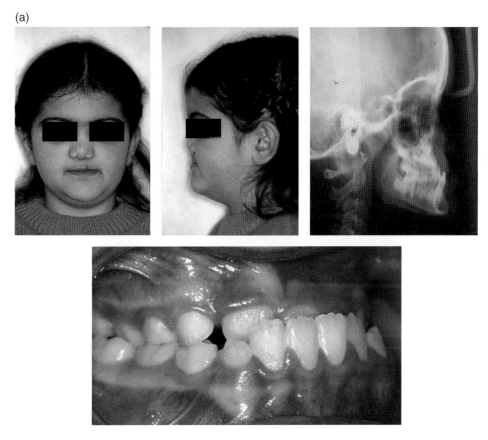

(b)

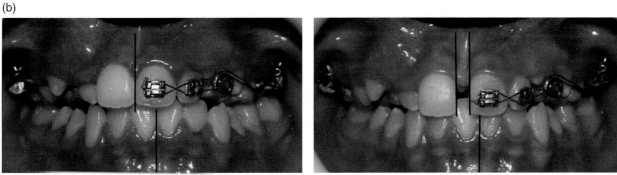

Figure 12.9.11 (a) Patient with Binder syndrome; (b) correction of the midline with rapid maxillary expansion and the upper left bite block; (c) final result.

(c)

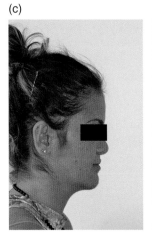
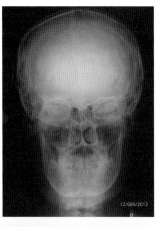
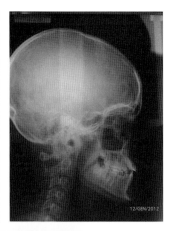

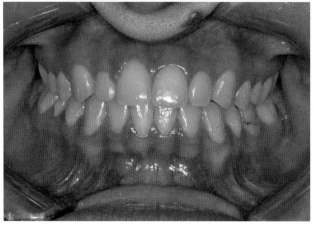

Figure 12.9.11 (Continued)

growth is demonstrated the less it is associated with severe manifestations of facial asymmetry. Sagittally and vertically exuberant mandibular growth easily associates with severe asymmetrical forms (Figure 12.9.12).

It is particularly useful and justified for diagnostic purposes in such dysgnathic forms to use CBCT according to ALADAIP criteria (Oenning et al. 2021). It allows the extent and direction of the alteration to be highlighted with great precision. It is particularly useful to distinguish malfunctions that occur in one plane, in two planes, and in three planes with deviations from the norm of linear, rotational, and linear and rotational types.

In late-growing subjects, correction of skeletal changes involves a therapeutic surgical course. Treatment typically involves presurgical orthodontic treatment, surgical correction, and postsurgical orthodontic treatment. Surgical correction should be planned and scheduled from the earliest diagnostic stages by defining exactly the position that the dental elements should assume to allow osteotomies

and surgical displacements that the jaws require. Therefore, the aforementioned detailed classification of one plane, two planes, three planes, linear, and rotational is useful, keeping well in mind the favorable or unfavorable synergism does exist between the various alterations (Maspero et al. 2012).

For example in the skeletal Class II with open bite with asymmetry, synergism is favorable because by correcting the open bite and asymmetry Class II becomes less severe.

The most complex picture that produces the absolute most unfavorable synergism is the skeletal Class III with open bite and asymmetry because by correcting open bite and asymmetry the Class III becomes worse. This clinical situation represents high complexity and requires close collaboration between orthodontist and surgeon.

The three different clinical situations of progressive diagnostic-therapeutic complexity that are presented below represent the above-mentioned scenarios.

Case 1

This case presents at the level of the dental arches an obvious left lower midline deviation. From the sagittal and vertical skeletal point of view, nothing remarkable is noted and a skeletal Class I with normal overbite is

present. In the frontal plane, the mandible is deviated to the left with an augmented mandibular body on the right and normal on the left. Thus, there is evidence of a single plane (frontal) displacement of a linear type from right to left. After presurgical orthodontic preparation, an

(a)

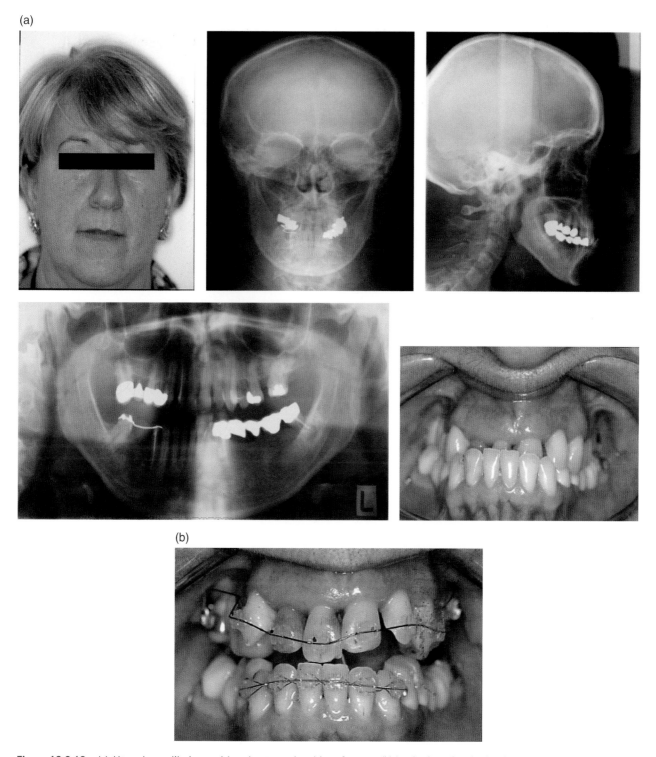

(b)

Figure 12.9.12 (a) Altered mandibular position due to occlusal interference; (b) beginning of orthodontic therapy; (c) end of orthodontic and restorative prosthetic treatment.

(c)

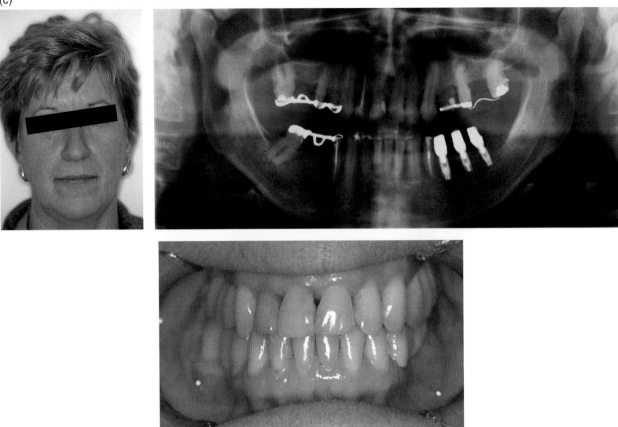

Figure 12.9.12   (Continued)

osteotomy was performed according to Obwegeser–Dal Pont at the mandibular angle with setback osteoctomy on the right and augmentation sliding on the left. Treatment continued with postsurgical orthodontics and retention (Figure 12.9.13).

Case 2

This case shows at the level of the dental arches a left lower midline deviation. The skeletal structures examined in the sagittal plane show a protruded and post-rotated mandible. In the frontal plane, the mandible is displaced from right to left. Thus, two planes with rotational and linear displacements are affected. The treatment plan involves the rotation of the mandible from left to right while at the same time retracting and antero-rotating the mandibular body. The three displacements are unfavorably synergistic with each other: if movement of the mandible from left to right takes place while at the same time antero-rotating, the mandibular body will be more advanced and it will be necessary to retract it more. The orthodontic postsurgical treatment made possible to set up the arches in such a way that the planned surgical shifts

could be properly performed thus achieving proper repositioning of the osteotomized bodies with osteotomy according to Obwegeser–Dal Pont at the mandibular angles. The orthodontic postsurgical treatment allowed excellent occlusal stabilization with restoration of a stable morphofunctional harmony (Figure 12.9.14).

Case 3

This case presents the highest complexity in orthodontic–surgical treatment. The subject has severe asymmetry clearly evident on clinical examination involving middle and lower thirds of the face. The dental arches are oblique in the frontal plane and she presents a marked Class III malocclusion with a large open bite. The dental arches midlines do not coincide with the one of the face and with each other. The maxilla is advanced, antero-rotated, deviated to the right, and oblique. The mandible is protruded, post-rotated, deviated to the left and oblique. This case presents a dysgnathia that has been disrupted in the three planes of space with marked linear and rotational type of displacements. It may be hypothesized as the etiologic factor a trauma at an early age to the nasal septum that

(a)

(b)

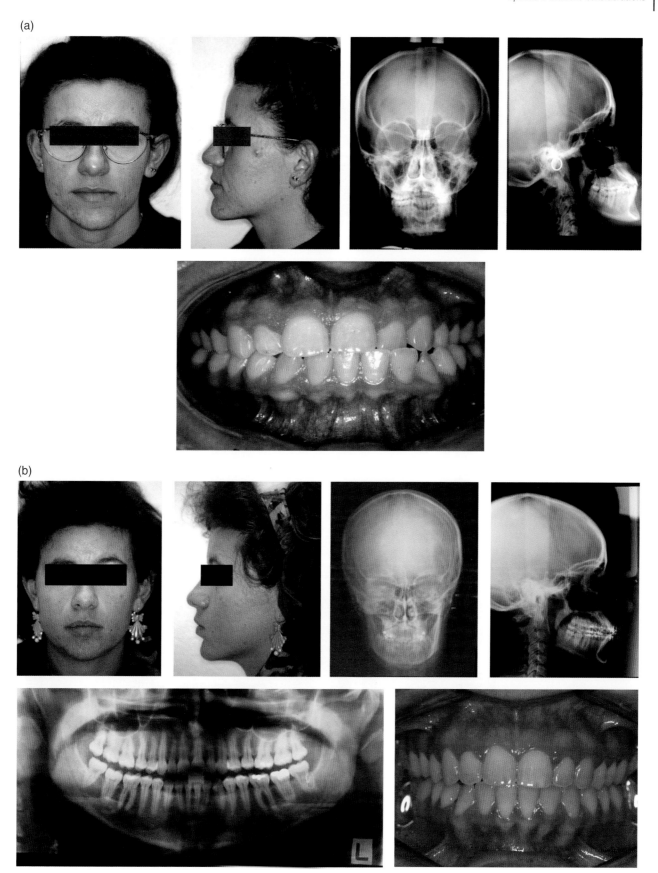

Figure 12.9.13 (a) Skeletal discrepancy on one plane. The mandible is displaced to the left; (b) the final result after orthodontic-surgical treatment including bilateral sagittal split osteotomy according to Obwegeser–Dal Pont; (c) the linear shift in the horizontal plane; (d) Follow-up after 10 years.

(c)

(d)

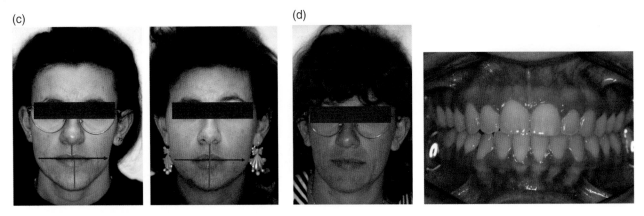

Figure 12.9.13 (Continued)

(a)

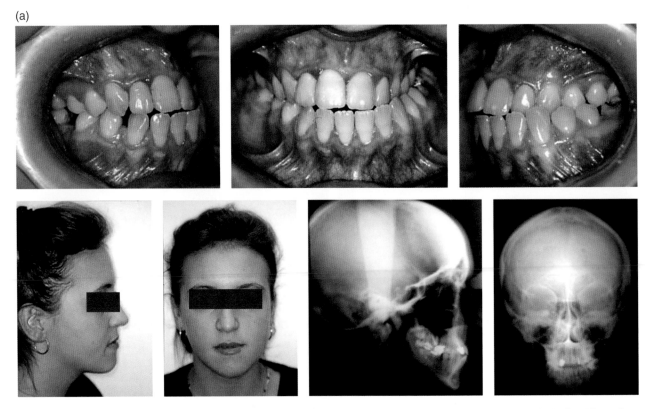

Figure 12.9.14 (a) Skeletal discrepancy on two planes; (b) the final result after orthodontic-surgical treatment including bilateral sagittal split osteotomy according to Obwegeser–Dal Pont; (c) the corrective movements that have affected the horizontal and vertical planes.

(b)

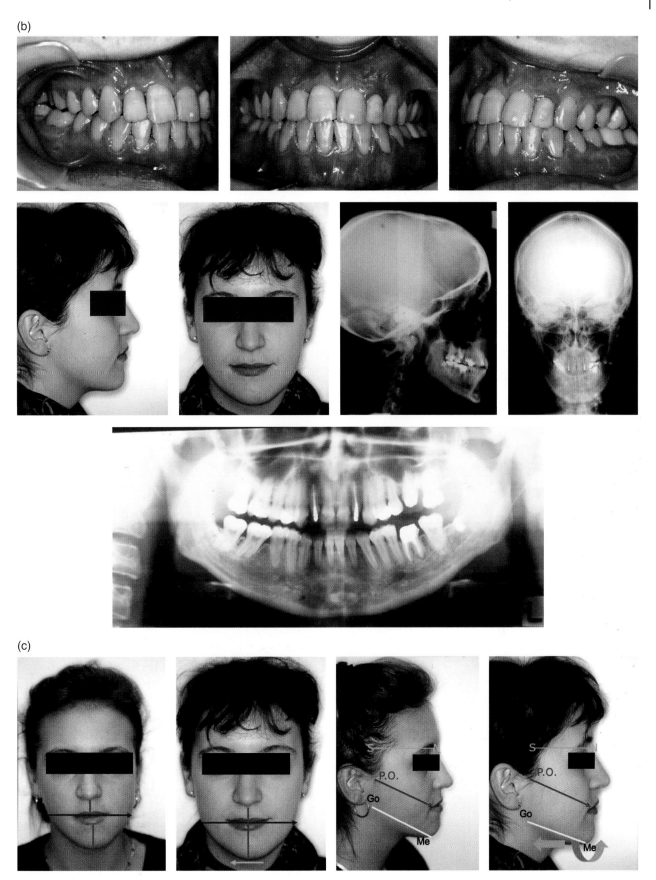

(c)

Figure 12.9.14 (Continued)

is widely deviated, which led to an alteration of respiratory function (forced oral breathing), swallowing (tongue interposition), on a family genetic substrate of severe Class III malocclusion. In addition, altered occlusal proprioceptive influence and altered mandibular kinesiology may be considered to complete the severely dysfunctional characteristics of this patient. Surgical correction involved a Le Fort I type osteotomy of the maxilla with advancement, postrotation in the sagittal plane, rotation to the right, and asymmetric elevation to make the upper arch horizontal. The upper jaw surgery facilitated the osteotomy at the mandibular angle according to Obwegeser–Dal Pont with retraction, antero-otation in the sagittal plane, rotation to the left, and rotation in the frontal plane to horizontally change the

occlusal plane. Only an extremely precise presurgical orthodontic treatment plan can enable compliance with the requirements of the surgical treatment plan in this case. In particular, the upper and lower midlines must align exactly with the maxillary and mandibular jaws midlines. Dental open bite will need to be increased to allow for maxillary post-rotation and mandibular antero-rotation. Rhino-septal surgery practiced at the same time with the osteotomies allowed restoration of proper respiratory function which is a prerequisite for stability of outcome. Also speech therapy facilitated and consolidated normal tongue posture. The stability of the result more than 10 years posttreatment confirms the success of the treatment (Figures 12.9.15 and 12.9.16).

(a)

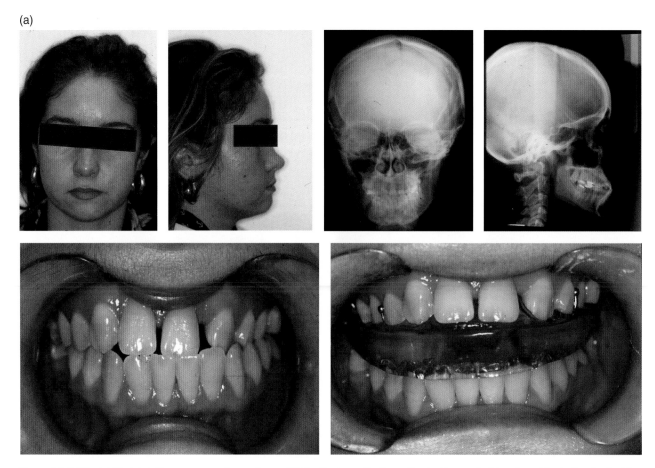

Figure 12.9.15 (a) Skeletal discrepancy on three planes; (b) the final result after orthodontic-surgical treatment including Le Fort I maxillary osteotomy and bilateral sagittal split osteotomy according to Obwegeser–Dal Pont; (c) movements that affect the three planes of space with linear and rotational movements; (d) 10 years Follow-up.

(b)

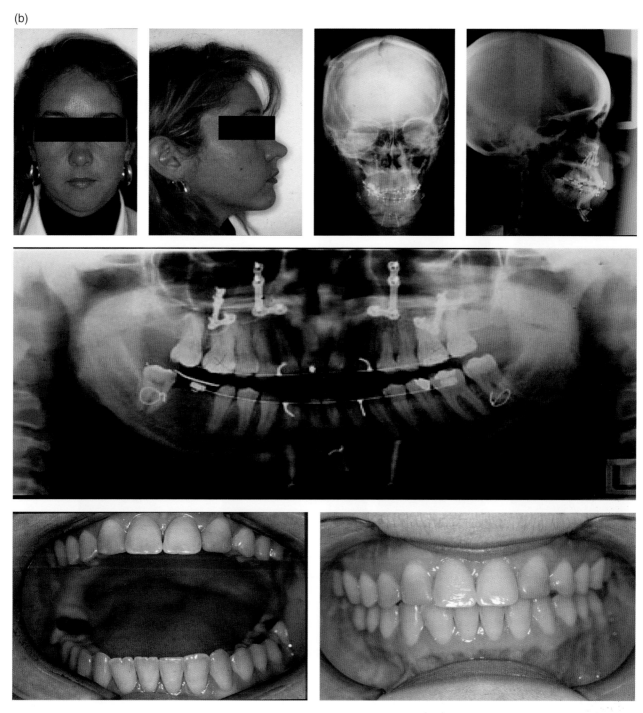

Figure 12.9.15 (Continued)

(c)

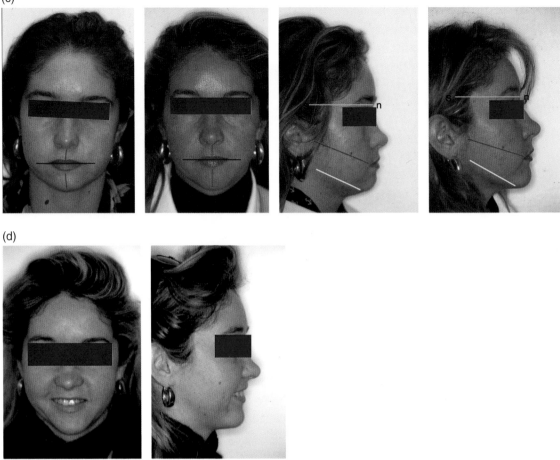

(d)

Figure 12.9.15 (Continued)

(a)

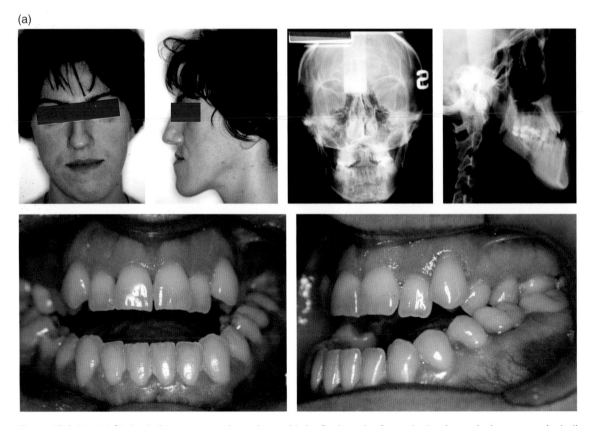

Figure 12.9.16 (a) Skeletal discrepancy on three planes; (b) the final result after orthodontic-surgical treatment including Le Fort I maxillary osteotomy and bilateral sagittal split osteotomy according to Obwegeser–Dal Pont; (c) movements that corrected the three planes of space with linear and rotational repositioning; (d) 10 years follow-up.

(b)

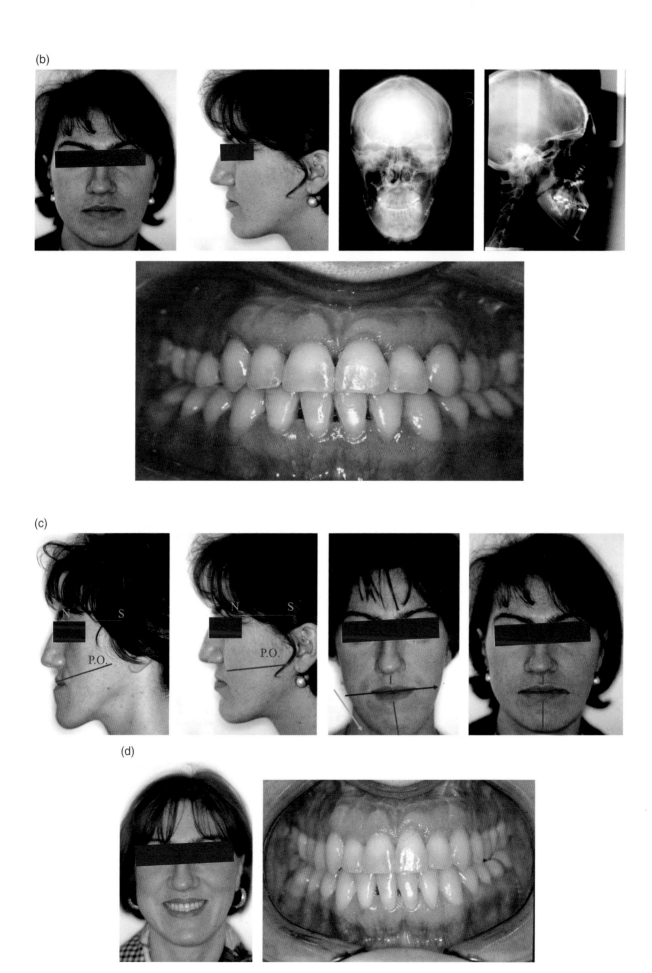

(c)

(d)

Figure 12.9.16 (Continued)

References

Andresen V. Bio-mekanisk ortodonti. Et ortodontisk system for privatpraksis og skole-tannklinikker. Norsk Tannlaegefor Tid. 1932;4:131–138.

Arvidsson LZ, Smith HJ, Flatø B, Larheim TA. Temporomandibular joint findings in adults with long-standing juvenile idiopathic arthritis: CT and MR imaging assessment. Radiology. 2010;256:191–200.

Bellintani C, Carletti V, Farronato G, Mastaglio C, Gattinara M, Gerloni V. Classification criteria of juvenile idiopathic arthritis and temporomandibular involvement. Ann Rheum Dis. 2005a;64:196.

Bellintani C, Garagiola U, Farronato G. ATM danno articolare nelle forme di artrite idiopatica giovanile, prevenzione e cura. Institutional Research Information System, Universita degli Studi di Milano, 2002.

Bellintani C, Ghiringhelli P, Gerloni V, Gattinara M, Farronato G, Fantini F. Temporomandibular joint involvement in juvenile idiopathic arthritis: treatment with an orthodontic appliance. Reumatismo. 2005b;57:201–207.

Bertram S, Rudisch A, Innerhofer K, Pümpel E, Grub-Wieser G, Emshoff R. Diagnosing TMJ internal derangement and osteoarthritis with magnetic resonance imaging. J Am Dent Assoc. 2001;132:753–761.

Bombeccari GP, Farronato G, Ganni AB, Spadari F. Diagnostic accuracy of cone beam computed tomography (CBCT) to detect bone invasion by oral carcinoma. Dent Cadmos. 2015;83:518–527.

Brusati R, Chiapasco M. Elementi di Chirurgia Oro-Maxillo-Facciale. Issy-Les-Moulineaux: Elsevier-Masson, 1999.

Chummun S, McLean NR, Nugent M, Anderson PJ, David DJ. Binder syndrome. J Craniofac Surg. 2012;23:986–990.

Ciancaglini R. Gnatologia e Dolori Oro-Facciali. Problemi e Soluzioni. Issy-Les-Moulineaux: Elsevier-Masson, 2007.

Cossellu G, Biagi R, Faggioni G, Farronato G. Orthodontic treatment of Binder syndrome: a case report with 5 years of follow-up. Cleft Palate Craniofac J. 2015;52:484–488.

Cozza P, Baccetti T, Franchi L, De Toffol L, McNamara JA Jr. Mandibular changes produced by functional appliances in Class II malocclusion: a systematic review. Am J Orthod Dentofac Orthop. 2006;129(599):e1–e12.

Cozza P, De Toffol L, Colagrossi S. Dentoskeletal effects and facial profile changes during activator therapy. Eur J Orthod. 2004;26:293–302.

Defraia E, Camporesi M, Conti G, Zoni V, Marinelli A. Oral and craniofacial findings of Binder syndrome: two case reports. Cleft Palate Craniofac J. 2012;49:498–503.

Draf W, Bockmühl U, Hoffmann B. Nasal correction in maxillonasal dysplasia (Binder's syndrome): a long term follow-up study. Br J Plast Surg. 2003;56:199–204.

Farronato G, Bellintani C, Garagiola U, Cressoni P, Puttini PS, Atzeni F, Cazzola M. Three-dimensional morphological condylar and mandibular changes in a patient with juvenile idiopathic arthritis: interdisciplinary treatment. Reumatismo. 2014a;66:254–257.

Farronato G, Carletti V, Giannini L, Farronato D, Maspero C. Juvenile idiopathic arthritis with temporomandibular joint involvement: functional treatment. Eur J Paediatr Dent. 2011a;12:131–134.

Farronato G, Carletti V, Maspero C, Farronato D, Giannini L, Bellintani C. Craniofacial growth in children affected by juvenile idiopathic arthritis involving the temporomandibular joint: functional therapy management. J Clin Pediatr Dent. 2009;33:351–357.

Farronato G, Farronato D, Toma L, Bellincioni F. A synthetic three-dimensional craniofacial analysis. J Clin Orthod. 2010a;44:673–678.

Farronato G, Folegatti C, Giannini L, Galbiati G, Pelo S, Maspero C. Sindrome di Binder: caso clinico. Dent Cadmos. 2014c;82:205–215.

Farronato G, Garagiola U, Carletti V, Cressoni P, Bellintani C. Psoriatic arthritis: temporomandibular joint involvement as the first articular phenomenon. Quintessence Int. 2010c;41:395–398.

Farronato G, Garagiola U, Carletti V, Cressoni P, Bellintani C. Juvenile idiopathic arthritis: condylar and mandibular morphologic and volumetric changes. Inflamm Res. 2011b;60(suppl. 1):287.

Farronato G, Garagiola U, Carletti V, Cressoni P, Mercatali L, Farronato D. Change in condylar and mandibular morphology in juvenile idiopathic arthritis: cone beam volumetric imaging. Minerva Stomatol. 2010d;59:519–534.

Farronato G, Garagiola U, Dominici A, Periti G, de Nardi S, Carletti V, Farronato D. "Ten-point" 3D cephalometric analysis using low-dosage cone beam computed tomography. Prog Orthod. 2010b;11:2–12.

Farronato G, Giannini L, Galbiati G, Mortellaro C, Maspero C. Presurgical orthodontic planning: predictability. J Craniofac Surg. 2013;24:e184–e186.

Farronato G, Giannini L, Galbiati G, Mortellaro C, Maspero C. Presurgical virtual three-dimensional treatment planning. J Craniofac Surg. 2015a;26:820–823.

Farronato G, Giannini L, Galbiati G, Pisani L, Mortellaro C, Maspero C. Verification of the reliability of the three-dimensional virtual presurgical orthodontic diagnostic protocol. J Craniofac Surg. 2014b;25:2013–2016.

Farronato G, Grillo ME, Giannini L, Farronato D, Maspero C. Long-term results of early condylar fracture correction: case report. Dent Traumatol. 2009a;25:e37–e42.

Farronato G, Periti G, Giannini L, Farronato D, Maspero C. Straight-wire appliances: standard versus individual prescription. Prog Orthod. 2009b;10:58–71.

Farronato G, Porro A, Pisani L, Magni A, Esposito L, Maspero C. Ortho-surgical treatment: 3D virtual protocol using CBCT. Dent Cadmos. 2015b;83:550–558.

Farronato G, Santamaria G, Cressoni P, Falzone D, Colombo M. The digital-titanium Herbst. J Clin Orthod. 2011c;45:263–288.

Firetto MC, Abbinante A, Barbato E, Bellomi M, Biondetti P, Borghesi A, Bossu' M, Cascone P, Corbella D, Di Candido V, Diotallevi P, Farronato G, Federici A, Gagliani M, Granata C, Guerra M, Magi A, Maggio MC, Mirenghi S, Nardone M, Origgi D, Paglia L, Preda L, Rampado O, Rubino L, Salerno S, Sodano A, Torresin A, Strohmenger L. National guidelines for dental diagnostic imaging in the developmental age. Radiol Med. 2019;124:887–916.

Garagiola U, Mercatali L, Bellintani C, Fodor A, Farronato G, Lőrincz A. Change in condylar and mandibular morphology in juvenile idiopathic arthritis: cone beam volumetric imaging. Fogorv Sz. 2013;106:27–31.

Garagiola U, Piancino MG, Naini FB, Cressoni P, Moro A, Gasparini G, Saponaro G, Nishiyama K, Farronato G. Damage quantification of mandibular condyle in juvenile idiopathic arthritis: 3D morphological study by cone beam computed tomography. J Biol Regul Homeost Agents. 2019;33:1269–1274.

Greenberg SA. Binder's syndrome (nasomaxillary dysplasia): an uncommonly common disorder. J La State Med Soc. 1991;143:27–33.

Holmström H. Clinical and pathologic features of maxillonasal dysplasia (Binder's syndrome): significance of the prenasal fossa on etiology. Plast Reconstr Surg. 1986;78:559–567.

Kreiborg S, Bakke M, Kirkeby S, Michler L, Vedtofte P, Seidler B, Møller E. Facial growth and oral function in a case of juvenile rheumatoid arthritis during an 8-year period. Eur J Orthod. 1990;12:119–134.

Maspero C, Galbiati G, Giannini L, Farronato G. Programmazione ortodontica-prechirurgica. Dent Cadmos. 2011;79:149–154.

Maspero C, Giannini L, Galbiati G, Farronato G. Programmazione ortodontica-prechirurgica tramite allestimento di mascherine termostampate. Mondo Ortod. 2012;37:3–12.

Meazzini MC, Caprioglio A, Garattini G, Lenatti L, Poggio CE. Hemandibular hypoplasia successfully treated with functional appliances: is it truly hemifacial microsomia? Cleft Palate Craniofac J. 2008;45:50–56.

Oenning AC, Jacobs R, Salmon B. ALADAIP, beyond ALARA and towards personalized optimization for paediatric cone-beam CT. Int J Paediatr Dent. 2021;31:676–678.

Pancherz H, Ruf S, Kohlhas P. "Effective condylar growth" and chin position changes in Herbst treatment: a cephalometric roentgenographic long-term study. Am J Orthod Dentofac Orthop. 1998;114:437–446.

12.10

The Vertical Component of Asymmetry: Etiology and Treatment

Joseph G. Ghafari

Depictions of differential vertical asymmetry have been related to specific congenital or pathologic symptoms, such as hemifacial microsomia and condylar hyperplasia. Vertical maxillary asymmetry (VMA) is a condition localized to the nasal/maxillary/occlusal region, characterized by dentoalveolar asymmetry, canted nasal floor and occlusal plane, and asymmetric lip elevation. The asymmetry does not affect the orbits and the mandible. The potential etiology includes dentoalveolar compensation to localized skeletal or dental disturbances and possibly neuromuscular origins. Early treatment is recommended if the condition is properly diagnosed clinically and on the posteroanterior cephalography.

> *Asymmetry is the rhythmic expression of functional design.*
> – Jan Tschischold
> German calligrapher,
> typographer and book designer

The Three-dimensional Nature of Asymmetry

The tenet that facial asymmetry is a common trait has been demonstrated in the cliché representation of differing appearance when the two rights and two lefts of a face are mirrored in the midline. Thus, a degree of asymmetry is acceptable in every face. Often, a small amount of asymmetry exists that may not influence the appraisal of facial attractiveness (Kaipainen et al. 2016). Treatment is often sought when a "measurable" asymmetry "disrupts" the general facial harmony.

Facial asymmetry has been reported extensively and mostly in the transverse dimension, ranging from mild midline deviations to extreme irregularities associated with recognized syndromes. However, its configuration in all planes of space is best captured by the spatial orientation of dentofacial traits in the three aeronautic rotational descriptors: pitch (posteroanterior up/down tip around a horizontal axis), roll (lateral up/down tip), and yaw (right/left rotation) (Ackerman et al. 2007; Ghafari 2012). Conceptually, pitch and roll comprise a vertical component and yaw predominantly includes a right/left discrepancy, such as midline deviations and subdivision malocclusions. The vertical component of pitch is revealed with the up and down position of posterior and anterior components of the occlusion relative to each other, often simplified in the relation of maxillary incisors and anterior gingival display to upper lip position at rest and in function. The normal inclination of the occlusal plane in the pitch direction favors a more downward tip of the anterior part, based on the normal inclination of the occlusal plane (9.5 degrees [range, 1.5–14.5 degrees]) (Downs 1952). Accordingly, deviations from this range do not begin at a flat (0 degrees) plane. Yaw and roll denote the more commonly defined dentofacial asymmetries.

The three rotational descriptors highlight the importance of their simultaneous assessment in various arrangements of malocclusion. More accurate evaluation is obtained with cone beam computed tomography (CBCT) images than traditional 2D lateral and posteroanterior cephalograms. Panoramic radiographs mainly illustrate roll, without inferences on pitch and only partial information on yaw.

Attempts have been made at quantifying the amount of deviation, including angular, linear, and proportional analyses that could "objectively" scrutinize such disruption. Non-radiographic instruments have been developed that readily assess shifts from the norm, such as the deviation from the divine proportions [Ricketts' "golden divider" (Ricketts 1982), Marquardt "golden decagon mask" (Marquardt 2002)].

Acceptable levels of midline deviation have been studied among laypeople, dentists, or orthodontics (Kokich et al. 1999). However, outside of the obvious asymmetry characteristic of pathologic syndromes, quantifying "acceptable" skeletal deviations may not be generalized. A hypothesis yet to be tested stipulates that less severe or mild asymmetries would be within one standard deviation, asymmetry becoming a significant dysmorphology beyond one standard deviation of a measurement. This premise must be balanced with the personal boundaries of comfort with and acceptance of asymmetric features.

A major shortcoming of a transverse cephalometric assessment in comparison with the sagittal evaluation is determining the potential concealment or exaggeration of the underlying skeletal discrepancy by the covering soft tissue thickness. Such assessment is possible on lateral cephalographs because soft tissue landmarks are properly defined and tegumental variations with hard tissue outlines are available.

Interaction between Maxillary and Mandibular Asymmetries

The association of maxillary and mandibular morphology has been reported during growth (Ghafari and Macari 2023) and treatment (Efstratiadis et al. 2005). Macari and Ghafari (2023) have demonstrated that not only mandibular position is affected by maxillary changes following sustained mouth breathing in young children, but also mandibular size. In craniofacial pathology, conditions have been classified under congenital (e.g. oral clefting, hemifacial microsomia, craniosynostoses) and acquired etiology (e.g. unilateral condylar hyperplasia, temporomandibular joint ankylosis or resorption, facial trauma or tumor). Regardless of the origin, considered in this review are commonly described maxillary asymmetries associated with mandibular asymmetry that involve the contribution of the orthodontist in their multidisciplinary treatment. They are classified in two basic types: maxillary asymmetry secondary to mandibular asymmetry, such as condylar hyperplasia and hemifacial microsomia, and mandibular asymmetry secondary to maxillary asymmetry, found with cleft lip and palate.

Maxillary Asymmetry Secondary to Mandibular Asymmetry

Condylar hyperplasia is a pathologic condition that usually sets in adolescence and may involve "normal" bilateral or unilateral condylar growth or abnormal enlargement of the condylar head (Machoň et al. 2023). Whereas bilateral hyperplasia has been hypothesized to occur in symmetrical Class III malocclusions (Genno et al. 2019), unilateral condylar growth causes mandibular asymmetry and compensatory maxillary asymmetry and progresses with rotational deviations in all planes, notably roll and yaw. The mandibular teeth, particularly the incisors, characteristically incline to the side of the hyperplastic condyle (Figure 12.10.1). Treatment of this condition involves high or total condylectomy (Wolford et al. 2002), more recently electrocautery of the condyle (Hashemi and Amirzargar 2022), and/or orthognathic surgery, depending on the time of diagnosis, severity of the facial dysmorphology, and the surgeon's experience (Machoň et al. 2023; Wolford et al. 2002). Often, bone scintigraphy using the isotope technetium (Tc-99m) is used to determine the active state or cessation of condylar cell proliferation (López et al. 2021). Frequently, the object of early orthodontic intervention is to maintain the symmetry in maxilla before further compensatory changes to the developing mandibular asymmetry.

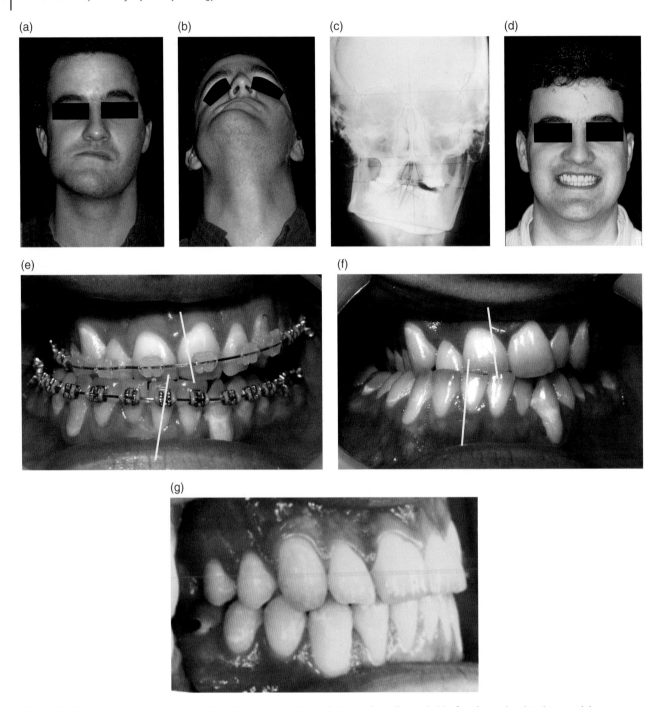

Figure 12.10.1 Facial photographs (a, b) and posteroanterior cephalometric radiograph (c) of patient who develop condylar hyperplasia showing overgrowth of the left condyle leading to mandibular and maxillary asymmetry and dentoalveolar compensation (e). Treatment included an orthodontic phase (f) prior to orthognathic surgery. Posttreatment facial (d) and occlusal (g) photographs reveal correction of asymmetry.

Hemifacial microsomia is characterized by a deficient or missing mandibular ramus, lack of tissue on the affected side of the face, and microtia (total or partial absence of the external ear). The mandibular asymmetry is related to the severity of condylar and ramal defect, which ranges from mild with a small ramus but normal temporomandibular joint (level 1 of Pruzansky's classification) (Figure 12.10.2) to the more severe pathology in which the joint and ramus are reduced or absent (Pruzansky's classification 2 and 3) (Roberts 2000).

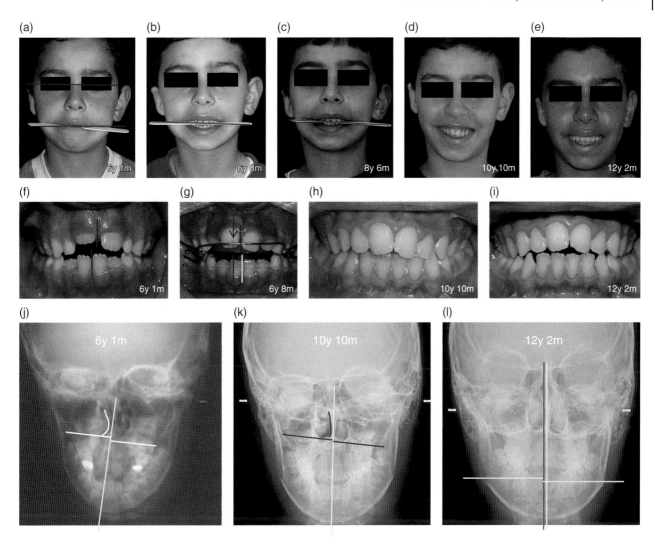

Figure 12.10.2 Hemifacial microsomia in a boy before treatment (a) with a functional appliance and in successive posttreatment stages (b–e) until nearly 6 years later (e). Corresponding intraoral photographs (f–i) and posteroanterior radiographs (j–l). A gradual decrease in asymmetry at the nasal, occlusal, and mandibular levels suggests an orthopedic effect of treatment.

Possible etiologies include a hemorrhage from the stapedial artery (about 6 weeks after conception) and the early loss of neural crest cells. Mandibular hypoplasia inhibits the symmetrical vertical growth of the maxilla, leading to a canted occlusal plane. Available studies indicate that the maxilla adapts to mandibular changes through dentoalveolar rather than skeletal compensation. In mild conditions, symmetry may be acceptable with sustained treatment (Figure 12.10.2). Early intervention with distraction osteogenesis in more severe conditions significantly improved the vertical maxillary asymmetry (VMA) 1 year post distraction through dentoalveolar modifications (Meazzini et al. 2012). On the other hand, in long-term follow-up of distraction osteogenesis until the completion of growth, treatment significantly improved vertical ramal asymmetry, but the results were gradually lost in time (Meazzini et al. 2005). Untreated patients maintained during growth the same ratio of affected/non affected ramal length as those who were treated. Thus, maxillary adjustments would also be influenced.

Mandibular Asymmetry Secondary to Maxillary Asymmetry

Representative of these conditions is the cleft lip and palate (CL/P) in which mandibular morphology, including asymmetry, adapts to the prevailing maxillary asymmetry. Studies of vertical mandibular asymmetry in patients with CL/P compared with control subjects who had malocclusions revealed greater mandibular asymmetry in the cleft patients, increasing with growth and peaking postpuberty (Figure 12.10.3) (Laspos et al. 1997; Kyrkanides

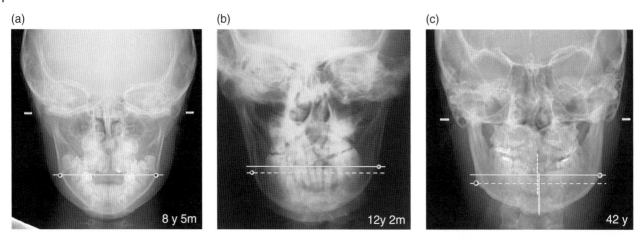

Figure 12.10.3 Posteroanterior cephalometric images of children aged 8 years, 5 months (a) and 12 years, 2 months (b), and a 42 years old man (c), with unilateral cleft lip/palate. Note symmetrical positions of gonions in the younger patient (a) and the discrepant vertical position of gonion in the other patients.

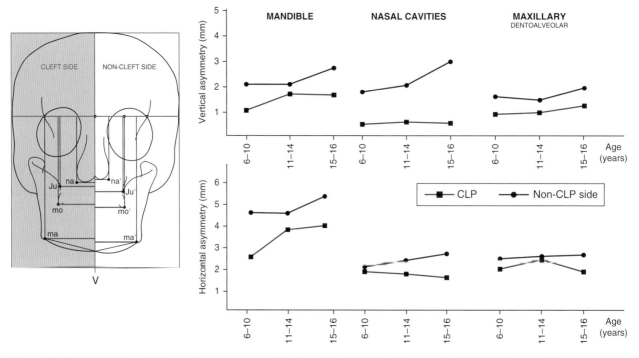

Figure 12.10.4 Vertical and horizontal asymmetry over time in unilateral cleft patients on the cleft side (blue color) compared with the control side (red) at the level of the mandible, nasal cavities, and maxillary molars (dentolaveolar), measured on posteroanterior cephalometric ragiographs. Each graph represents right and left deviations relative to the midline vertical (V) drawn as the perpendicular to the horizontal plane through right and left latero-orbitale. Note greatest vertical deviations at the level of the nasal cavities and horizontal deviations in the mandible. *Source:* Adapted from Laspos et al. (1997).

et al. 2000). However, the reported average differences were within 2–3 mm (Figure 12.10.4), not necessarily clinically significant to warrant orthognathic surgery, which is often needed in the maxilla. Such decision is usually weighed by the severity of horizontal rather than vertical mandibular asymmetry. In addition, the reported statistically significant correlations in the vertical plane between the asymmetric growths of the jaws, and between vertical lower facial asymmetry and the vertical maxillary dentoalveolar measurements (Kyrkanides et al. 2000; Laspos et al. 1997) suggest that lower facial asymmetries develop in a pattern parallel with the dentolaveolar structures (Figure 12.10.3). The development of mandibular asymmetry may also be related to age and consequently to the timing and success of treatment for cleft-associated maxillary problems.

"Field" Interactions

The described conditions, whether generated by a dysmorphology of the maxilla or mandible, reinforce the concept of symbiotic field interaction between skeletal and dentoalveolar structures whereby during development, an adaptive "domino" effect is sustained until homeostasis is reached defining the final malrelationship. Hypothetically, the skeletal component may be the dominant "culprit" that "orchestrates" the dynamic interplay between the skeletal and dentoalveolar components. However, it is conceivable that the latter may trigger the abnormal interplay, such as the development of Class II, division 2 malocclusion (Ghafari and Haddad 2014). In this malocclusion with predominant vertical deviations (decreased lower facial height, hypodivergence, deep overbite), a seemingly self-restrictive dentoalveolar complex through underoccluded posterior teeth and supraerupted anterior teeth dictates a more

mesial development of the mandible away from the dentition, accentuating the prominence of the chin.

Unimaxillary Vertical Asymmetry not Affecting the Symmetry of the Other Jaw

Localized maxillary or mandibular asymmetries have been reported, often of idiopathic origin. VMA falls in this category.

Vertical Maxillary Asymmetry (VMA)

This condition involves the predominance of VMA at various levels, mainly the different heights of the right and left images of the nasal floor and levels of the occlusal plane, which were initially observed in the same direction (up or down on the same side), and the lack of apparent and significant mandibular asymmetry. Open bite is not usually observed with the dentoalveolar discrepancy (Ghafari 2012). Also, asymmetric lip elevation is observed, disclosing more gingival display unilaterally. VMA is observed clinically and on the panoramic and lateral cephalographs (Figures 12.10.5–12.10.9). References to vertical asymmetry

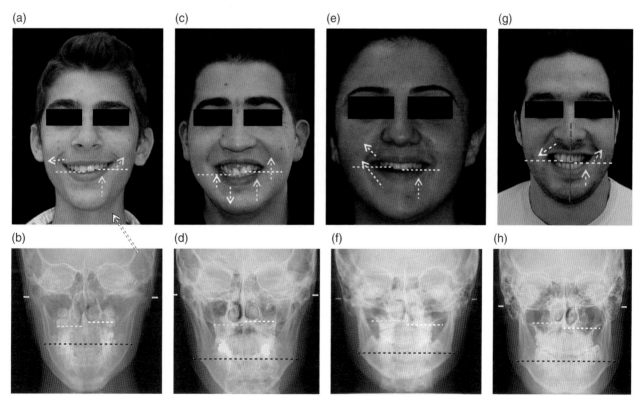

Figure 12.10.5 Patients with VMA. Horizontal lines on facial photographs indicate differential occlusal levels and arrows point to asymmetric lip elevation. On posteroanterior cephalographs, different nasal levels are indicated by horizontal lines; mandibular symmetrical vertical levels are reflected by a horizontal line through gonions. (a, b) VMA in a 13.8-year-old boy. (c, d) VMA in a 22.3-year-old man. (e, f) VMA in a 23.2-year-old woman. (g, h) VMA in a 23.7-year-old man.

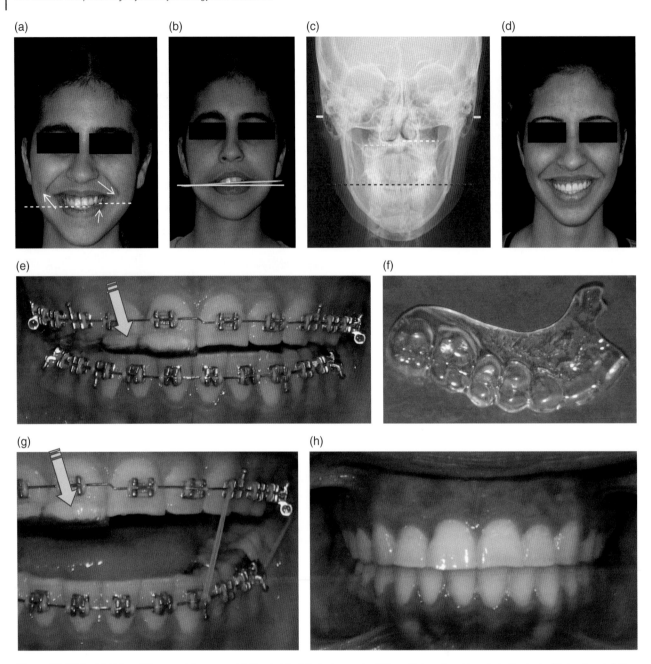

Figure 12.10.6 VMA in a 19-year-old woman. (a) Frontal facial photograph, differential occlusal levels indicated with horizontal lines and varied lip elevation by arrows; (b) tongue blade between the teeth underscores the level of occlusal asymmetry relative to horizontal (yellow) line; (c) posteroanterior cephalometric radiograph; horizontal lines show different vertical nasal levels but symmetrical mandibular gonial heights; (d) facial photograph after treatment shows asymmetric lip elevation; (e) unilateral removable appliance inserted on right side disoccludes the left side; (f) unilateral removable appliance made of clear acrylic; (g) unilateral vertical elastics were worn by the patient to extrude the maxillary left teeth against a heavier wire in mandibular arch; (h) occlusion after removal of fixed appliances.

in the literature are combined with dominant transverse discrepancies, primarily within the described congenital and pathologic entities.

In a pilot retrospective case series study, 781 digital posteroanterior cephalographs were screened for VMA, 28 (3.46%) of which (belonging to 18 females, 10 males) met the main inclusion criterion of a minimal difference of 2 mm between the right and left nasal floors (Figure 12.10.10). Findings did not reveal significant differences between mean orbital and ramal right and left heights, indicating symmetry of these structures (Tables 12.10.1 and 12.10.2). The significant differences between

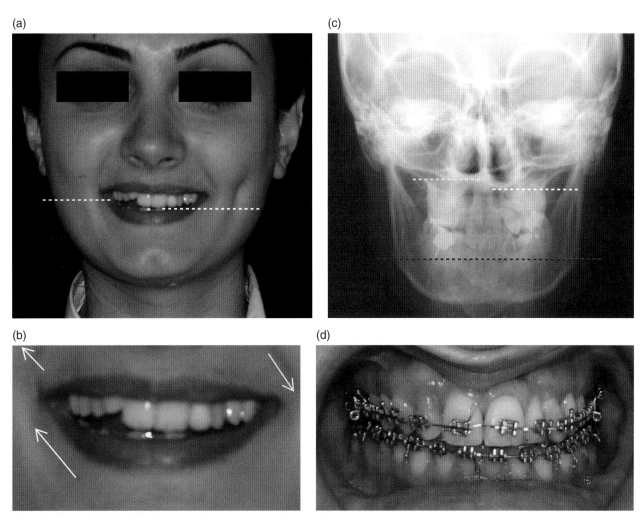

Figure 12.10.7 (a) Frontal facial photograph reveals differential occlusal levels indicated with horizontal lines; (b) asymmetric lip elevation; (c) posteroanterior cephalometric radiograph, two horizontal lines are drawn at differential nasal levels and one straight line through the symmetrical mandibular gonial levels; (d) occlusion leveled through differential extrusion of maxillary right and mandibular left teeth.

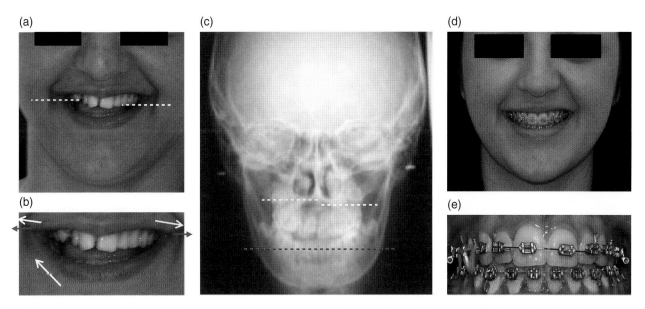

Figure 12.10.8 VMA in a 18.5-year-old girl. (a) Frontal facial photograph, horizontal lines indicate differential occlusal levels; (b) asymmetric lip elevation; (c) posteroanterior cephalometric radiograph, horizontal lines drawn at different nasal levels and straight line indicates symmetry of gonial mandibular levels; (d, e) facial and occlusal photographs after vertical leveling of occlusion.

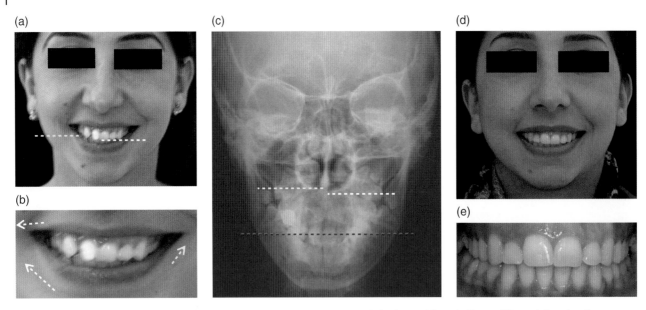

Figure 12.10.9 VMA in a 25.7-year-old woman. (a) Frontal facial photograph: horizontal lines indicate differential occlusal levels; (b) asymmetric lip elevation discloses more mandibular teeth on right than left side; (c) posteroanterior cephalometric radiograph: horizontal lines illustrate different nasal levels and a straight-line highlights symmetry of gonial mandibular heights; (d, e) facial and occlusal photographs after treatment reveal occlusal improvement.

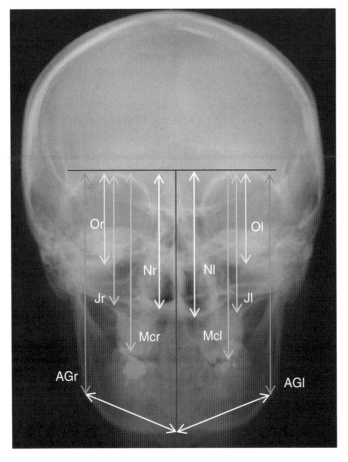

Figure 12.10.10 The following bilateral landmarks (r: right, l: left) were measured on the posteroanterior radiograph from a horizontal line perpendicular to the midline vertical drawn through the crista galli and anterior nasal spine: O- most inferior point on orbital contour, N- lowest point on inferior nasal contour, J- jugale (J, at the jugal process, the intersection of the outline of the maxillary tuberosity and the zygomatic buttress), AG- antegonion (AG, at the antegonial notch, the lateral inferior margin of the antegonial protuberances), and M- molar point (intersection between maxillary and mandibular first molars). Bilateral transverse symmetry was gauged by measuring the difference between the right and left corpus length (distances AG to menton). In addition, the contour of the septum was evaluated to determine the presence or absence of septal deviation, confirmed by an otolaryngologist.

Table 12.10.1 Vertical differences (mm) between right and left sides at the levels of the orbit, nose, maxilla, molars, and mandible.

	Age (yr)	Orbit	Nose	Maxilla	Occlusion	Ramus	AG-Me
Mean	21.64	0.39	3.24	3.23	3.17	0.62	1.33
SD	4.84	0.39	1.24	0.84	1.31	0.39	0.67

Table 12.10.2 Difference between mandibular corpus lengths in younger and older patients.

	AG-Me left	AG-Me right	Difference	P
Younger	52.23 ± 2.49	51.62 ± 2.36	1.38 ± 0.87	0.52
Older	54.47 ± 5.82	5.13 ± 4.84	1.53 ± 0.64	0.87

Table 12.10.3 Correlations among measurements of heights at the level of the nose, maxilla, occlusal plane, and ramus in younger and older patients.

Older/Younger	Orbit	Nose	Maxilla at jugale	Molar level	Ramus
Orbit		−0.12	−0.16	−0.20	−0.13
Nose	−0.58		0.61	0.62	0.33
Maxilla	−0.60	0.85		0.65	0.31
Occl plane	−0.56	0.94	0.92		0.78
Ramus	−0.60	0.55	0.40	0.53	

nasal, maxillary, and occlusal levels (about 3 mm) confirmed the observed synergy in vertical discrepancy between nasal floor and occlusion and reflected a localized skeletal asymmetry with apparent dentoalveolar adaptation to nasal asymmetry (or vice versa). In the same context, the correlations among nasal, maxillary, occlusal, and nasal heights were the highest, the vertical level of the dentition being commensurate with the nasal/maxillary levels (Figures 12.10.5–12.10.9). The correlations among the older patients ($0.85 < r < 0.94$; $n = 13$; ages 11–16.9 years) were stronger than in the younger patients ($0.65 < r > 0.65$; $n = 15$; ages 17–41 years) (Table 12.10.3), indicating a developmental nature of the condition. The small mandibular differences suggested that the effect on the ramal heights was not significant enough to reach clinical manifestation. Septal deviation was observed in nearly half (54%) of the patients (69% of younger, 40% of older) (Ghafari 2012).

Based on these findings, a roll factor would be prevalent because of the predominant vertical asymmetry between right and left sides, although the occlusal surfaces may be straight and not necessarily obliquely inclined. Therefore, a translational vertical movement may be speculated as the position of the dentition was parallel to the nasal levels. The lack of statistically significant differences between right and left corpus lengths suggests that the "roll" did not affect the gonial heights.

Treatment in most patients may be limited to orthodontics through differential unilateral bite opening performed sequentially on one side before the other to produce the pertinent and indicated differential intrusion and extrusion of the supraerupted and infraerupted quadrant, respectively (Figure 12.10.6). Depending on diagnostic features, particularly in the presence of differential excessive gingival display (EGD – "gummy" smile), differential intrusion against miniscrews may be indicated. In the presence of a severe generalized EGD, intrusion against miniscrews, or orthognathic surgery may be considered.

Possible Etiologies of VMA

The etiology of VMA remains idiopathic, but morphologic, syndromic, and neuromuscular causes are possible. The original symptom may be septal deviation, which usually refers to unilateral bony, cartilaginous, or combined convexities of the septum with accompanying irregularities of midline structures. Although occurring in 80% of people in varying degrees (Hong et al. 2016; Uygur et al. 2003), a deviated septum is considered of clinical significance when associated with difficulty breathing, usually worse on the side of the deviation, or other nasal troubles such as sinus infections or nose bleeds.

Septal deviation can be congenital or acquired, such as through trauma, including birth trauma, unequal growth, uneven infections, congenital deformities (cleft palate), and minor overlooked childhood injuries that are difficult to track later (Reitzen et al. 2011). Compensatory growth occurs in the adjacent nasal structures, notably the middle chonca on the concave side. Similarly, the association between septal deviation and VMA would be developmental among the nasal, maxillary, and occlusal heights, with the compensatory potential occurring at the level of the dentition, apparently unilaterally accounting for the vertical asymmetry. The prevalence of septal deviation in the pilot study (about 50%) was based on posteroanterior cephalographs that disclosed only bony alterations. Cartilaginous deformities may elevate this incidence.

In contrast, it would be conceivable that nasal floor adaptation is secondary to a dentoalveolar origin, such as the compensation for a unilateral delayed emergence of mandibular (or maxillary) teeth by the extrusion of opposing maxillary (or mandibular) teeth on the affected side, or the induction by early eruption of mandibular (or maxillary) teeth on a contralateral side of infraeruption of maxillary (mandibular) teeth on the same side.

The mechanism of induction of the VMA by septal deviation and dentoalveolar etiologic paths would involve a downward compensatory progression of the condition generated by septal deviation and an upward compensatory process generated at the level of the dentition. Extended research is needed to affirm these speculations.

The differential elevation of the lips and in some patients asymmetric nasolabial crease during smiling suggest a potential neuromuscular contribution. VMA could possibly reflect a subclinical form of, or a long-term phenotypic compensation to a primary syndrome, not reaching the severity level of the pathology. Recognized syndromes with asymmetric lip elevation include the asymmetric crying (baby) facies (ACF), reported in less than 1% (0.63%) of live births. In this neonate or infant condition, the face is asymmetric during crying, when the corner of the mouth is pulled downward on one side because of hypoplasia or agenesis of the depressor anguli oris (DAO) muscle or compression of one of the facial nerve branches, which may occur during birth (Pape and Pickering 1972; Shapira and Borochowitz 2009). The mouth appears symmetric at rest, and other functions of the facial muscles are also symmetric, including sucking (with no drooling), nasolabial fold depth, respiratory nostril dilatation, forehead wrinkling, frowning, closure of eyelids, and tearing.

ACF becomes less evident with age, as functions of other facial muscles and smiling dominate the child's facial expressions (Bawle et al. 1998; Lahat et al. 2000). It may be associated with other anomalies, commonly in the cardiovascular system and notably the Cayler cardiofacial syndrome, characterized by chromosome 22q11.2 deletion (Bawle et al. 1998; Cayler 1969).

Clinical and Research Considerations

If VMA is diagnosed and treated early enough in its development, the impact would be evident on the occlusion and associated dental and facial esthetics before the condition worsens with age. Various levels of asymmetry have been shown to negatively influence these esthetics (Kokich et al. 1999). Prevention or early correction also may address the differential emergence of permanent teeth during their eruption in the oral cavity.

Research is warranted to ascertain the validity of VMA as a separate entity or sequence through 3D (CBCT) assessment of facial characteristics. Also needing study is the variation in its components and means to predict and prevent the occlusal asymmetry. The potential etiology should be determined whether VMA is a series of morphologic adaptations to other primary causes, possibly secondary to a vertical muscular asymmetry that generates corresponding underlying vertical discrepancies or representing a subclinical variation of another condition of neuromuscular origin in which maxillary-nasal and occlusal adjustments are part of a compensatory process. Facial muscular (transverse) asymmetry has been described in patients with posterior crossbite before treatment, eventually switching to symmetry comparable to that observed in control patients (Kiliaridis et al. 2007).

Conclusion

Vertical facial asymmetry may be of congenital or environmental etiology. VMA predominantly affects the heights of maxillary structures, namely the nasal floor and dentoalveolar/occlusal level, but not those of the orbit and mandible, and is associated with asymmetric lip elevation. Speculation on etiology ranges from compensatory changes to a local etiology to subclinical expression of other syndromes. Frontal facial imaging is necessary to confirm the diagnosis of VMA. Excluding the prevention or an earlier correction of the vertical occlusal asymmetry, treatment varies with the severity of the asymmetry and extent of "gummy" smile, from mostly orthodontic compensation to possible surgical intervention.

References

Ackerman JL, Proffit WR, Sarver DM, Ackerman MB, Kean MR. Pitch, roll, and yaw: describing the spatial orientation of dentofacial traits. Am J Orthod Dentofac Orthop. 2007;131:305–310.

Bawle EV, Conard J, Van Dyke DL, Czarnecki P, Driscoll DA. Seven new cases of Cayler cardiofacial syndrome with chromosome 22q11.2 deletion, including a familial case. Am J Med Genet. 1998;79:406–410.

Cayler GG. Cardiofacial syndrome. Congenital heart disease and facial weakness, a hitherto unrecognized association. Arch Dis Child. 1969;44:69–75.

Downs WB. The role of cephalometrics in orthodontic case analysis and diagnosis. Am J Orthod. 1952;38:162–182.

Efstratiadis S, Baumrind S, Shofer F, Jacobsson-Hunt U, Laster L, Ghafari J. Evaluation of Class II treatment by cephalometric regional superimpositions versus conventional measurements. Am J Orthod Dentofac Orthop. 2005;128:607–618.

Genno PG, Nemer GM, BouZeineddine S, Macari AM, Ghafari JG. 3 novel genes tied to mandibular prognathism in East-Mediterranean families. Am J Orthod Dentofac Orthop. 2019;156:104–112.

Ghafari JG. Vertical maxillary asymmetry: a prevalent lateral roll in spatial orientation. Orthodontics (Chic). 2012;13:e127–e139.

Ghafari JG, Haddad RV. Cephalometric and dental analysis of Class II, division 2 reveals various sub-types of the malocclusion and the primacy of dentoalveolar components. Semin Orthod. 2014;20:272–286.

Ghafari JG, Macari AT. Interaction between the orthodontist and medical airway specialists on respiratory and non-respiratory disturbances. In: Krishnan V, Kuijpers-Jagtman AM, eds. Integrated Clinical Orthodontics. London: Wiley-Blackwell, 2023:248–271.

Hashemi HM, Amirzargar R. Can electrocautery of the mandibular condyle effectively treat condylar hyperplasia? J Cranio-Maxillofacial Surg. 2022;50:785–789.

Hong CJ, Monteiro E, Badhiwala J, Lee J, de Almeida JR, Vescan A, Witterick IJ. Open versus endoscopic septoplasty techniques: a systematic review and meta-analysis. Am J Rhinol Allergy. 2016;30:436–442.

Kaipainen AE, Sieber KR, Nada RM, Maal TJ, Katsaros C, Fudalej PS. Regional facial asymmetries and attractiveness of the face. Eur J Orthod. 2016;38:602–608.

Kiliaridis S, Mahboubi PH, Raadsheer MC, Katsaros C. Ultrasonographic thickness of the masseter muscle in growing individuals with unilateral crossbite. Angle Orthod. 2007;77:607–611.

Kokich VO Jr, Kiyak HA, Shapiro PA. Comparing the perception of dentists and laypeople to altered dental esthetics. J Esthet Dent. 1999;11:311–324.

Kyrkanides S, Klambani M, Subtelny JD. Cranial base and facial skeleton asymmetries in individuals with unilateral cleft lip and palate. Cleft Palate Craniofac J. 2000;37:556–561.

Lahat E, Heyman E, Barkay A, Goldberg M. Asymmetric crying facies and associated congenital anomalies: prospective study and review of the literature. J Child Neurol. 2000;15:808–810.

Laspos CP, Kyrkanides S, Tallents RH, Moss ME, Subtelny JD. Mandibular and maxillary asymmetry in individuals with unilateral cleft lip and palate. Cleft Palate Craniofac J. 1997;34:232–239.

López DF, Castro MA, Muñoz JM, Cárdenas-Perilla R. Reference values of mandibular condyles metabolic activity: a study using ^{99m}Tc-MDP single-photon emission computed tomography. Orthod Craniofac Res. 2021;24:328–334.

Macari AT, Ghafari JG. Secondary analysis of airway obstruction in children with adenoid hypertrophy: Association with jaw size and position. Semin Orthod. 2023;29:264–270.

Machoň V, Bartoš M, Suchý T, Levorová J, Foltán R. Micro-computed tomography evaluation of bone architecture in various forms of unilateral condylar hyperplasia. Int J Oral Maxillofac Surg. 2023;52:44–50.

Marquardt SR. Stephen R. Marquardt on the Golden Decagon and human facial beauty. Interview by Dr. Gottlieb. J Clin Orthod. 2002;36:339–347.

Meazzini MC, Mazzoleni F, Bozzetti A, Brusati R. Comparison of mandibular vertical growth in hemifacial microsomia patients treated with early distraction or not treated: follow up till the completion of growth. J Craniomaxillofac Surg. 2012;40:105–111.

Meazzini MC, Mazzoleni F, Gabriele C, Bozzetti A. Mandibular distraction osteogenesis in hemifacial microsomia: long-term follow-up. J Craniomaxillofac Surg. 2005;33:370–376.

Pape KE, Pickering D. Asymmetric crying facies: an index of other congenital anomalies. J Pediatr. 1972;81:21–30.

Reitzen SD, Chung W, Shah AR. Nasal septal deviation in the pediatric and adult populations. Ear Nose Throat J. 2011;90:112–115.

Ricketts RM. The biologic significance of the divine proportion and Fibonacci series. Am J Orthod. 1982;81:351–370.

Roberts D. Hemifacial microsomia. In: Fonseca RJ, Baker SB, Wolford LM, eds. Fonseca Oral Maxillofacial Surgery. Philadelphia: WB Saunders, 2000:239–270.

Shapira M, Borochowitz ZU. Asymmetric crying facies. NeoReviews. 2009;10:e502–e509.

Uygur K, Tüz M, Dogru H. The correlation between septal deviation and concha bullosa. Otolaryngol Head Neck Surg. 2003;129:33–36.

Wolford LM, Mehra P, Reiche-Fischel O, Morales-Ryan CA, Garcia-Morales P. Efficacy of high condylectomy for management of condylar hyperplasia. Am J Orthod Dentofac Orthop. 2002;121:136–150.

12.11

Helping Children and Their Families with Facial Differences – Patient Centered Outcomes and Experiences

Eleftherios G. Kaklamanos

CHAPTER MENU

Introduction

People exhibit differences in personality, attitudes, preferences, or looks, which are essential in providing one's unique identity so that no two people are the same or behave in an identical manner. Contemporary societies place particular emphasis on physical appearance and concerns about "image" might affect a substantial portion of the general population (Gilbert and Thompson 2002; Rumsey and Harcourt 2004). Some people are born with conditions that affect the appearance of the body or the characteristics of the face; other develop deformative changes during the lifetime, which can be acceptable to a greater or a lesser extent (Newell 2000).

Mild degrees of asymmetry are present in ostensibly symmetric faces (Proffit et al. 2019). More severe asymmetry affecting the appearance of an individual's face and creating a visible facial difference, might be the result of a combination of inherited tendencies and environmental influences on growth of the jaws, that in some cases cannot be treated with conventional orthodontic treatment only and require surgical intervention as well (Severt and Proffit 1997). Such conditions might affect quality of life

(QoL) and self-esteem, especially in females (Agırnaslıgıl et al. 2019; Frejman et al. 2013; Jung 2016; Kurabe et al. 2016; Meger et al. 2021; Ribeiro-Neto et al. 2018; Sun et al. 2018; Yi et al. 2019).

However, other conditions leading to facial asymmetries and differences, present increased complexity in their structural and functional characteristics creating a significant burden on patients and families not only from the condition itself, but also from its profound psychosocial impacts as well. Such face asymmetries can be congenital or acquired affecting individuals and creating visible differences at any time point in their life. Orofacial clefts are among the most common birth defects worldwide (Mossey and Catilla 2003; Shaw 2004), are fully visible at birth, and represent a spectrum of disorders referring to any cleft affecting the mouth and/or other areas of the face. Clefting has an average incidence of 1:700 births (with significant geographical and ethnical variability), reflecting the intricate and sensitive nature of the mechanisms associated with the early development of the head and neck region (Wilderman et al. 2018). Seventy percent of registered orofacial cleft cases are non-syndromic, while the remainder develops in the context of various congenital syndromes

---

(Mossey and Catilla 2003; Shaw 2004). Since such disorders are often associated with an asymmetry in the upper dental arch, they might result in a concomitant facial asymmetry. Other congenital conditions leading to facial asymmetry, include hemifacial microsomia (Horgan et al. 1995), craniosynostoses (Mathijssen 2015), hemangiomata (Harris 1997), neurofibromatosis (Cohen 1995), etc. Acquired face asymmetries include those attributed to trauma (Lund 1974), diseases (e.g. juvenile rheumatoid arthritis) (Ince et al. 2000), and other causes (Proffit et al. 2019).

The current chapter will present the concerns, arising from conditions of increased complexity leading to asymmetry and facial difference, regarding parameters known only to the patient, like self-image, social difficulties, QoL, and other patient-centered domains. Patient-centered outcomes provide a context to advance evidence-based care by considering a wide range set of condition and management-related parameters that contribute to an individual's physical, mental, and social well-being, with the focus being placed on a hierarchy of concerns as determined by patients (DeBronkart 2015; Lavallee et al. 2016). Patient-centered outcomes involve self-reports concerning physical, psychological, and social interaction status at various time points and complement clinical assessment in population and individual health needs appraisal, as well as the evaluation of individual and public health interventions (Albrecht and Devlieger 1999; Gimprich and Paterson 2002). The variety of information provided by patient-centered outcomes contributes to the assessment of the impacts of diseases and treatments on the physical, psychological, and social spheres, sheds light on the reasons individuals react differently to similar conditions or management strategies, and informs the development of clinical strategies and services (Fontaine and Barofsky 2001). Such a perspective might be particularly informative to foster improvement of care for individuals with complex facial differences across a multifactorial model, since their experiences might be different conceptually different from the perceptions of others including clinicians (Valladares-Neto et al. 2014; Feu et al. 2013).

The Face as a Functional Structure and as an Element of Identity

The head region is characterized by unique anatomical structures and physiological processes fulfilling specialized functional requirements and acting as the origin of various sensory pathways (Siemionow and Sonmez 2008).

The entrance to the airway, which is necessary for the function of breathing and smelling, resides in the nose and the nostrils (Hornung 2006; Kastoer et al. 2016). The visual tract begins with the eyelids and the orbits (Huff and Austin 2016). The orbicularis oris muscle, the tongue, and the oral cavity contribute to the functions of swallowing and speech (Siemionow and Sonmez 2008). The external ear leads to the auditory tube and contributes to sound reception (Kastoer et al. 2016). The skin of the face forms a protecting barrier regulating body temperature and sweating (Casey 2002). Moreover, it contains nociceptors and free nerve endings detecting alterations in the mechanical environment that convey proprioceptive stimuli necessary for the function of speech and the coordination of the muscles of facial expression (Connor and Abbs 1998; Johansson et al. 1999; Kawakami et al. 2001; Schulze et al. 1997).

Besides its physiological functions and sensorial capacities, the face plays a cardinal role in determining an individual's identity and self-concept. During the course of life, we usually try to improve our facial appearance in order to enhance the presentation of ourselves, acknowledging its importance for social perceptions (Rumsey and Harcourt 2004).

The face is the key for the recognition of other human beings and our interactions with them, by being the primary area for expressing ourselves and demonstrating our emotions (Siemionow and Sonmez 2008). The facial area is also important for body image and self-perception, through the well-described interrelationship between appearance and self-concept (Harter 1999). Moreover, it influences how others perceive and evaluate us, affecting their assessments and subsequent inferences. The selection of a partner for life can be modified by facial and skin characteristics (Jones and Kramer 2015; McNulty et al. 2008; Montoya 2008; Samson et al. 2010; Zebrowitz 1997). Professional decisions, court rulings, and electoral behaviors are partly dependent on similar parameters (Barry 2020; Finkeldey and Demuth 2021; Todorov et al. 2005). Especially the characteristic of attractiveness of the appearance has received particular attention in relation to the psychosocial perception of the face (Zebrowitz and Montepare 2008). Individuals with attractive facial appearance enjoy greater approval and are considered to show greater abilities, characteristics that can constitute advantages in the social sphere (Bashour 2006; Lemay et al. 2010; Maner et al. 2008; Persichetti et al. 2019; Rhodes 2006). Thus, it does not come as a surprise that facial appearance and perceived attractiveness, are important for the construction of one's self-image (Chatterjee et al. 2009).

The Facial Difference from the Patient's Perspective

As the face is central to an individual's self-image and the primary area of social demonstration of various personality traits, expressions, and emotions, facial appearance can potentially affect one's self-concept, as well as the perceptions and behaviors of others (Grogan 1999; Harter 1997). Even less severe issues of facial appearance, like most malocclusion problems, have been shown to impact the everyday life and activities of young individuals (Bernabé et al. 2008; Foster Page et al. 2005; Johal et al. 2007; O'Brien et al. 2006, 2007). Children needing orthodontic intervention report twice as many impacts than those with little or no need (Bernabé et al. 2008). Reduced oral health-related quality of life (OHRQoL) has been observed in children as well (Do and Spencer 2008). Similar findings have been reported in young adults; maxillary and mandibular crowding more than two mm in the incisor area increases the chance of issues with "smiling, laughing, and showing teeth without embarrassment." When overjet is more than five mm, emotional impacts have been observed (Traebert and Peres 2007). Overall, the self-reported impact of malocclusion and dental appearance encompasses the psychological and social functions, including domains such as smiling, emotional state, and social encounters (Bernabé et al. 2008; Traebert and Peres 2007).

In individuals with significant facial differences, the interrelationship of the constructs of appearance and self-image is probably stronger than in the rest of the population (Kent and Thompson 2002). Although, perfect facial symmetry is rare when asymmetry is an individual's main concern it might become very significant as the patient encounters the problem every time one looks in the mirror (Severt and Proffit 1997). Irrespective of the time point a visible facial difference is being recognized, at birth or later in life, it might affect an individual's psychosocial sphere and lead to alterations in body image, impaired self-esteem, and QoL (Rumsey and Harcourt 2004). However, it is not possible to identify a priori the individuals with significant impairments (Feragen et al. 2009, 2015; Hunt et al. 2007). Resilient individuals manage to cope effectively and downgrade the impacts of their difference (Rumsey 2002). Resilience can be influenced by a person's subjective perception of how noticeable their difference is to others (Harris 1997), sociocultural factors (Rumsey 1997), coping styles (Moss 1997), social interaction skills (Kapp-Simon 1995), as well as family environment and social support (Lansdown et al. 1997).

Psychological Implications

Whether congenital or acquired, facial differences may have important psychological implications, including altered body image and poor self-esteem (Rumsey et al. 2002, 2003, 2004). Children with cleft tend to be less satisfied with their appearance and exhibit body image problems, especially with features in the area of the nose, mouth, and teeth (Feragen et al. 2015; Hunt et al. 2006, 2007; Slifer et al. 2004). In a Swedish nationwide register cohort with orofacial clefts, children presented with increased risk for personality disorders (Tillman et al. 2018) although major problems are not experienced usually (Hunt et al. 2005). Children with cleft lip and palate have been reported to have a more external locus of control, feel more dependent, present higher hostility, and demonstrate depressive symptoms and negative outlooks. Moreover, they are prone to feel less accepted by their parents, who are considered to show negative feelings and worry a lot (Berger and Dalton 2009; Collett et al. 2012; Feragen and Borge 2010; Feragen et al. 2015).

Craniofacial conditions are often associated with negative self-image and lower self-confidence that might last for many years (Crerand et al. 2017; Rumsey and Harcourt 2004). Almost three-quarters of a group of 15-year-old adolescents and 20-year-old adults with clefts felt that their self-confidence was impaired by their condition (Turner et al. 1997). Self-described low self-esteem, depressive symptoms, and anxiety in children with unilateral and bilateral cleft lip and palate are related to the facial appearance difference, with greater problems observed in the bilateral cleft lip and palate group that expectedly shows greater facial difference (Demir et al. 2011; Hunt et al. 2007). Danish adults with clefts have been reported to have double suicide rate (Herskind et al. 1993), however, investigations in Sweden did not produce corroborating results (Tillman et al. 2018). The degree of the effect of a facial difference on psychological parameters might be moderated by various factors, as research has shown that reports of self-esteem in affected children might be similar or even higher than those of non-affected groups (Mink van der Molen et al. 2021; Walters 1997). Psychosocial resilience has been associated with acceptable emotional functioning, appearance satisfaction, and a low exposure to teasing events (Feragen et al. 2009, 2010).

Social Interaction Implications

Any visible facial difference might also include a social handicap parameter, as, additionally to the impact on one's emotions, thoughts, and behaviors, it can be noticed by others as well (Macgregor 1989). Moreover, facial differences that affect the muscles of the face and problems with hearing, vision, or speech, might result in unusual verbal and nonverbal communication and prevent the interpretation of expressions and emotions of affected individuals during social encounters leading to difficulties in liaising with others (Brown et al. 1997; Fellinger et al. 2009; Macgregor 1989; McAlpine and Moore 1993; van Daal et al. 2007). For example, nerve deficits in some patients with craniofacial microsomia might lead to similar problems (Rives Bogart and Matsumoto 2010). The extent of the impact, however, depends on the complex interrelationship of various social and personal parameters (Rumsey and Harcourt 2004).

Social interaction impairments such as anxiety and inferences of negative evaluation by others have also been frequently reported (Rumsey and Harcourt 2004). The impediments to social interaction and the avoidance of social relationships are secondary to the reported difficulties in meeting people, making new friends, and maintaining long-term relationships (Robinson 1997). The social entourage, family, and peers can complicate the psychosocial impairment by comments, harassment, and teasing (Feragen and Borge 2010; Feragen et al. 2009; Rumsey 2002). Children with a facial difference are at higher risk of social stigmatization (Masnari et al. 2012). Sixty percent of a sample of children with a cleft condition reported being subjected to teasing, an event that caused excessive anxiety to a quarter of them (Turner et al. 1997). Patients with craniofacial microsomia experience also bullying and have low self-esteem (Johns et al. 2018; Luquetti et al. 2018; Padwa et al. 1991).

As a consequence, negative attitudes and a feeling of reduced control in social encounters might result in prepossession with one's appearance and a vicious circle of further social avoidance, reduced social support, and increased psychosocial impacts (Rumsey and Harcourt 2004). Children with unilateral and bilateral cleft lip and palate have been reported to demonstrate adjustment problems, as judged by teachers and parents (Murray et al. 2010), or other behavioral problems especially if they are dissatisfied with their appearance (Hunt et al. 2006, 2007; Wehby et al. 2014). However, contrasting findings have been reported as well (Brand et al. 2009). Adaptation of patients to facial disfigurement seems to be enhanced in patients before or during adolescence. Acquiring a visible facial difference later than adolescence leads to greater disparity with the pre-existing self-concept, significant challenges in coping with the new situation, and increased consciousness of self-image and social perceptions (Rumsey 2004). Such adverse consequences are independent of gender and the magnitude of the defects (Fingeret et al. 2010, 2012; Katz et al. 2003; Rumsey et al. 2003). It is interesting to note that the range of

concerns, emotional reactions, and behavioral patterns exhibited by individuals with visible differences can be similar to those observed by some individuals dissatisfied with specific traits of their apparently "ordinary" appearance (Rumsey 2002).

Quality of Life Implications

Established on the multidimensional concept of health as "a state of complete physical, mental, and social well-being and not merely the absence of disease or infirmity," the notion of QoL is described as "an individual's perception of their position in life in the context of the culture and value systems in which they live and in relation to their goals, expectations, standards and concerns" (World Health Organization 1995). A direct implication of this description is that perception of QoL may differ in relation to the historical period, the cultural norms, and individual experiences. Within this multifactorial framework, the aspects of QoL specializing on how individuals understand their general health and oral health level refer to the terms health-related quality of life (HRQoL) and OHRQoL (Inglehart and Bagramian 2002).

HRQoL encompasses the physical, psychological, and social aspects of health, perceived as distinguishable domains moderated by individual experiences, beliefs, expectations, and perceptions (Testa and Simonson 1996). The aspects most frequently included in HRQoL definitions involve physical, emotional, psychological, social, spiritual, and functional parameters (Gimprich and Paterson 2002). Consequently, assessing HRQoL presupposes a holistic understanding of health beyond physical condition assessment to include the constructs of psychological status, social interaction, and self-realization (Atchison et al. 2006; Slade 2002). Typically, HRQoL appraisal focuses on constructs of the physical, functional, social, and psychological domains (Inglehart and Bagramian 2002). Other significant aspects include individual opportunities (e.g. school, work, social environment, etc.), health expectations, and satisfaction from disease management (Sischo and Broder 2011).

In the sense that oral health affects general health perception, daily functioning of individuals, and overall QoL (Naito et al. 2006), OHRQoL has been described as "the absence of negative impacts of oral conditions on social life and a positive sense of dentofacial self-confidence" (Inglehart and Bagramian 2002), representing a multifactorial construct, that focuses on individuals' reflections for physical functions like eating, etc., social encounters, self-esteem, and satisfaction with oral health (United States Department of Health and Human Services 2000). Therefore, OHRQoL results from the intriguing interaction between conditions and diseases of the mouth and face, and the parameters pertaining to general health and social entourage, during the life course of an individual (Atchison et al. 2006; Locker et al. 2005; Sischo and Broder 2011).

Within the context of OHRQoL, facial differences and social anxiety characterizing some patients with conditions like orofacial clefts, craniofacial microsomia, synostosis, and other craniofacial anomalies leading to facial differences, have been shown to impact children (Antonarakis et al. 2013; Bennett and Phillips 1999; Klassen et al. 2012; Queiroz Herkrath et al. 2015; Topolski et al. 2005). OHRQoL has been lower in children with cleft lip and palate with increased need for treatment (Broder et al. 2014a). QoL impacts involve mostly the social role (Kramer et al. 2009). Self-concept is positively associated with QoL reports and resilience mitigates the negative effects of the condition (Broder et al. 2014b). Following surgery, children report significant improvements in overall QoL scores including functional and emotional well-being, as well as self-esteem (Broder et al. 2017). Females report decreased QoL corroborating appearance research considering girls at higher risk for body image dissatisfaction (Crerand et al. 2017).

While patients with isolated craniosynostosis do not seem to have impacts on HRQoL (Boltshauser et al. 2003), patients with syndromic and complex craniosynostosis report lower scores (de Jong et al. 2012). The affected aspects include primarily the physical function and mental domains (Bannink et al. 2010). Those Apert and Crouzon syndrome patients with adequate functioning present a satisfactory QoL, demonstrating the acquisition of the necessary personality tools to mitigate the impacts from their conditions (Lloyd et al. 2016; Raposo-Amaral et al. 2014). Children with hemifacial microsomia report HRQoL impacts in the domains of physical, social, and school functioning (Hamilton et al. 2018; Khetani et al. 2013).

The Facial Difference from the Family Perspective

To raise a child with a craniofacial anomaly is challenging and stresses parents because of factors like repeated medical appointments, functional and psychosocial issues, bullying, as well as other difficulties (Mathijssen 2015; Nelson et al. 2012; Sarimski 1998; Speltz et al. 2000). At the same time, families play a crucial role in shaping children's experience with the conditions (Baker et al. 2009).

In most cases, the diagnosis period constitutes a highly demanding experience, characterized by despair, grief, the element of shock, and emotions of guilt (Vanz and Ribeiro 2011). Parents express a multitude of concerns,

with the way relative information is shared having significant impact on the overall experience and the ability to cope (Chuacharoen et al. 2009; Hodgkinson et al. 2005; Nelson et al. 2012; Vanz and Ribeiro 2011). Despite some concerns, no differences regarding mother–child attachment have been observed in comparison to control populations (Collett and Speltz 2007; Hunt et al. 2005; Murray et al. 2008). In general, the family impact is greater while the child is young and in the presence of other medical problems (Baker et al. 2009). Inversely, family variables can influence the psychosocial development of the child, like parenting skills (Murray et al. 2010), parental stress (Endriga et al. 2003), and the interaction between the mother and the child (Collett et al. 2012; Speltz et al. 2000).

Parents of patients experience social stigmatization as well. Their stress is linked mainly to the patient's learning difficulties and the issue of acceptance. However, facial appearance does not seem to be a significant determinant of stress (Johns et al. 2018; Luquetti et al. 2018; Ongkosuwito et al. 2018; Padwa et al. 1991). Parents of children with syndromic craniosynostosis may suffer from the increased medical needs and the possibility of a significant disruption in the mother–infant attachment and bonding process, with early correction possibly helping in minimizing disruptions (Kluba et al. 2016; Rogers-Salyer et al. 1987).

Psychosocial Support for Children and Families

Current systems of care for individuals with facial differences are predominantly focused on a biomedical model of care. Cosmetic surgery might decrease stress over a particular feature but does not change overall body image (Sarwer 2002). Increased importance should be placed on the factors affecting resilience to the psychosocial implications arising from a visible facial difference like a person's subjective perception of one's difference (Harris 1997), sociocultural factors (Rumsey 1997), social interaction skills (Kapp-Simon 1995), as well as family environment and social support (Lansdown et al. 1997). All health professionals involved in the care of patients with visible facial differences play an important role to foster psychological coping and positive adjustment of patients and families.

Patients should be regularly approached and consulted in order to identify threats to their well-being (Mink van der Molen et al. 2021). Particular attention should be given to problems arising from teasing or bullying (Hunt et al. 2007), issues relevant to self-esteem, or the adequacy of social skills (Feragen et al. 2009). The use of instruments in the psychodiagnostics process like the Strengths and Difficulties Questionnaire (Goodman 2001), has been advocated as well (Mink van der Molen et al. 2021). Particular attention should be placed to the interaction between parents and the affected child. Children with clefts and impairment of their interaction with their parents are at risk of unfavorable psychosocial development (Hentges et al. 2011). Meeting with parents should include discussions on perceived stress, skills, and acceptance of the problem (Mink van der Molen et al. 2021). Although every possible opportunity to discuss the above issues should be used, screening for possible threats to psychological coping and adjustment of patients and families should include birth and cardinal transition moments in the life of the child: before starting school (2–3 years), before primary education (5–6 years), before secondary education (10–11 years) and before adulthood (17 years). During these interactions, factors relative to the child (social skills, well-being, bullying, acceptance, learning problems, etc.) and the family (perceived stress, skills, acceptance of the problem, etc.) should take place (Mink van der Molen et al. 2021).

As social anxiety constitutes an important difficulty encountered by individuals with visible differences, various forms of psychosocial interventions have been proposed to be beneficial (Norman et al. 2015). Such interventions for children include social skills training (Collett and Speltz 2007; Kapp-Simon 1995), cognitive behavioral therapy (Maddern et al. 2006; Newell and Clarke 2000; Robinson et al. 1996), or coping strategies training (Baker et al. 2009). For parents, it has been recommended to discuss their fears and concerns (Pelchat et al. 2004) and to train them to accept the condition, express their grief, and learn to cope (Endriga et al. 2003). In the context of reducing societal pressure on individuals with facial differences, some lay-led organizations (e.g. Changing Faces: www.changingfaces.org) have developed clinical services for children and families (Kish and Lansdown 2000) and have also organized "camps" and forums offering a secure and positive environment (Tiemens et al. 2006).

References

Agırnaslıgıl MO, Gul Amuk N, Kılıc E, Kutuk N, Demırbas AE, Alkan A. The changes of self-esteem, sensitivity to criticism, and social appearance anxiety in orthognathic surgery patients: a controlled study. Am J Orthod Dentofac Orthop. 2019;155:482–489.e2.

Albrecht GL, Devlieger PJ. The disability paradox: high quality of life against all odds. Soc Sci Med. 1999:977–988.

Antonarakis GS, Patel RN, Tompson B. Oral health-related quality of life in non-syndromic cleft lip and/or palate patients: a systematic review. Community Dent Health. 2013;30:189–195.

Atchison KA, Shetty V, Belin TR, Der-Martirosian C, Leathers R, Black E, Wang J. Using patient self-report data to evaluate orofacial surgical outcomes. Community Dent Oral Epidemiol. 2006;34:93–102.

Baker SR, Owens J, Stern M, Willmot D. Coping strategies and social support in the family impact of cleft lip and palate and parents' adjustment and psychological distress. Cleft Palate Craniofac J. 2009;46:229–236.

Bannink N, Maliepaard M, Raat H, Joosten KF, Mathijssen IM. Health-related quality of life in children and adolescents with syndromic craniosynostosis. J Plast Reconstr Aesthet Surg. 2010;63:1972–1981.

Barry BM. How Judges Judge: Empirical Insights into Judicial Decision-Making. London: Informa Law from Routledge, 2020.

Bashour M. History and current concepts in the analysis of facial attractiveness. Plast Reconstr Surg. 2006;118:741–756.

Bennett ME, Phillips CL. Assessment of health-related quality of life for patients with severe skeletal disharmony: a review of the issues. Int J Adult Orthodon Orthogn Surg. 1999;14:65–75.

Berger ZE, Dalton LJ. Coping with a cleft: psychosocial adjustment of adolescents with a cleft lip and palate and their parents. Cleft Palate Craniofac J. 2009;46:435–443.

Bernabé E, Sheiham A, de Oliveira CM. Condition-specific impacts on quality of life attributed to malocclusion by adolescents with normal occlusion and Class I, II and III malocclusion. Angle Orthod. 2008;78:977–982.

Boltshauser E, Ludwig S, Dietrich F, Landolt MA. Sagittal craniosynostosis: cognitive development, behaviour, and quality of life in unoperated children. Neuropediatrics. 2003;34:293–300.

Brand S, Blechschmidt A, Müller A, Sader R, Schwenzer-Zimmerer K, Zeilhofer HF, Holsboer-Trachsler E. Psychosocial functioning and sleep patterns in children and adolescents with cleft lip and palate (CLP) compared with healthy controls. Cleft Palate Craniofac J. 2009;46:124–135.

Broder HL, Wilson-Genderson M, Sischo L. Examination of a theoretical model for oral health-related quality of life among youths with cleft. Am J Public Health. 2014b;104:865–871.

Broder HL, Wilson-Genderson M, Sischo L. Oral health-related quality of life in youth receiving cleft-related surgery: self-report and proxy ratings. Qual Life Res. 2017;26:859–867.

Broder HL, Wilson-Genderson M, Sischo L, Norman RG. Examining factors associated with oral health-related quality of life for youth with cleft. Plast Reconstr Surg. 2014a;133:828e–834e.

Brown R, Hobson RP, Lee A, Stevenson J. Are there "autisticlike" features in congenitally blind children? J Child Psychol Psychiatry. 1997;38:693–703.

Casey G. Physiology of the skin. Nurs Stand. 2002;16:47–51.

Chatterjee A, Thomas A, Smith SE, Aguirre GK. The neural response to facial attractiveness. Neuropsychology. 2009;23:135–143.

Chuacharoen R, Ritthagol W, Hunsrisakhun J, Nilmanat K. Felt needs of parents who have a 0- to 3-month-old child with a cleft lip and palate. Cleft Palate Craniofac J. 2009;46:252–257.

Cohen MM Jr. Perspectives on craniofacial asymmetry. VI. The hamartoses. Int J Oral Maxillofac Surg. 1995;24:195–200.

Collett BR, Cloonan YK, Speltz ML, Anderka M, Werler MM. Psychosocial functioning in children with and without orofacial clefts and their parents. Cleft Palate Craniofac J. 2012;49:397–405.

Collett BR, Speltz ML. A developmental approach to mental health for children and adolescents with orofacial clefts. Orthod Craniofacial Res. 2007;10:138–148.

Connor NP, Abbs JH. Orofacial proprioception: analyses of cutaneous mechanoreceptor population properties using artificial neural networks. J Commun Disord. 1998;31:535–542,553.

Crerand CE, Sarwer DB, Kazak AE, Clarke A, Rumsey N. Body image and quality of life in adolescents with craniofacial conditions. Cleft Palate Craniofac J. 2017;54:2–12.

de Jong T, Maliepaard M, Bannink N, Raat H, Mathijssen IM. Health-related problems and quality of life in patients with syndromic and complex craniosynostosis. Childs Nerv Syst. 2012;28:879–882.

DeBronkart D. From patient centred to people powered: autonomy on the rise. Br Med J. 2015;350:h148.

Demir T, Karacetin G, Baghaki S, Aydin Y. Psychiatric assessment of children with nonsyndromic cleft lip and palate. Gen Hosp Psychiatry. 2011;33:594–603.

Do LG, Spencer AJ. Evaluation of oral health-related quality of life questionnaires in a general child population. Community Dent Health. 2008;25:205–210.

Endriga MC, Jordan JR, Speltz ML. Emotion self-regulation in preschool-aged children with and without orofacial clefts. J Dev Behav Pediatr. 2003;24:336–344.

Fellinger J, Holzinger D, Sattel H, Laucht M, Goldberg D. Correlates of mental health disorders among children with hearing impairments. Dev Med Child Neurol. 2009;51:635–641.

Feragen KB, Borge AI. Peer harassment and satisfaction with appearance in children with and without a facial difference. Body Image. 2010;7:97–105.

Feragen KB, Borge AI, Rumsey N. Social experience in 10-year-old children born with a cleft: exploring psychosocial resilience. Cleft Palate Craniofac J. 2009;46:65–74.

Feragen KB, Kvalem IL, Rumsey N, Borge AI. Adolescents with and without a facial difference: the role of friendships and social acceptance in perceptions of appearance and emotional resilience. Body Image. 2010;7:271–279.

Feragen KB, Stock NM, Kvalem IL. Risk and protective factors at age 16: psychological adjustment in children with a cleft lip and/or palate. Cleft Palate Craniofac J. 2015;52:555–573.

Feu D, Miguel JA, Celeste RK, Oliveira BH. Effect of orthodontic treatment on oral health-related quality of life. Angle Orthod. 2013;83:892–898.

Fingeret MC, Vidrine DJ, Reece GP, Gillenwater AM, Gritz ER. Multidimensional analysis of body image concerns among newly diagnosed patients with oral cavity cancer. Head Neck. 2010;32:301–309.

Fingeret MC, Yuan Y, Urbauer D, Weston J, Nipomnick S, Weber R. The nature and extent of body image concerns among surgically treated patients with head and neck cancer. Psychooncology. 2012;21:836–844.

Finkeldey JG, Demuth S. Race/ethnicity, perceived skin color, and the likelihood of adult arrest. Race Justice. 2021;11:567–591.

Fontaine KR, Barofsky I. Obesity and health-related quality of life: review. Obes Rev. 2001;2:173–182.

Foster Page LA, Thomson WM, Jokovic A, Locker D. Validation of the child perceptions questionnaire (CPQ 11-14). J Dent Res. 2005;84:649–652.

Frejman MW, Vargas IA, Rösing CK, Closs LQ. Dentofacial deformities are associated with lower degrees of self-esteem and higher impact on oral health-related quality of life: results from an observational study involving adults. J Oral Maxillofac Surg. 2013;71:763–767.

Gilbert S, Thompson J. Body shame in childhood & adolescence. In: Gilbert P, Miles J, eds. Body Shame. Hove: Brunner-Routledge, 2002.

Gimprich B, Paterson AG. Health-related quality of life: conceptual issues and research applications. In: Inglehart MR, Bagramian RA, eds. Oral Health-Related Quality of Life. Carol Stream: Quintessence, 2002.

Goodman R. Psychometric properties of the strengths and difficulties questionnaire. J Am Acad Child Adolesc Psychiatry. 2001;40:1337–1345.

Grogan S. Body Image. Hove: Routledge, 1999.

Hamilton KV, Ormond KE, Moscarello T, Bruce JS, Bereknyei Merrell S, Chang KW, Bernstein JA. Exploring the medical and psychosocial concerns of adolescents and young adults with craniofacial microsomia: a qualitative study. Cleft Palate Craniofac J. 2018;55:1430–1439.

Harris D. Types, causes and physical treatment of visible differences. In: Lansdown R, Rumsey N, Bradbury R, Carr T, Partridge J, eds. Visibly Different: Coping with Disfigurement. Oxford: Butterworth-Heinemann, 1997.

Harter S. The Construction of the Self: A Developmental Perspective. New York: Guilford, 1999.

Hentges F, Hill J, Bishop DV, Goodacre T, Moss T, Murray L. The effect of cleft lip on cognitive development in school-aged children: a paradigm for examining sensitive period effects. J Child Psychol Psychiatry. 2011;52:704–712.

Herskind A, Christensen K, Juel K, Fogh-Anderson P. Cleft lip: a risk factor for suicide. 7th International Congress on Cleft Palate and Related Craniofacial Anomalies, Broadbeach, Australia, Queensland, 1993.

Hodgkinson PD, Brown S, Duncan D, Grant C, McNaughton A, Thomas P, Mattick CR. Management of children with cleft lip and palate: a review describing the application of multidisciplinary team working in this condition based upon the experiences of a regional cleft lip and palate centre in the United Kingdom. Fetal Matern Med Rev. 2005;16:1–27.

Horgan JE, Padwa BL, LaBrie RA, Mulliken JB. OMENSPlus: analysis of craniofacial and extracraniofacial anomalies in hemifacial microsomia. Cleft Palate Craniofac J. 1995;32:405–412.

Hornung DE. Nasal anatomy and the sense of smell. Adv Otorhinolaryngol. 2006;63:1–22.

Huff JS, Austin EW. Neuro-ophthalmology in emergency medicine. Emerg Med Clin North Am. 2016;34:967–986.

Hunt O, Burden D, Hepper P, Johnston C. The psychosocial effects of cleft lip and palate: a systematic review. Eur J Orthod. 2005;27:274–285.

Hunt O, Burden D, Hepper P, Stevenson M, Johnston C. Self-reports of psychosocial functioning among children and young adults with cleft lip and palate. Cleft Palate Craniofac J. 2006;43:598–605.

Hunt O, Burden D, Hepper P, Stevenson M, Johnston C. Parent reports of the psychosocial functioning of children with cleft lip and/or palate. Cleft Palate Craniofac J. 2007;44:304–311.

Ince DO, Ince A, Moore TL. Effect of methotrexate on the temporomandibular joint and facial morphology in juvenile rheumatoid arthritis patients. Am J Orthod Dentofac Orthop. 2000;118:75–83.

Inglehart MR, Bagramian RA. Oral health-related quality of life: an introduction. In: Inglehart MR, Bagramian RA, eds. Oral Health-Related Quality of Life. Carol Stream: Quintessence, 2002.

Johal A, Cheung MY, Marcene W. The impact of two different malocclusion traits on quality of life. Br Dent J. 2007;202:E2.

Johansson O, Wang L, Hilliges M, Liang Y. Intraepidermal nerves in human skin: PGP 9.5 immunohistochemistry with special reference to the nerve density in skin from different body regions. J Peripher Nerv Syst. 1999;4:43–52.

Johns AL, Luquetti DV, Brajcich MR, Heike CL, Stock NM. In their own words: caregiver and patient perspectives on stressors, resources, and recommendations in craniofacial microsomia care. J Craniofac Surg. 2018;29:2198–2205.

Jones AL, Kramer SS. Facial cosmetics have little effect on attractiveness judgments compared with identity. Perception. 2015;44:79–86.

Jung MH. Quality of life and self-esteem of female orthognathic surgery patients. J Oral Maxillofac Surg. 2016;74:e1–e7.

Kapp-Simon KA. Psychological interventions for the adolescent with cleft lip and palate. Cleft Palate Craniofac J. 1995;32:104–108.

Kastoer C, Leach R, Vandervcken O. Face and neck: airway and sensorial capacities. B-ENT. 2016;Suppl 26:11–19.

Katz MR, Irish JC, Devins GM, Rodin GM, Gullane PJ. Psychosocial adjustment in head and neck cancer: the impact of disfigurement, gender and social support. Head Neck. 2003;25:103–112.

Kawakami T, Ishihara M, Mihara M. Distribution density of intraepidermal nerve fibers in normal human skin. J Dermatol. 2001;28:63–70.

Kent G, Thompson A. The development and maintenance of shame in disfigurement: implications for treatment. In: Gilbert P, Miles J, eds. Body Shame: Conceptualisation, Research and Treatment. Hove: Brunner-Routledge, 2002.

Khetani MA, Collett BR, Speltz ML, Werler MM. Health-related quality of life in children with hemifacial microsomia: parent and child perspectives. J Dev Behav Pediatr. 2013;34:661–668.

Kish V, Lansdown R. Meeting the psychosocial impact of facial disfigurement: developing a clinical service for children & families. Clin Child Psychology Psychiatry. 2000;5:497–512.

Klassen AF, Tsangaris E, Forrest CR, Wong KW, Pusic AL, Cano SJ, Syed I, Dua M, Kainth S, Johnson J, Goodacre T. Quality of life of children treated for cleft lip and/or palate: a systematic review. J Plast Reconstr Aesthet Surg. 2012;65:547–557.

Kluba S, Rohleder S, Wolff M, Haas-Lude K, Schuhmann MU, Will BE, Reinert S, Krimmel M. Parental perception of treatment and medical care in children with craniosynostosis. Int J Oral Maxillofac Surg. 2016;45:1341–1346.

Kramer FJ, Gruber R, Fialka F, Sinikovic B, Hahn W, Schliephake H. Quality of life in school-age children with orofacial clefts and their families. J Craniofac Surg. 2009;20:2061–2066.

Kurabe K, Kojima T, Kato Y, Saito I, Kobayashi T. Impact of orthognathic surgery on oral health-related quality of life in patients with jaw deformities. Int J Oral Maxillofac Surg. 2016;45:1513–1519.

Lansdown R, Rumsey N, Bradbury E, Carr A, Partridge J, eds. Visibly Different: Coping with Disfigurement. Oxford: Butterworth-Heinemann, 1997.

Lavallee DC, Chenok KE, Love RM, Petersen C, Holve E, Segal CD, Franklin PD. Incorporating patient-reported outcomes into health care to engage patients and enhance care. Health Aff (Millwood). 2016;35:575–582.

Lemay EP Jr, Clark MS, Greenberg A. What is beautiful is good because what is beautiful is desired: physical attractiveness stereotyping as projection of interpersonal goals. Personal Soc Psychol Bull. 2010;36:339–353.

Lloyd MS, Venugopal A, Horton J, Rodrigues D, Nishikawa H, White N, Solanki G, Noons P, Evans M, Dover S. The quality of life in adult patients with syndromic craniosynostosis from their perspective. J Craniofac Surg. 2016;27:1510–1514.

Locker D, Jokovic A, Tompson B. Health-related quality of life of children aged 11 to 14 years with orofacial conditions. Cleft Palate Craniofac J. 2005;42: 260–266.

Lund K. Mandibular growth and remodelling processes after condylar fracture. A longitudinal roentgencephalometric study. Acta Odontol Scand Suppl. 1974;32:3–117.

Luquetti DV, Brajcich MR, Stock NM, Heike CL, Johns AL. Healthcare and psychosocial experiences of individuals with craniofacial microsomia: patient and caregivers perspectives. Int J Pediatr Otorhinolaryngol. 2018;107:164–175.

Macgregor FC. Social, psychological and cultural dimensions of cosmetic and reconstructive plastic surgery. Aesthet Plast Surg. 1989;13:1–8.

Maddern LH, Cadogan JC, Emerson MP. 'Outlook': a psychological service for children with a different appearance. Clin Child Psychol Psychiatry. 2006;11:431–443.

Maner JK, DeWall CN, Gailliot MT. Selective attention to signs of success: social dominance and early stage interpersonal perception. Personal Soc Psychol Bull. 2008;34:488–501.

Masnari O, Landolt MA, Roessler J, Weingaertner SK, Neuhaus K, Meuli M, Schiestl C. Self- and parent-perceived stigmatisation in children and adolescents with congenital or acquired facial differences. J Plast Reconstr Aesthet Surg. 2012;65:1664–1670.

Mathijssen IM. Guideline for care of patients with the diagnoses of craniosynostosis: working group on craniosynostosis. J Craniofac Surg. 2015;26:1735–1807.

McAlpine LM, Moore C. The development of social understanding in children with visual impairments. J Vis Impair Blind. 1993;89:349–358.

McNulty JK, Neff LA, Karney BR. Beyond initial attraction: physical attractiveness in newlywed marriage. J Fam Psychol. 2008;22:135–143.

Meger MN, Fatturi AL, Gerber JT, Weiss SG, Rocha JS, Scariot R, Wambier LM. Impact of orthognathic surgery on quality of life of patients with dentofacial deformity: a systematic review and meta-analysis. Br J Oral Maxillofac Surg. 2021;59:265–271.

Mink van der Molen AB, van Breugel JMM, Janssen NG, RJC A, van Adrichem LNA, Bierenbroodspot F, Bittermann D, van den Boogaard MH, Broos PH, Dijkstra-Putkamer JJM, van Gemert-Schriks MCM, Kortlever ALJ, Mouës-Vink CM, Swanenburg de Veye HFN, van Tol-Verbeek N, Vermeij-Keers C, de Wilde H, Kuijpers-Jagtman AM. Clinical practice guidelines on the treatment of patients with cleft lip, alveolus, and palate: an executive summary. J Clin Med. 2021;10:4813.

Montoya RM. I'm hot, so I'd say you're not: the influence of objective physical attractiveness on mate selection. Personal Soc Psychol Bull. 2008;34:1315–1331.

Moss T. Individual variation in adjusting to visible differences. In: Lansdown R, Rumsey N, Bradbury E, Carr A, Partridge J, eds. Visibly Different: Coping with Disfigurement. Oxford: Butterworth-Heinemann, 1997.

Mossey PA, Catilla EE. Global Registry and Database on Craniofacial Anomalies: Report of a WHO Registry Meeting on Craniofacial Anomalies. Geneva: World Health Organization, 2003.

Murray L, Arteche A, Bingley C, Hentges F, Bishop DVM, Dalton L, Goodacre T, Hill J, Cleft Lip and Palate Study Team. The effect of cleft lip on socio-emotional functioning in school-aged children. J Child Psychol Psychiatry. 2010;51:94–103.

Murray L, Hentges F, Hill J, Karpf J, Mistry B, Kreutz M, Woodall P, Moss T, Goodacre T, Cleft Lip and Palate Study Team. The effect of cleft lip and palate, and the timing of lip repair on mother-infant interactions and infant development. J Child Psychol Psychiatry. 2008;49: 115–123.

Naito M, Yuasa H, Nomura Y, Nakayama T, Hamajima N, Hanada N. Oral health status and health-related quality of life: a systematic review. J Oral Sci. 2006;48:1–7.

Nelson P, Glenny AM, Kirk S, Caress AL. Parents' experiences of caring for a child with a cleft lip and/or palate: a review of the literature. Child Care Health Dev. 2012;38:6–20.

Newell R. Body Image and Disfigurement Care. London: Routledge, 2000.

Newell R, Clarke M. Evaluation of a self-help leaflet in treatment of social difficulties following facial disfigurement. Int J Nurs Stud. 2000;37:381–388.

Norman A, Persson M, Stock N, Rumsey N, Sandy J, Waylen A, Edwards Z, Hammond V, Partridge L, Ness A. The effectiveness of psychosocial intervention for individuals with cleft lip and/or palate. Cleft Palate Craniofac J. 2015;52:301–310.

O'Brien C, Benson PE, Marshman Z. Evaluation of a quality of life measure for children with malocclusion. J Orthod. 2007;34:185–193.

O'Brien K, Wright JL, Conboy F, Macfarlane T, Mandall N. The child perception questionnaire is valid for malocclusions in the United Kingdom. Am J Orthod Dentofac Orthop. 2006;129:536–540.

Ongkosuwito E, van der Vlies L, Kraaij V, Garnefski N, van Neck H, Kuijpers-Jagtman AM, Hovius S. Stress in parents of a child with hemifacial microsomia: the role of child characteristics and parental coping strategies. Cleft Palate Craniofac J. 2018;55:959–965.

Padwa BL, Evans CA, Pillemer FC. Psychosocial adjustment in children with hemifacial microsomia and other craniofacial deformities. Cleft Palate Craniofac J. 1991;28:354–359.

Pelchat D, Lefebvre H, Proulx M, Reidy M. Parental satisfaction with an early family intervention program. J Perinat Neonatal Nurs. 2004;18:128–144.

Persichetti P, Barone M, Cogliandro A, Di Stefano N, Tambone V. Can philosophical aesthetics be useful for plastic surgery? The subjective, objective and relational view of beauty. J Plast Reconstr Aesthet Surg. 2019;72:1856–1871.

Proffit WR, Fields HW Jr, Larson BE, Sarver DM. Contemporary Orthodontics. Philadelphia: Elsevier, 2019.

Queiroz Herkrath AP, Herkrath FJ, Rebelo MA, Vettore MV. Measurement of health-related and oral health-related quality of life among individuals with nonsyndromic orofacial clefts: a systematic review and meta-analysis. Cleft Palate Craniofac J. 2015;52:157–172.

Raposo-Amaral CE, Neto JGJ, Denadai R, Raposo-Amaral CM, Raposo-Amaral CA. Patient-reported quality of life in highest-functioning Apert and Crouzon syndromes: a comparative study. Plast Reconstr Surg. 2014;133:182e–191e.

Rhodes G. The evolutionary psychology of facial beauty. Annu Rev Psychol. 2006;57:199–226.

Ribeiro-Neto CA, Ferreira G, Monnazzi GCB, Gabrielli MFR, Monnazzi MS. Dentofacial deformities and the quality of life of patients with these conditions: a comparative study. Oral Surg Oral Med Oral Pathol Oral Radiol. 2018;126:457–462.

Rives Bogart K, Matsumoto D. Facial mimicry is not necessary to recognize emotion: Facial expression recognition by people with Moebius syndrome. Soc Neurosci. 2010;5:241–251.

Robinson E. Pyschological research on visible differences in adults. In: Lansdown R, Rumsey N, Bradbury E, Carr A, Partridge J, eds. Visibly Different: Coping with Disfigurement. Oxford: Butterworth-Heinemann, 1997.

Robinson E, Rumsey N, Partridge J. An evaluation of the impact of social interaction skills training for facially disfigured people. Br J Plast Surg. 1996;49:281–289.

Rogers-Salyer M, Jensen AG, Barden RC. Effects of facial deformities and physical attractiveness on mother-infant bonding. In: Marchac D, ed. Craniofacial Surgery. Berlin: Springer, 1987.

Rumsey N. Historical and anthropological perspectives on appearance. In: Lansdown R, Rumsey N, Bradbury E, Carr A, Partridge J, eds. Visibly Different: Coping with Disfigurement. Oxford: Butterworth-Heinemann, 1997.

Rumsey N. Body image and congenital conditions with visible differences. In: Cash T, Pruzinsky T, eds. Body Image: A Handbook of Theory, Research and Clinical Practice. New York: Guilford, 2002.

Rumsey N. Psychological aspects of face transplantation: read the small print carefully. Am J Bioeth. 2004;4:22–25.

Rumsey N, Clarke A, Musa M. Altered body image: the psychosocial needs of patients. Br J Community Nurs. 2002;7:563–566.

Rumsey N, Clarke A, White P. Exploring the psychosocial concerns of outpatients with disfiguring conditions. J Wound Care. 2003;12:247–252.

Rumsey N, Clarke A, White P, Wyn-Williams M, Garlick W. Altered body image: appearance-related concerns of people with visible disfigurement. J Adv Nurs. 2004;48:443–453.

Rumsey N, Harcourt D. Body image and disfigurement: issues and interventions. Body Image. 2004;1:83–97.

Samson N, Fink B, Matts PJ. Visible skin condition and perception of human facial appearance. Int J Cosmet Sci. 2010;32:167–184.

Sarimski K. Children with Apert syndrome: behavioural problems and family stress. Dev Med Child Neurol. 1998;40:44–49.

Sarwer DB. Cosmetic surgery and changes in body image. In: Cash TF, Pruzinsky T, eds. Body Image: A Handbook of Theory, Research, and Clinical Practice. New York: Guilford, 2002.

Schulze E, Witt M, Fink T, Hofer A, Funk RH. Immunohistochemical detection of human skin nerve fibers. Acta Histochem. 1997;99:301–309.

Severt TR, Proffit WR. The prevalence of facial asymmetry in the dentofacial deformities population at the University of North Carolina. Int J Adult Orthodon Orthognath Surg. 1997;12:171–176.

Shaw DW. Global strategies to reduce the health care burden of craniofacial anomalies: report of WHO meetings on international collaborative research on craniofacial anomalies. Cleft Palate Craniofac J. 2004;41:238–243.

Siemionow M, Sonmez E. Face as an organ. Ann Plast Surg. 2008;61:345–352.

Sischo L, Broder HL. Oral health-related quality of life: what, why, how, and future implications. J Dent Res. 2011;90:1264–1270.

Slade DG. Assessment of oral-health-related quality of life. In: Inglehart MR, Bagramian RA, eds. Oral Health-Related Quality of Life. Carol Stream: Quintessence Publishing Co Inc, 2002.

Slifer KJ, Amari A, Diver T, Hilley L, Beck M, Kane A, McDonnell S. Social interaction patterns of children and adolescents with and without oral clefts during a videotaped analogue social encounter. Cleft Palate Craniofac J. 2004;41:175–184.

Speltz ML, Endriga MC, Hill S, Maris CL, Jones K, Omnell ML. Cognitive and psychomotor development of infants with orofacial clefts. J Pediatr Psychol. 2000;25:185–190.

Sun H, Shang HT, He LS, Ding MC, Su ZP, Shi YL. Assessing the quality of life in patients with dentofacial deformities before and after orthognathic surgery. J Oral Maxillofac Surg. 2018;76:2192–2201.

Testa MA, Simonson DC. Assessment of quality-of-life outcomes. N Engl J Med. 1996;334:835–840.

Tiemens K, Beveridge HL, Nicholas DB. A therapeutic camp weekend for adolescents with craniofacial differences. Cleft Palate Craniofac J. 2006;43:44–46.

Tillman KK, Hakelius M, Höijer J, Ramklint M, Ekselius L, Nowinski D, Papadopoulos FC. Increased risk for neurodevelopmental disorders in children with orofacial clefts. J Am Acad Child Adolesc Psychiatry. 2018;57:876–883.

Todorov A, Mandisodza AN, Goren A, Hall CC. Inferences of competence from faces predict election outcomes. Science. 2005;308:1623–1626.

Topolski TD, Edwards TC, Patrick DL. Quality of life: how do adolescents with facial differences compare with other adolescents? Cleft Palate Craniofac J. 2005;42:25–32.

Traebert ES, Peres MA. Do malocclusions affect the individual's oral health-related quality of life? Oral Health Prev Dent. 2007;5:3–12.

Turner SR, Thomas PW, Dowell T, Rumsey N, Sandy JR. Psychological outcomes amongst cleft patients and their families. Br J Plast Surg. 1997;50:1–9.

United States Department of Health and Human Services. Oral health in America: A Report of the Surgeon General. Rockville: National Institutes of Health, 2000.

Valladares-Neto J, Biazevic MG, Paiva JB, Rino-Neto J. Oral health-related quality of life in patients with dentofacial deformity: a new concept in decision-making treatment? Oral Maxillofac Surg. 2014;18:265–270.

van Daal J, Verhoeven L, van Balkom H. Behaviour problems in children with language impairment. J Child Psychol Psychiatry. 2007;48:1139–1147.

Vanz AP, Ribeiro NR. Listening to the mothers of individuals with oral fissures. Rev Esc Enferm USP. 2011;45:596–602.

Walters E. Problems faced by children and families living with visible differences. In: Lansdown R, Rumsey N, Bradbury E, Carr T, Partridge J, eds. Visibly Different: Coping with Disfigurement. Oxford: Butterworth-Heinemann, 1997.

Wehby GL, Collet B, Barron S, Romitti PA, Ansley TN, Speltz M. Academic achievement of children and adolescents with oral clefts. Pediatrics. 2014;133:785–792.

Wilderman A, Van Oudenhove J, Kron J, Noonan JP, Cotney J. High-resolution epigenomic atlas of human embryonic craniofacial development. Cell Rep. 2018;23:1581–1597.

World Health Organization. The World Health Organization quality of life assessment (WHOQOL): position paper from the World Health Organization. Soc Sci Med. 1995;41:1403–1409.

Yi J, Lu W, Xiao J, Li X, Li Y, Zhao Z. Effect of conventional combined orthodontic-surgical treatment on oral health-related quality of life: a systematic review and meta-analysis. Am J Orthod Dentofac Orthop. 2019;156:29–43.e5.

Zebrowitz L. Reading Faces: Window to the Soul? Boulder: Westview Press, 1997.

Zebrowitz LA, Montepare JM. Social psychological face perception: why appearance matters. Soc Personal Psychol Compass. 2008;2:1497.

Index

Note: *Italicized* and **bold** page numbers refer to figures and tables, respectively.

Dentofacial and Occlusal Asymmetries, First Edition. Edited by Birte Melsen and Athanasios E. Athanasiou.
© 2025 John Wiley & Sons Ltd. Published 2025 by John Wiley & Sons Ltd.